Nutrition, Aging, and the Elderly

Human Nutrition
A COMPREHENSIVE TREATISE

General Editors:
Roslyn B. Alfin-Slater, *University of California, Los Angeles*
David Kritchevsky, *The Wistar Institute, Philadelphia*

Volume 1	*Nutrition: Pre- and Postnatal Development* *Edited by Myron Winick*
Volume 2	*Nutrition and Growth* *Edited by Derrick B. Jelliffe and E. F. Patrice Jelliffe*
Volume 3A	*Nutrition and the Adult: Macronutrients* *Edited by Roslyn B. Alfin-Slater and David Kritchevsky*
Volume 3B	*Nutrition and the Adult: Micronutrients* *Edited by Roslyn B. Alfin-Slater and David Kritchevsky*
Volume 4	*Nutrition: Metabolic and Clinical Applications* *Edited by Robert E. Hodges*
Volume 5	*Nutrition and Behavior* *Edited by Janina R. Galler*
Volume 6	*Nutrition, Aging, and the Elderly* *Edited by Hamish N. Munro and Darla E. Danford*

A Continuation Order Plan is available for this series. A continuation order will bring delivery of each new volume immediately upon publication. Volumes are billed only upon actual shipment. For further information please contact the publisher.

Nutrition, Aging, and the Elderly

Edited by
Hamish N. Munro
USDA Human Nutrition Research Center on Aging
Tufts University
Boston, Massachusetts

and

Darla E. Danford
National Institutes of Health
Bethesda, Maryland

Springer Science+Business Media, LLC

Library of Congress Cataloging in Publication Data

Nutrition, aging, and the elderly / edited by Hamish N. Munro and Darla E. Danford.
p. cm. — (Human nutrition; v. 6)
Includes bibliographies and index.
ISBN 978-1-4899-2539-8

1. Aged — Nutrition. 2. Aging — Physiological aspects. I. Munro, Hamish N. (Hamish Nisbet) II. Danford, Darla E. III. Series. [DNLM: 1. Aging. 2. Nutrition — in old age. QU 145 H9183 v.6] QP141.A1H84 vol. 6
612'.3s — dc19
[613.2'0880565]
DNLM/DLC 88-39816
for Library of Congress CIP

ISBN 978-1-4899-2539-8 ISBN 978-1-4899-2537-4 (eBook)
DOI 10.1007/978-1-4899-2537-4

Originally published by Plenum Press, New York in 1989
Softcover reprint of the hardcover 1st edition 1989

Contributors

Richard A. Anderson • U.S. Department of Agriculture, ARS, Beltsville Human Nutrition Research Center, Beltsville, Maryland 20705

Jeffrey B. Blumberg • USDA Human Nutrition Research Center on Aging, Tufts University, Boston, Massachusetts 02111

Barbara B. Bowman • Department of Biochemistry, Emory University School of Medicine, Atlanta, Georgia 30322

William Cameron Chumlea • Division of Human Biology, Department of Pediatrics, Wright State University School of Medicine, Dayton, Ohio 45435

Dorice M. Czajka-Narins • Department of Physiology and Biophysics, University of Health Sciences/Chicago Medical School, North Chicago, Illinois 60064

William J. Evans • USDA Human Nutrition Research Center on Aging, Tufts University, Boston, Massachusetts 02111

Anna Ferro-Luzzi • National Institute on Nutrition, 00179 Rome, Italy

Meira Fields • Georgetown University, Washington, D.C. 20007

Robert P. Heaney • Creighton University, Omaha, Nebraska 68178

W. P. T. James • Rowett Research Institute, Bucksburn, Aberdeen AB2 9SB, Scotland, United Kingdom

Mary Bess Kohrs • Department of Community Health Sciences, University of Illinois–Chicago, Chicago, Illinois 60612

David Kritchevsky • The Wistar Institute of Anatomy and Biology, Philadelphia, Pennsylvania 19104

Orville A. Levander • U.S. Department of Agriculture, ARS, Beltsville Human Nutrition Research Center, Beltsville, Maryland 20705

Edward J. Masoro • Department of Physiology, The University of Texas Health Science Center at San Antonio, San Antonio, Texas 78284-7756

Carol N. Meredith • USDA Human Nutrition Research on Aging, Tufts University, Boston, Massachusetts 02111

Walter Mertz • U.S. Department of Agriculture, ARS, Beltsville Human Nutrition Research Center, Beltsville, Maryland 20705

Simin Nikbin Meydani • USDA Human Nutrition Research Center on Aging, Tufts University, Boston, Massachusetts 02111

Eugene R. Morris • U.S. Department of Agriculture, ARS, Beltsville Human Nutrition Research Center, Beltsville, Maryland 20705

Hamish N. Munro • USDA Human Nutrition Research Center on Aging, Tufts University, Boston, Massachusetts 02111

James W. Nordstrom • Human Nutrition Research Program, Lincoln University, Jefferson City, Missouri 65101

Ann Ralph • Rowett Research Institute, Bucksburn, Aberdeen AB2 9SB, Scotland, United Kingdom

Robert R. Recker • Creighton University School of Medicine, Omaha, Nebraska 68178

Alex F. Roche • Division of Human Biology, Department of Pediatrics, Wright State University School of Medicine, Dayton, Ohio 45435

Daphne A. Roe • Division of Nutritional Sciences, Cornell University, Ithaca, New York 14853

Irwin H. Rosenberg • USDA Human Nutrition Research Center on Aging, Tufts University, Boston, Massachusetts 02111

Robert M. Russell • USDA Human Nutrition Research Center on Aging, Tufts University, Boston, Massachusetts 02111

J. Cecil Smith, Jr. • U.S. Department of Agriculture, ARS, Beltsville Human Nutrition Research Center, Beltsville, Maryland 20705

Maria L. Steinbaugh • Nutrition Education, Ross Laboratories, Columbus, Ohio 43216

Paulo M. Suter • USDA Human Nutrition Research Center on Aging, Tufts University, Boston, Massachusetts 02111

Emorn Udomkesmalee • Visiting Scientist from Institute of Nutrition, Mahidol University, Research Center, Ramathibodi Hospital, Bangkok 10400, Thailand

Preface

The proportion of the population over 65 years of age is increasing steadily in most industrialized countries. In the United States the proportion of elderly people has risen from four percent in 1900 to 11% in 1978, and is projected to be 14% by the year 2000. The occurrence of debilitating chronic diseases in the elderly increases with each additional year. These diseases, along with the natural loss of tissue function that occurs throughout adult life, impose a heavy burden on the health care system. Nutrition plays an important etiologic role in many of these degenerative changes. Consequently, the aging segment of the population presents a challenge to the nutrition scientist, who should be able to recommend optimal intakes of nutrients to minimize the functional losses associated with aging and to optimize the health of those already elderly.

This sixth volume in the series *Human Nutrition: A Comprehensive Treatise* provides a conspectus of the various interactions of nutrition with the aging process and a comprehensive survey of current knowledge of the amounts of individual nutrients needed by the elderly. The volume begins with a general survey of the multifaceted relationship of nutrition to aging, followed by four chapters on how nutrition can affect age-related changes in selected body functions. The next six chapters cover the available evidence regarding the needs of the elderly for dietary energy, protein, calcium, trace elements, vitamins, and fiber. The final three chapters deal with other factors relevant to the nutritional status of the elderly. This volume provides a reference source for those working in the field of gerontology as well as in nutrition.

We are grateful to all those who have contributed to this volume. We are especially indebted to the authors of the chapters for having provided authoritative and lucid presentations of their areas of expertise. We also wish to acknowledge Mary Phillips Born and Steven Melvin of Plenum for guiding the volume through the publication process so expeditiously. We hope that the book arising from the efforts of these many people will be of benefit in improving the health status of people as they age and in their later years.

Hamish N. Munro
Darla E. Danford

Contents

Chapter 5

Exercise and Nutrition in the Elderly

William J. Evans and Carol N. Meredith

Part II • Nutrient Needs of the Elderly

Chapter 6

Energy Needs of the Elderly: A New Approach

W. P. T. James, Ann Ralph, and Anna Ferro-Luzzi

Chapter 10

Vitamin Nutriture and Requirements of the Elderly

Paulo M. Suter and Robert M. Russell

Chapter 11

Role of Fiber in the Diet of the Elderly

David Kritchevsky

Part III • Other Aspects of the Nutrient Status of the Elderly

Chapter 12

Factors Affecting Nutritional Status of the Elderly

Mary Bess Kohrs, Dorice M. Czajka-Narins, and James W. Nordstrom

Chapter 13

Anthropometric Approaches to the Nutritional Assessment of the Elderly

William Cameron Chumlea, Alex F. Roche, and Maria L. Steinbaugh

1

The Challenges of Research into Nutrition and Aging

Introduction to a Multifaceted Problem

Hamish N. Munro

1. Introduction

The role of nutrition in the process of aging has been receiving progressively more attention in recent years, reflecting the increasing numbers of old people in the population and the disproportionate demands they make on health care (Rowe, 1985). The proportion of people over 65 years of age varies from less than 5% in some underdeveloped areas of the world to over 16% in many parts of Western Europe. In the United States the proportion of elderly people has increased from 4% in 1900 to 11% in 1978 and is projected to be close to 14% by the end of the century (Brody and Brock, 1985). The impact of this on health care services can be appreciated from estimates made in Massachusetts (Katz *et al.*, 1983) of the number of years after 65 that remain for independent living followed by the number of years of assisted living, the latter category meaning the need for help in rising from bed, bathing, dressing, or eating (Table I). Thus, for men aged 65–69 years, these periods average 9.3 years of independent living followed by 3.8 years of dependence; for women of 65–69 years, the projected periods are 10.6 and 8.9 years, respectively. The end of the period of independent living is presumably determined by degenerative changes in nervous system function, and the much longer survival of women in an assisted state probably represents the slower development of cardiovascular disease in the female because of the years of estrogen protection.

This suggested division into aging of systems (here, the nervous system) and the impact of chronic disease (e.g., atherosclerosis) have been further emphasized by Fries (1980). He points out that chronic diseases are potentially susceptible to prevention

Hamish N. Munro • USDA Human Nutrition Research Center on Aging, Tufts University, Boston, Massachusetts 02111.

Table I. Active and Total Life Expectancy in Massachusetts[a]

Age and sex	Average remaining active years	Average remaining total years	Years of dependency[b]
Men			
65–69	9.3	13.1	3.8
70–74	8.2	11.9	3.7
75–79	6.5	9.6	3.1
80–84	4.8	7.4	2.6
85+	3.3	6.5	3.2
Women			
65–69	10.6	19.5	8.9
70–74	8.0	15.9	7.9
75–79	7.1	13.2	6.1
80–84	4.8	9.8	5.0
85+	2.8	7.7	4.9

[a]Data derived from Katz *et al.* (1983).
[b]Years of dependency for rising, bathing, dressing, or feeding, represented by the difference between the total and active years remaining, obtained by subtracting the two previous columns.

through identification of life-style factors in their etiology, and he suggests that, in their absence, mortality would occur over a narrow range (e.g., 75–85 years) from "natural" aging through progressive and inevitable loss of function ending in terminal organ failure. However, organ failure at a narrow age range is precluded by genetic variation in the population, so that the consequent compression of morbidity over a short period around the 80th to 90th year is probably unattainable. Indeed, the evidence shows that cardiovascular disease becomes an increasingly common cause of death as age advances (Brody and Brock, 1985). At age 65–69, this family of diseases accounts for 47% of deaths, and the proportion rises progressively to 70% over the age of 85 years.

Nutrition may interact with the aging process in three ways. First, most tissue functions decrease during adult life, and we can ask whether nutrition and other features of adult life style contribute to or ameliorate this age-related loss of tissue substance and function. Second, the frequency of many chronic diseases, such as cardiovascular diseases and cancer, increases with advancing age, and indeed, there is a large body of evidence relating to the role of nutrition in the etiology of these conditions. Third, adults usually eat less as they grow old, and in consequence the nutrient intakes of elderly adults can fall below the recommended dietary allowances (National Academy of Sciences, 1980). In all these three aspects of aging, the changes are progressive throughout adult life, so that an arbitrary definition of aging as those over 65 years obscures the fact that senior citizenship represents the terminal years of a continuum of diminishing tissue function, in the development of chronic disease, and in reductions in nutrient intake. In all three areas, nutrition may play a role that is part of the aging continuum. As Exton-Smith (1977) remarks, "the individual dietary patterns in the majority of old people remain similar to those which have been acquired by habits established at a younger age."

2. *Age-Related Body Changes and Nutrition*

As pointed out above, aging is a continuous process throughout adult life. In this section, we review the progressive changes taking place in body composition, metabolism, and tissue function and the evidence of a role of nutrition in modulating the rates of change. This is followed by a brief section dealing with the role of long-term nutrition in the etiology of chronic age-related disease.

2.1. *Body Composition, Metabolism, and Tissue Function*

The continuous nature of the changes occurring throughout adult life is well illustrated by body composition, which undergoes a loss of lean body mass accompanied by a gain in body fat (Cohn *et al.*, 1980). The loss of body protein affects particularly skeletal muscle, as evidenced by 40% reduction in urinary output of the muscle-derived metabolites creatinine and 3-methylhistidine between the ages of 20 and 70 years (Munro and Young, 1978). This erosion in body protein throughout adult life is discussed in greater detail in Chapter 7, Section 2.1.

Aging also affects metabolism. The progressive impairment in tolerance for a dose of glucose (Fig. 1) is discussed in detail by Silverberg (1983) and results from diminished sensitivity of the peripheral tissues to insulin (Rowe *et al.*, 1983). In a comprehensive review, Kritchevsky (1979) has concluded that aging reduces the capacity of the individual to remove lipids from the circulation, so that they accumulate in the tissues. The differential action of aging on plasma lipoproteins is shown in Fig. 2, which displays an age-related fall in high-density lipoproteins (HDLs) of men while

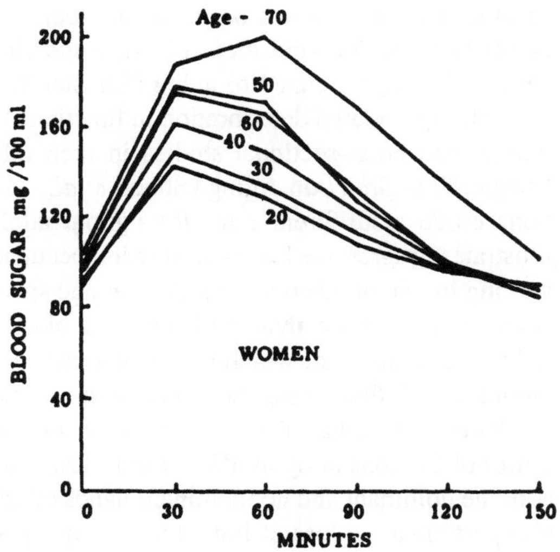

Fig. 1. Effect of age on mean blood sugar levels fasting (0) and at 30, 60, 90, 120, and 150 min after oral intake of 50 g of glucose. (From Keen and Fuller, 1980, with permission.)

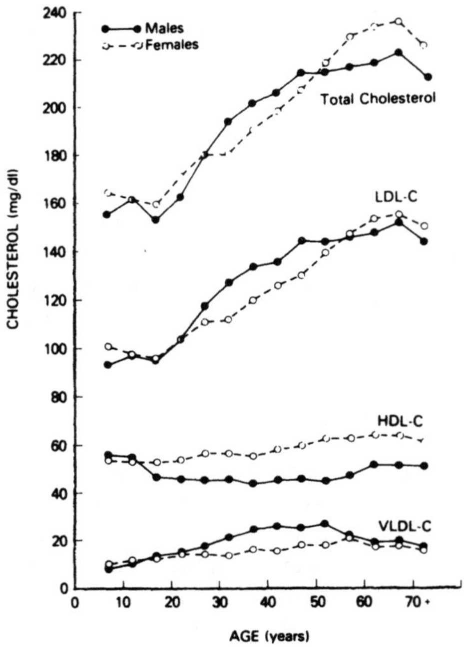

Fig. 2. Age-related changes in the concentrations of cholesterol in different classes of plasma lipoproteins in the blood of men and women in the United States. (Drawn by Dr. E. A. Shafer from Lipid Research Clinics, 1980, *Population Studies Data Book*.)

low-density lipoproteins (LDL) continue to climb. This is relevant to the earlier onset and severity of cardiovascular disease in men. Age-related changes in protein metabolism are detailed in Chapter 7 (Section 2.2). In old age, there is a small reduction in body protein turnover reflecting chiefly the smaller muscle mass of the elderly. In addition, the regulation of protein synthesis in response to dietary supply of protein may change. In the case of plasma albumin, synthesis of this protein by elderly subjects fails to replicate the increase seen in young subjects when the intake of protein is raised from low to adequate levels (Gersovitz *et al.*, 1980). They argue that this is because a lower cap has been set on albumin synthesis in the elderly. Finally, data gathered on amino acid metabolism in the elderly have not provided consistent evidence of changes related to aging (Chapter 7, Section 2).

The age-related deterioration in function is extensively documented by both longitudinal and cross-sectional studies in men followed over decades by the Baltimore Longitudinal Study on Aging (Shock *et al.*, 1984). These data show that organ functions erode at different rates throughout adult life (Shock *et al.*, 1972). Figure 3 illustrates progressive losses in function occurring over the range 30 to 80 years of age, varying in magnitude over this 50-year age span from a reduction of only 15% in nerve conduction to more than 50% in renal blood flow. Loss of muscle mass involves reduction in strength, which has been ascribed by some to diminishing exercise as age progresses. Although regular exercise may ameliorate loss of muscle strength, there is no doubt that aging takes an inevitable toll, as seen in the progressive reduction in power of the constantly used hand muscles, evidenced by the declining grip strength of both the dominant and nondominant hands of adults as they age (Fig. 4). Other systems also participate in loss of function with aging, notably the nervous system (see *Hand-*

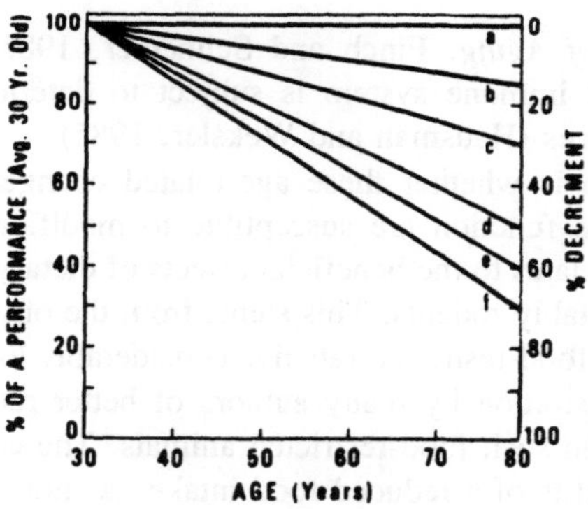

Fig. 3. Age-related decrements in physiological functions of men, expressed as percentage of function remaining at different ages: a, fasting blood glucose; b, nerve conduction velocity; c, resting cardiac index; d, vital capacity, renal blood flow; e, maximum breathing capacity; f, maximum work rate, maximum oxygen uptake. (From Shock, 1972, with permission.)

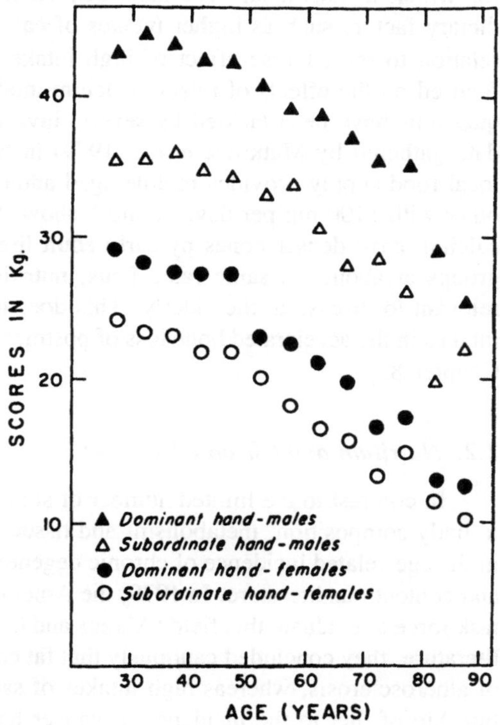

Fig. 4. Age-related decrement in muscle strength for dominant and subordinate hands of men and women. (Reproduced from Miles, 1950, and Shock, 1972, with permission.)

book of the Biology of Aging, Finch and Schneider, 1985, for several chapters). Finally, the important immune system is subject to deterioration with aging with widespread consequences (Hausman and Weksler, 1985).

A major question is whether these age-related changes in body composition, metabolism, and tissue function are susceptible to modification by diet. The most compelling evidence relates to the beneficial affects of dietary restriction on the aging process in animals, notably rodents. This stems from the observations of McCay and colleagues (1935) that food-restricted rats live considerably longer and is amplified by the subsequent demonstration by many authors of better retention of essentially all body functions tested in such food-restricted animals. The contribution of individual nutrients to these benefits of a reduced food intake has not been exhaustively examined, but the review in Chapter 2 of this technique for extending life and prolonging organ functions makes a persuasive case for the reduced intake of energy as being the primary factor in conferring these benefits associated with long-term reduction in food intake. The caged rat eating *ad libitum* is probably equivalent to an indolent adult. Although the application of this animal model of delayed aging may thus not easily be transferred to man, it does provide an important tool for investigating the variable factors involved in the aging process. In studies on mice, Liu *et al.* (1984) have shown that weekly injections of mice with an antibody to T-suppressor cells prolonged their lives, suggesting that the mechanism by which calorie restriction increases the life span may be through improved functioning of the immune system.

Osteoporosis represents another progressive, age-related loss of tissue substance for which a nutritional base has been vigorously explored in relation to retarding dietary factors such as higher intakes of calcium, vitamin D, and of fluoride and in relation to the adverse effect of high intakes of protein. Much of this research has focused on the effects of raising calcium intake and when it is most effective. These questions have been tackled by several investigators. Figure 5 presents bone density data gathered by Matkovic *et al.* (1979) in two areas of Yugoslavia, one where the local food supply provides middle-aged adults with 500 mg calcium per day and the other with 1100 mg per day. Figure 5 shows that those receiving the higher intake of calcium have denser bones by early adult life and that bone density declines in both groups at about the same rate. Thus, nutritional factors in early adult life become relevant to disease in the elderly. This does not preclude benefits from high calcium intakes in the accelerated bone loss of postmenopausal women, as discussed in detail in Chapter 8.

2.2. *Nutrition and Chronic Diseases*

In contrast to the limited number of studies on the effects of nutrition on changes in body composition, metabolism, and tissue function, the role of long-term nutrition in the age-related incidence of chronic degenerative disease has generated an extensive and contentious literature. In 1979, the American Society of Clinical Nutrition set up a task force to evaluate this field (Ahrens and Connor, 1979). After careful review of the literature, they concluded cautiously that fat consumption is related to the development of atherosclerosis, whereas high intakes of salt play a role in hypertension. The relationship of diet to the incidence of cancer has been evaluated in depth in a detailed

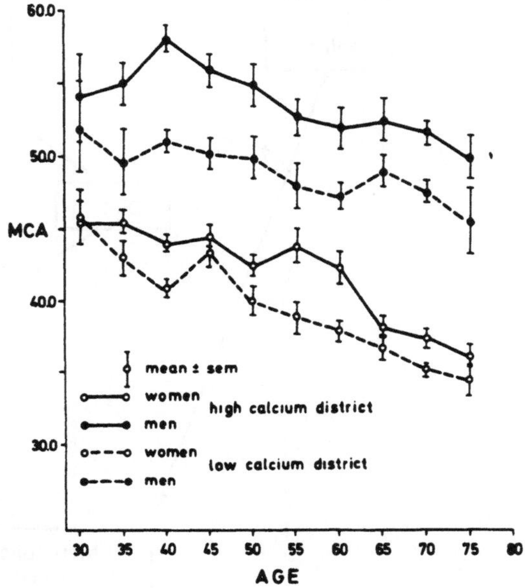

Fig. 5. Age-related changes in metacarpal bone density in men and women in two districts in Yugoslavia, one providing a high calcium intake, the other a low intake. (From Markovic *et al.*, 1979, with permission.)

report by the National Academy of Sciences (1982), which evaluates the relationship of individual nutrients to the incidence of various cancers. Finally, all areas with a potential interaction between long-term nutrition and disease are the subject of a forthcoming lengthy investigation by a committee of the National Research Council (*Diet and Health Report*), which will provide a perspective on the relationship of long-term nutritional habits on the incidence of chronic diseases, most of them much more frequent in older people.

The complexity of the relationships between various life-style factors and the incidence of chronic disease is best illustrated by a diagram (Fig. 6) showing the interactions between primary aging factors (age-related loss of metabolic control) and secondary aging (diet and exercise), the latter affecting obesity, which in the course of time interacts with the age-related impairment of glucose metabolism and thus leads to diabetes and additionally acts adversely on lipid metabolism with consequent atherosclerosis. It is of interest in this context that the McCay animal model of life extension and retention of organ function through caloric restriction has been extended to prolonging the survival of inbred rodents with high incidences of cancer, hypertension, autoimmune diseases, etc. (Good and Gajjar, 1986).

3. *Nutrient Needs and Intakes of the Elderly*

Here we consider the basis on which the requirements for essential nutrients have been determined for older adults, how their nutrient intakes are assessed, and, finally, the actual intakes of essential nutrients by adults as they age and what factors affect these intakes.

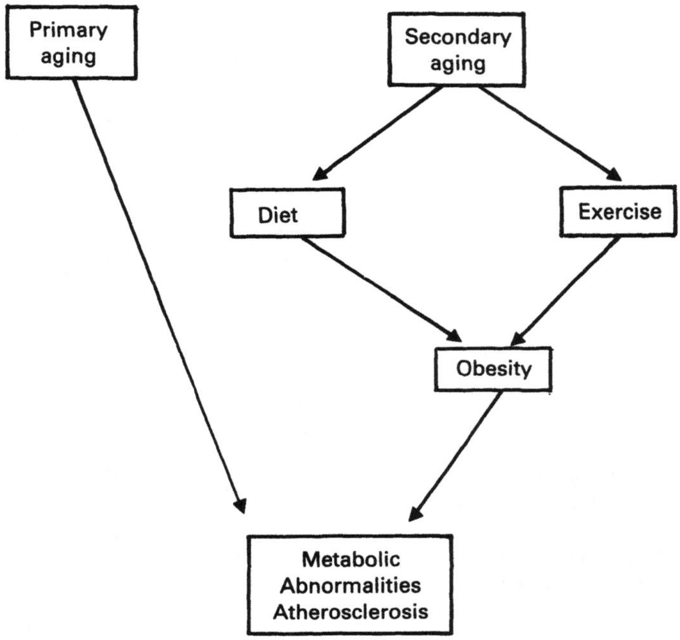

Fig. 6. Interaction of primary aging and secondary aging factors (diet, exercise) on metabolic abnormalities. (From a diagram by A. Goldberg, National Institute on Aging Center at Baltimore.)

3.1. Assessment of Nutrient Requirements

Nutritional status and requirements are determined at both international and national levels. At the international level, the needs of people for individual nutrients are determined by expert committees of the Food and Agricultural Organization (FAO) and the World Health Organization (WHO). For individual countries, this important service is performed by national committees such as the National Academy of Sciences of the United States through its Committee on Dietary Allowances, who periodically issue revised editions of *Recommended Dietary Allowances,* now in its ninth edition (National Academy of Sciences, 1980). In that volume, the recommended dietary allowances are defined as "the levels of intake of essential nutrients considered, in the judgment of the Committee on Dietary Allowances of the Food and Nutrition Board on the basis of available scientific knowledge, to be adequate to meet the known nutritional needs of practically all healthy persons." In estimating allowances, the Committee recognized that individuals vary in their requirements for each nutrient. Accordingly, they used an accepted procedure in which the mean of the needs for each nutrient by individuals within a specific sex and age range is first obtained from published evidence. The variability of individual requirements is then expressed as a standard deviation around the mean, assuming the distribution of individual requirements to be Gaussian (Fig. 7). From this, one can identify the intake needed to satisfy individuals whose requirements are two standard deviations above the mean. By using two stan-

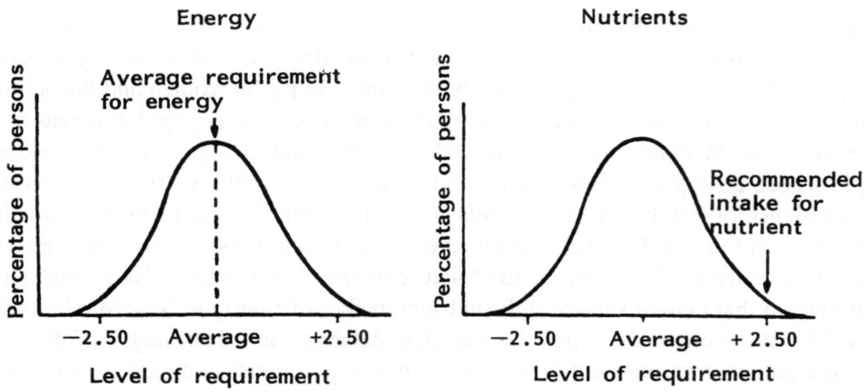

Fig. 7. Distribution of requirements for energy and for a nutrient illustrating the current conventions of describing the average requirement for energy and the average +2 S.D. for nutrients. (From Beaton, 1985, with permission.)

dard deviations above the mean as the requirement, the needs of all but 2.5% of people of that age and sex should be covered.

This procedure has been applied to essential nutrients in general. In the case of energy needs, however, it is obvious that recommending the intakes that cover 97.5% of the population would lead to obesity for those with lesser caloric requirements. Accordingly, the average need of the age and sex group is recommended as the energy allowance. In the ninth edition of the *RDA* (National Academy of Sciences, 1980), the recommended energy levels are provided with ranges as well as mean levels in order to emphasize the considerable variation between individuals. In addition, the ninth edition includes estimates of allowances for three vitamins (vitamin K, biotin, and pantothenic acid), six trace elements (copper, chromium, fluoride, manganese, molybdenum, and selenium), and three electrolytes (sodium, potassium, and chloride) for which the evidence is much less complete. Accordingly, these are presented as ranges of intakes recommended as safe and adequate. In the case of trace elements, persistently exceeding the upper limit of the range may lead to toxic effects.

Relevant to the dietary allowances for the elderly is the classification of adults in the *RDA* (National Academy of Sciences, 1980) into only three groups, namely, 19–22 years, 23–50 years, and 51 years upwards. The last of these groups covers the spectrum from the active middle-aged man with a daily energy intake of 2500 kcal to the 90-year-old case in a nursing home consuming less than 1250 kcal. A similar though less severe change applies to women. The consequent reduction in intake of nutrients contained in the energy sources is discussed later in this chapter. It should be noted that the nutrient needs prescribed in the *RDA* (National Academy of Sciences, 1980) for those 51 years and over are in general the same as those for younger adults, although we shall see in Section 3.3 that their actual intakes of essential nutrients diminish progressively with age.

The difficulties in arriving at plausible estimates of dietary allowances for some nutrients is illustrated by the case of folic acid. According to the *RDA* (National Academy of Sciences, 1980), adults of all ages are recommended to consume an average daily intake of 400 μg. This is criticized in a report on the folate status of the elderly (Rosenberg *et al.*, 1982), which points out that a Canadian survey reported average daily intakes of 150 μg by elderly men and 130 μg by women and that similar estimates were obtained in a dietary survey in Sweden. In neither population was there evidence of megaloblastic anemia attributable to folate deficiency. Even those elderly people whose absorption of dietary folate is impaired by achlorhydria fail to show a high incidence of low blood folate levels (Russell, 1986). The decision as to whether the RDA is set too high or the consumption of folate is underreported is complicated by incomplete analysis of foodstuffs for folate content. For example, Garry and Hunt (1986) report that in their survey of the nutrient intakes of elderly in New Mexico, 40% of the 2400 items on their computerized nutrient database lacked an entry for folic acid. A similar picture presents itself in the case of zinc requirements and intakes (Sandstead *et al.*, 1982).

The concepts and applications of the recommended dietary allowances are constantly under review and undergo an evolutionary process. Some of these proposed changes are particularly relevant to aging and to the elderly. In a recent published lecture, Beaton (1986) has discussed the meaning of nutritional requirements in relation to nutritional status. He looks on estimated requirements of essential nutrients as meeting two levels of objectives. First, he identifies a basal requirement that is needed to prevent any clinically demonstrable impairment of function. Second, he recognizes a second level he calls a normative storage requirement in order to provide and maintain a reserve of the nutrient in the body. This allows a supply of the nutrient that can be mobilized under stressful conditions without impairing function. In addition to defined nutrient requirements, he goes on to recognize that diet has a much less quantifiable relationship to many chronic diseases that usually declare themselves in older adults. From this he concludes that the end product of assessing nutrient requirements should include the form of recommended dietary patterns of foods and food mixtures to meet requirements for essential nutrients and at the same time minimize the risk of developing chronic disease. This appears to be a prescription for optimizing the dietary habits of the aging adult.

3.2. Assessment of Adequacy of Nutrient Intakes of Populations

In evaluating the nutritional status of the elderly in a population, it is important to know their average daily intakes of individual nutrients and to compare these with the estimated requirements for persons of the same age and sex. In the United States, the main national surveys of nutrient intakes are the Health and Nutrition Examination Surveys (HANES I and II) of the National Center for Health Statistics and the Nation-wide Food Consumption Surveys (NFCS) of the U.S. Department of Agriculture. To obtain maximum information about nutritional adequacy from dietary intake data, it is desirable to supplement the survey findings with biomedical and clinical examinations on the individuals surveyed. The HANES provides some such information, but not the NFCS series of studies. Unfortunately, the HANES data do not extend beyond 74 years of age, thus cutting off the elderly most likely to suffer from nutritional deficiencies. In addition to the HANES and NFCS nutritional surveys, specific studies have been made of localized groups of elderly (e.g., Garry *et al.*, 1982a,b,c; Hunt *et al.*, 1983; McGandy *et al.*, 1986).

In order to interpret the frequency of inadequate intakes in the population surveyed, it has been customary to compare the nutrient intakes of individual members of the population with the recommended dietary allowances for the same nutrients for people of that sex and age. This allows one to state how many in the group have intakes falling below the standard set by the RDAs. However, the RDAs have built-in safety margins for most nutrients so that many people receiving less than the RDA for a nutrient are not necessarily deficient. Accordingly, it has become the practice to reduce the cut-off point to two-thirds or three-quarters of the RDA in order to identify those with inadequate intakes. In a recent National Research Council report entitled *Nutrient Adequacy: Assessment Using Food Consumption Surveys* (NRC, 1986), it is suggested that a new approach should be developed to detect nutrient deficiencies in a population. It is based on the probability of an individual's requirement for a nutrient being above or below the average for persons of his or her age and sex. This can be compared with an estimate, also determined by probability analysis, of his or her customary intake of the nutrient obtained from intakes reported over a few days. By applying a statistical approach to these two estimates, it is possible to compute how many people in a population are likely to be at risk of deficiency of the nutrient and what the reliability of that estimate is.

Two factors limit this approach. One is the paucity of reliable information for each essential nutrient regarding the mean requirement and the range of its requirements within the population. This becomes even more restrictive when applied to the elderly, for whom both mean nutrient requirements and their variability have been much less investigated than is the case for young adults. The estimates of variability in requirements should also take account of other dietary factors that affect the utilization of a nutrient, such as the impact of energy intake on the amount of protein needed to achieve nitrogen balance (Chapter 7, Section 3.1) and the effect of dietary protein level on calcium balance (Chapter 8). The second limiting factor is the uncertainty of estimates of nutrient intake. These estimates usually depend on the accurate cooperation of the subject who either recalls food consumed, makes records in a diary at the time of eating, or even sets aside equal portions of the food for subsequent analysis. The variability introduced by having to deal with a combination of working days and weekend days has been explored by van Staveren *et al.* (1985) and others, who show the necessity to take into account this schism in our eating patterns. Another factor distorting normal food consumption is the self-consciousness induced by being an experimental subject, a topic extensively explored in a study published by Kim *et al.* (1983a). In a companion paper reporting a 1-year study of intakes, Kim *et al.* (1983b) confirm the reduced energy intake of those over 35 years old.

In all these approaches to accurate assessment of the food intakes of individuals in groups or populations, it is desirable to have some guarantee of the precision of the individual estimates. On a limited scale it is possible to compare estimated energy intakes with energy expenditures using dissociation of $D_2{}^{18}O$ as an integrating measure of energy expenditure over several weeks. Using this to examine the energy expenditures of young adult women, Prentice *et al.* (1985) have confirmed their low energy intakes recorded in dietary surveys. Less demanding is the use of urinary N output to compare with protein intake (Isaksson, 1980; van Staveren *et al.*, 1985). Finally, the use of blood levels of vitamins is good confirmation of the frequency of inadequate intakes measured from dietary histories. Thus, Garry and Hunt (1986) show good correlations between blood levels of vitamin C (0.59), B_2 (0.55), B_{12} (0.45), folate (0.50), and α-tocopherol (0.64) and their assessed total intakes by an elderly population.

A further restriction on the methodology of dietary intake assessment is the limitations of the food composition database that is applied to a person's consumption of foodstuffs in order to obtain intakes of individual nutrients. Food composition has been inadequately extended to the full range of foods for folic acid, zinc, and trace metals, largely because of limitations in analytical methodology. This may result in underestimation of intakes of these nutrients. Another factor lies in differences in the nutrient composition of foodstuffs encoded in different databases. Danford (1981) submitted the food items listed for a single day's diet to 11 different computer programs for calculation of nutrient content. The coefficients of variation between programs were considerable, from 4% around the mean estimate for the calcium content of the day's diet through 12% each for energy and for protein content, 29% for thiamin, 41% for vitamin B_{12}, 42% for vitamin B_6 and for zinc, 70% for vitamin E, and 96% for copper.

In view of these sources of uncertainty about RDAs and about nutrient consumption, it seems premature to apply the methods advocated in the NRC (1985) report until better basic data on requirements and on dietary survey methodology are guaranteed. An initial step would be to apply measurements of $D_2{}^{18}O$ dissociation and urinary N output to selected subjects from the HANES and NFCS dietary intake surveys in order to test the precision of these measures of energy and protein intakes. An additional precaution would be the inclusion of biochemical indices of deficiency, such as the plasma levels of certain plasma proteins for confirmation of protein–calorie malnutrition and similarly for intakes of many of the vitamins. Finally, clinical examination for nutrient deficiencies would provide additional guarantees of the incidence of malnutrition independent of dietary surveys. In this respect, inclusion of clinical examinations also allows the investigator to determine whether other diseases are responsible for precipitating any nutritional deficiencies found in the population. This last feature is especially important in nutritional surveys of the elderly, as discussed in the next section of this chapter.

3.3. *Age-Related Changes in Nutrient Intake*

As people grow older, they experience changes in food consumption patterns. First, aging reduces appetite for food. Second, changes in food preferences occur in the population in general over the decades. Last, the food supply changes. Each of these will now be illustrated.

Much evidence testifies to the conclusion that total food consumption declines progressively from early adult life through to old age. Nowhere is this more compellingly demonstrated than in the Baltimore Longitudinal Study of Aging (BLSA). This group of upper-middle-class men was carefully evaluated during 1961–1965 for their

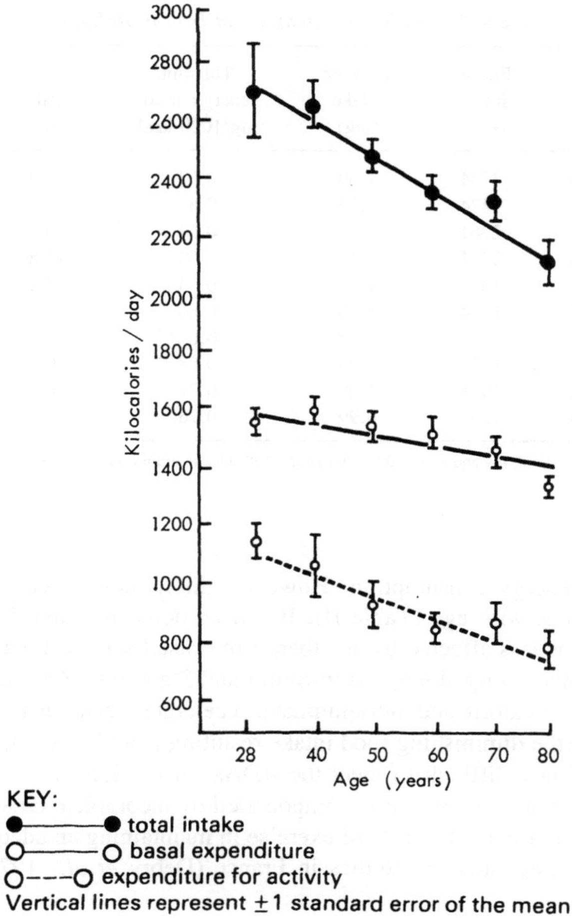

Fig. 8. Daily intake and expenditure of energy in men of different ages. (From Shock, 1972, with permission.)

intakes of energy and of selected nutrients (McGandy *et al.*, 1966). Figure 8 shows these cross-sectional data for energy intake and confirms the decline occurring decade by decade, a minor part of which can be ascribed to reduced basal energy metabolism, whereas a major cause is the steadily diminishing physical activity associated with aging. With this reduction in energy consumption goes a general diminution in intakes of nutrients present in the caloric source. In the case of the Baltimore study, aging was associated with declining intakes of iron, thiamin, riboflavin, and niacin. This is confirmed by data from national surveys such as HANES II, which show a progressive age-related reduction in the thiamin and iron intakes of adults from age 25 to 74 years in parallel with energy intakes (Table II). In the case of thiamin, the need for this vitamin is linked to energy intake, so that the reduction with aging is compensated by

Table II. Dietary Intake by Adults of Thiamin and Iron in Relation to Energy Intake[a]

Sex	Age (yr)	Energy intake (kcal)	Thiamin intake (mg)	Thiamin energy ratio (mg/1000 kcal)	Iron intake (mg)	Iron energy ratio (mg/1000 kcal)
Males	25–34	2734	1.69	0.62	17.3	6.3
	35–44	2424	1.55	0.64	16.1	6.6
	45–54	2361	1.51	0.64	16.2	6.9
	55–64	2071	1.40	0.68	14.8	7.1
	65–74	1828	1.33	0.73	14.1	7.7
Females	25–34	1634	1.08	0.66	10.9	6.6
	35–44	1579	1.05	0.66	11.2	7.1
	45–54	1439	0.98	0.68	10.4	7.3
	55–64	1401	1.00	0.71	10.7	7.6
	65–74	1295	0.99	0.76	10.2	7.9

[a]Data taken from HANES-II survey and reported by Iber *et al.* (1982) for thiamin intake and by Lynch *et al.* (1982) for iron intake.

the diminishing energy consumption. However, this is not the case for iron intake, which also declines with age (Table II). It can be noted in Table II that the energy intake of women is less affected by age than is the case for men. Finally, in an elderly subgroup of women living alone, Exton-Smith and Stanton (1965) have demonstrated that the reduction in caloric and nutrient intake accelerates between age 70 and 80 years (Table III). With the diminishing food intake resulting from less demand for energy, it becomes increasingly difficult to meet the RDAs for calcium, iron, zinc, folic acid, vitamin B_6, and vitamin E, which is compounded by incomplete data on food content of some of these nutrients. The role of exercise in maintaining an adequate food intake by the elderly is illustrated by studies in France (Debry *et al.*, 1977) showing that

Table III. Nutrient Intakes of Older Women Living Alone and Changes between Age 70 and 80 Years[a]

Nutrient	Mean daily intake	Percentage reduction (70–80 yrs)
Calories	1890	19
Protein (g)	57	24
Fat (g)	74	30
Carbohydrate (g)	221	8
Calcium (mg)	860	18
Iron (mg)	9.9	29
Vitamin C (mg)	37	31
Vitamin D (i.u.)	135	—

[a]Abstracted from Exton-Smith (1980b).

Table IV. Effect of Age on Attempted Weight Loss by Obese Adults in a Representative U.S. Population[a]

Age group (yr)	Proportion attempting weight loss (%)	Choice of weight loss procedure	
		Eating less (%)	Exercise (%)
18–29	32	75	69
30–44	39	81	59
45–64	40	84	49
65+	24	83	40

[a]Abstracted from Thornberry *et al.* (1986).

elderly women in an urban setting had daily energy intakes averaging 1710 kcal, whereas those in the countryside had intakes of 2170 kcal, presumably related to greater physical activity in rural areas. However, adults become less inclined to exercise as age advances, as illustrated by the data in Table IV for people losing excess weight either by dietary means or by exercise. As age advanced, progressively fewer of the subjects chose exercise.

The conclusions drawn from cross-sectional studies are strengthened by longitudinal studies on the Baltimore cohort of men. Elahi *et al.* (1983) have followed the food intakes of 180 survivors of the initial dietary studies made during 1961–1965. During the subsequent 15 years, two additional measurements of the food consumption of this population were made. From these three assessments of dietary intake spread out over this period, the investigators were able to use regression analysis to dissect out the effects of age, of cohort, and of elapsed time on intakes of calories, carbohydrate, total fat, saturated and unsaturated fatty acids, and cholesterol. They confirmed that advancing age is the main factor associated with the reduction in intake of energy (expressed as total intake or intake per kilogram body weight) and in total fat. On the other hand, the intake of polyunsaturated fats and the polyunsaturated/saturated ratio were unaffected by the subject's age but increased over the 15-year period of the study at all ages. Thus, the elderly share in the trendiness of the rest of the population, being just as susceptible to nutritional changes as are younger adults.

Finally, have there been significant changes in the pattern of available nutrients in the American food supply as consumed over the life span of individuals who are now over the age of 65 years? This is answered by the daily supply of nutrients per individual in the population, a computation made annually by the U.S. Department of Agriculture since 1907. These figures represent the amount of food purchased from suppliers divided by the U.S. population and are probably exaggerated because of the use of food for domestic animals and because of food wastage. Nevertheless, the data do provide trends. Table V abstracts the data for each decade between 1910 and 1980 and shows that total caloric and protein intakes have changed little over this period but that carbohydrate as a source of calories has diminished 20% while fat intake has increased by 30%. More detailed analysis of this trend shows that this change has occurred mainly since 1960 and has taken the form of greater consumption of unsatu-

Table V. Food Energy and Nutrient Content per Capita per Day[a]

Nutrient	1910	1920	1930	1940	1950	1960	1970	1980	RDAs (51+ yr)[b]	
									Males	Females
Energy (kcal)	3460	3270	3430	3340	3250	3160	3300	3410	2200	1700
Protein (g)	100	92	91	93	94	96	100	100	56	44
Carbohydrate (g)	493	456	472	428	400	373	379	392	—	—
Fat (g)	124	122	134	143	145	147	160	163	—	—
Cholesterol (mg)	504	490	517	524	578	544	526	490	—	—
Fiber (g)	6.2	5.7	5.7	5.5	4.8	4.3	4.1	4.1	—	—
Vit. A (I.U.)	8000	8400	8700	9100	8900	8000	7900	7600	5000	4000
Thiamin (mg)	1.62	1.51	1.53	1.54	1.90	1.91	1.95	2.16	1.2	1.0
Riboflavin (mg)	1.77	1.76	1.80	1.88	2.28	2.25	2.26	2.36	1.4	1.2
Niacin (mg)	19.2	17.5	17.2	17.8	20.4	21.6	24.0	25.7	16.0	13.0
Vit. B_6 (mg)	2.20	1.96	1.92	1.92	1.84	1.85	1.97	2.00	2.2	2.0
Vit. B_{12} (μg)	8.1	8.0	7.6	8.1	8.7	8.9	9.6	9.0	3.0	3.0
Folacin (μg)	318	300	302	304	293	281	275	284	400	400
Vit. C (mg)	109	108	103	114	104	103	107	120	60	60
Calcium (mg)	740	790	820	890	970	930	900	900	800	800
Phosphorus (mg)	1510	1440	1450	1490	1530	1510	1510	1500	800	800
Magnesium (mg)	405	378	380	381	360	340	336	333	350	300
Iron (mg)	15.1	14.2	13.8	13.7	15.9	15.8	16.9	16.8	10	10
Zinc (mg)	12.5	11.4	10.9	11.1	11.3	11.6	12.3	12.1	15	15

[a]U.S. Food Supply Historical Series, summarized in U.S. Dept. of Health and Human Services and U.S. Dept. of Agriculture (1986) report.
[b]From *Recommended Dietary Allowances*, 9th ed. (National Academy of Sciences, 1980).

rated fats (Munro, 1975). Another change, this time dating from 1940, has been a sharp increase in available thiamin, riboflavin, and niacin and coincides with fortification of cereal products with these vitamins. On the other hand, there has been an 18% decline in magnesium intake, and in addition, consumption of more refined cereals during the century has resulted in a 34% decrease in fiber intake. Finally, the zinc and the folate content of the national diet has always been less than the recommended adult intakes of 15 mg and 400 μg, respectively (National Academy of Sciences, 1980). As discussed in Chapter 11, there is some evidence that consumption of more fiber can decrease the incidence of diverticulosis and diverticulitis of the large intestine. Such a relationship does not prove that the active agent in the diets of vegetarians is necessarily fiber; it could be other factors (nutrients) in the foods containing fiber. These various trends are relevant to the long-term exposure of adults to dietary factors affecting aging.

4. *Other Factors Affecting Nutritional Status of the Elderly*

The nutritional status of the elderly is more varied than that of younger adults because of a variety of age-related changes in social, physiological, and pathological status. Exton-Smith (1980b) has listed cases of malnutrition among the elderly according to cause.

First, there are adverse social and environmental factors as primary causes of malnutrition. These include ignorance of the basic facts of nutrition, men who have never cooked being especially vulnerable when they are widowed. Poverty restricts the range of foods available to the elderly person. Physical disability also limits the capacity of some elderly people to get around to a variety of food stores. Social isolation causes the elderly single person to lose interest in food, a problem that can be averted by participating in congregate feeding programs (see Chapter 12). Depressive mental illness and confusional states occur more frequently among old people, all of which are incompatible with well-balanced nutrition.

Secondly, elderly people have malnutrition secondary to pathological conditions. This group includes malabsorption because of previous gastrectomy and gastrointestinal dysfunctions from bacterial overgrowth; major nutrients affected are fat-soluble vitamins, folic acid, and vitamin B_{12}. Inefficient mastication from ill-fitting dentures (or none) can restrict food choices. Alcoholism and therapeutic drugs can affect nutrition in various ways. Alcohol substitutes empty calories for foods containing a variety of nutrients and can also interfere with absorption, particularly of folic acid (see Chapter 10). Drugs such as barbiturates can also impair absorption of folic acid, and other drugs impair nutrient utilization in other ways, making it desirable to supplement dietary vitamin intakes when these drugs are being administered (Chapter 14). Disease processes can increase requirements for nutrients while also impairing appetite, either from the disease process itself or because of medications (see Chapter 14).

This last factor of disease has to be considered an increasing feature affecting the nutritional status of the elderly as age advances. In a survey representative of the British elderly population (Department of Health and Social Security, 1979), the frequency of malnutrition as judged from intake, biochemical assessment, and clinical evaluation was 6% for men and 5% for women between 70 and 80 years and 12% and 8%, respectively, after that age. Malnutrition was mostly diagnosed as protein–calorie malnutrition and anemia. Essentially all undernourished subjects had a primary illness (chronic bronchitis, emphysema, dementia, postgastrectomy syndrome, etc.) that accounted for their lower food intake and also contributed tissue losses through the disease process. In contrast, a Boston survey (Munro *et al.*, 1987) that excluded elderly with wasting illnesses provided no evidence of protein–calorie malnutrition as evidenced by lack of diet-related changes in plasma proteins and in muscle mass. The effect of chronic disease on nutritional status may also account for the varied number of elderly people with unacceptably low blood values for certain vitamins, depending on whether they lived at home or in a nursing home (Baker *et al.*, 1979; Vir and Love, 1979).

Finally, there is some evidence suggesting that the elderly can more easily become nutrient deficient in response to stressful illnesses. Exton-Smith (1980a) cites instances in which acute intercurrent infections can precipitate Wernicke's encephalopathy because of insufficiency of thiamin or Jolliffe's encephalopathy from lack of niacin. Lipschitz (1986) has identified reduced capacity of the elderly to form blood cells under conditions of stress when compromised by nutritional deficiencies. This combination of age-related deterioration in response mechanisms together with impaired nutritional status is also seen in the lack of capacity of the elderly to increase albumin synthesis when protein intake is raised from a suboptimal to a high level (Gersovitz *et al.*, 1980).

In conclusion, the study of nutritional status and requirements of the elderly is complicated by many factors that do not significantly affect nutritional studies in the young adults. These should be recognized if the nutrition of the elderly is to receive adequate evaluation.

5. References

Ahrens, E. H., and Connor, W. E., 1979, The evidence relating six dietary factors to the nation's health, *Am. J. Clin. Nutr.* **32**:2621–2748.

Baker, H., Frank, O., Thind, I. S., Jaslow, S. P., and Louria, D. B., 1979, Vitamin profiles in elderly persons living at home or in nursing homes versus profiles in healthy young subjects, *J. Am. Geriatr. Soc.* **27**:444–450.

Beaton, G. H., 1985, Uses and limits of the use of the Recommended Dietary Allowances for evaluating dietary intake data, *Am. J. Clin. Nutr.* **41**:155–164.

Beaton, G. H., 1986, Toward harmonization of dietary, biochemical and clinical assessments: The meaning of nutritional status and requirements, *Nutr. Rev.* **44**:349–360.

Brody, J. A., and Brock, D. B., 1985, Epidemiologic and statistical characteristics of the United States elderly population, in: *Handbook of the Biology of Aging,* 2nd ed. (C. E. Finch and E. L. Schneider, eds.), Van Nostrand-Rheinhold, New York, pp. 3–26.

Cohn, S. H., Vartsky, D., Yasumura, S., Sawitsky, A., Zanzi, I., Vaswani, A., and Ellis, K. J., 1980, Compartmental body composition based on total body nitrogen, potassium and calcium, *Am. J. Physiol.* **239**:E524–530.

Danford, D. E., 1981, Computer applications to medical nutrition problems, *J. Parenteral Enteral Nutr.* **5**:441–446.

Debry, G., Bleyer, R., and Martin, J. M., 1977, Nutrition of the elderly, *J. Hum. Nutr.* **31**:195–204.

Department of Health and Social Security, 1979, *A Nutrition Survey of the Elderly, Reports on Health Social Subjects No. 16,* Her Majesty's Stationery Office, London.

Elahi, V. K., Elahi, D., Andres, R., Tobin, J. D., Butler, M. G., and Norris, A. H., 1983, A longitudinal study of nutritional intake in men, *J. Gerontol.* **38:**162–180.

Exton-Smith, A. N., 1977, Malnutrition in the elderly, *Proc. R. Soc. Med.* **70:**615–619.

Exton-Smith, A. N., 1980a, Vitamins, in: *Metabolic and Nutritional Disorders in the Elderly* (A. N. Exton-Smith and F. I. Caird, eds.), Wright, Bristol, pp. 26–38.

Exton-Smith, A. N., 1980b, Nutritional status: Diagnosis and prevention of malnutrition, in: *Metabolic and Nutritional Disorders in the Elderly* (A. N. Exton-Smith and F. I. Caird, eds.), Wright, Bristol, pp. 66–76.

Exton-Smith, A. N., and Stanton, B. R., 1965, *Report of an Investigation into the Dietary of Elderly Women Living Alone,* King Edward's Hospital Fund, London.

Finch, C. E., and Schneider, E. L., eds., 1985, *Handbook of the Biology of Aging,* 2nd ed., Van Nostrand-Rheinhold, New York.

Fries, J. F., 1980, Aging natural death and the compression of morbidity, *N. Engl. J. Med.* **303:**130–135.

Garry, P. J., and Hunt, W. C., 1986, Biochemical assessment of vitamin status in the elderly: Effects of dietary and supplemental intakes, in: *Nutrition and Aging* (M. L. Hutchinson and H. N. Munro, eds.), Academic Press, Orlando, FL, pp. 117–137.

Garry, P. J., Goodwin, J. S., and Hunt, W. C., 1982a, Nutritional status in a healthy population: Riboflavin, *Am. J. Clin. Nutr.* **36:**902–909.

Garry, P. J., Goodwin, J. S., Hunt, W. C., Hooper, E. M., and Leonard, A. G., 1982b, Nutritional status in a healthy elderly population: Dietary and supplemental intakes, *Am. J. Clin. Nutr.* **36:**319–331.

Garry, P. J., Goodwin, J. S., Hunt, W. C., and Gilbert, B. A., 1982c, Nutritional status in a healthy elderly population: Vitamin C, *Am. J. Clin. Nutr.* **36:**332–339.

Gersovitz, M., Munro, H. N., Udall, J., and Young, V. R., 1980, Albumin synthesis in young and elderly subjects using a new stable isotope methodology: Response to level of protein intake, *Metabolism* **29:**1075–1086.

Good, R. A., and Gajjar, A. J., 1986, Diet, immunity, and longevity, in: *Nutrition and Aging* (M. L. Hutchinson and H. N. Munro, eds.), Academic Press, Orlando, FL, pp. 235–249.

Hausman, P. B., and Weksler, M. E., 1985, Changes in the immune response with age, in: *Handbook of the Biology of Aging,* 2nd ed. (C. E. Finch and E. L. Schneider, eds.), Van Nostrand-Rheinhold, New York, pp. 414–432.

Hunt, W. C., Leonard, A. G., Garry, P. J., and Goodwin, J. S., 1983, Components of variance of dietary data for an elderly population, *Nutr. Res.* **3:**433–444.

Iber, F. L., Blass, J. P., Brin, M., and Leevy, C. M., 1982, Thiamin in the elderly—relation to alcoholism and to neurological degenerative disease, *Am. J. Clin. Nutr.* **36:**1067–1082.

Isaksson, B., 1980, Urinary nitrogen output as a validity test in dietary surveys, *Am. J. Clin. Nutr.* **33:**4–5.

Katz, S., Branch, L. G., Branson, M. H., Papsidero, J. H., Beck, J. C., and Greer, D. S., 1983, Active life expectancy, *N. Engl. J. Med.* **309:**1218–1224.

Keen, H., and Fuller, J. H., 1980, The epidemiology of diabetes, in: *Metabolic and Nutritional Disorders in the Elderly* (A. N. Exton-Smith and F. C. Caird, eds.), Wright, Bristol, pp. 146–160.

Kim, W. W., Mertz, W., Judd, J. T., Marshall, M. W., Kelsay, J. L., and Prather, E. S., 1984a, Effect of making duplicate food collections on nutrient intakes calculated from diet records, *Am. J. Clin. Nutr.* **40:**1333–1337.

Kim, W. W., Kelsay, J. L., Judd, J. T., Marshall, M. W., Mertz, W., and Prather, E. S., 1984b, Evaluation of long-term dietary intakes of adults consuming self-selected diets, *Am. J. Clin. Nutr.* **40:**1327–1332.

Kritchevsky, D., 1979, Diet, lipid metabolism and aging, *Fed. Proc.* **38:**2001–2006.

Lipid Research Clinics, 1980, *Population Studies Data Book,* Volume I, *The Prevalence Study* (NIH Publication no. 80-1527), U.S. Dept. of Health and Human Services, Washington, pp. 28–81.

Liu, J. J., Segre, D., Gelberg, H. B., Fudenberg, H. H., Tsang, K. Y., Khansari, N., Waltenbaugh, C. R., and Segre, M., 1984, Effects of long-term treatment of mice with anti-I-J-monoclonal antibody and dialyzable leukocyte extract on immune function and life-span, *Mech. Aging Dev.* **27:**359–372.

Lipschitz, D. A., 1986, Nutrition and the aging hematopoietic system, in: *Nutrition and Aging* (M. L. Hutchinson and H. N. Munro, eds.), Academic Press, Orlando, FL, pp. 251–262.

Lynch, S. R., Finch, C. A., Monsen, E. R., and Cook, J. D., 1982, Iron status of elderly Americans, *Am. J. Clin. Nutr.* **36:**1032–1045.

Matkovic, V., Kostial, K., Simonovic, I., Buzina, R., Brodarec, A., and Nordin, B. E. C., 1979, Bone status and fracture rates in two regions of Yugoslavia, *Am. J. Clin. Nutr.* **32:**540–549.

McCay, C. M., Crowell, M. F., and Maynard, L. A., 1935, The effect of retarded growth upon the length of the life-span and upon ultimate body size, *J. Nutr.* **10:**63–79.

McGandy, R. B., Barrows, C. H., Spanias, A., Meredith, A., Stone, J. L., and Norris, A. H., 1966, Nutrient intakes and energy expenditure in men of different ages, *J. Gerontol.* **21:**581–587.

McGandy, R. B., Russell, R. M., Hartz, S. C., Jacob, R. A., Tannenbaum, S., Peters, H., Sahyoun, N., and Otradovec, C., 1986, Nutritional status survey of healthy non-institutionalized elderly: Nutrient intakes from 3-day diet records and nutrient supplements, *Nutr. Res.* **6:**785–798.

Miles, W. R., 1950, Simultaneous right and left hand grip, in: *Methods in Medical Research*, Vol. 3 (R. N. Gerard, ed.), Yearbook Medical Publishers, Chicago, pp. 154–156.

Munro, H. N., 1975, Health-related aspects of animal products for the human, in: *Fat Content and Composition of Animal Products,* National Academy of Sciences, Washington, pp. 24–44.

Munro, H. N., and Young, V. R., 1978, Urinary excretion of N^{T}-methylhistidine (3-methylhistidine): A tool to study metabolic responses in relation to nutrient and hormonal status in health and disease in man, *Am. J. Clin. Nutr.* **31:**1608–1614.

Munro, H. N., McGandy, R. B., Hartz, S. C., Russell, R. M., Jacob, R. A., and Otradovec, C. L., 1987, Protein nutriture of a group of free-living elderly, *Am. J. Clin. Nutr.* **46:**586–592.

National Academy of Sciences, 1980, *Recommended Dietary Allowances,* 9th rev. ed., National Academy Press, Washington.

National Academy of Sciences, 1982, *Diet, Nutrition and Cancer Report,* National Academy Press, Washington.

NRC, 1986, *Nutrient Adequacy: Assessment Using Food Consumption Surveys,* National Academy Press, Washington.

Prentice, A. M., Coward, W. A., Davies, H. L., Murgatroyd, P. R., Black, A. E., Goldberg, G. R., Ashford, J., Sawyer, M., and Whitehead, R. G., 1985, Unexpectedly low levels of energy expenditure in healthy women, *Lancet* **1:**1419–1422.

Rosenberg, I. H., Bowman, B. B., Cooper, B. A., Halsted, C. H., and Lindenbaum, J., 1982, Folate nutrition in the elderly, *Am. J. Clin. Nutr.* **36:**1060–1066.

Rowe, J. W., 1985, Health care of the elderly, *N. Engl. J. Med.* **312:**827–835.

Rowe, J. W., Minaker, K. L., Pallotta, J. A., and Flier, J. S., 1983, Characterization of the insulin resistance of aging, *J. Clin. Invest.* **71:**1581–1587.

Russell, R. M., 1986, Implications of gastric atrophy for vitamin and mineral nutriture, in: *Nutrition and Aging* (M. L. Hutchinson and H. N. Munro, eds.), Academic Press, Orlando, FL, pp. 59–69.

Sandstead, H. H., Henriksen, L. K., Greger, J. L., Prasad, A. D., and Good, R. A., 1982, Zinc nutriture in the elderly in relation to taste acuity, immune response, and wound healing, *Am. J. Clin. Nutr.* **36:**1046–1059.

Shock, N. W., 1972, Energy metabolism, caloric intake, and physical activity of the aging, in: *Nutrition in Old Age (Xth Symposium of the Swedish Nutrition Foundation* (L. A. Carlson, ed.), Almqvist & Wiksell, Uppsala, pp. 12–23.

Shock, N., Greulich, R. C., Andres, R, Arenberg, D., Costa, P. T., Lakatta, E. G., and Tobin, J. D., 1984, *Normal Human Aging: The Baltimore Longitudinal Study of Aging,* NIH Publication no. 84-2450, U.S. Government Printing Office, Washington.

Silverberg, A. B., 1984, Carbohydrate metabolism and diabetes in the aged, in: *Nutritional Intervention in the Aging Process* (H. J. Ambrecht, J. M. Prendergast, and R. M. Coe, eds.), Springer, New York, pp. 191–208.

Thornberry, O. T., Wilson, R. W., and Golden, P. M., 1986, *Health Promotion Data for the 1990 Objectives: Estimates from the National Health Interview Survey of Health Promotion and Disease Prevention: United States, 1985, Advance Data from Vital and Health Statistics, No. 126,* DHHS Pub No. (PHS) 86-1250, Public Health Service, Hyattsville, MD.

U.S. Department of Health and Human Services and U.S. Department of Agriculture, 1986, *Nutrition Monitoring in the United States—A Report from the Joint Nutrition Monitoring Evaluation Committee,* DHHS Publication No. (PHS) 86-1255, Public Health Service, Washington.

van Staveren, W. A., de Boer, J. O., and Burema, J., 1985, Validity and reproducibility of a dietary history method estimating the usual food intake during one month, *Am. J. Clin. Nutr.* **42**:554–559.
Vir, S. C., and Love, A. H. G., 1979, Nutritional status of institutionalized and non-institutionalized aged in Belfast, Northern Ireland, *Am. J. Clin. Nutr.* **32**:1934–1947.

I

Nutrition and Age-Related Changes in Body Function

2

Nutrition and Aging in Animal Models

Edward J. Masoro

1. Introduction

Nutrition is frequently claimed to be an important factor influencing the aging processes of humans and other animals (Porta, 1980). In part, this belief is based on nothing more than faith in the "fountain of youth" and in nutrition as a path to it. However, in fact, there are some data in the literature that indicate that nutrition holds promise as a basis for interventions that modulate the adverse effects of aging, thereby enhancing the quality of life at advanced age (Masoro, 1985). By the same token, there are also data that suggest that certain nutritional regimens or dietary components promote the aging process or at least promote age-associated disease or deterioration (Guigoz and Munro, 1985).

What is currently needed is the development of research strategies that can rigorously define the nutritional factors that modulate the aging processes as well as strategies for the determination of the mechanism by which they do so. It would be extremely difficult, probably impossible, to accomplish these goals in studies using human subjects. The most promising avenue is the development and use of animal models for this purpose. Indeed, a significant data base exists on nutrition and aging in animal models (Munro, 1981).

2. Criteria

What criterion or criteria establish that a nutritional manipulation has influenced the aging processes? The difficulties encountered in determining adequate criteria are the major reasons for our slow progress in learning about nutrition as a modulator of aging.

Changes in longevity have been a widely used criterion. However, there are

Edward J. Masoro • Department of Physiology, The University of Texas Health Science Center at San Antonio, San Antonio, Texas 78284-7756.

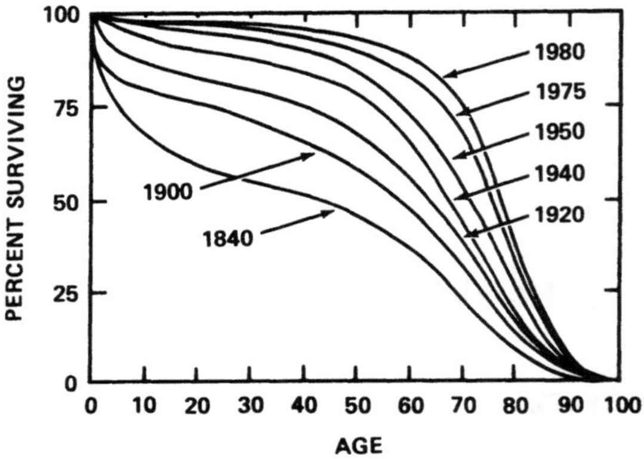

Fig. 1. Survival curves for the United States population for the year 1840 and projected for the years 1900, 1920, 1940, 1950, 1975, and 1980. (From Fries and Crapo, 1981, from data of the National Bureau of Health Statistics.)

problems with this criterion. For instance, over the last 140 years there has been a marked increase in the life expectancy of Americans from about 40 years of age in 1840 to over 70 years of age in 1980 (Hazzard, 1983). This increase in life expectancy has probably not resulted from factors influencing the aging processes *per se* but rather primarily from protecting the population from premature death from specific disease. Indeed, the maximum life-span potential of humans has remained at about 100 years since at least the time of the ancient Romans. The increase in life expectancy with no change in maximum life-span potential is clearly evident in the survival curves for the U.S. population over the time span of 1840 to 1980 shown in Fig. 1. Indeed, a change in the maximum life-span potential of a species is a much better criterion that aging has been influenced than is a change in life expectancy. A nutritional manipulation that increases the maximum life-span potential probably does so by slowing the rate of aging. However, conversely, a manipulation that decreases the maximum life-span potential may have done so by accelerating the aging process or through a number of other possible mechanisms such as a specific toxic action.

A major problem with the use of longevity as a criterion that a manipulation has influenced aging is the length of time needed to make this assessment. Indeed, for practical purposes, this criterion can only be used with short-lived animal models such as rodents. It is for this reason that there has been much effort towards developing reliable biomarkers of aging (Reff and Schneider, 1982). However, it has been difficult to be certain that a particular functional or morphological measurement is a reliable biomarker of aging because it is not possible to define aging in the fundamental biological terms that could serve as a primary standard. Of course, changes in many functional activities and the occurrence of many disease processes are associated with aging, and it is of importance to learn about nutritional manipulations that influence these age-associated events. However, the influencing of such age-associated events should not be taken as evidence that a nutritional manipulation has modulated the aging processes. For instance, it appears that nutritional programs in the United States may be retarding the progression of atherosclerosis. Even if this possibility becomes established fact, it provides no evidence that these nutritional programs have retarded an aging process. Our current evidence does not permit a distinction between the possibilities that (1) atherosclerosis and aging are unrelated events that merely share the same time frame or (2) there is a causal interaction between aging and atherosclerosis.

3. *Food Restriction*

If increasing the maximum life-span potential is used as the criterion that the aging processes have been slowed, the only nutritional manipulation that has been shown to do so in mammals is food restriction in laboratory rodents. This was first clearly shown by McCay and Crowell (1934) and has been confirmed by many other workers (Barrows and Kokkonen, 1977). The dietary protocols used have varied, with some low-calorie diets being supplemented with vitamins or minerals or protein and others not, but all limiting caloric intake by 20 to 60% (Weindruch, 1985). In the initial studies, food restriction was started at weaning, but in several subsequent studies it was found that maximum life-span potential also increased when food restriction was initiated during adult life (Goodrick *et al.*, 1983; Weindruch and Walford, 1982; Stuchliková *et al.*, 1975; Cheney *et al.*, 1983; Yu *et al.*, 1985; Beauchenne *et al.*, 1986). Indeed, Yu *et al.* (1985) found that food restriction initiated in early adult life was as effective in extending the maximum life-span potential of rats as that started soon after weaning (see Fig. 2 for survival curves). This action of food restriction has not been shown for other mammals; in particular, careful research has not been done on long-lived mammals. It should be noted that in nonmammalian species findings similar to those with rodents have been obtained: protozoa (Rudzinka, 1952), rotifers (Fanestil and Barrows, 1965), *Daphnia* (Ingle *et al.*, 1937), *Drosophila* (Loeb and Northrop, 1917), and fish (Comfort, 1963).

Food restriction not only influences longevity but also delays or prevents many age-related functional changes. These include blunting of the age-related increases in serum lipids (Liepa *et al.*, 1980; Masoro *et al.*, 1983), blunting of the age-related increase in parathyroid hormone and calcitonin concentrations (Kalu *et al.*, 1983, 1984), modulating the age-related loss in the response of adipocytes to hormones (Reaven *et al.*, 1983; Bertrand *et al.*, 1980b; Yu *et al.*, 1980; Voss *et al.*, 1982), modulating the change in central nervous system function including retarding the loss with advancing age of neurotransmitter receptors and other neurochemical markers of senescence (Joseph *et al.*, 1983; Levin *et al.*, 1982; London *et al.*, 1985), slowing the age-related loss of soluble γ-crystallins from the lens of the eye (Leveille *et al.*, 1984), delaying reproductive senescence (Merry and Holehan, 1979; Holehan and Merry, 1985), slowing age-related change in skeletal muscle structure and functions (McCarter *et al.*, 1982), preventing the age-related decrease in spontaneous locomotor activity (Yu *et al.*, 1985), and slowing age-related alterations in immune function including the maintenance of the production of and response to interleukin-2 (Fernandes, 1984; Cheney *et al.*, 1983; Fernandes *et al.*, 1978; Jung *et al.*, 1982; Weindruch *et al.*, 1983; Kubos *et al.*, 1984b). The age-related increase in circulating immune complexes in the (NZB × NZW)F_1 mouse is also decreased by food restriction (Safai-Kutti *et al.*, 1980).

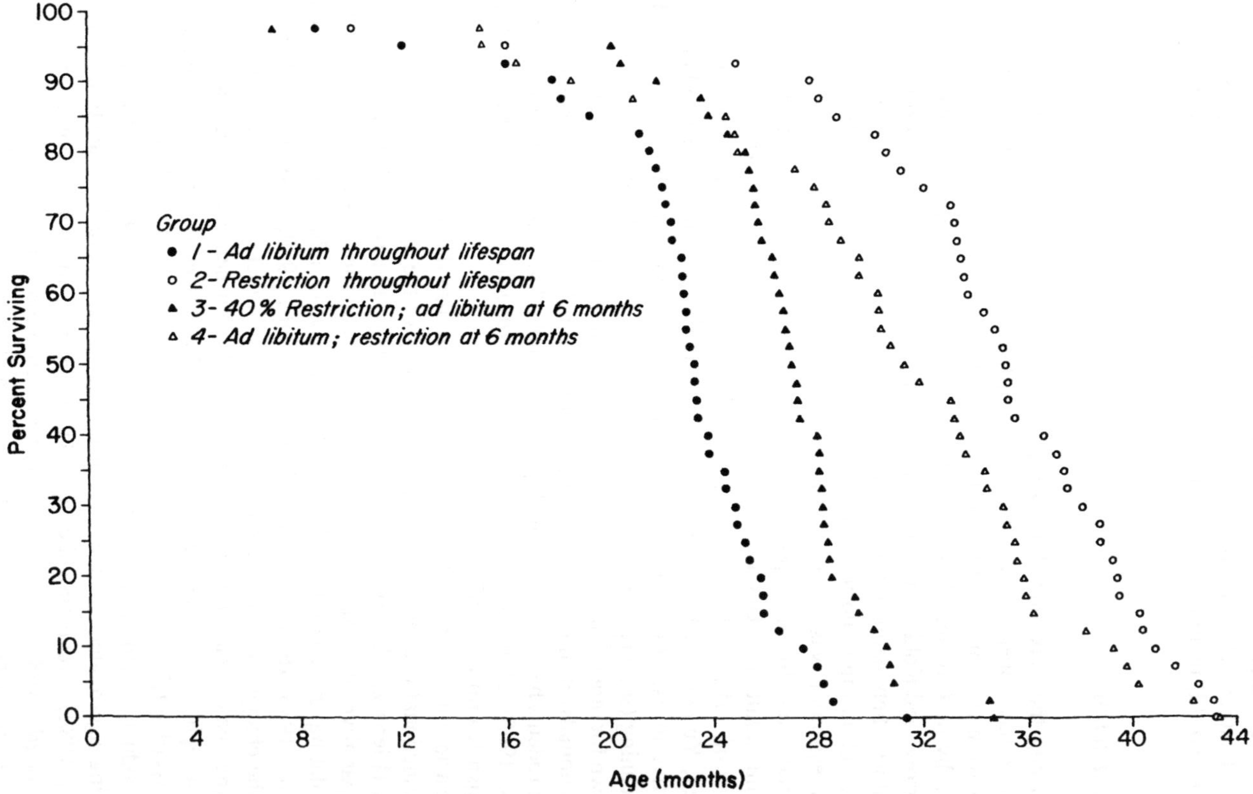

Fig. 2. Survival curves for *ad-libitum*-fed rats and for rats food-restricted for various parts of life. Group 1, *ad libitum* fed throughout life; group 2, *ad libitum* fed until 6 weeks of age and food-restricted thereafter; group 3, *ad libitum* fed until 6 weeks of age, food-restricted from 6 weeks until 6 months of age, and *ad libitum* fed thereafter; group 4, *ad libitum* fed until 6 months of age and food-restricted thereafter. Food restriction consisted of 60% of the mean food intake of the *ad-libitum*-fed rats. (From Yu *et al.*, 1985.)

Food restriction also slows or prevents a broad spectrum of age-related diseases. The most striking is its ability to retard markedly the progression of chronic nephropathy in rats (Berg and Simms, 1960; Bras and Ross, 1964; Nolen, 1972; Saxton and Kimball, 1941; Tucker *et al.*, 1976; Yu *et al.*, 1982; Maeda *et al.*, 1985). Indeed, Maeda *et al.* (1985) found that so markedly was the progression of chronic nephropathy curtailed that almost none of the food-restricted rats were in renal failure at death even though most lived to a very advanced age. Kubos *et al.* (1984b) found that the onset of glomerulonephritis in (NZB × NZW)F_1 autoimmune-prone mice was also delayed by food restriction.

Food restriction in rats also decreased the progression of cardiomyopathy and the prevalence of gastric ulcers, osteodystrophy, metastatic calcifications, and parathyroid hyperplasia (Maeda *et al.*, 1985). Spontaneous neoplastic disease in mice and rats is delayed by food restriction, and in some cases the occurrence is prevented (Maeda *et al.*, 1985; Saxton and Kimball, 1941; Tannenbaum, 1943; Ross and Bras, 1965; Silberberg and Silberberg, 1955; Cheney *et al.*, 1983). Carcinogen-induced tumors can also be inhibited by food restriction (Pollard *et al.*, 1984). In addition, food restriction extends the life of genotypes with short life spans such as the (NZB × NZW)F_1 mouse, which suffers from renal disease from autoimmune processes (Fernandes *et al.*, 1978; Kubos *et al.*, 1984b), the SHR rat, which succumbs to hypertension-related problems (Lloyd, 1984), and the MRL/Mp-lpr/lpr mouse, which suffers from lymphoproliferative disease (Kubos *et al.*, 1984a; Mark *et al.*, 1984). In the case of the (NZB × NZW)F_1 mouse, food restriction reduces the hepatic production of the retroviral envelope glycoprotein gp70 (Izui *et al.*, 1981).

It was suggested by McCay *et al.* (1935) that food restriction delayed the aging process by slowing growth and development. The findings of Barrows and Roeder (1965) further supported this view. Indeed, for many years the view prevailed that retarding maturation, slowing the rate of growth, and prolonging its duration were at the basis of the effects of food restriction on longevity. However, since 1965, many studies have challenged this concept (Goodrick *et al.*, 1983; Weindruch and Walford, 1982; Stuchlikova *et al.*, 1975; Cheney *et al.*, 1983; Yu *et al.*, 1985). Moreover, Yu *et al.* (1985) found that food restriction limited to the developmental period was less effective than food restriction initiated in early adult life in regard to extending maximum life-span potential and retarding other age-associated processes. Also, Weindruch *et al.* (1982) reported that food restriction initiated in adulthood retards immunosenescence and spontaneous tumor incidence in a fashion not unlike that observed with weaning-initiated food restriction. These findings have redirected current views on the action of food restriction away from growth and development to a focus on mechanisms retarding the aging processes in the mature animal.

It was first proposed by Berg and Simms (1960) that food restriction may increase longevity by reducing the fat content of the body. Bertrand *et al.* (1980a) showed that food restriction not only decreased body fat content but also decreased the number of adipocytes in the fat depots. However, in that study they also concluded that the lower fat mass of the food-restricted rats did not appear to be involved in the life-prolonging action of food restriction. Within the *ad-libitum*-fed group of rats, there was no correlation between body fat content and length of life. However, in the case of the food-restricted rats, there was a significant positive correlation between length of life and body fat content; i.e., more fat was associated with a longer life. On the basis of data from a study in which the duration of food restriction and the part of the life span involved were varied, Stuchlikova *et al.* (1975) came to the same conclusion. Also, Harrison *et al.* (1984) found that food-restricted obese (*ob/ob*) mice were fatter but lived longer than *ad-libitum*-fed lean litter mates. They therefore concluded that reducing body fat content does not play a major role in the action of food restriction on longevity.

The proposal by Sacher (1977) that food restriction reduces the metabolic rate and by so doing retards the aging processes has been widely embraced. Indeed, Harman (1981) linked this hypothesis to the free-radical theory of aging. His view was the following: by reducing the rate of electron transport and thus O_2 utilization, the rate of generation of O_2 free radicals is reduced. Indeed, if these free radicals are important contributors to the aging process, then reducing their production should slow the aging process.

Sacher based his proposal on data and concepts in the literature. For example, early in this century Rubner (1908) proposed on the basis of his studies with domestic animals that vary in size that all species utilize a similar number of calories per unit of body mass per lifetime; i.e., the length of life is inversely related to the metabolic rate. Pearl (1928) generalized this line of thought in his "rate of living theory of aging" in which he proposed that the higher the metabolic rate per unit of body mass, the faster the rate of aging, and the shorter the length of life. Moreover, there are data showing that limiting food intake reduces the metabolic rate per unit metabolic mass (Forsum *et al.*, 1981; Apfelbaum, 1978). However, these studies were of short duration (weeks in the case of rats and months in humans). Sacher directly supported his hypothesis with calculations based on published data of Ross (1969) showing that food-restricted rats had the same intake of calories per gram body mass per lifetime as *ad-libitum*-fed rats.

Recently, McCarter *et al.* (1985) directly measured the metabolic rate of *ad-libitum*-fed rats and of rats undergoing prolonged, life-extending food restriction. They found that food restriction that markedly increases life-span potential and retards a spectrum of aging processes did not decrease metabolic rate per unit lean body mass or per unit "metabolic mass." Thus, the hypothesis that food restriction slows the aging processes by lowering the metabolic rate should be discarded, since its effects on aging can occur without a decrease in metabolic rate.

The classic view that food restriction acts by reducing the intake of calories or other nutrients per unit of "metabolic mass" is challenged in the report of Masoro *et al.* (1982). Specifically, the lean body mass of food-restricted rats is decreased in proportion to the decrease in caloric intake (see Table I). Since the composition of the diet fed the *ad-libitum*-fed rats and the food-restricted rats is similar, food restriction does not involve a decrease in nutrient or caloric input per unit lean body mass or per unit "metabolic mass." Thus, food restriction cannot be coupled to the aging process by a reduced input of calories or any other nutrient per unit of tissue mass. Rather, an event involving the total organism's response to food restriction must be involved. The most likely possibility is that food restriction influences the regulatory systems, endocrine or neural or both, and that it is through those regulatory systems that food restriction is coupled to the aging processes in the tissues and organs of the body. The nature of the specific regulatory systems involved remains to be defined.

Table I. Caloric Intake by Ad-Libitum-Fed and Food-Restricted Rats[a]

Age (months)	*Ad-libitum*-fed rats (kcal/g)		Food-restricted rats (kcal/g)	
	Per body mass	Per lean body mass	Per body mass	Per lean body mass
6	0.14	0.17	0.14	0.17
12	0.13	0.17	0.14	0.17
18	0.12	0.16	0.13	0.15

[a]This table is based on data published by Masoro *et al.* (1982) and on unpublished data on body fat content from which the lean body mass was calculated.

One possibility was suggested more than a decade ago by Everitt (1973), who proposed that food restriction decreases the secretion of an aging factor by the pituitary gland. He supported this view with the finding that the hypophysectomy of rats (given cortisone replacement therapy only) had actions in common with food restriction, such as increased life expectancy and maximum life-span potential, the inhibition of the onset of renal and neoplastic disease, and the retardation of the aging of collagen (Everitt *et al.*, 1980). The hypothesis was further developed by the following model (Everitt, 1982): food restriction alters neurotransmitter metabolism within the hypothalamus, which decreases the secretion of a hypothalmic releasing hormone and results in a decreased secretion of a pituitary hormone. Although this hypothesis is intriguing, it is not yet supported by a solid data base. A serious problem is that hypophysectomy inhibits food consumption, making it difficult to know to what extent the findings on aging are directly related to a direct endocrine influence on aging or to an indirect one secondary to the decreased food intake. Moreover, if it is directly related to an endocrine factor, the nature of the hormone system remains to be defined.

The hypothalamic–pituitary–adrenal cortical system is a possible candidate. The view that hyperadrenocorticism promotes the aging processes has a long history [see Finch and Landfield (1985) for a review of the evidence on which this belief is based]. A recent provocative version is the glucocorticoid cascade hypothesis of aging proposed by Sapolsky *et al.* (1986) in which a high level of glucocorticoids in time leads to inadequate functioning of the brain–pituitary–adrenal cortical regulatory system and thereby to hyperadrenocorticism with its pathological consequences. Indeed, there is evidence that indicates that hyperadrenocorticism at least in part underlies the occurrence of age-related disease in rodents (Riley, 1981; Sapolsky and Donnelly, 1985). However, as yet, experiments have not been done that show food restriction to couple to the aging process by modulating the hypothalamic–pituitary–adrenocortical system. Moreover, the pituitary system is so complex that it provides many possible candidates in addition to that of glucocorticoids. Unfortunately, little work has been done in this area to date.

In addition to modulating the hypothalamic–pituitary system, another way food restriction could influence aging is by affecting the control systems that regulate plasma glucose levels and glucose homeostasis. Cerami (1985) has proposed that glucose is a mediator of aging. He suggests that a loss of biological function through the nonenzymatic reaction of glucose with proteins and nucleic acids yielding advanced glycosylation end products is a basic aging mechanism. The nonenzymatic glycosylation of proteins and nucleic acids begins with reaction of an amino group with the aldehyde group of glucose to form a Schiff base. Once formed, the unstable Schiff base of glucose can undergo an Amadori rearrangement to form a more stable product, the Amadori product. The Amadori product can undergo a series of dehydration steps and rearrangements to yield brown, fluorescent pigments (called advanced glycosylation end products by Cerami). These end products cross link proteins and nucleic acids and in this way cause loss of biological function. The chemical nature of these advanced glycosylation end products has not been fully elucidated, but one appears to be 2-furoyl-4(5)-(2-furanyl)-1H-imidazole. The rate of formation of advanced glycosylation end products is increased as the concentration of glucose and the time of exposure to glucose increase. Cerami points out that the complications of diabetic patients are frequently put forth as a paradigm of aging. Of course, these complications could also relate to alterations in glucose metabolism or insulin action rather than to sustained high levels of extracellular fluid glucose *per se*. Nevertheless, glucose and the glucose–insulin system are clearly potential couplers between food restriction and the aging process and should be studied.

In summary, food restriction markedly retards the aging processes in rodents. It does not do so by reducing the input of a nutrient per unit of protoplasmic mass. It is likely that it acts via neural, endocrine, or neuroendocrine control systems. Almost no work has been done on the nature of the control systems involved.

Although food restriction probably does not act directly on most tissues and organs, their function must be influenced, albeit indirectly, through endocrine and neural signals in such a fashion as to retard the aging processes. The nature of this functional modification is not known. However, support is accumulating for the view of Lindell (1982) that food restriction acts by maintaining gene expression. He postulated that enhanced gene expression plays an important role in maintaining cellular homeostasis in the aging organism. Cheung and Richardson (1982) expanded this view by stressing the importance of maintaining protein turnover for adequate cellular homeostasis. Richardson's group (Birchenall-Sparks *et al.*, 1985; Ricketts *et al.*, 1985) has provided evidence that food restriction retards the age-related decrease in the rate of protein synthesis. Also, Lewis *et al.* (1985) showed that food restriction enhanced turnover of body proteins during most of the life span. Surprisingly, the work of the same group (Merry and Holehan, 1985) on the RNA/DNA ratio and the protein/RNA ratio does not seem consistent with the turnover findings. The capacity for protein synthesis (the RNA/DNA ratio) was decreased in several tissues and organs by food restriction, and translational activity per ribosome (protein/RNA ratio) was not influenced by food restriction.

4. Macronutrients

The effect of individual macronutrients on longevity and associated aging events has been explored by altering the dietary content of the macronutrient being assessed. A major problem with this type of analysis is the fact that such a change in dietary composition may influence the total amount of food eaten. Unfortunately, the food intake is often not measured or when measured is not taken into account when interpreting the findings. Since, as described in detail in this chapter, the amount of food eaten profoundly influences the aging processes, failure to address this issue renders the results of such studies of little value.

4.1. Protein

There have been studies (Goodrick, 1978; Leto *et al.*, 1976) that indicate that decreasing the intake of dietary protein increases longevity. Other studies (Ross and Bras, 1973; Nakagawa and Masana, 1971) do not support this view. This discrepancy may relate to food intake, which was either not carefully measured or the measurements not fully reported. Davis *et al.* (1983) studied food-restricted rats provided diets with varying protein content and concluded that decreasing the protein content of the diet in this circumstance decreased longevity. On the other hand, Yu *et al.* (1985) found that decreasing the casein content of the diet of *ad-libitum*-fed male Fischer 344 rats from 21% to 12.6% caused a small but significant increase in both life expectancy and maximal life-span potential. In that study caloric intakes of both groups of *ad-libitum*-fed rats were the same. The rats fed the protein-restricted diet had less severe chronic nephropathy than rats fed the 21% protein diet (Maeda *et al.*, 1985), and it is likely that it is because of this that the rats fed the 12.6% protein diet had an increased longevity. The rats with the lower protein intake also had a decreased severity of cardiomyopathy and a lower occurrence of calcification and degeneration of the skeletal muscle, but the occurrence of neoplastic disease was not influenced, nor were age changes in physiological processes such as the loss of hormone-stimulated lipolysis in adipocytes. Replacing the casein in the diet with soy protein with no reduction in dietary protein content was also found to increase life expectancy and maximum life-span potential of male Fischer 344 rats (Iwasaki *et al.*, 1986). The caloric intake was the same for rats fed the soy-protein-containing diet as for those fed the casein-containing diet. The major reason for the increase in longevity was a retardation in the age-related progression in severity of chronic nephropathy. Other age changes were not influenced by the soy protein diet other than the rise in serum parathyroid hormone levels, which was prevented by the soy protein diet, probably because of the prevention of severe renal disease.

Friend *et al.* (1978) reported protein restriction of the autoimmune-prone NZB × NZW mouse protected the mice from the development of immune nephritis. However, the lack of information on food intake makes it impossible to know if this is a result of protein restriction or caloric restriction. In the NZB mouse, protein restriction without caloric restriction was found to have slowed age-related immune system changes and delayed autoimmune hemolytic anemia but not to have influenced longevity (Fernandes *et al.*, 1976).

It has also been found that tryptophan-deficient diets increase longevity of Long–Evans female rats (Segall, 1979). However, this diet also reduces food intake, which may be responsible for the increased longevity rather than the tryptophan deficiency *per se*. Similarly, a diet low in phenylalanine and tyrosine increases the length of life and retards the development of nephropathy in (NZB × NZW) mice, but again this may be caused by a decreased food intake rather than by the amino acid deficiency *per se* (Dubois and Strain, 1973).

4.2. *Fat*

Early studies showed that increasing the fat content of the diet decreased the life span (French *et al.*, 1953; Silberberg and Silberberg, 1955). High levels of fat have also been found to result in the appearance of tumors at younger ages and to increase the incidence of certain tumors (Carroll, 1975; Clayson, 1975; Reddy *et al.*, 1976). Diets high in fat have also been found to accelerate the aging of collagen (Hruza and Chvapil, 1962; Everitt *et al.*, 1981) and to decrease cell-mediated immunity as well as promote autoimmune disease in NZB mice (Fernandes *et al.*, 1973b). Kelley and Izui (1983) found that a high-fat diet shortened the life of NZB × W mice by accelerating nephritis through a local vascular effect. Fernandes *et al.* (1973c) also reported that in NZB × W mice, high-fat diets promote the development of vascular lesions. The issue that has not been fully addressed in these studies is the extent to which the findings are related to fat *per se* rather than to a change in caloric intake.

Levy *et al.* (1982) investigated the influence of the diets varying in amount and kind of fat on the immune system, immune complex disease, and longevity of (NZB × NZW)F_1 mice. They found that high fat intake resulted in more severe immune complex nephritis and an earlier death. They concluded that the amount of dietary lipid influences cellular and humoral immune responses and the spontaneous development of immune complex disease. They provide some evidence that these findings are not caused by differences in caloric intake, but that aspect of the study was not thoroughly executed. Prickett *et al.* (1981, 1983) reported that the length of life of this strain of mice could be extended, and the occurrence of the autoimmune nephritis prevented, by enriching the diet with eicosapentaenoic acid. Related to this effect of eicosapentaenoic acid is the finding that fish oil containing this fatty acid has a similar action when added to the diet (Robinson *et al.*, 1985). Also, when the (NZB × NZW)F_1 mice are fed essential-fatty-acid-deficient diets, they live longer, and the severity of the autoimmune nephritis is decreased (Hurd *et al.*, 1981); unfortunately, no information was provided in regard to the amount of food eaten.

4.3. *Carbohydrates*

Little has been done on the effects of dietary carbohydrates on the aging process. Using the BHE strain and the Wistar strain, Durand *et al.* (1968) fed male rats diets in which 39% of diet was carbohydrate with either sucrose or glucose or corn starch as the source of carbohydrate. They found that with the Wistar rats life expectancy was not influenced by the source of carbohydrate but that the life expectancy of the BHE rats was reduced when sucrose was the source. Unfortunately, maximum life-span potential was not reported.

Dolderup and Visser (1969) reported that adding sucrose to a complete diet did not significantly influence caloric intake but nevertheless reduced the life expectancy of male Wistar rats. They also found that the development of chronic nephropathy was accelerated in these sucrose-fed rats. Again, data on maximum life-span potential were not reported. Recent studies by Shafrir and Adler (1984) have again shown that sucrose in the diet reduces the length of life compared to the same diet in which starch replaced sucrose. In this case, spiny mice were the animal model.

These studies on the effects of sucrose are provocative. Unfortunately, none involved the generation of detailed survival curves. The effects of sucrose in particular and carbohydrates in general on the aging processes deserve further study. In this regard, a recent report by Kasiske *et al.* (1986) indicated that carbohydrate restriction does not retard the progression of glomerular injury in obese female Zucker rats in spite of the fact that the procedure used to restrict carbohydrate intake in some instances decreased caloric intake somewhat. These findings indicate that food restriction does not retard the development of chronic nephropathy by restricting the intake of carbohydrates.

5. *Micronutrients*

The micronutrients, i.e., the minerals and vitamins, are a vast and difficult area to study in regard to aging because of the large number of components in each class of nutrients. Indeed, there is little information on their role in aging, although considerable study has been aimed at ascertaining the relationship of specific components to age-related pathological processes (e.g., calcium and vitamin D in relation to osteoporosis; calcium and sodium in relation to hypertension).

5.1. *Minerals*

The effects of reducing mineral intake (all components including trace minerals) to the same extent as in life-prolonging food restriction has been carried out in our laboratory with male Fischer 344 rats. The results have not yet been published but can be briefly summarized as follows. The restriction of the minerals did not influence life expectancy or maximum life-span potential. The restriction of sodium, chloride, calcium, and phosphorus to the same extent that they are restricted in a life-prolonging food restriction regimen also did not influence the life expectancy or maximum life-span potential of male Fischer 344 rats (Yu *et al.*, 1982, 1985).

A marked reduction in the zinc intake of NZB mice and NZB/W was found to retard the development of autoimmune disease and to increase longevity (Beach *et al.*, 1981, 1982). In part, this was related to the reduced food intake in the mice fed the zinc-deficient diets, but, in part, it appeared to be caused by the reduced zinc intake *per se*. Any relevance of this finding to aging of most mice strains and other species seems doubtful, but it does point out the need for the exploration of each mineral element in more than one animal model in relation to aging processes.

5.2. *Vitamins*

Kokkonen and Barrows (1985) reported a study in which male C57BL/6J mice were fed *ad libitum* diets that contained either the amount of vitamins recommended by the National Research Council or one-half this amount or four times this amount. Life expectancy was significantly reduced when the dietary vitamin content was one-half that recommended by the National Research Council, but the fourfold increase in dietary vitamin content did not influence longevity. The interpretation of this study is difficult because of possible differences in food intake. The complexity of this issue is emphasized by the report of Kayser *et al.* (1972) that the life span of rats is lengthened by vitamin restriction.

Porta *et al.* (1980) reported that high dietary vitamin E prolonged the life of rats fed diets containing high levels of unsaturated fat, but this finding is difficult to interpret because food intake was decreased in rats so treated. In general, antioxidants including those that are vitamins have frequently been found to increase life expectancy but not maximum life-span potential (Harman, 1978). Moreover, the role that changes in food intake may play has usually not been adequately addressed.

6. Summary

Food restriction slows the aging processes. This conclusion is based on the following: (1) it markedly increases the maximum life-span potential, and (2) it retards or prevents a broad spectrum of age-related physiological changes and disease processes. Food restriction does not do this by reducing the input of calories or any other nutrient per unit of metabolic mass or lean body mass. Rather, it appears that there is a total organism response resulting in changes in the functioning of neural or endocrine or neuroendocrine systems, which are the vehicles modulating aging in the tissues and organs of the body.

There is no conclusive evidence that increasing or decreasing the intake of a specific nutrient influences the aging process. The small increase in maximum life span noted when dietary protein is restricted appears to be caused by the retardation of the progression of chronic nephropathy and not by an influence on aging processes in general. The failure to find such effects of individual nutrients may not result from the absence of such actions but rather may reflect the inadequacy of the research done to date. The research effort in this area been not only scant but also often flawed. The major flaws have been (1) failure to determine the effect of the dietary manipulation under study on the maximum life-span potential and (2) failure to assess adequately the influence of the manipulation on total food and caloric intake.

7. References

Apfelbaum, M., 1978, Adaptation to changes in caloric intake, *Proc. Food Nutr. Sci.* **2**:543–559.

Barrows, C. H., Jr., and Kokkonen, G. C., 1977, Relationship between nutrition and aging, *Adv. Nutr. Res.* **1**:253–298.

Barrows, C. H., Jr., and Roeder, L. M., 1965, The effects of reduced dietary intake on enzymatic activities and life span of rats, *J. Gerontol.* **20**:69–71.

Beach, R. S., Gerschwin, M. E., and Hurley, L. S., 1981, Nutritional factors and autoimmunity. I. Immunopathology of zinc deprivation in New Zealand mice, *J. Immunol.* **126**:1999–2006.

Beach, R. S., Gerschwin, M. E., and Hurley, L. S., 1982, Nutritional factors and autoimmunity. II. Prolongation of survival of zinc-deprived NZB/W mice, *J. Immunol.* **128:**308–313.

Beauchenne, R. E., Bales, C. W., Bragg, C. S., Hawkins, S. T., and Mason, R. L., 1986, Effect of age of initiation of food restriction on growth, body composition, and longevity of rats, *J. Gerontol.* **41:**13–19.

Berg, B. N., and Simms, H. S., 1960, Nutrition and longevity in the rat. II. Longevity and onset of disease with different levels of intake, *J. Nutr.* **71:**255–263.

Bertrand, H. A., Lynd, F. T., Masoro, E. J., and Yu, B. P., 1980a, Changes in adipose mass and cellularity through the adult life of rats fed *ad libitum* or a life prolonging restricted diet, *J. Gerontol.* **35:**827–835.

Bertrand, H. A., Masoro, E. J., and Yu, B. P., 1980b, Maintenance of glucagon-promoted lipolysis in adipocytes by food restriction, *Endocrinology* **107:**591–595.

Birchenall-Sparks, M. G., Roberts, M. S., Staecker, J., Hardwick, J. P., and Richardson, A., 1985, Effect of dietary restriction on liver protein synthesis in rats, *J. Nutr.* **115:**944–950.

Bras, G., and Ross, M. H., 1964, Kidney disease and nutrition in the rat, *Toxicol. Pharmacol.* **6:**246–262.

Carroll, K. K., 1975, Experimental evidence of dietary factors and hormone dependent cancers, *Cancer Res.* **35:**3374–3383.

Cerami, A., 1985, Hypothesis: Glucose as a mediator of aging, *J. Am. Geriatr. Soc.* **33:**626–634.

Cheney, K. E., Liu, R. K., Smith, G. S., Meredith, P. J., Mickey, M. R., and Walford, R. L., 1983, The effect of dietary restriction of varying duration on survival, tumor patterns, immune function, and body temperature in $B10C3F_1$ female mice, *J. Gerontol.* **38:**420–430.

Cheung, H. T., and Richardson, A., 1982, The relationship between age-related changes in gene expression, protein turnover and the responsiveness of an organism to stimuli, *Life Sci.* **31:**605–613.

Clayson, D. B., 1975, Nutrition and experimental carcinogenesis: A review, *Cancer Res.* **35:**3292–3300.

Comfort, A., 1963, Effect of delayed and resumed growth on the longevity of a fish (*Lebistes reticulatus*, Peters) in captivity, *Gerontology* **8:**150–155.

Davis, T. A., Bales, C. W., and Beauchenne, R. E., 1983, Differential effects of dietary caloric and protein restriction in the aging rat, *Exp. Gerontol.* **18:**427–435.

Dolderup, L. M., and Visser, W., 1969, Influence of extra sucrose in the daily food on the life-span of Wistar albino rats, *Nature* **222:**1050–1052.

Dubois, E. L., and Strain, L., 1973, Effect of diet on survival and nephropathy of NZB/NZW hybrid mice, *Biochem. Med.* **7:**336–342.

Durand, A., Fischer, M., and Adams, M., 1968, The influence of types of dietary carbohydrates, *Arch. Pathol.* **85:**318–324.

Everitt, A. V., 1973, The hypothalamic–pituitary control of aging and age-related pathology, *Exp. Gerontol.* **8:**265–277.

Everitt, A. V., 1982, Nutrition and the hypothalamic pituitary influence on aging, in: *Nutritional Approaches to Aging* (G. B. Moment, ed.), CRC Press, Boca Raton, FL, pp. 245–256.

Everitt, A. V., Seedsman, N. J., and Jones, F., 1980, The effects of hypophysectomy and continuous food restriction begun at age 70 and 400 days on collagen aging, proteinuria, incidence of pathology and longevity in the male rat, *Mech. Aging Dev.* **12:**161–172.

Everitt, A. V., Porter, B. D., and Steele, M., 1981, Dietary, caging and temperature factors in the aging of collagen fibers in rat tail tendon, *Gerontology* **27:**37–41.

Fanestil, D. P., and Barrows, G. H., Jr., 1965, Aging in the rotifer, *J. Gerontol.* **20:**462–469.

Fernandes, G., 1984, Nutritional factors: Modulating effects on immune function and aging, *Pharmacol. Rev.* **36:**1235–1295.

Fernandes, G., Yunis, E. J., Jose, D. G., and Good, R. A., 1973a, Dietary influence on breeding behavior, hemolytic anemia and longevity in NZB mice, *Proc. Soc. Exp. Biol. Med.* **139:**1189–1196.

Fernandes, G., Yunis, E. J., Jose, D. G., and Good, R. A., 1973b, Dietary influence on antinuclear antibodies and cell-mediated immunity in NZB mice, *Int. Arch. Allergy Appl. Immunol.* **44:**770–782.

Fernandes, G., Alsonso, D. R., Tanaka, T., Thaler, H. T., Yunis, E. J., and Good, R. A., 1973c, Influence of diet on vascular lesions in autoimmune-prone B/W mice, *Proc. Natl. Acad. Sci. U.S.A.* **80:**874–877.

Fernandes, G., Yunis, E. J., and Good, R. A., 1976, Influence of protein restriction on immune function in NZB mice, *J. Immunol.* **116:**782–790.

Fernandes, G., Friend, P., Yunis, E. J., and Good, R. A., 1978, Influence of dietary restriction on immunologic function and renal disease in (NZB × NZW)F_1 mice, *Proc. Natl. Acad. Sci. U.S.A.* **75:**1500–1504.

Finch, C. E., and Landfield, P. W., 1985, Neuroendocrine and autonomic functions in aging mammals, in: *Handbook of Biology of Aging,* 2nd ed. (C. E. Finch and E. L. Schneider, eds.), Van Nostrand-Reinhold, New York, pp. 567–594.

Forsum, E., Hillman, P. E., and Nesheim, M. C., 1981, Effect of energy restriction on total heat production, basal metabolic rate and specific dynamic action of food in rats, *J. Nutr.* **111:**1691–1697.

French, C. E., Ingram, R. H., Unram, J. A., Barron, G. P., and Swift, R. W., 1953, The influence of dietary fat and carbohydrates on growth and longevity in rats, *J. Nutr.* **51:**329–339.

Friend, P. S., Fernandes, G., Good, R. A., Michael, A. F., and Yunis, E. J., 1978, Dietary restrictions early and late effects on the nephropathy of the NZB × NZW mouse, *Lab. Invest.* **38:**629–632.

Fries, J. F., and Crapo, L. M., 1981, *Vitality and Aging,* W. H. Freeman, San Francisco.

Goodrick, C. L., 1978, Body weight-increment and length of life: The effect of genetic constitution and dietary proteins, *J. Gerontol.* **33:**104–190.

Goodrick, C. L., Ingram, D. K., Reynolds, M. A., Freeman, J. R., and Cider, H. L., 1983, Differential effects of intermittent feeding and voluntary exercise on body weight and life span in adult rats, *J. Gerontol.* **38:**36–45.

Guigoz, Y., and Munro, H. N., 1985, Nutrition and aging, in: *Handbook of the Biology of Aging,* 2nd ed. (C. E. Finch and E. L. Schneider, eds.), Von Nostrand-Reinhold, New York, pp. 878–893.

Harman, D., 1978, Free radical theory of aging: Nutritional implications, *Age* **1:**143–150.

Harman, D., 1981, The aging process, *Proc. Natl. Acad. Sci. U.S.A.* **78:**7124–7128.

Harrison, D. E., Archer, J. R., and Astole, C. M., 1984, Effects of food restriction on aging: Separation of food intake and adiposity. *Proc. Natl. Acad. Sci. U.S.A.* **81:**1835–1838.

Hazzard, W. R., 1983, Clinical rationales for the inclusion of geriatrics in medical education, in: *Proceedings of the Regional Institutes of Geriatric and Medical Education,* Association of American Medical Colleges, Washington, pp. 23–52.

Holehan, A. M., and Merry, B. J., 1985, Lifetime breeding studies in fully fed and dietary restricted female CFY Sprague–Dawley rats. 1. Effects of age, housing conditions and diet on fecundity, *Mech. Aging Dev.* **33:**19–28.

Hruza, Z., and Chvapil, M., 1972, Collagen characteristics in skin, tail tendons and lungs in experimental atherosclerosis in the rat, *Physiol. Bohemoslav.* **11:**423–429.

Hurd, E. R., Johnston, J. M., Okita, J. R., MacDonald, P. C., Ziff, M., and Gilliam, J. N., 1981, Prevention of glomerulonephritis and prolonged survival in New Zealand black/New Zealand white F_1 hybrid mice fed an essential fatty acid-deficient diet, *J. Clin. Invest.* **67:**476–485.

Ingle, L., Wood, T. R., and Banta, A. M., 1937, A study of longevity, growth, reproduction and heart rate in *Daphnia longispina* as influenced by limitations in quantity of food, *J. Exp. Zool.* **76:**325–352.

Iwasaki, K., Gleiser, C. A., Masoro, E. J., and Yu, B. P., 1986, Dietary protein and chronic nephropathy in the rat, *Fed. Proc.* **45:**829.

Izui, S., Fernandes, G., Hara, I., McConahey, P. J., Jensen, F. C., Dixon, F. J., and Good, R. A., 1981, Low-calorie diet selectively reduces expression of retroviral envelope glycoprotein gp 70 in sera of NZB × NZW F_1 hybrid mice, *J. Exp. Med.* **154:**1116–1124.

Joseph, J. A., Witaker, J., Roth, G. S., and Ingram, D. K., 1983, Life-long dietary restriction affects striatially-mediated behavioral responses in aged rats, *Neurobiol. Aging* **4:**191–196.

Jung, L. K. L., Palladino, M. A., Calvano, S., Mark, D. A., Good, R. A., and Fernandes, G., 1982, Effect of caloric restriction on the production and responsiveness to interleukin-2 in (NZB × NZW)F_1 mice, *Clin. Immunol. Immunopathol.* **25:**291–301.

Kalu, D. N., Cockerham, R., Yu, B. P., and Roos, B. A., 1983, Lifelong dietary modulation of calcitonin levels in rats, *Endocrinology* **113:**2010–2016.

Kalu, D. N., Hardin, R. R., Cockerham, R., Yu, B. P., Norling, B. K., and Egan, J., 1984, Lifelong food restriction prevents senile osteoporosis and hyperparathyroidism in rats, *Mech. Aging Dev.* **26:**103–112.

Kasiske, B. L., Cleary, M. P., O'Donnell, M. P., and Keane, W. F., 1986, Effects of carbohydrate restriction on renal injury in the obese Zucker rat, *Am. J. Clin. Nutr.* **44:**56–65.

Kayser, J., Neumann, J., and Lavolley, J., 1972, Effets favorables exercés sur la longvité du rat Wistar per divers types de restrictions vitaminiques, *C. R. Acad. Sci. [D] (Paris)* **274**:3593–3596.

Kelley, V. E., and Izui, S., 1983, Enriched lipid diet accelerates lupus nephritis in NZB × W mice, *Am. J. Pathol.* **111**:288–297.

Kokkonen, G. C., and Barrows, C. H., 1985, The effect of dietary vitamin, protein and intake levels on the life span of mice of different ages, *Age* **8**:13–17.

Kubos, C., Day, N. K., and Good, R. A., 1984a, Influence of early or late dietary restriction on life span and immunological parameters in MRL/Mp-1pr/1pr mice, *Proc. Natl. Acad. Sci. U.S.A.* **81**:5831–5835.

Kubos, C., Johnson, B. C., Day, N. K., and Good, R. A., 1984b, Calorie source, calorie restriction, immunity and aging of (NZB/NZW)F_1 mice, *J. Nutr.* **114**:1884–1899.

Leto, S., Kokkonen, G., and Barrows, C., 1976, Dietary proteins, life spans, biochemical variables in female mice, *J. Gerontol.* **31**:144–148.

Leveille, P. J., Weindruch, R., Walford, R. L., Bok, I., and Horwitz, J., 1984, Dietary restriction retards age-related loss of gamma crystallins in mouse lens, *Science* **224**:1247–1249.

Levin, P., Janda, J. K., Joseph, J. A., Ingram, P. K., and Roth, G. S., 1982, Dietary restriction retards the age-associated loss of rat striatal dopaminergic receptors, *Science* **214**:561–562.

Levy, J. A., Ibrahim, A. B., Shirai, T., Ohta, K., Nagasawa, R., Yoshida, H., Estes, J. R., and Gardner, M., 1982, Dietary fat affects immune responses, production of antiviral factors, and immune complex disease in NZB/NZW mice, *Proc. Natl. Acad. Sci. U.S.A.* **79**:1974–1978.

Lewis, S. E. M., Goldspink, D. F., Phillips, J. G., Merry, B. J., and Holehan, A. M., 1985, The effects of aging and chronic dietary restriction on whole body growth and protein turnover in the rat, *Exp. Gerontol.* **20**:253–263.

Liepa, G. U., Masoro, E. J., Bertrand, H. A., and Yu, B. P., 1980, Food restriction as a modulator of age-related changes in serum lipids, *Am. J. Physiol.* **238**:E253–E257.

Lindell, T. J., 1982, Molecular aspects of dietary modulation of transcription and enhanced longevity, *Life Sci.* **31**:625–635.

Lloyd, T., 1984, Food restriction increases life span of hypertensive rats, *Life Sci.* **34**:401–407.

Loeb, J., and Northrop, J. H., 1917, On the influence of food and temperature upon the duration of life, *J. Biol. Chem.* **32**:102–121.

London, E. D., Waller, S. B., Ellis, A. T., and Ingram, D. K., 1985, Effect of intermittent feeding on neurochemical makers in aging rat brain, *Neurobiol. Aging* **6**:199–204.

Maeda, H., Gleiser, C. A., Masoro, E. J., Murata, I., McMahan, C. A., and Yu, B. P., 1985, Nutritional influences on aging of Fischer 344 rats: II. Pathology, *J. Gerontol.* **40**:671–688.

Mark, D. A., Alsonso, D. R., Quimby, F., Thaler, H. T., Kiru, Y. T., Fernandes, G., Good, R. A., and Weksler, M. E., 1984, Effects of nutrition on disease and life span, *Am. J. Pathol.* **117**:110–124.

Masoro, E. J., 1985, Nutrition and aging—a current assessment, *J. Nutr.* **115**:842–848.

Masoro, E. J., Yu, B. P., and Bertrand, H. A., 1982, Action of food restriction in delaying the aging process, *Proc. Natl. Acad. Sci. U.S.A.* **79**:4239–4241.

Masoro, E. J., Compton, C., Yu, B. P., and Bertrand, H., 1983, Temporal and compositional dietary restrictions modulate age-related changes in serum lipids, *J. Nutr.* **113**:880–892.

McCarter, R. J. M., Masoro, E. J., and Yu, B. P., 1982, Rat muscle structure and metabolism in relation to age and food intake, *Am. J. Physiol.* **242**:R89–R93.

McCarter, R., Masoro, E. J., and Yu, B. P., 1985, Does food restriction retard aging by reducing the metabolic rate? *Am. J. Physiol.* **248**:E488–E490.

McCay, C. M., and Crowell, M. F., 1934, Prolonging the life span, *Sci. Monthly* **39**:405–414.

McCay, C., Crowell, M., and Maynard, L., 1935, The effect of retarded growth upon the length of life span and upon ultimate size, *J. Nutr.* **10**:63–79.

Merry, B. J., and Holehan, A. M., 1979, Onset of puberty and duration of fertility in rats fed restricted diet, *J. Reprod. Fertil.* **57**:253–259.

Merry, B. J., and Holehan, A. M., 1985, *In vivo* DNA synthesis in the dietary restricted long-lived rat, *Exp. Gerontol.* **20**:15–18.

Munro, H. N., 1981, Nutrition and aging, *Br. Med. Bull.* **37**:83–88.

Nakagawa, I., and Masana, Y., 1971, Effect of protein nutrition on growth and life span in the rat, *J. Nutr.* **101**:613–620.

Nolen, G. A., 1972, Effect of various restricted dietary regimens on the growth, health and longevity of albino rats, *J. Nutr.* **102:**1477–1494.

Pearl, R., 1928. *The Rate of Living,* Alfred Knopf, New York.

Pollard, M., Luckerts, P. H., and Pan, G. Y., 1984, Inhibition of intestinal tumorigenesis in methylazoxymethanol-treated rats by dietary restriction, *Cancer Treat. Rep.* **68:**405–408.

Porta, E. A., 1980, Nutritional factors and aging, in: *Advances in Modern Human Nutrition,* Volume I (R. B. Tobin and M. A. Mehlman, eds.), Pathotox Publishers, Park Forest South, IL, pp. 55–119.

Porta, E. A., Joun, N. S., and Nitta, R. T., 1980, Effects of the type of dietary fat at two levels of vitamin E in Wistar male rats during development and aging. I. Lifespan, serum biochemical parameters and pathological changes, *Mech. Aging Dev.* **13:**1–39.

Prickett, J. D., Robinson, D. R., and Steinberg, A. D., 1981, Dietary enrichment with the polyunsaturated fatty acid eicosapentaenoic acid prevents proteinuria and prolongs survival in NZB × NZW F_1 mice, *J. Clin. Invest.* **68:**556–559.

Prickett, J. D., Robinson, D. R., and Steinberg, A., 1983, Effects of dietary enrichment with eicosapentaenoic acid upon autoimmune nephritis in female NZB × NZW/F_1 mice, *Arthritis Rheum.* **26:**133–139.

Reaven, E., Wright, D., Mondon, C. E., Salomon, R., Ho, H., and Reaven, G. M., 1983, Effect of age and diet on insulin secretion and insulin action in the rat, *Diabetes* **23:**175–180.

Reddy, B. S., Narisawa, T., Vokusich, D., Weisburger, J. H., and Wynder, E., 1976, Effect of quality and quantity of dietary fat and dimethylhydrazine in colon carcinogenesis in rats, *Proc. Soc. Exp. Biol. Med.* **151:**237–239.

Reff, M. E., and Schneider, E. L., 1982, *Biological Markers of Aging,* National Institutes of Health, Bethesda.

Ricketts, W. G., Birchenall-Sparks, M. C., Hardwick, J. P., and Richardson, A., 1985, Effect of age and dietary restriction on protein synthesis by isolated kidney cells, *J. Cell. Physiol.* **125:**492–498.

Riley, V., 1981, Psychoneuroendocrine influences on immunocompetence and neoplasma, *Science* **212:**1100–1109.

Robinson, D. R., Prickett, J. D., Pollison, R., Steinberg, A. D., and Levine, L., 1985, The protective effect of dietary fish oil on murine lupus, *Prostaglandins* **30:**51–75.

Ross, M. H., 1969, Aging, nutrition and hepatic enzyme activity in the rat, *J. Nutr.* **97**(Suppl. Part II)**:**563–602.

Ross, M. H., and Bras, G., 1965, Tumor incidence patterns and nutrition in the rat, *J. Nutr.* **87:**245–260.

Ross, M., and Bras, G., 1973, Influence of protein under- and overnutrition on spontaneous tumor prevalence in the rat, *J. Nutr.* **103:**944–963.

Rubner, M., 1908, *Das Problem der Lebensdauer und seine Beziehungen zum Wachstum und Ernabrung,* Oldenbourg, Munich.

Rudzinska, M. A., 1952, Overfeeding and lifespan in *Tokophyra infusiom, J. Gerontol.* **7:**544–548.

Sacher, G. A., 1977, Life table modification and life prolongation, in: *Handbook of Biology of Aging* (C. E. Finch and L. Hayflick, eds.), Van Nostrand-Reinhold, New York, pp. 582–638.

Safai-Kutti, S., Fernandes, G., Wang, Y., Safai, B., Good, R. A., and Day, N. K., 1980, Reduction of circulating immune complexes by caloric restriction in (NZB × NZW) F_1 mice, *Clin. Immunol. Immunopathol.* **15:**293–300.

Sapolsky, R., and Donnelly, T., 1985, Vulnerability to stress-induced tumor growth increases with age in the rat: Role of glucocorticoid hypersecretion, *Endocrinology* **117:**662–666.

Sapolsky, R., Krey, L. C., and McEwen, B. S., 1986, The neuroendocrinology of stress and aging: The glucocorticoid cascade hypothesis, *Endocrinol. Rev.* **7:**284–301.

Saxton, J. A., and Kimball, G. C., 1941, Relation to nephrosis and other diseases of albino rats to age and to modifications of diet, *Arch. Pathol.* **32:**951–965.

Segall, P. E., 1979, Interrelations of dietary and hormonal effects in aging, *Mech. Aging Dev.* **9:**515–525.

Shafrir, E., and Adler, J. H., 1984, Effect of long-term sucrose diet on the reproduction and survival of spiny mice (*Acomys cahirinus*), *Nutr. Res.* **4:**495–501.

Silberberg, M., and Silberberg, R., 1955, Diet and life span, *Physiol. Res.* **35:**347–362.

Stuchliková, E., Juricová-Horáková, M., and Deyl, Z., 1975, New aspects of dietary effect of life prolongation in rodents. What is the role of obesity in aging? *Exp. Gerontol.* **10:**141–144.

Tannenbaum, A., 1945, The dependence of tumor formation on the composition of the calorie-restricted diet as well as on the degree of restriction, *Cancer Res.* **5**:616–625.

Tucker, S. M., Mason, R. I., and Beauchenne, R. E., 1976, Influence of diet and food restriction on kidney function of aging male rats, *J. Gerontol.* **31**:264–270.

Voss, K. H., Masoro, E. J., and Anderson, W., 1982, Modulation of age-related loss of glucagon promoted lipolysis by food restriction, *Mech. Aging Dev.* **18**:135–149.

Weindruch, R., 1985, Aging rodents fed restricted diets, *J. Am. Geriatr. Soc.* **33**:125–132.

Weindruch, R., and Walford, R. L., 1982, Dietary restriction in mice beginning at 1 year of age: Effect on life-span and spontaneous cancer incidence, *Science* **215**:1415–1418.

Weindruch, R., Gottesman, S. R. S., and Walford, K. L., 1982, Modification of age-related immune decline in mice dietarily restricted from or after midadulthood, *Proc. Natl. Acad. Sci. U.S.A.* **79**:898–902.

Weindruch, R., Devens, B. H., Raff, H. U., and Walford, R., 1983, Influence of aging and diet restriction on natural killer cell activity in mice, *J. Immunol.* **130**:993–996.

Yu, B. P., Bertrand, H. A., and Masoro, E. J., 1980, Nutrition–aging influences of catecholamine-promoted lipolysis, *Metabolism* **29**:438–444.

Yu, B. P., Masoro, E. J., Murata, I., Bertrand, H. A., and Lynd, F. T., 1982, Life span study of SPF Fischer 344 male rats fed *ad libitum* or restricted diets: Longevity, growth, lean body mass and disease, *J. Gerontol.* **37**:130–141.

Yu, B. P., Masoro, E. J., and McMahan, C. A., 1985, Nutritional influences on aging of Fischer 344 rats: I. Physical, metabolic and longevity characteristics, *J. Gerontol.* **40**:657–670.

3

Aging and the Digestive System

Irwin H. Rosenberg, Robert M. Russell, and Barbara B. Bowman

1. *Introduction*

The decline in organ function that accompanies normal aging, especially at the extremities of age, includes digestive functions selectively. In this chapter we address the functions of the various organs of the human digestive tract and those studies in man that examine the effects of aging. Insofar as possible, we examine the changes associated with normal aging as distinguished from those changes that result from diseases of the digestive tract. This chapter updates a consideration of this topic, which has been subject of previous reviews in the recent past (Bowman and Rosenberg, 1983; Thompson and Keelan, 1986; Russell, 1987).

2. *Taste and Smell*

Physiological changes in taste and smell, although not digestive functions *per se*, can certainly influence food intake and alimentation. Aging is associated with increased thresholds for taste and smell; olfaction is affected to a greater extent than taste (Stevens *et al.*, 1984). With aging, both the number of taste buds per papilla and the number of papillae decrease; also, the numbers of both taste and olfactory nerve endings are said to decrease (Schiffman and Pasternak, 1979). The loss of taste buds occurs in the anterior part of the tongue initially, so that the ability to detect sweet and salty tastes is affected first; this is consistent with the complaint by some older people that all foods taste bitter or sour (Busse, 1978). Although there is controversy about the magnitude of the change in taste thresholds with aging (Grzegorczyk *et al.*, 1979), it has been demonstrated that improved oral hygiene (Langan and Yearick, 1976), but

Irwin H. Rosenberg and Robert M. Russell • USDA Human Nutrition Research Center on Aging, Tufts University, Boston, Massachusetts 02111. **Barbara B. Bowman** • Department of Biochemistry, Emory University, School of Medicine, Atlanta, Georgia 30322.

neither supplemental zinc (Greger and Geissler, 1978) nor B-vitamin supplementation (Langer, 1976), can significantly enhance taste activity in elderly people.

3. *Function of Alimentary Organs during Aging*

3.1. *Salivary Secretion*

The relationship between age-related changes in human salivary gland morphology and function (saliva production) has been uncertain. The stimulated parotid saliva flow rate in 208 subjects in the Baltimore Longitudinal Study of Aging was not affected by age, although the rate of saliva production was lower in postmenopausal women who were taking medications (Baum, 1981).

3.2. *Esophageal Function and Swallowing*

Esophageal motility studies demonstrate some abnormalities, including disordered contractions and spontaneous gastroesophageal reflux, that are detected more frequently in asymptomatic elderly persons, particularly in those older than age 70 (Khan *et al.*, 1977; Hollis and Castell, 1974). However, the basic swallowing pattern is maintained in older subjects: in at least 75% of the swallows observed, peristaltic contractions and the expected response of the lower esophageal sphincter occurred following swallowing (Khan *et al.*, 1977). The demonstration of these relatively minor abnormalities of esophageal function requires considerable diagnostic effort. It is probable that clinically significant symptoms rarely result. Age-related changes in motility have not been well documented in the remaining portions of the gastrointestinal tract.

3.3. *Gastric Function and Emptying*

Age-related changes in gastric physiology include decreased secretions of hydrochloric acid, intrinsic factor, and pepsin. According to calculations by Blackman *et al.* (1970), normal mean values for peak acid output adjusted for sex and body weight decrease by as much as 40% between ages 45 and 65. This decline is apparently caused by the increasing prevalence of atrophic gastritis with advancing age. The type of atrophic gastritis that is found in aging is not related to autoimmune phenomena (e.g., anti-intrinsic-factor antibodies, anti-parietal-cell antibodies), and its etiology is unclear (Strickland and MacKay, 1973). The majority of elderly who do not have atrophic gastritis continue to secrete hydrochloric acid in normal amounts.

In epidemiologic studies, the prevalence of atrophic gastritis has been estimated by serum pepsinogen I and II values (Samloff *et al.*, 1982). Pepsinogen I and pepsinogen II are both secreted by the chief and mucous neck cells of the fundic gland mucosa, but pepsinogen II also is derived from the pyloric glands in the gastric antrum, an area of the stomach that is often histologically normal in patients with fundic atrophic gastritis. Because of the discordant involvement of the fundic and pyloric gland areas of the stomach in atrophic gastritis, there are nonparallel changes in serum pepsinogen I and pepsinogen II levels that result in a progressive decrease in the pepsinogen I and pepsinogen II ratio with increasing severity of atrophic gastritis of the fundic gland mucosa. A serum ratio of pepsinogen I to II of less than 2.9 is predictive of atrophic gastritis (Samloff *et al.*, 1982). On the basis of this ratio, the prevalence of atrophic gastritis among people over the age of 60 in a healthy Bostonian population is approximately 20% (Krasinski *et al.*, 1986). However, in healthy elderly of age 80 and above, the prevalence approaches 40%. Among the sick elderly patients, the prevalence of atrophic gastritis may be higher. For example, 68% of 657 consecutive patients admitted to a geriatric unit have been reported to be hypo- or achlorhydric (Bird *et al.*, 1977).

Physiological changes that occur with atrophic gastritis include more rapid emptying of liquids, slower emptying of mixed solid–liquid diets (Davies *et al.*, 1971; Halvorsen *et al.*, 1973), a rise in the stomach and proximal small bowel pH (Russell *et al.*, 1986), and increased numbers of bacteria growing in the stomach and proximal small intestine. Changes in gastric secretion of acid and pepsin could result in impaired digestion and/or absorption of certain nutrients, including iron, calcium, copper, zinc, folic acid, vitamin B_{12}, and protein (Russell, 1986). For example, divalent cations are released from fiber in an acid milieu (James *et al.*, 1978). Therefore, it is possible that there is decreased biovailability of zinc and calcium when these minerals are eaten with a high-fiber diet in the presence of atrophic gastritis. The "simple colonization" by bacteria that occurs in atrophic gastritis is made up of rare anaerobes (Tabaqchali, 1970). The role of such bacteria in causing nutrient malabsorption or, alternatively, in making up for absorptive defects resulting from atrophic gastritis (e.g., by synthesis of certain vitamins) has yet to be determined. The implications of atrophic gastritis for the absorption of specific nutrients are discussed later.

Studies of gastric motility and emptying in the elderly have not been frequently reported. The weight of evidence is such that the most important regulator of liquid emptying from the stomach is the gastric–duodenal pressure gradient (Schiller, 1983). The emptying of mixed meals or of solid foods, however, is more complicated and is intimately connected with the processes of mixing and grinding. Several different techniques have been used to measure gastric emptying. For liquid meals, the most frequently used and reliable method has been that of intubation and aspiration using a nonabsorbable marker to correct for gastric secretion. However, the most popular method because of the ease in getting a quantitative estimate of gastric emptying is scintigraphics, a method based on radionuclide scanning after administration of radioisotopically labeled test compounds. The emptying of mixed diets, liquids, or solid meals can all be assessed by scintigraphic means.

In general, liquid meals empty more rapidly from normal stomachs than do ingested solids, and gastric emptying slows as acidity increases (Schiller, 1983). Depending on the method used and whether emptying of a liquid or a solid meal was studied, aging has been shown to speed gastric emptying, retard gastric emptying, or have no effect (Van Liere and Northrup, 1941; Evans *et al.*, 1981; Horowitz *et al.*, 1984; Kupfer *et al.*, 1985). In a recent study of gastric emptying in 10 elderly persons without gastrointestinal disease and not using medications known to affect gastrointestinal motility, the stomach emptying time was significantly longer than in young controls (123 min in the elderly versus 50 min in young volunteers) (Evans *et al.*, 1981). In passing, it should be noted that studies of intestinal transit time in the elderly are also rare. However, Brauer *et al.* (1981) found no difference in intestinal transit time in young versus elderly subjects.

Since the pH of the stomach is higher in hypochlorhydria, gastric emptying should theoretically be quicker. Davies *et al.* (1971) studied the disappearance of solid–liquid meals in 16 patients with atrophic gastritis or gastric atrophy. The method used was scintigraphy. It was found that the half-time in normal subjects was 35.6 min versus 67.9 min in patients with atrophic gastritis or gastric atrophy. This result is the opposite of the theoretical prediction. However, when gastric emptying of a liquid meal was studied in atrophic gastritis subjects by intubation in a Swedish study by Halvorsen *et al.* (1973), patients with hypochlorhydria did have faster gastric emptying of a liquid meal than control subjects. Thus, other factors associated with aging may determine the outcome.

3.4. Liver and Biliary Function

Although structural and biochemical changes have been well documented in aging liver, and the ratio of liver weight to body weight decreases after about age 50, there seem to be no age-related changes in liver function in persons with histologically normal livers. A 10% reduction in serum albumin concentrations was noted in a study of 11,000 adults above age 80 without disorders known to affect albumin metabolism (Greenblatt, 1979). Other work indicates that the rate of albumin synthesis in the elderly is not influenced by protein intake, in contrast to the situation in young adults, and may be regulated at a lower set point (Gersovitz *et al.*, 1980). In the face of this evidence of generally well-retained function of the liver during the aging process, it is understandable that age restrictions on donors for liver transplant have been removed. The evidence thus far is that donor livers from elderly patients perform as well as livers from younger donors.

3.5. Pancreatic Secretion

In the older literature, there are scattered reports of decreased secretion of some, but not all, pancreatic digestive enzymes in elderly humans (Meyer *et al.*, 1940; Necheles *et al.*, 1942). Using the fluorescein dilaurate pancreolaurel test, Gullo *et al.* (1986) examined pancreatic function in elderly people aged 66 to 88. Fluorescein dilaurate is hydrolyzed by pancreatic arylesterases into lauric acid and water-soluble fluorescein. The free fluorescein is absorbed, congugated in the liver, and excreted rapidly in the urine. The urinary output of fluorescein is thus a measure of pancreatic function. No difference was seen in the excretion of fluorescein among 60 elderly versus 36 healthy younger subjects. Further, no difference in pancreatic function was observed when comparing elderly under 80 years old with those over 80 years old. On repeated pancreatic stimulation with cholecystokinin and secretin, lower bicarbonate and enzyme outputs were observed in elderly than in young men (Bartos and Groh, 1969). However, although these changes were statistically significant, the absolute changes were small, and it is unlikely that they are clinically significant. Pitchumoni *et al.* (1984) have reported increased fibrosis of the pancreas in nonalcoholic elderly individuals. However, it is unlikely that such histological changes are functionally important.

3.6. Intestinal Morphology and Function

There is little literature on age-related morphological changes in the human intestine. Histologically normal upper jejunal biopsy specimens were compared between ten young and ten elderly subjects, and the average villous heights were not significantly reduced and enterocyte height was the same (Warren *et al.*, 1978). None of the histological changes described in aging mice (e.g., amyloid, collagen infiltration of the lamina propria) were present (Warren *et al.*, 1978). Webster and Leeming (1975a) studied jejunal mucosa from necropsies on 32 young victims of sudden death and 39 geriatric patients undergoing rehabilitation after a stroke or for arthritis (age range 67 to 90 years). There were only minor differences in morphology between the young control group and the geriatric patients, the most striking being a shorter villous height in elderly subjects. A more recent study compared elderly subjects more carefully screened for malabsorption or malnutrition with younger controls. This study by Corazza *et al.* (1986) found no significant deficits in surface area-to-volume ratio or enterocyte height in the elderly.

3.7. Intestinal Microflora

From studies on a small number of elderly patients without atrophic gastritis, it appears that only limited numbers of bacteria (less than 10^3/ml) normally inhabit the proximal small bowel (Russell *et al.*, 1986). However, in elderly subjects with atrophic gastritis, bacterial numbers increase to levels of 10^6–10^9. The bacterial overgrowth in atrophic gastritis has been termed "simple colonization," being made up largely of streptococci, lactobacilli, and bacteria found in the oral cavity (Drasar *et al.*, 1969). Few of these bacteria are able to deconjugate bile salts, so that fat malabsorption is rarely seen in atrophic gastritis. However, simple colonization may affect the absorption of certain micronutrients such as vitamin B_{12} (see Section 5.1.2). Thus, the functional significance of such colonizing bacteria remains uncertain. It should be pointed out that when significant malabsorption is present in an elderly person, bacterial overgrowth with anerobic, bile-salt-splitting bacteria is the most frequent cause (McEvoy *et al.*, 1983; Montgomery *et al.*, 1986).

The [^{14}C]-glycocholate breath test has been employed to screen for abnormal intestinal bacterial colonization. Hellemans *et al.* (1984) fed [^{14}C]-glycocholate to 25 elderly subjects in good health, 22 hospitalized geriatric patients presenting with weight loss, and 42 normal young volunteers acting as controls. Fifty-six percent of the healthy elderly and 50% of the elderly patients with weight loss had high radioactive CO_2 excretion in the breath at the end of 3 hr, indicating abnormal bacterial deconjugation of the test dose. Among the patients with weight loss, a course of antibiotics was given, and seven of 11 breath tests returned to normal. Later studies by Arora *et al.* (1987) found no significant differences in bile salt breath test results in normal healthy elderly versus younger controls. Thus, the prevalence of bile-salt-splitting bacterial overgrowth of the small bowel in the elderly remains an open question.

4. Digestion and Absorption of Macronutrients

Since studies of absorption in elderly humans have rarely been designed to differentiate digestion from absorptive processes, digestion and absorption are considered together in this review. In addition, we concentrate as far as possible on changes in healthy, free-living elderly. Those elderly who are hospitalized and diseased present a different picture in regard to absorption and malabsorption (Webster, 1980).

4.1. Fat

The most recent and probably definitive work on fat absorption in normal aging has been reported by Arora *et al.* (1987). One hundred four healthy subjects underwent fecal fat collections after being on a 100-g fat diet for 3 days before and during 3 days of fecal collection. It was found that there was no increase in fat malabsorption with age. Mean daily fecal fat was 2.8 ± 0.5 g in those aged 19–44, 2.5 ± 0.3 g in 45- to 69-year-olds, and 2.9 ± 0.3 g in the population from 70 to 91 years. However, if dietary fat is raised to higher levels, fecal fat excretion has been shown to rise in elderly subjects, whereas in younger controls it remains constant (Werner and Hambraeus, 1972). For example, in this Swedish study, the range of fecal fat excretion on a steady 85- to 90-g fat diet was the same (3 to 7 g/day) for eight asymptomatic elderly subjects aged 67 to 72 as for six subjects aged 34–42. However, when the fat content of the diet was increased to 115 to 120 g/day, mean fecal fat excretion in the elderly rose to 7–12 g/day, whereas in the younger subjects it remained at 3 to 9 g/day. All but two of the elderly subjects excreted 12 g of fat per day or more. In another study on two elderly women, fat excretion was within normal limits when fat was distributed among four to six meals but excessive when most of the fat was taken in with one meal. This observation may have implications for design of appropriate feeding practices for the elderly.

Among institutionalized elderly, fecal fat levels frequently have been found to be high. For example, in 17 of 43 elderly institutionalized persons, fecal fat was found to be greater than 20% of dry weight, and fecal free fatty acids were low in 10 of the 17 samples (Peltz *et al.*, 1968). This is consistent with decreased pancreatic lipase activity. Southgate and Durnin (1970) have reported a very small but significant difference in the apparent digestibility of fat between young and elderly women (96.4% versus 94.7%) on a fat intake of 80–95 g/day. Since dietary fiber has been shown to adsorb pancreatic enzymes and possibly make them unavailable for participation in digestion, it is possible that the high-fiber diets that are frequently prescribed for the elderly could result in increased amounts of fat excretion if pancreatic reserve were lessened in elderly people (Dutta and Hlaski, 1985). However, results from the detailed balance studies on the effects of dietary fiber and energy utilization do not support the concept that fiber has a significant effect.

Webster *et al.* (1977) studied chylomicron appearance in blood after consumption of a meal containing 100 g of fat. Chylomicron levels at 3 and 4 hr were significantly higher in young controls than in elderly subjects (average age 82). When 3 g of pancreatic extract was added to the fatty meal, the difference became smaller and was no longer significant. A limitation of the study is that gastric emptying was not complete by 4 hr in over 80% of the elderly subjects compared to 50% of young controls. It is possible that slow gastric emptying flattened the chylomicron curve in the elderly. Among 70 patients over the age of 65 admitted to a metabolic unit for chronic bowel disorders, malabsorption (based on high fecal fat and/or an abnormal Schilling test and an abnormal 1-hr blood D-xylose test) was found in 56 individuals (Montgomery *et al.*, 1986). Bacterial overgrowth was found to be a predominant feature among these patients; small bowel diverticulosis and postgastrectomy syndrome were the most predominant causes.

4.2. Protein

Protein and amino acid absorption studies in elderly humans are rare. The results of nitrogen balance studies to evaluate protein requirements in the elderly are conflicting. Nitrogen balance is a function of protein intake, digestion, absorption, metabolism, utilization, and excretion. Thus, an understanding of protein digestion and absorption is essential in evaluating protein requirements of the elderly. In a Swedish study of protein tolerance, fecal nitrogen doubled to 4.0 g in five of seven elderly subjects given diets containing 1.4 to 1.5 g/kg of protein per day versus 0.9 to 1.0 g/kg per day (Werner and Hambraeus, 1972). Fecal nitrogen did not rise to the same level in younger adults when on the high-protein diet. Thus, high-protein diets may be less well tolerated by elderly persons. However, only a very few elderly subjects have been studied.

4.3. Carbohydrate

There is little evidence that glucose absorption is impaired in elderly people. Beaumont *et al.* (1987) studied in young and elderly subjects the absorption of 3-O-methylglucose, a nonmetabolized sugar, as well as the absorption of mannitol, which is thought to diffuse passively through the small intestinal wall. Although urinary recovery of both substances declined with age, when recovery was corrected for renal function no differences were seen between younger and elderly subjects. However, when the solutions were made hypertonic, the ratio of percentage recovery of 3-O-methylglucose to the percentage recovery of mannitol was significantly reduced in elderly subjects compared to middle-aged and young adult controls, suggesting a possible defect in active sugar transport in the elderly. A similar change was not seen in malnourished elderly patients; thus, the interpretation of this finding is at present uncertain.

Absorption of D-xylose, a pentose sugar, which is absorbed predominantly from the jejunum, has not been shown to be impaired with age. The D-xylose absorption test is considered to be an index of adequacy of the small intestinal mucosal absorptive surface. It has been observed that the average urinary excretion of D-xylose after an administered test dose is decreased in persons older than 65 years. However, other studies have established that the inverse relationship between age and D-xylose urinary excretion is primarily caused by deteriorating renal function at least up to age 80 (Guth, 1968; Kendall, 1970). Arora *et al.* (1987), by partial correlation analysis, have shown that the decline in D-xylose urinary excretion with age after a 25-g oral load can be totally accounted for by a decrease in creatinine clearance. Using a combination of oral and intravenous D-xylose doses, Webster and Leeming (1975b) found no evidence of impaired gastrointestinal absorption except in very old persons (average age 81 years).

In humans, jejunal lactase activity decreases with advancing age, although the activities of other disaccharidases remain constant throughout adult life (Welsh *et al.*, 1974, 1978). Although many adults maintain high brush border lactase levels, some degree of lactose intolerance is the rule rather than the exception in all racial groups save Caucasians (Caskey *et al.*, 1977; Bayless *et al.*, 1975). Although the amount of lactose needed to produce symptoms varies, most studies indicate that the amount of lactose contained in one glass of milk (approximately 12.5 g) can be tolerated by most lactase-deficient individuals (Debongnie *et al.*, 1979). However, many elderly persons avoid milk and milk products because they associate consumption of these foods with the development of cramps, bloating, and abdominal discomfort. In a double-blind comparison of tolerance among 87 healthy elderly persons using lactose-containing and lactose-free drinks, Rorick and Scrimshaw (1979) found that lactose malabsorption was probably not responsible for the symptoms of intolerance experienced by the elderly. Around 30% of those able and unable to absorb lactose were symptomatic with either drink. Some of the intolerance may be related to the image of milk as a "child's food."

One of the more interesting studies on the effects of age on intestinal carbohydrate metabolism was carried out by Feibusch and Holt (1982). These investigators fed elderly and young individuals meals of increasing carbohydrate content and measured breath hydrogen output as a measure of unabsorbed carbohydrate. Whereas young individuals did not show an increase in breath hydrogen levels even after meals with carbohydrate contents as high as 200 g, elderly individuals showed a high prevalence of abnormal breath hydrogen tests. With a 200-g dose of carbohydrate, only 20% of elderly individuals had normal breath hydrogen test results. This could be because of carbohydrate malabsorption with increased exposure of the unabsorbed carbohydrate to colonic bacteria or of normal absorption but exposure of the carbohydrate to greater numbers of bacteria in the proximal small intestine (either anaerobic or aerobic).

In summary, there is little evidence of malabsorption of simple sugars with advanced age. However, there does appear to be an increased prevalence of maldigestion of lactose and possibly of high doses of complex carbohydrates.

4.4. Calcium

Osteoporosis is one bone disease whose incidence increases with age, particularly in Caucasian women after the menopause (Chapter 8). Although the etiology of osteoporosis is not understood, calcium and vitamin D and hormone interrelationships are considered important. Studies using several different approaches indicate that intestinal calcium absorption decreases with aging in both men and women, particularly after age 70 (Bullamore *et al.*, 1970; Gallagher *et al.*, 1979). All 30 patients over age 80 studied by Bullamore's group in Leeds had significant malabsorption of calcium. However, calcium absorption was reported to be normal in 18 elderly institutionalized women in Montreal (Somerville *et al.*, 1977).

Gallagher *et al.* (1979) have examined the interrelationships of age, calcium intake and absorption, and vitamin D metabolism in 94 normal volunteers (aged 30–

90) and 52 untreated women with postmenopausal osteoporosis. Fractional calcium absorption decreased significantly with age but was not significantly correlated with dietary calcium intake in the elderly subjects, with the correlation approaching significance in subjects under age 65. There was no significant age-related difference in serum 25-OHD levels; however, average 1,25-$(OH)_2D$ levels and intestinal calcium absorption were significantly lower in the elderly group, suggesting less effective renal conversion. Finally serum 1,25-$(OH)_2D$ levels and intestinal calcium absorption were significantly correlated, implying at all ages that intestinal absorption is determined by 1,25-$(OH)_2D$. A comparison of these relationships in 27 elderly patients with osteoporosis and 20 normal subjects indicated no significant differences in 25-OHD or dietary calcium intake but significant differences in calcium absorption and in circulating 1,25-$(OH)_2D$.

Other work indicates that adaptation to a lower calcium intake is impaired in elderly subjects. Ireland and Fordtran (1973) used a triple-lumen perfusion system to study calcium absorption from the proximal jejunum in healthy young and elderly adults (average age 68 years) who were adapted for 1–2 months to diets containing 300 or 2000 mg of calcium daily. Calcium absorption after adaptation to the low-calcium diet was significantly increased in the young subjects, and the adapted young subjects consistently absorbed more calcium than older people, who appeared to have a blunted adaptive response to the low calcium intake.

Noted earlier was the possibility that calcium absorption may be influenced by the loss of stomach acid in those elderly with hypo- or achlorhydria. A deficit in absorption of calcium carbonate was demonstrated in elderly patients with achlorhydria by Recker (1985), but these same patients absorbed calcium normally in a meal.

Further research is needed to define the cause of the age-related decrease in intestinal calcium absorption and in adaptation to decreased intakes, to establish its role in postmenopausal and osteoporotic bone loss, and to elucidate the mechanism(s) responsible for the decreased serum concentration of 1,25-$(OH)_2D$ observed in elderly persons. Loss of renal 1-hydroxylase reserve as a reflection of loss of renal functional mass, although likely, has yet to be proven in man. Similarly, the possibility that end-organ (intestine) responsiveness is lost with aging is unproved in man (Francis *et al.*, 1983). These possibilities deserve further study.

5. *Absorption of Micronutrients*

Low levels of circulating vitamins and minerals have been demonstrated in casual surveys of elderly populations, although relatively few studies have attempted to differentiate effects at the stages of dietary intake, absorption, metabolism, utilization, and excretion. We have chosen to focus on studies relating to the absorption of vitamins, minerals, and trace elements by elderly people in the following sections.

5.1. *Water-Soluble Vitamins*

5.1.1. *Thiamin*

There is no evidence for defective thiamin absorption in the elderly (Thomson, 1966). Twenty-four elderly convalescent inpatients (average age of 82) and 21 younger subjects were given oral doses of 1, 5, and 20 mg of thiamin. After an intravenous flushing dose, there were no differences in the subsequent urinary excretion of thiamin between the two groups (Thomson, 1966).

5.1.2. Vitamin B_{12}

The elderly may be at particular risk of vitamin B_{12} deficiency in that the dietary intake of vitamin B_{12} is often low, especially among poor elderly people. In different surveys, up to 23% of elderly showed low serum or plasma vitamin B_{12} levels (Elwood *et al.*, 1971; Garry *et al.*, 1984; Magnus *et al.*, 1982; Bailey *et al.*, 1980). However, Bailey *et al.* (1979) reported normal serum vitamin B_{12} levels in a group of low-income elderly that was 80% black and 20% Spanish-American. The average serum vitamin B_{12} concentration in this study was 700 pg/ml, which is well above the lower limit of normal.

Impaired secretion of intrinsic factor is a problem in some elderly, but more commonly the degree of atrophic gastritis seen in elderly people is not sufficient to result in severely lowered intrinsic factor secretion. Moreover, autoimmune phenomena such as intrinsic factor antibodies are usually lacking in the elderly people with atrophic gastritis (Krasinski *et al.*, 1986). However, in atrophic gastritis, two physiological consequences may result in impaired vitamin B_{12} absorption other than by the mechanism of impaired intrinsic factor secretion: (1) decreased digestive release of vitamin B_{12} from food–protein complexes and (2) increased bacterial overgrowth in the proximal small bowel leading to competition with the intestinal epithelial cells for vitamin B_{12} (Russell, 1986).

In a survey among elderly subjects with or without atrophic gastritis, serum vitamin B_{12} levels were found to be significantly lower in those with atrophic gastritis (Krasinski *et al.*, 1986). In the same survey, it was found that the prevalence of low serum vitamin B_{12} levels, (i.e., <120 pg/ml) increased with increasing severity of the atrophic gastritis. Low serum vitamin B_{12} levels were found in eight of 15 (53%) subjects with severe atrophic gastritis and in 9% of subjects with mild to moderate atrophic gastritis. Only five of 134 (4%) subjects without atrophic gastritis had low serum vitamin B_{12} levels.

Although Schilling tests using crystalline vitamin B_{12} have been shown to be normal in several series of elderly patients (Schepp *et al.*, 1980; Nilsson-Ehle *et al.*, 1986), absorption of vitamin B_{12} bound to chicken serum protein or incorporated into egg has been found to be considerably less efficient among patients with hypochlorhydria (Doscherholmen and Swaim, 1973; Steinberg *et al.*, 1980; Carmel *et al.*, 1987). Carmel *et al.* (1987) studied 25 patients with low serum vitamin B_{12} levels who were without clinical or hematological findings of cobalamin deficiency. Of these, seven patients displayed malabsorption of protein-bound cobalamin despite normal absorption of free cobalamin by Schilling tests. These observations are clinically significant because patients who have achlorhydria or who are receiving antacid or histamine H_2-receptor antagonist therapy may absorb food-bound vitamin B_{12} inefficiently despite normal Schilling tests employing crystalline vitamin B_{12}. In such cases, appropriate therapy may be oral cyanocobalamin (Toskes, 1980). With regard to the role of bacteria in the elderly, Russell *et al.* (1987) have described a series of patients with atrophic gastritis who had a return from abnormal to normal protein-bound vitamin B_{12} absorption tests on oral tetracycline therapy. They attributed this reversal to diminished numbers of small intestinal bacteria after tetracycline and hence to less bacterial uptake of the very small amount of free cobalamin that is released from dietary protein in hypochlorhydric states.

5.1.3. Folic Acid

The reported prevalence of folate deficiency among the elderly has varied widely. In general, only 3 to 7% of free-living elderly have been found to have low serum and/or plasma folate levels (i.e., <3 ng/ml) (Elwood *et al.*, 1971; Garry *et al.*, 1984). Among well-to-do New Mexican elderly, 8% had low serum folates, and 3% had low red blood cell folates (i.e., <140 ng/ml) (Garry *et al.*, 1984). In contrast, 70% of low-income black or Spanish-American elderly populations have been shown to have erythrocyte folate levels less than 160 ng/ml (Bailey *et al.*, 1979).

Potential causes of folate deficiency in the elderly include dietary deficiency, malabsorption, and drug–folate antagonism (Rosenberg *et al.*, 1982). Baker *et al.* (1978) hypothesized that age-related changes in the gut could lead to impaired absorption of dietary folate (polyglutamyl folates). They based this on differences in circulating blood folate levels between elderly and young subjects after ingestion of yeast polyglutamyl folates. This question was later addressed directly by Bailey *et al.* (1984), who showed that luminal disappearance and urinary recovery of folate from synthetic pteroyl heptaglutamate was identical in elderly and young subjects. In this same study monoglutamyl folate absorption was also the same in elderly and young subjects. Finally, direct measurement of folyl polyglutamate hydrolase in intestinal biopsies showed no evidence of a decline with age. Elsborg (1976) showed that folic acid (pteroylmonoglutamic acid) absorption estimated by urinary excretion of tritiated folic acid was not significantly affected by age or sex in 64 randomly selected subjects (age 23 to 70) who were not deficient in folate. Elderly patients (average age 72) with nutritional folate deficiency initially showed impaired absorption, which returned to normal after 1 month of folate supplementation. Thus, the balance of data indicates that aging does not impair absorption of either mono- or polyglutamyl folate.

In vitro studies using rat intestinal rings and Caco-2 cells, a colon cancer-derived intestinal cell line, have shown that folic acid uptake was markedly influenced by pH, maximal folic acid uptake occurring at approximately pH 6.3 (Russell *et al.*, 1979; Vincent *et al.*, 1985). Folic acid absorption was studied in 12 elderly subjects with atrophic gastritis and ten elderly normal controls using pteroylmononoglutamic acid (Russell *et al.*, 1986). As expected, proximal small intestinal pH was higher in atrophic gastritis subjects than in controls (7.1 and 6.7, respectively; $P < 0.05$). It was hypothesized that folate absorption might be impaired in atrophic gastritis subjects because of a rise in the intraluminal pH of the proximal small bowel from the lack of gastric acid. Two folic absorption tests were carried out on each subject given either water or 0.1 N hydrochloric acid. Folic acid absorption was found to be significantly lower in subjects with atrophic gastritis than in normal controls (31% versus 51%, respectively). In subjects with atrophic gastritis, folic acid absorption rose significantly to 54% when administered with acid. Nevertheless, in spite of this demonstrated folate malabsorption in atrophic gastritis subjects, in surveys of elderly subjects with atrophic gastritis, serum folate levels were actually found to be higher than in elderly without atrophic gastritis (Krasinski *et al.*, 1986). In explaining this paradox, Russell *et al.* (1986) showed bacterial counts to be higher in the small intestinal fluid of atrophic gastritis subjects than in normal controls and, further, that the bacteria cultured from the intestinal aspirates of subjects with atrophic gastritis were able to synthesize folate *in vitro* when incubated in a folate-free medium. In conclusion, the modest deficit in folate absorption attributable to atrophic gastritis and achlorhydria appears to be offset by folate synthesis by the increased bacterial mass in the small intestine. In elderly without achlorhydria or other gastrointestinal disease, there is no evidence of folate malabsorption.

5.1.4. Ascorbic Acid

In humans, the concentration of ascorbic acid in several tissues reportedly declines with age, but because these concentrations can be increased by oral supplementation, the reduced levels probably reflect low intake rather than impaired absorption of the vitamin (Kirk and Chieffi, 1953; Loh, 1972; Cheng *et al.*, 1985). The only direct studies comparing vitamin C absorption in young and old subjects compare healthy young with hospitalized nonscorbutic elderly. Such studies demonstrate lower elevations of serum ascorbate after oral doses in elderly and lower urinary excretion (Davies *et al.*, 1984). The applicability of these studies to healthy free-living elderly is uncertain.

5.1.5. Other Water-Soluble Vitamins

In a nutritional survey of almost 200 institutionalized elderly persons (average age 79), biochemical evidence of vitamin and mineral deficiency was observed in 91% of a nonsupplemented group and 64% of a multivitamin-supplemented group (Vir and Love, 1979). Multivitamin supplements normalized the blood assays for ascorbic acid, thiamin, and riboflavin in all or nearly all subjects but failed to normalize the red cell vitamin B_6 assay in 20% of them. Similarly, Hoorn *et al.* (1975) failed to normalize the erythrocyte glutamic oxalacetic transaminase activity coefficient in about 10% of B_6-deficient elderly with a daily vitamin B_6 supplement given for 12 days. On the basis of this evidence, Vir and Love suggested that an increased dietary need of vitamin B_6 might be considered for the elderly, possibly as a result of malabsorption of the vitamin. No other studies on the absorption of vitamin B_6 in the elderly have been reported.

Intake, urinary excretion, and blood concentrations of pantothenic acid were similar in free-living and institutionalized elderly (Srinivasan *et al.*, 1981). In those taking pantothenic acid supplements, blood levels remained unchanged, but urinary excretion was increased. These results suggest that age *per se* is unlikely to compromise one's panothenic acid status.

5.2. Fat-Soluble Vitamins

5.2.1. Vitamin A

Yiengst and Shock (1949) found no age differences in the peak plasma concentration of vitamin A after a pharmacological dose of 100,000 IU of the vitamin. However, it was noted that the peak rise occurred earlier in men under age 70 than in elderly individuals, probably as a result of faster gastric emptying. Using physiological doses of vitamin A, Krasinski *et al.* (1985), however, showed no time difference for the peak rise of vitamin A in blood; rather, they showed that elderly individuals had higher peak rises and areas under the tolerance curves than did normal young controls. This could be the result of either increased absorption or decreased liver clearance of vitamin A with age.

5.2.2. *Vitamin D*

Many studies have reported age-related declines of serum 25-OH vitamin D levels in blood, although these levels are mostly maintained within the normal range (Vir and Love, 1979; Corless *et al.*, 1979; Dattani *et al.*, 1984). Vir and Love (1979) reported concentrations of 25-OH vitamin D below 3.8 ng/dl among almost half of 49 geriatric patients tested. The marked seasonal variation of serum 25-OH vitamin D levels in elderly as compared to younger controls is, in part, caused by less ultraviolet light exposure and/or decreased synthesis of vitamin D in the skin with age (Lund and Sorensen, 1979; Stamp and Round, 1974; MacLaughlin and Holick, 1985). Because of the paucity of sunlight to which the elderly are exposed, particularly if institutionalized, a full understanding of how age affects vitamin D absorption and metabolism is necessary. Somerville *et al.* (1977) observed identical serum levels of 25-OH vitamin D in young controls and in 18 elderly women (average age 83) after 2 weeks of oral therapy with 10,000 IU per day of cholecalciferol. This would tend to mitigate against an absorptive defect. However, other data on age-related changes in vitamin D absorption are contradictory (Barragry *et al.*, 1978). The differences in results may possibly be explained by different body stores of vitamin D to begin with or different compositions of the administered diet with which vitamin D was given.

5.3. *Trace Elements*

Marx (1979) compared iron absorption in active elderly persons and young adults, all with normal iron status, using a double-isotope technique that allowed the differentiation of mucosal uptake, mucosal transfer, and retention of iron. There was no age difference in iron absorption, but red cell iron uptake of retained iron was about one-third lower in the elderly subjects. Young and old patients with uncomplicated iron deficiency had increased iron absorption to a similar extent. In this study, absorption of iron from ferrous ammonium sulfate was not impaired in the elderly; bioavailability of the forms of iron found in food is unknown, however. The bulk of evidence, including the study by Bunker *et al.* (1984) that demonstrated that healthy elderly can remain in iron balance on intakes even below the RDA, is that iron absorption does not decline significantly with normal aging. Possible causes of the iron deficiency observed in elderly persons include inadequate intake, blood loss, and changes in iron absorption secondary to atrophic gastritis (Lynch *et al.*, 1982). In achlorhydria the absorption of nonheme iron is reduced, but the absorption of heme iron is not affected (Jacobs *et al.*, 1964). Similarly, inhibition of acid secretion by cimetidine or antacids results in significantly impaired absorption of nonheme iron (Skikne *et al.*, 1981).

Data on absorption of other trace minerals in the elderly are limited. Turnlund and her co-workers (1986) used stable isotopic zinc to confirm earlier studies on man with radioisotopes and showed a decreased zinc absorption with age. In contrast, using stable isotopes of copper, Turnlund and her colleagues (1982) found absorption in seven elderly men comparable to that reported in young adults with radioisotopic copper.

6. Conclusion

As with other organ systems, certain of the digestive tract organs experience some diminution of function with age. Decrements in taste and smell may affect gustatory enthusiasm and thus food intake. Changes in esophageal motility, unless severe, probably do not interfere with alimentation. Gastric atrophy may have variable effects on absorption of vitamin B_{12}, folate, calcium, and iron, but the extent of these changes in absorption from meals deserves further study. Efficient digestion and absorption of macronutrients, fat, starches, sugars, and protein, appear to be retained during normal aging. More work is needed on the exploration of aging effects on the absorption of vitamins and minerals, but, with the possible exception of calcium, changes in the aging digestive tract have not yet been shown to influence recommendations regarding requirements of vitamins and minerals in the elderly.

7. References

Arora, S., Russell, R. M., Kassarjian, Z., Krasinski, S., and Kaplan, M. M., 1987, Evaluation of absorptive and hepatobiliary function in the aging digestive tract, *J. Am. Clin. Nutr.* **6**(5):434.

Bailey, L. B., Wagner, P. A., Christakis, G. J., Araujo, P. E., Appledorf, H., Davis, C. G., Masteryanni, J., and Dinning, J. S., 1979, Folacin and iron status and hematological findings in predominantly black elderly persons from urban low income households, *Am. J. Clin. Nutr.* **32**:2346–2353.

Bailey, L. B., Wagner, P. A., Christakis, G. J., Araujo, P. E., Appledorf, H., Davis, C. G., Dorsey, E., and Dinning, J. S., 1980, Vitamin B_{12} status of elderly persons from urban low-income households, *J. Am. Geriatr. Soc.* **28**:276–278.

Bailey, L. B., Cerda, J. J., Brandon, S., Block, M., Busby, J., Vargas, L., Chandler, C. J., and Halsted, C. H., 1984, Effect of age on poly- and monoglutamyl folacin absorption in human subjects, *J. Nutr.* **114**:1770–1776.

Baker, H., Jaslow, S. P., and Frank, O., 1978, Severe impairment of dietary folate utilization in the elderly, *J. Am. Geriatr. Soc.* **26**:218.

Barragry, J. M., France, M. Q., Corless, D., Gupta, S., Switala, P., Boucher, B. J., and Cohen, R. D., 1978, Intestinal cholecalciferol absorption in the elderly and in younger adults, *Clin. Sci. Mol. Med.* **5**:213–220.

Bartos, V., and Groh, J., 1969, The effect of repeated stimulation of the pancreas on the pancreatic secretion in young and aged men, *Gerontol. Clin.* **11**:56–62.

Baum, B. J., 1981, Evaluation of stimulated parotid saliva flow rate in different age groups, *J. Dent. Res.* **60**(7):1292–1296.

Bayless, T. M., Rothfeld, B., Massa, C., Wise, L., Paige, D., and Bedine, M. S., 1975, Lactose and milk intolerance: Clinical implications, *N. Engl. J. Med.* **292**:1156–1159.

Beaumont, D. M., Cobden, I., Sheldon, W. L., Laker, M. F., and James, O. F. W., 1987, Passive and active carbohydrate absorption by the ageing gut, *Age and Ageing* **16**:294–300.

Bird, T., Hall, M. R. P., and Schade, R. O. K., 1977, Gastric histology and its relation to anaemia in the elderly, *Gerontology* **23**:309–321.

Blackman, A. H., Lambert, D. L., Thayer, W. R., and Martin, H. F., 1970, Computed normal values for peak acid output based on age, sex and body weight, *Am. J. Dig. Dis.* **15**:783–789.

Bowman, B. B., and Rosenberg, I. H., 1983, Digestive function and aging, *Hum. Nutr. Clin. Nutr.* **37C**:75–89.

Brauer, P. M., Slavin, J. J., and Marlett, J. A., 1981, Apparent digestibility of neutral detergent fiber in elderly and young adults, *Am. J. Clin. Nutr.* **34**:1061–1070.

Bullamore, J. R., Wilkinson, R., Gallagher, J. C., and Nordin, B. E. C., 1970, Effect of age on calcium absorption, *Lancet* **2**:535–537.

Bunker, V. W., Lawson, M. S., and Clayton, B. E., 1984, Uptake and excretion of iron by healthy elderly subjects, *J. Clin. Pathol.* **37**:1353–1357.

Busse, E. W., 1978, How mind, body, and environment influence nutrition in the elderly, *Postgrad. Med.* **63**:118–125.

Carmel, R., Sinow, R. M., and Karnaze, D. S., 1987, Atypical cobalamin deficency, *J. Lab. Clin. Med.* **109**:454–463.

Caskey, D. A., Payne-Bose, D., Welsh, J. D., Gearhart, H. L., Nance, M. K., Morrison, R. D., 1977, Effects of age on lactose malabsorption in Oklahoma Native Americans as determined by breath H_2 analysis, *Dig. Dis. Sci.* **22**:113–116.

Cheng, L., Cohen, M., and Bhagavan, H. N., 1985, Vitamin C and the elderly, in: *Handbook of Nutrition in the Aged* (R. R. Watson, ed.), CRC Press, Boca Raton, FL, pp. 157–185.

Corazza, G. R., Frazzoni, M., Gatto, M. R. A., and Gasbarrini, G., 1986, Ageing and small-bowel mucosa: A morphometric study, *Gerontology* **321**:60–65.

Corless, D., Gupta, S. P., Sattar, D. A., Switala, S., and Boucher, B. J., 1979, Vitamin D status of residents of an old people's home and long-stay patients, *Gerontology* **25**:350–355.

Dattani, J. T., Exton-Smith, A. N., and Stephen, M. L., 1984, Vitamin D status of the elderly in relation to age and exposure to sunlight, *Hum. Nutr. Clin. Nutr.* **38C**:131–137.

Davies, H. E. F., Davies, J. E. W., Hughes, R. E., and Jones, E., 1984, Studies on the absorption of L-xyloascorbic acid (vitamin C) in young and elderly subjects, *Hum. Nutr. Clin. Nutr.* **38**:463–471.

Davies, W. T., Kirkpatrick, J. R., Owen, G. M., and Shields, R., 1971, Gastric emptying in atrophic gastritis and carcinoma of the stomach, *Scand. J. Gastroenterol.* **6**:297–301.

Debongnie, J. C., Newcomer, A. D., McGill, D. B., and Phillips, S. F., 1979, Absorption of nutrients in lactase deficiency, *Dig. Dis. Sci.* **24**:225–231.

Doscherholmen, A., and Swaim, W. R., 1973, Impaired assimilation of egg ^{57}Co vitamin B_{12} in patients with hypochlorhydria and achlorhydria and after gastric resection, *Gastroenterology* **64**:913–919.

Drasar, B. S., Shiner, M., and McLeod, G. M., 1969, Studies on the intestinal flora, *Gastroenterology* **56**(1):71–79.

Dutta, S. K., and Hlaski, J., 1985, Dietary fiber in pancreatic disease: Effect of high fiber diet on fat malabsorption in pancreatic insufficiency and *in vitro* study of the interaction of dietary fiber with pancreatic enzymes, *Am. J. Clin. Nutr.* **41**:517–525.

Elsborg, L., 1976, Reversible malabsorption of folic acid in the elderly with nutritional folate deficiency, *Acta Haematol.* **55**:140–147.

Elwood, P. C., Shinton, N. K., Wilson, C. I. D., Sweetnam, P., and Frazer, A. C., 1971, Haemoglobin, vitamin B_{12} and folate levels in the elderly, *Br. J. Haematol.* **21**:557–563.

Evans, M. A., Triggs, E. J., Cheung, M., Broe, G. A., and Creasey, H., 1981, Gastric emptying rate in the elderly: Implications for drug therapy, *J. Am. Geriatr. Soc.* **29**(5):201–205.

Feibusch, J. M., and Holt, P. R., 1982, Impaired absorptive capacity for carbohydrate in the aging human, *Dig. Dis. Sci.* **27**:1095–1100.

Francis, R. M., Peacock, M., Storer, J. H., Davies, A. E. J., Brown, W. B., and Nordin, B. H. C., 1983, Calcium malabsorption in the elderly: The effect of treatment with oral 25-hydroxyvitamin D_3, *Eur. J. Clin. Invest.* **13**:391–396.

Gallagher, J. C., Riggs, B. L., Eisman, J., Hamstra, A., Arnaud, S. B., and DeLuca, H. F., 1979, Intestinal calcium absorption and serum vitamin D metabolites in normal subjects and osteoporotic patients, *J. Clin. Invest.* **64**:729–736.

Garry, P. J., Goodwin, J. S., and Hunt, W. C., 1984, Folate and vitamin B-12 status in a healthy elderly population, *J. Am. Geriatr. Soc.* **32**:719–726.

Gersovitz, M., Munro, H. N., Udall, J., and Young, V. R., 1980, Albumin synthesis in young and elderly subjects using a new stable isotope methodology: Responses to level of protein intake, *Metabolism* **29:**1075–1086.

Greenblatt, D. J., 1979, Reduced serum albumin concentration in the elderly: A report from the Boston Collaborative Drug Surveillance Program, *J. Am. Geriatr. Soc.* **27:**20–22.

Greger, J. L., and Geissler, A. H., 1978, Effect of zinc supplementation on taste acuity of the aged, *Am. J. Clin. Nutr.* **31:**633–637.

Grzegorczyk, P. B., Jones, S. W., and Mistretta, C. M., 1979, Age related differences in salt taste acuity, *J. Gerontol.* **34:**834–840.

Gullo, L., Ventrucci, M., Naldoni, P., and Pezzilli, R., 1986, Aging and pancreatic function, *J. Am. Geriatr. Soc.* **34:**790–792.

Guth, P. H., 1968, Physiologic alterations in small bowel function with age: The absorption of D-xylose, *Am. J. Dig. Dis.* **13:**565–571.

Halvorsen, I., Dotevall, G., and Walan, A., 1973, Gastric emptying in patients with achlorhydria or hyposecretion of hydrochloric acid, *Scand. J. Gastroenterol.* **8:**395–399.

Hellemans, J., Joosten, E., Ghoos, Y., Carchon, H., Vantrappen, G., Pelemans, W., and Rutgeerts, P., 1984, Positive $^{14}CO_2$ bile acid breath test in elderly people, *Age Ageing* **13:**138–143.

Hollis, J. B., and Castell, D. O., 1974, Esophageal function in elderly men, *Ann. Intern. Med.* **80:**371–374.

Hoorn, R. K. H., Flikweert, J. P., and Westerink, D., 1975, Vitamin B_1, B_2, and B_6 deficiencies in geriatric patients, measured by coenzyme stimulation of enzymatic activities, *Clin. Chem. Acta* **61:**151–162.

Horowitz, M., Maddern, G. J., Chatterton, B. E., Collins, P. J., Harding, P. E., and Shearman, D. J. C., 1984, Changes in gastric emptying rates with age, *Clin. Sci.* **67:**213–218.

Ireland, P., and Fordtran, J. S., 1973, Effect of dietary calcium and age on jejunal calcium absorption in humans studied by intestinal perfusion. *J. Clin. Invest.* **52:**2672–2681.

Jacobs, P., Bothwell, T., and Charlton, R. W., 1964, Role of hydrochloric acid in iron absorption, *J. Appl. Physiol.* **19:**187–188.

James, W. P. T., Branch, W. J., and Southgate, D. A. T., 1978, Calcium binding by dietary fibre, *Lancet* **1:**638–639.

Kendall, M. J., 1970, The influence of age on the xylose absorption test, *Gut* **11:**498–501.

Khan, T. A., Shragge, B. W., Crispin, J. S., and Lind, J. F., 1977, Esophageal motility in the elderly, *Am. J. Dig. Dis.* **22:**1049–1054.

Kirk, J. E., and Chieffi, M., 1953, Vitamin studies in middle-aged and old individuals, XII. Hypovitaminemia C, *J. Gerontol.* **8:**305–311.

Krasinski, S. D., Russell, R. M., and Dallal, G. E., 1985, Aging changes vitamin A absorption characteristics, *Gastroenterology* **88:**1563.

Krasinski, S. D., Russell, R. M., Samloff, I. M., Jacob, R. A., Dallal, G. E., McGandy, R. B., and Hartz, S. C., 1986, Fundic atrophic gastritis in an elderly population: Effect on hemoglobin and several serum nutritional indicators, *J. Am. Geriatr. Soc.* **34:**800–806.

Kupfer, R. M., Heppell, M., Haggith, J. W., and Bateman, D. N., 1985, Gastric emptying and small-bowel transit rate in the elderly, *J. Am. Geriatr. Soc.* **33**(5):340–343.

Langan, M. J., and Yearick, E. S., 1976, The effects of improved oral hygiene in taste perception and nutrition of the elderly, *J. Gerontol.* **31:**413–418.

Langer, A., 1976, Oral signs of aging and their clinical significance, *Geriatrics* **31:**63–69.

Loh, H. S., 1972, The relationship between dietary ascorbic acid intake and buffy coat and plasma ascorbic acid concentrations at different ages, *Int. J. Vitam. Nutr. Res.* **42:**80–85.

Lund, B., and Sorensen, O. H., 1979, Measurement of 25-hydroxyvitamin D in serum and its relation to sunshine, age and vitamin D intake in the Danish population, *Scand. J. Clin. Lab. Invest.* **39:**23–30.

Lynch, S. R., Finch, C. A., Monsen, E. R., and Cook, J. D., 1982, Iron status of elderly Americans, *Am. J. Clin. Nutr.* **36:**1032–1045.

MacLaughlin, J., and Holick, M. F., 1985, Aging decreases the capacity of human skin to produce vitamin D_3, *J. Clin. Invest.* **76:**1536–1538.

Magnus, E. M., Bache-Wiig, J. E., Aanderson, T. R., and Melbostad, E., 1982, Folate and vitamin B_{12} (cobalamin) blood levels in elderly persons in geriatric homes, *Scand. J. Haematol.* **28:**360–366.

Marx, J. J. M., 1979, Normal iron absorption and decreased red cell iron uptake in the aged, *Blood* **53:**204–211.

McEvoy, A., Dutton, J., and James, O. F. W., 1983, Bacterial contamination of the small intestine is an important cause of occult malabsorption in the elderly, *Br. Med. J.* **287**:789–793.

Meyer, J., Spier, E., and Neuwelt, F., 1940, Basal secretion of digestive enzymes in old age, *Arch. Intern. Med.* **65**:171–174.

Montgomery, R. D., Haboubi, N. Y., Mike, N. H., Chesner, I. M., and Asquith, P., 1986, Causes of malabsorption in the elderly, *Age Ageing* **15**:235–240.

Necheles, H., Plotke, F., and Meyer, J., 1942, Studies on old age, *Am. J. Dig. Dis.* **9**(5):157–159.

Nilsson-Ehle, H., Jagenburg, R., Landahl, S., Lindstedt, G., Swolin, B., and Westin, J., 1986, Cyanocobalamin absorption in the elderly: Results for healthy subjects and for subjects with low serum cobalamin concentration, *Clin. Chem.* **32**(7):1368–1371.

Pelz, K. S., Goffried, S. P., and Sooes, E., 1968, Intestinal absorption studies in the aged, *Geriatrics* **23**:149–153.

Pitchumoni, C. S., Glasser, M., Saran, R. M., Panchacharam, P., and Thelmo, W., 1984, Pancreatic fibrosis in chronic alcoholics and nonalcoholics without clinical pancreatitis, *Am. J. Gastroenterol.* **79**(5):382–388.

Recker, R. M., 1985, Calcium absorption and achlorhydria, *N. Engl. J. Med.* **313**:70–73.

Rorick, M. H., and Scrimshaw, N. S., 1979, Comparative tolerance of elderly from differing backgrounds to lactose-containing and lactose-free dairy drinks: A double-blind study, *J. Gerontol.* **34**:191–196.

Rosenberg, I. H., Bowman, B. B., Cooper, B. A., Halsted, C. H., and Lindenbaum, J., 1982, Folate nutrition in the elderly, *Am. J. Clin. Nutr.* **36**:1060–1066.

Russell, R. M., 1986, Implications of gastric atrophy for vitamin and mineral nutriture, in: *Nutrition and Aging, Bristol Meyers Nutrition Symposia* (M. L. Hutchinson and H. N. Munro, eds.), Academic Press, Orlando, FL, pp. 59–69.

Russell, R. M., 1987, Nutritional implications of the aging gastrointestinal tract, *J. Am. Coll. Nutr.* **6**:421.

Russell, R. M., Dhar, G. J., Dutta, S. K., and Rosenberg, I. H., 1979, Influence of intraluminal pH on folate absorption: studies in control subjects and in patients with pancreatic insufficiency, *J. Lab. Clin. Med.* **93**:428–436.

Russell, R. M., Krasinski, S. D., Samloff, I. M., Jacob, R. A., Hartz, S. C., and Brovender, S. R., 1986, Folic acid malabsorption in atrophic gastritis, *Gastroenterology* **91**:1476–1482.

Russell, R. M., Suter, P. M., and Golner, B., 1987, Decreased bioavailability of protein bound vitamin B_{12} in mild atrophic gastritis: Reversal by antibiotics, *Gastroenterology* **92**(5):1606.

Samloff, I. M., Varis, K., Ihamaki, T., Siurala, M., and Rotter, J. I., 1982, Relationships among serum pepsinogen I, serum pepsinogen II, and gastric mucosal histology. *Gastroenterology* **83**:204–209.

Schepp, W., Lindstaedt, H., Miederer, S. E., and Elster, K., 1980, No influence of age and gastric acid secretion on serum vitamin B_{12} concentration, *Hepatogastroenterology* **27**:294–299.

Schiffman, S., and Pasternak, M., 1979, Decreased discrimination of food odors in the elderly, *J. Gerontol.* **34**:73–79.

Schiller, L. R., 1983, Motor function of the stomach, in: *Gastrointestinal Disease,* 3rd ed. (M. H. Sleisenger and J. S. Fordtran, eds.), W. B. Saunders, Philadelphia, pp. 521–541.

Schmucker, D. L., and Daniels, C. K., 1986, Aging, gastrointestinal infections, and mucosal immunity, *J. Am. Geriatr. Soc.* **34**:377–384.

Skikne, B. S., Lynch, S. R., and Cook, J. D., 1981, Role of gastric acid in food iron absorption, *Gastroenterology* **81**:1068–1071.

Somerville, P. J., Lien, J. W. K., and Kaye, M., 1977, The calcium and vitamin D status in an elderly population and their response to administered supplemental vitamin D_3, *J. Gerontol.* **32**:659–663.

Southgate, D. A. T., and Durnin, J. V. G. A., 1970, Calorie conversion factors. An experimental reassessment of the factors used in the calculation of the energy value of human diets, *Br. J. Nutr.* **24**:517–535.

Srinivasan, V., Christensen, N., Wyse, B., and Hansen, R. G., 1981, Pantothenic acid nutritional status in the elderly—institutionalized and noninstitutionalized, *Am. J. Clin. Nutr.* **34**:1736–1742.

Stamp, T. C. B., and Round, J. M., 1974, Seasonal changes in human plasma levels of 25-hydroxyvitamin D_3, *J. Clin. Invest.* **76**:1536–1538.

Steinberg, W. M., King, C. E., and Toskes, P. P., 1980, Malabsorption of protein-bound cobalamin but not unbound cobalamin during cimetidine administration, *Dig. Dis. Sci.* **25**:188–191.

Stevens, J. C., Bartoshuk, L. M., and Cain, W. S., 1984, Chemical senses and aging: Taste versus smell, *Chem. Sens.* **9**:167–179.

Strickland, R. G., and MacKay, I. R., 1973, A reappraisal of the nature and significance of chronic atrophic gastritis, *Dig. Dis. Sci.* **18:**426–440.

Tabaqchali, S., 1970, The pathophysiologic role of small intestinal bacterial flora, *Scand. J. Gastroenterol.* **6:**139–163.

Thompson, A. B. R., and Keelan, M., 1986, The aging gut, *Can. J. Physiol. Pharmacol.* **64:**30–38.

Thomson, A. D., 1966, Thiamine absorption in old age, *Gerontol. Clin.* **8:**354–361.

Toskes, P. P., 1980, Current concepts of cobalamin (vitamin B_{12}) absorption and malabsorption, *J. Clin. Gastroenterol.* **2:**287–297.

Turnlund, J. R., Michel, M. C., Keyes, W. R., Schutz, Y., and Margen, S., 1982, Copper absorption in elderly men determined by using stable ^{65}Cu, *Am. J. Clin. Nutr.* **36:**587–591.

Turnlund, J. R., Durkin, N., Costa, F., and Margen, S., 1986, Stable isotope studies of zinc absorption and retention in young and elderly men, *J. Nutr.* **116:**1239–1247.

Van Liere, E. J., and Northup, D. W., 1941, The emptying time of the stomach of old people, *Am. J. Physiol.* **134:**719–722.

Vincent, M. L., Russell, R. M., and Sasak, V., 1985, Folic acid uptake characteristics of a human colon carcinoma cell line, Caco-2, *Hum. Nutr. Clin. Nutr.* **39C:**355–360.

Vir, S. C., and Love, A. H. G., 1979, Nutritional status of institutionalized and non-institutionalized aged in Belfast, Northern Ireland, *Am. J. Clin. Nutr.* **32:**1934–1947.

Warren, P. M., Pepperman, M. A., and Montgomery, R. D., 1978, Age changes in small-intestinal mucosa, *Lancet* **2:**849–850.

Webster, S. G. P., 1980, Gastrointestinal function and absorption of nutrients, in: *Metabolic and Nutritional Disorders in the Elderly* (A. N. Exton-Smith, ed.), John Wright & Sons, Bristol, pp. 87–99.

Webster, S. G. P., and Leeming, J. T., 1975a, The appearance of the small bowel mucosa in old age, *Age Ageing* **4:**168–174.

Webster, S. G. P., and Leeming, J. T., 1975b, Assessment of small bowel function in the elderly using a modified xylose tolerance test, *Gut* **16:**109–113.

Webster, S. G. P., Wilkinson, E. M., and Gowland, E., 1977, A comparison of fat absorption in young and old subjects, *Age Ageing* **6:**113–117.

Welsh, J. D., Russell, L. C., and Walker, A. W., Jr., 1974, Changes in intestinal lactase and alkaline phosphatase activity levels with age in the baboon (*Papio papio*), *Gastroenterology* **66:**993–997.

Welsh, J. D., Poley, J. R., Bhatia, M., and Stevenson, D. E., 1978, Intestinal disaccharidase activities in relation to age, race, and mucosal damage, *Gastroenterology* **75:**847–855.

Werner, I., and Hambraeus, L., 1972, The digestive capacity of elderly people, in: *Nutrition in Old Age* (L. A. Carlson, ed.), Almquist and Wiksell, Uppsala, pp. 55–60.

Yiengst, M. J., and Shock, N. W., 1949, Effect of oral administration of vitamin A and carotene in aged males, *J. Gerontol.* **4:**205–211.

4

Nutrition and Immune Function in the Elderly

Simin Nikbin Meydani and Jeffrey B. Blumberg

1. Introduction

There is a growing recognition that nutrition influences immune function not only in young populations with severe malnutrition and a high incidence of infectious disease but also in groups with relatively mild or single nutrient deficiencies (Chandra and Chandra, 1986; James and Makinodan, 1984). Several comprehensive reviews in this area have been published recently (Stinnett, 1983; Gershwin *et al.*, 1985; Fernandes, 1984; Beisel, 1982; Keusch *et al.*, 1983). The elderly represent a large and expanding group with a significant number of individuals noted to possess poor nutritional status in the face of potentially increasing nutrient requirements and decreasing immunocompetence. Thus, as malnutrition impairs immunity, nutritional problems may contribute to declining immunity in old age, and appropriate dietary intervention may improve immune responsiveness and reduce the burden of illness in the elderly. Recently, attention has been focused on the possibility of utilizing selective nutritional manipulations to regulate the aberrant response of diseases associated with immune disorders (Chandra, 1985; Corman, 1985).

Scrimshaw *et al.* (1959) and Scrimshaw (1964) were the first to review early scientific findings and present the concept of a synergistic interaction between nutrition and the immune response to infectious disease. This interaction is bidirectional: nutritional status influences host immunologic responsiveness, and infectious disease has a detrimental influence on the nutritional status. In an ecological milieu characterized by frequent illness and poor nutrition, the age-related decline in immune responsiveness may result in many of the chronic diseases associated with morbidity and mortality in the elderly. It also appears that conditions associated with chronic overnutrition, e.g., obesity, cardiovascular disease, and adult-onset diabetes, significantly modulate im-

Simin Nikbin Meydani and Jeffrey B. Blumberg • USDA Human Nutrition Research Center on Aging, Tufts University, Boston, Massachusetts 02111.

mune function; the diets employed to treat these afflictions may have a far-ranging influence on host defense against infectious challenge.

Little is known about the mechanisms by which nutritional factors affect immune function and the ontogeny of the immune response. However, the general nature of this influence has been shown to be both qualitative and quantitative, varying with the individual nutrients. Diet may act specifically on the lymphoid system and immune cell function or nonspecifically on associated factors. Nutrient availability could also impact on metabolic, neurological, or endocrine parameters that influence immunologic function. Further, essential nutrients are involved in the stability of the plasma membrane and the differentiation and expression of cell surface characteristics. Thus, nutritional factors could affect the development and maintenance of immunocompetence through multiple pathways.

As immunologic vigor decreases with age, the incidence among the elderly of infections, autoimmune and immune-complex diseases, and cancer increases. It is well established that food intake diminishes as adults age (Chapter 1, Fig. 8), causing reduced consumption of nutrients that may be critical to sustaining immune function. Malnutrition is a frequent concomitant among the elderly, caused partially by chronic disease and economic, psychosocial, dental, and drug-related problems. Nutritional status surveys of the elderly have shown a low to moderate prevalence of frank nutrient deficiencies and a markedly increased risk of deficiencies in both institutionalized and noninstitutionalized groups (McGandy *et al.*, 1986). Moreover, degenerative physiological changes during the aging process may give rise to altered nutrient requirements (Munro *et al.*, 1987). Age-associated changes in body composition, e.g., loss of lean body mass and bone density, and nutritional status, e.g., lower levels of plasma albumin and pyridoxal phosphate, further complicate clinical nutritional assessment of the elderly.

It is not yet established whether the slow progressive decline in immunity associated with aging results in part from nutritional deficiencies. Few studies have considered nutrition and immune function simultaneously in elderly subjects or senescent animal models. There is some indication of a causal relationship between undernutrition and impaired immunity in elderly subjects, but whether maintenance of good nutrition will assure immunologic vigor and prevent some of the diseases associated with aging is not known.

2. *Immunologic Effects of Aging*

Alterations in immune function with age have been well documented in humans and experimental models (Makinodan, 1976; Hausman and Weksler, 1985). Those components of the immune system discussed in this chapter are illustrated in Fig. 1. Such diverse defects as dysfunction of T and B lymphocytes, elevated levels of circulating immune complexes, an increase in autoantibodies, and monoclonal gammopathies have been described (DeKruyff *et al.*, 1980). Many of these changes in immune function have been correlated with involution of the thymus gland, which begins at puberty and is complete by middle age (Weksler, 1981). Several investigators have proposed immunologic theories of aging in which one or more deficits in immune

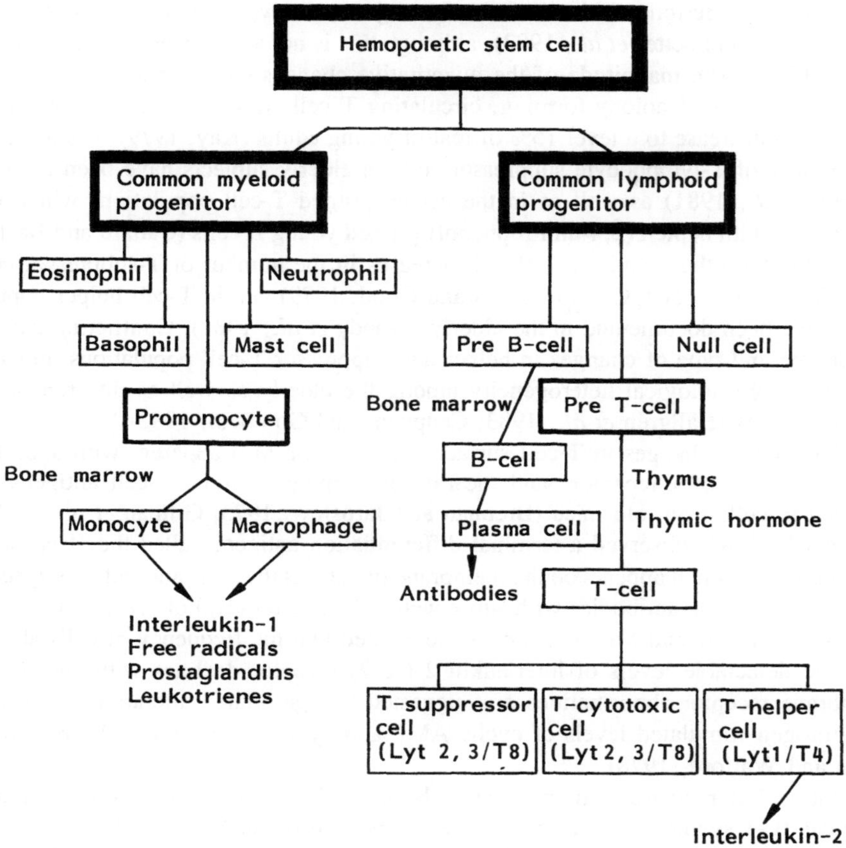

Fig. 1. Schematic presentation of immune system components. The immune system consists of several different cell types, each derived from hemopoietic stem cells. The stem cells give rise to two distinct progenitors, one for lymphoid cells and the other for myeloid cells. The lymphoid lineage produces lymphocytes, while the myeloid lineage yields phagocytes (polymorphonuclear granulocytes), mast cells, and platelets. The lymphocytes differentiate to either T cells or B cells depending on whether they home into thymus or fetal liver/bone marrow. T cells are further divided into suppressor, helper, or cytotoxic cells, each with distinct functions and cell surface markers. The null cells lack characteristics which correspond with either T or B cells, and their differentiation sequence is not clear.

function underlie the physiological changes of the aging process (Schofield and Davies, 1978; Weitekamp and Aber, 1984; Williams, 1980).

2.1. Cell-Mediated Immunity in Aging

Cell-mediated immunity is that specific immune response to antigens mediated by lymphocytes and macrophages with minor participation by other cell types. Cellular immunity is responsible for delayed cutaneous hypersensitivity (DCH), foreign graft rejection, resistance to many pathogenic microorganisms, and tumor immunosurveillance.

There is generally a decrease in the absolute number and percentage of total T lymphocytes in peripheral blood of elderly subjects relative to young adults (Nagel *et al.*, 1983; Rosenkoetter *et al.*, 1983), although this is not a consistent finding (Barrett *et al.*, 1980). The magnitude of the quantitative changes can be dramatic; e.g., the absolute number of colony-forming, circulating T cells in elderly subjects has been reported to decrease to a level 15% of that of young adults (Kay, 1979). Decreases in the number of T-lymphocyte suppressor cells in elderly subjects have been reported (Nagel *et al.*, 1981) as well as in the carrier-primed T-cell population, which can collaborate with hapten (2,4-dinitrophenol)-primed young B cells (Callard and Basten, 1978). On the other hand, age-related increases in the number of T-suppressor cells with Fc receptors for IgG (T_γ) (Gupta and Good, 1979) and in T-cell helper populations have been documented in the elderly (Moody *et al.*, 1981). Conflicting data on the degree and type of changes in helper and suppressor T-cell populations probably reflect the physiological heterogeneity among the elderly as well as different assay methodologies (Hallgren *et al.*, 1983; Ceuppens and Goodwin, 1982).

Qualitative changes in T-cell surface receptors are also apparent with age. The surface density of τ receptors and the rate of capping of some T-cell antigens are reduced in cells from old mice (Brennan and Jaroslow, 1975; Gilman *et al.*, 1981). Kay *et al.* (1983) observed a terminal differentiation antigen, called the "senescent cell antigen," which appears on the membrane of cells as they age and initiates specific binding of IgG autoantibodies with subsequent selective removal of senescent cells by macrophages. Vie and Miller (1986) demonstrated that the frequency of cells able to generate detectable levels of interleukin 2 (IL-2) receptor declines with age. Other membrane receptor abnormalities are suggested by age-related alterations in resting and mitogen-stimulated levels of cyclic AMP and cyclic GMP in T cells from mice (Tam and Walford, 1978).

Intracellular changes in immune cells have also been detected during aging. Whereas IL-1 synthesis and responsiveness appear to be unaltered or decreased with age, defects in the synthesis and utilization of IL-2 have been reported in aged rodents (Thoman and Weigle, 1982; Meydani *et al.*, 1986a; Chang *et al.*, 1982). The IL-2 synthetic defect is stimulus dependent, but the deficient IL-2 responsiveness is independent of the type of stimulus and the amount of exogenous IL-2, suggesting that IL-2 receptor generation does not proceed normally in activated T cells. Similar IL-2 defects have been reported in humans (Joncourt *et al.*, 1982). Morphologically, swollen mitochondria containing myelinlike structures with reduced numbers of cristae in sheep red blood cell (SRBC)-rosetting T cells of old but not young humans have been noted.

In general, there is a functional deficit in T-cell-dependent cell-mediated responses with age. Most, but not all, investigators have reported diminished DCH reactions in the elderly (Delafuente *et al.*, 1983; Dworsky *et al.*, 1983; Knicker *et al.*, 1984). Negative DCH in the elderly, however, may result from lack of recent antigen exposure and not necessarily a state of anergy; repeated testing of negative test subjects frequently converts them to positive through an enhanced antigen sensitivity (Delafuente *et al.*, 1983; Keystone *et al.*, 1980). The DCH correlates well with *in vitro* lymphocyte proliferation assays (Delafuente *et al.*, 1981). *In vitro*, an impaired proliferative capacity of T cells is observed in elderly humans and senescent rodents in response to mitogens such as phytohemagglutinin (PHA) and concanavalin A (Con A), antigens such as *Mycobacterium tuberculosis* and varicella virus, and allogeneic target cells (Miller, 1980; Licastro *et al.*, 1983; Bach, 1979; Abraham *et al.*, 1977). Interestingly, lymphocytes from elderly subjects appear to require more calcium to restore their proliferative response after inhibition and are more sensitive to chelating agents (Kennes *et al.*, 1981). Segal (1986) demonstrated that the age-related decline in the responsiveness of rat thymocytes to Con A was caused in part by decreased cellular stimulation by calcium and sugar uptake. The autologous mixed lymphocyte reaction of T cells to autologous non-T mononuclear cells also decreases with age in humans (Fernandez and Macsween, 1980).

T-cell suppressor function is not well defined, and both age-related increases and decreases in Con-A-stimulated suppressor activity have been reported (Hallgren and Yunis, 1977; Antel *et al.*, 1978). Other studies reveal that most healthy aged subjects maintain their ability to generate suppressor activity in autologous suppressor cell assays but not in tests with allogeneic cells (Schulof *et al.*, 1980; Barrett *et al.*, 1980). Blunted autologous mixed lymphocyte reactions noted in some elderly subjects have been associated with an inability of old lymphocytes to express HLA-Dr (Ia) cell surface antigens properly (Indiveri *et al.*, 1983).

Age-related immunologic declines have been ascribed to diminished helper T-lymphocyte function (Krogsrud and Perkins, 1977; Price and Makinodan, 1972a), but others report no alterations (Barrett *et al.*, 1980; Delfraissy *et al.*, 1982). Miller (1983), using a limited dilution assay, found a significant decrease in precursor frequencies of helper and cytolytic T cells with age. On the other hand, more helper T cells are generated during *in vitro* mitogen stimulation in elderly than young subjects (Otte *et al.*, 1983), and when suppressor cells are removed, aged helper T cells produce more activity than younger ones. Ceuppens and Goodwin (1982) suggest that this age-related increase in helper T-cell responsiveness may be a compensatory mechanism for maintaining an adequate immune status.

2.2. Humoral Immunity in Aging

The humoral immune system primarily involves plasma cell production of immunoglobulins. In general, there are fewer and less marked changes in humoral immunity than in cellular immunity with age. However, abnormal regulation of antibody production is a common finding in the elderly as evidenced by a high incidence of autoantibody production, decreased ability to produce antibodies to antigens, and the occurrence of benign monoclonal gammopathies.

The total number of circulating B cells in human populations has been observed to remain relatively constant (Becker *et al.*, 1979) or to decrease with age (Cobleigh *et al.*, 1980). The number of colony-forming B cells in peripheral blood of human subjects decreases with age (Kay, 1979). The number of B cells in the spleen and lymph nodes has been reported to increase in several mouse strains (Kay *et al.*, 1979). In long-lived mouse strains, however, these tissues show a decrease in B cells that is offset by a proportional increase in bone marrow B cells (Haaijman and Hijmans, 1978). Indirect observations suggest that the sizes of B-cell subpopulations change with age. Several human studies reveal that serum and cerebrospinal fluid IgG and IgA and benign monoclonal gammopathies increase with age (Radl *et al.*, 1975; Nerenberg and Prasad, 1975). During aging in mice, decreases in the number of B cells responsive to certain antigens (Price and Makinodan, 1972b), increases in IgG_1 and IgG_2 levels (Haaijman *et al.*, 1977), and decreases in IgM levels (Radl *et al.*, 1975) have been reported.

In rodents, indices of B-cell function such as mitogenic response of lymph node and spleen cells to T-independent antigens such as type 3 II pneumococcal polysaccharide and lipopolysaccharide have been variously reported to change or remain constant with age depending on the species, strain, or hybrid tested (Kay *et al.*, 1979). It has been demonstrated that recruitment of active B cells from old mice in a primary antibody response by allogeneically stimulated T cells is not as effective as recruitment in young mice (Popp and Francis, 1979). Senescent B cells lose their ability to function and respond normally in some tests; e.g., given the same amount of helper stimulus (pokeweed mitogen), isolated B cells from elderly subjects produce less antibody than those from young adults (Ceuppens and Goodwin, 1982). The antibody response to foreign antigens such as parainfluenza virus vaccine and tetanus toxoid is lower in elderly than in younger subjects (Kishimoto *et al.*, 1980). Although high levels of antibodies are not necessarily an indicator of good health, sex differences among the elderly appear to persist in response to multivalent pneumococcal vaccine, with women having lower antibody levels than men (Roghmann *et al.*, 1987). Conversely, autoantibody production is greater in the elderly, accounting for the high prevalence of false-positive serological tests among this population (Hallgren *et al.*, 1973). It has been suggested that in the elderly there is an increased activity of suppressor T cells regulating antibody production to foreign antigens with a concomitant decreased activity of a suppressor T-cell subpopulation regulating autoantibody production (Weksler, 1981). Thus, defects in immunoglobulin production reflect disorders in both immunoregulatory T and B lymphocytes.

2.3. *Other Aspects of Immunoregulation of the Elderly*

The number of pluripotent stem cells decreases slightly in some senescent mouse strains, but several of their functions decline more markedly with age, e.g., their ability to expand clonally, repair x-ray-induced damage, and home into the thymus and their rate of division and B-cell formation (Kay, 1985). Further, kinetic limitations on stem-cell reserves in elderly subjects may contribute to age-related immunodeficiencies such as the absence of elevated white cell counts in some geriatric patients with sepsis. No differences in neutrophil function or chemotaxis have been observed between young and old adults (Kessler, 1979). Null cells tend to increase with age (Twomey *et al.*, 1982). The ability to generate cytotoxic T lymphocytes and natural killer cells diminishes with age in animal models (Effros and Walford, 1983), but conflicting data have been reported in humans (Fernandes and Gupta, 1981; Penschow and Mackay, 1980).

The ability of macrophages to process antigens, phagocytose and destroy infectious agents, or support proliferation of lymphocytes does not appear to change significantly in the elderly (Gardner *et al.*, 1981; Weksler, 1983). However, Chang *et al.* (1982) showed that changes in both murine macrophages and T lymphocytes were responsible for decreased IL-2 production. Rosenberg *et al.* (1983) demonstrated that cell–cell interaction and cooperation via lymphokine and other regulatory molecules are impaired in aged mice and that increased macrophage numbers in aged rat spleen might have a suppressive effect. Chang *et al.* (1982) also showed that macrophages from old mice decreased IL-2 production by spleen nonadherent cells (NAC) from young mice and that culturing NAC from old mice with macrophages from young mice improved lymphocyte proliferation and IL-2 production. Bash (1983) showed that macrophages from young rats in numbers up to 5% of NAC cells enhanced lymphocyte proliferation and IL-2 formation, whereas macrophages from old rats caused profound suppression at 2.5% or above; the number of macrophages in spleen increased threefold during aging. However, profound differences in the regulatory capacity of macrophages from young and old animals were observed despite an equal number of macrophages.

The suppressive effect of macrophages from aged mice has been attributed to either a decrease in IL-1 production (Chang *et al.*, 1982) or an increase in suppressive factors. Increased prostaglandin E_2 (PGE_2) production by macrophages from aged rats (Bash, 1983) and mice (Bartocci *et al.*, 1982) has been reported. Furthermore, Rosenstein and Strauser (1980) were able to achieve substantial enhancement of aged spleen cell responsiveness *in vitro* and *in vivo* with indomethacin, a cyclooxygenase inhibitor. Bartocci *et al.* (1982) also showed that decreasing macrophage PGE_2 production with aspirin results in enhanced tumor rejection in aged mice. Splenocytes from aged mice synthesize more PGE_2 and accumulate less IL-2 in Con-A-stimulated cultures than do those from young mice (Meydani *et al.*, 1986a).

Although there is now abundant evidence confirming a decline in immunologic responsiveness with advancing age, the molecular mechanisms underlying these changes remain to be elucidated. The involution of the thymus, occurring during sexual maturity, precedes and may be responsible for the age-related decline in T-cell-dependent immune responses. However, the complex interactions among immune, neuroendocrine, and other systems make identification of the key events, and those susceptible to nutritional modulation, in immunosenescence difficult.

3. Nutritional Manipulation of the Aging Immune System

The importance of nutritional deficiencies in the maintenance of the immune system in young and adult animals and humans is widely recognized. However, very few studies have been conducted to examine the possible beneficial or adverse effects of nutrient supplementation on the immune responsiveness of the elderly. Those studies that have directly addressed these issues in senescent animal models or in humans are reviewed here. It will be readily noted that only a few nutrients have received such attention. The role of nutritional factors in the immune response of specially bred short-lived autoimmune-prone mice is not addressed below, as several recent reviews have covered this aspect of the topic (e.g., Good and Gajjar, 1986).

3.1. Malnutrition

In animal models, food restriction enhances immune responsiveness (Chapter 2), although in man malnutrition, and especially protein–energy malnutrition (PEM), is associated with a compromised immune function. Anergy to a battery of antigens used in DCH has been shown to occur with development of PEM and to resolve when the patients were treated (Smythe *et al.*, 1971; Moldawer *et al.*, 1979). Deficiencies in secretory IgA, complement, and phagocytic activity have been reported in PEM (McMurray *et al.*, 1977; Keusch *et al.*, 1983). Human subjects with PEM were found to have decreased lymphocyte proliferation to PHA (Chandra, 1972). The immunologic changes occurring in both humans and animals have been reviewed by Keusch *et al.* (1983).

Many elderly are at high risk of malnutrition because of their limited income, food preference, and overall health status resulting from chronic disease. Linn and Jensen (1984) studied the prevalence of malnutrition in young (<65) and old (>65) outpatients in an ambulatory care unit excluding those with infection, autoimmune diseases, and major medical diseases. Malnutrition was more prevalent in the older than in the younger group. Malnourished subjects in both age groups had less lymphocyte response to allogeneic cells and to PHA but greater response to pokeweed mitogen (PWM) and higher IgA levels. Polymorphonuclear cells (PMN) from malnourished elderly patients had lower stimulated chemotaxis than those from well-nourished individuals as assessed by migration of neutrophils through a Boyden chamber with or without zymosan-activated serum.

Chandra and Puri (1985) showed that nutritional supplementation of 30 malnourished elderly men aged 70–84 improved their antibody response to influenza vaccine. Hamm *et al.* (1985) examined the effect of protein level (6% versus 25%) in the diet on Fc and C3b receptor-mediated phagocytosis of elicited peritoneal macrophages of young (6 months) and old (24 months) C57BL/6Nia mice. They found that Fc receptor-mediated phagocytosis was depressed after 5 weeks of feeding a 6% protein diet in 24-month-old mice but not in 6-month-old animals. Furthermore, old mice fed the 25% protein diet had augmented C3b receptor-mediated phagocytosis. These effects were not explained by changes in membrane fluidity.

The respiratory burst activity of neutrophils, as well as the level of the various neutrophil enzymes secreted during degranulation, from elderly individuals is decreased in response to a wide variety of stimuli (McLaughlin *et al.*, 1986; Nagel *et al.*, 1982; Suzuki *et al.*, 1982). These changes in function were not sufficient to cause a measurable decrease in the ability of neutrophils from the elderly subjects to phagocytize or kill bacteria. Nonetheless, infections are more common among the elderly, especially when they are malnourished (Gladstone and Recco, 1976). Lipschitz and Udupa (1986) examined the combined effect of aging and protein deficiency on neutrophil function in mice. Six-month- or 24- to 26-month-old C57BL/6Nia mice were fed isocaloric diets containing 2% or 20% casein for 3 weeks. The old mice fed the 20% protein diet had significantly less PMA-induced superoxide generation than young mice fed the same diet. Neutrophils from both young and old mice fed the 2% protein diet produced less O_2 than those from mice fed the 20% protein diet. Neutrophils from old mice also had significantly lower base-line and PMA-stimulated lysozyme, myeloperoxidase, and glucuronidase levels than those from young mice. Lower levels of these enzymes were detected in the mice fed the 2% protein diet compared to those fed the 20% protein diet. There was no difference between young and old mice fed the 20% protein diet in their phagocytic or bacteriocidal activity.

However, neutrophils from young mice fed the 2% protein diet killed a higher percentage of the ingested bacteria than those from old mice fed the same diet. Thus, although neutrophil activity is compromised by aging, in the absence of additional environmental stress such as protein deficiency, these changes do not necessarily affect their functional capacity. These studies emphasize the importance of protein–calorie malnutrition on changes in host-defense mechanisms in the elderly.

3.2. Food Restriction

As discussed in Chapter 2, food restriction without malnutrition, initiated at weaning or even by midadulthood and maintained until death, increases mean and maximal life spans in rodents and several other species (Yu *et al.*, 1982; Cheney *et al.*, 1980; Weindruch and Walford, 1982). This extension of maximal survivorship by reducing the total input of calories or nutrient per animal appears to involve an unidentified interaction with mechanisms basic to the aging process (Chapter 2). Food restriction has thus far proven to be the most potent and consistent intervention in experimental animals to prolong life expectancy and life span and to reduce the incidence and delay the onset of age-related loss of organ function and diseases including spontaneous cancers. Underfeeding protocols also profoundly influence age-sensitive immunologic indices.

The early food restriction studies of Jose and Good (1971, 1973) showed that cellular and particularly humoral immune responses to malignant tumors in allogeneic, syngeneic, and autochthonous murine systems were adversely affected. However, these adverse effects were largely on the primary immune response and could be overcome by repeated exposure to antigenic challenge, i.e., by the tertiary immune response. Inhibition of the tumor growth appeared to occur through an immune-mediated phenomenon rather than simply a slowdown of tumor growth from lack of essential nutrients. Caloric restriction is also effective in preventing the development of spontaneous mammary adenocarcinoma in mice (Fernandes *et al.*, 1976); along with the diminished incidence of cancer was an enhanced responsiveness to T-lymphocyte mitogens and a depressed plaque-forming cell (PFC) response to SRBC administration in the low-calorie mice. These mice also exhibited increased lytic activity, suggesting that increased suppressor cell activity may be an underlying mechanism in reducing the incidence of adenocarcinoma among mice fed the low-calorie diet. Endocrine hypofunction may contribute to such altered immune parameters. Coincident with the preservation of immune function with dietary restriction is the decrease in spontaneous tumors observed in strains of mice subject to autoimmune disease, e.g., New Zealand and MRL/1 mice (Beach *et al.*, 1982; Fernandes *et al.*, 1978).

When otherwise adequate diets containing 60% of the total energy found in control diets are fed just prior to or after weaning, PFC responsiveness, T- and B-cell mitogen-stimulated lymphocyte proliferation, and rates of skin allograft rejection are compromised in young and early adult mice (Walford *et al.*, 1973; Gebrase-DeLima *et al.*, 1975). However, at later stages of life (>22 months), calorically restricted animals showed significantly enhanced immune responsiveness relative to the well-fed mice. Although the older restricted mice possess fewer nucleated cells per spleen, their proliferative response is generally increased at both optimal and lower cell densities

(Weindruch *et al.*, 1982a). An increase in splenic T-cell PHA responsiveness from dietary restriction has been partially attributed to an increased proportion of T cells that are responsive to this mitogen (Weindruch *et al.*, 1982b). This effect of dietary restriction is consistent with an increasing proportion of the less mature, PHA-sensitive Lyt-$1^+2^+3^+$ lymphocytes relative to Con-A-responsive Lyt-$1^+2^-3^-$ lymphocytes (Nakayama *et al.*, 1980; Ledbetter *et al.*, 1980). On the other hand, dietary restriction has also been associated with a reversal of the age-associated decrease in thymic cortex : medulla ratios and T-cell migration from the thymus (Walford *et al.*, 1981); these changes are correlated with elevated lymphocyte blast transformation in response to both PHA and Con A (Weindruch *et al.*, 1979; Weindruch and Suffin, 1980). Therefore, increased proportions of Lyt-$1^+2^-3^-$ cells, as reflected by elevated Con A responsiveness, could also result from dietary restriction in some mouse strains (Weindruch *et al.*, 1979). Thus, the ultimate enhancement of immunologic function by dietary restriction in aged mice may be mediated in part by alterations in specific T-cell subpopulations, rates of thymocyte death, or alterations in lymphocyte migratory behavior.

There is an age-related decline in basal natural killer (NK) cell activity with age in mice that is accentuated by dietary restriction (Weindruch *et al.*, 1983). However, NK cells of old restricted mice respond more vigorously than those of controls to the potentiating stimulus of polyinosinic : polycytidylic acid. Further, the decline of cytotoxic T-lymphocyte generation is less marked in restricted mice. Weindruch *et al.* (1983) suggest that restricted mice have a higher resistance to tumorigenic influences because of the accentuated responsiveness of NK cells to induction signals and the more efficient cytotoxic T lymphocytes.

Graded variations of the caloric content and source fed to laboratory animals have not been extensively examined. In general, when mice were fed diets ranging from 25% to 65% caloric restriction, there was a dose-dependent effect with an increasingly beneficial influences on PHA and Con-A-induced splenic lymphocyte proliferation in adult and old subjects; responses to purified protein derivative (PPD) were not influenced by aging or diet (Weindruch *et al.*, 1986). When variations of calorie sources have been compared, e.g., sucrose–glycerol versus lard as the source of nonprotein calories, results suggested that caloric intake and not source of calories is the most critical dietary variable for most immune function parameters. For example, parameters noted to be affected strictly by restricted caloric intake included decreased circulating immune complexes, decreased production of anti-DNA antibodies, increased thymocyte proliferation in response to exogenous IL-2, increased Con-A-stimulated IL-2 production, and increased mixed lymphocyte reaction of spleen cells (Kubo *et al.*, 1984). Two *in vitro* parameters affected by both caloric restriction and high sucrose content were response to SRBC and cytotoxic cell-mediated immune response to allogeneic antigen. Furthermore, Kubo *et al.* (1987) found that the source of nonprotein energy influences longevity in food-restricted (NZB $\times$ NZW)F_1 mice such that longer life spans were seen when the nonprotein energy source was carbohydrate than when it was fat.

There are no controlled clinical correlates of caloric restriction without malnutrition. A series of experiments employing acute total energy deprivation (for 10 days in adult subjects who used fasting as part of their pattern of behavior) found decreases in some acute-phase reactants, an increase in IgM antibodies, decreases in PWM and PPD mitogen stimulation of peripheral lymphocytes, and a depression of *in vitro* neutrophil bactericidal capacity; most other immune parameters remained unchanged (Palmblad, 1976; Palmblad *et al.*, 1977).

The impact of self-induced semistarvation (anorexia nervosa) on immunocompetence has been investigated (Dowd and Eckert, 1984). Aberrant immunohematological parameters are common in anorexia nervosa, including leukopenia, lymphocytosis, neutropenia, and thrombocytopenia (Bowers and Eckert, 1978). However, despite their altered immunologic status, patients with anorexia nervosa seldom exhibit a marked increase in infectious disease. Both humoral and cell-mediated immune functions in these patients appears within normal ranges and, under some conditions (particularly by when body weight remains above 60% of ideal body weight), may actually be enhanced (Bowers and Eckert, 1978; Golla *et al.*, 1981). Murray and Murray (1981) have proposed that immunologic mechanisms adjust quite well to starvation and that during periods of famine, disease may be significantly curtailed. They suggest that decreased food intake may alter hormone levels and other mediators to slow the rate of cell growth of both host tissues and the infectious and malignant pathogenic influences on those cells. However, most such information regarding human populations consuming limited amounts of food is not relevant to the antiaging effect of calorie restriction, as these groups suffer from malnutrition and poor environmental conditions. It is of interest though to note that a greater concentration of centenarians survive in Okinawa than in the rest of Japan. Okinawans are reported to have a lower intake of energy and sugar and a higher intake of green–yellow vegetables and meat than the average Japanese (Kagawa, 1978); however, since other genetic and environmental differences exist between these populations, diet may not be the only factor responsible for the longevity of the Okinawans.

3.3. Vitamin C

The low intake and poor nutritional status of vitamin C among the elderly in Great Britain have been suggested as a significant contributory factor to the group's high disease prevalence (Kataria *et al.*, 1965; Taylor, 1966). Burr *et al.* (1974) studied residents over 65 years of age in a British village and found that women had higher plasma and leukocyte ascorbate content than men and that subjects over 75 years of age, regardless of sex, had significantly lower plasma and leukocyte vitamin C levels. Furthermore, these values declined with increasing age. The lower plasma and leukocyte levels appeared to be caused by a lower dietary intake of ascorbate since there was a significant correlation between frequency of fruit and green vegetable consumption and plasma and leukocyte ascorbate concentration.

Several studies have indicated that a low vitamin C intake (Hodkinson and Exton-Smith, 1976) or blood level (Wilson *et al.*, 1972, 1973) is associated with increased risk of death. However, in two randomized controlled trials, vitamin C supplementation of elderly people with low blood ascorbate levels did not decrease the mortality rate (Wilson *et al.*, 1973; Burr *et al.*, 1975). The failure of supplementation trials to show any beneficial effect may be because irreversible damage had occurred as a result of a longstanding vitamin C deficiency, and supplementation should have started earlier in life. On the other hand, low vitamin C status may have occurred as a consequence of poor health, which ultimately caused death.

More direct evidence for a beneficial effect of vitamin C has been obtained by studying the effect of vitamin C supplementation on the immune response of elderly individuals. Kennes *et al.* (1983) examined the effect of intramuscular injections of vitamin C (500 mg/day for 1 month) on proliferative response of lymphocytes to PHA and Con A and DCH response to tuberculin in 20 elderly subjects over the age of 70. A significant increase in [^{3}H]thymidine incorporation stimulated by PHA and Con A was observed after 30 days of supplementation. Vitamin-C-supplemented subjects also had an increase in the mean DCH induration diameter to tuberculin relative to placebo-treated subjects. As vitamin C status was not determined, it is not clear whether the observed improvement was caused by correction of a vitamin C deficiency state or by a direct immunostimulatory action of injected vitamin C. An immunostimulatory effect of vitamin C has been claimed in young people with presumably normal vitamin C levels (Anderson *et al.*, 1980).

The mechanism of the immunostimulatory effect of vitamin C is not known. However, the serum level of lipid peroxides rises in healthy subjects with increasing age (Satoh, 1978; Svematsu *et al.*, 1977), suggesting that the immunostimulatory effect of vitamin C might be mediated through its antioxidant function. The concentration of certain antioxidants such as vitamin C, selenium, and superoxide dismutase decreases with advancing age (Leibovitz and Siegel, 1980). Supplementation of elderly women with vitamin C or vitamin E for 12 months decreased serum peroxide levels by 13% and 26%, respectively (Wartanowicz *et al.*, 1984). On the other hand vitamin C has been reported to increase *in vivo* generation of cyclic GMP (Atkinson *et al.*, 1978), a signal for cell commitment into S phase (Katz *et al.*, 1978).

Delafuente *et al.* (1986) studied a group of elderly patients over 65 years with chronic cardiovascular diseases receiving a variety of medications and examined the effect of *in vitro* and *in vivo* supplementation of vitamin C on lymphocyte proliferation and DCH to *Candida albicans* and mumps skin test antigen. They found that although *in vitro* addition of vitamin C to lymphocytes from elderly subjects increased their Con-A-stimulated proliferation to levels comparable to those of young subjects, *in vivo* supplementation with 2 g/day vitamin C for 3 weeks did not significantly affect mitogenic responses or reverse anergy. These *in vivo* results are in contrast to those of Kennes *et al.* (1983) described above who employed healthy elderly subjects receiving 500 mg/day of vitamin C intramuscularly with no other medication and found improvement in the immunologic parameters measured following supplementation. Unfortunately, plasma or white blood cell vitamin C levels were not measured in these studies.

Ziemlanski *et al.* (1986) found significantly increased serum IgG, IgM, and complement C3 levels in 158 women over 78 years old receiving 400 mg ascrobic acid supplements. Goodwin and Garry (1983) found that the healthy elderly subjects within the top 10% for plasma vitamin C concentration had significantly fewer anergic subjects in response to four different antigens and higher mean DCH scores. However, no difference in mitogenic response to PHA was observed between those with high and low vitamin C status.

In summary, lower plasma and leukocyte levels of vitamin C and age-related increases in serum lipid peroxides have been reported in the elderly. Compromised vitamin C status appears to contribute to the decreased immune responsiveness observed in the elderly, although conflicting reports on the beneficial effects of high-dose supplementation with this vitamin make unequivocal recommendations impossible.

3.4. Vitamin E

Vitamin E is involved in normal immune function. Tengerdy and Brown (1977) first reported that chickens given 100 mg/kg vitamin E had significantly increased generation of anti-SRBC PFC. Mice fed 60–100 mg/kg of vitamin E had significantly increased humoral immune responses as measured by PFC and antibody responses to SRBC and tetanus toxoid (Tengerdy, 1980). Vitamin E deficiency decreased the PFC response to SRBC in mice, an effect restored to normal by vitamin E but not by the antioxidant N,N-diphenyl-*p*-phenylenediamine (Tengerdy, 1980). Corwin and Shloss (1980a,b) found that vitamin E and 2-mercaptoethanolamine were both mitogenic. Vitamin E supplementation in mice enhanced the proliferative response of lymphocytes to suboptimal doses of Con A. Pigs supplemented with vitamin E showed enhanced proliferation of the peripheral blastogenic response of lymphocytes to PHA (Larsen and Tollersrud, 1981). Vitamin E deficiency in dogs decreased the blastogenic response to Con A attributable to a serum factor that could be washed from the cell surface of depressed lymphocytes (Tanka *et al.*, 1979). In mice, dietary vitamin E was shown to enhance helper T-cell activity. Bendich *et al.* (1983) reported that low splenic vitamin E levels in spontaneously hypertensive rats (SHR) were correlated with depressed splenic mitogen responses; tocopherol supplementation enhanced immune responsiveness in SHR and normotensive rats. Bendich *et al.* (1986) later demonstrated that 15 mg/kg diet per day of vitamin E was adequate to prevent myopathy in SHR rats, but optimal lymphocyte proliferation to PHA and Con A was obtained only at vitamin E levels of 50 mg/kg diet per day. These studies indicate that the dietary tocopherol requirement for maintenance of optimal immune responsiveness may be higher than the levels recommended for normal growth and reproduction.

The mechanism of the immunostimulatory effect of vitamin E is not understood. Vitamin E may exert its effect by inhibiting prostaglandin synthesis and/or decreasing free radical formation. Vitamin E can affect the lipoxygenase and cyclooxygenase pathways of arachidonic acid metabolism. One of the biological changes associated with aging is increased free radical formation with subsequent damage to cellular processes. Numerous studies have expounded on the free radical theory of aging and the role of antioxidants, including vitamin E, on the life expectancy of rodents (reviewed by Blumberg and Meydani, 1986). Oxygen metabolites, especially H_2O_2, produced by activated macrophages, depress lymphocyte proliferation. Free radical formation associated with aging may be an underlying factor in the depressed immune response observed in aged rodents. Tocopherol has been shown to decrease H_2O_2 formation by polymorphonuclear cells.

Garry *et al.* (1982), in assessing the nutritional status of a healthy elderly population, found that 25% consumed less than 50% of the RDA for tocopherol, although most other reports do not indicate inadequate intake or status of vitamin E among the elderly (Leichter *et al.*, 1978). Several studies have demonstrated an age-related increase in total serum tocopherol through middle age (Chen *et al.*, 1977; Wei Wo and Draper, 1975; Kelleher and Losowsky, 1978) followed by a decline after age 65 (Wei Wo and Draper, 1975; Barnes and Chen, 1981), which probably reflects similar changes in plasma lipid profiles (Horowitt *et al.*, 1972). Although Vatassery *et al.* (1983) found that platelet vitamin E concentrations decline with age, Underwood *et al.* (1970) found no age-related change in liver tocopherol concentrations of people who died accidentally. Meydani *et al.* (1986) observed in rats that cerebellum and brainstem show selective decreases in tocopherol content with age. Lower serum tocopherol levels have been found in aged relative to young mice (Meydani *et al.*, 1986a).

It has been suggested by Harman (1982) that vitamin E and other antioxidants may increase longevity by influencing the immune system and reducing age-related diseases. An immunologic basis for many of the age-associated diseases such as amyloidosis, atherosclerosis, and cancer has been proposed by Walford (1982). An increase in average life span of short-lived autoimmune-prone NZB/NZW mice receiving vitamin E supplements was reported by Harman (1980). Furthermore, Meydani *et al.* (1986a) found 500 ppm dietary vitamin E supplementation of 24-month-old C57BL/6j mice for 6 weeks significantly increased splenocyte proliferation to Con A and lipopolysaccharide but not to PHA relative to control animals fed 30 ppm of the vitamin. In addition, vitamin E supplementation significantly increased DCH to 2,4-dinitro-7-fluorobenzene. This immunostimulatory effect of vitamin E was associated with an increased production of IL-2 and a decreased production of PGE_2 (Table I). No stimulatory effect of vitamin E was noted on NK-mediated cytotoxicity of old C57BL/6Nia mice. However, if the mice were immunized with SRBC prior to assessment, the supplemented mice had higher NK-mediated cytotoxicity than nonsupplemented mice receiving the standard 30-ppm dietary level of vitamin E (Meydani *et al.*, 1988). Interestingly, pathological examination of these mice revealed that 40% of old mice fed 30 ppm vitamin E had kidney amyloidosis, a common age-related pathological feature, whereas none of the old mice fed 500 ppm vitamin E had such amyloid deposits (Meydani *et al.*, 1986b).

Regarding clinical evidence, Goodwin and Garry (1983) in their study of elderly subjects consuming megadoses of vitamin supplements did not see any correlation between vitamin E intake and tests of lymphocyte proliferation and DCH. However, the study was complicated by the fact that several vitamin supplements were used by each subject and the interaction between different nutrients present confounding variables. Harman and Miller (1986) supplemented 103 patients from a chronic care facility with 200 or 400 mg/day α-tocopherol acetate but did not see any beneficial effect on antibody development against influenza virus vaccine. Unfortunately, data on the health status, medication use, antibody levels, and other relevant parameters were not reported. Chavance *et al.* (1985) conducted an epidemiologic survey on the relationship between nutritional and immunologic status in healthy French subjects over 60 years of age. They reported that plasma vitamin E levels were positively correlated with the number of positive DCH responses to diphtheria toxoid, *Candida*, and trichophyton. In men only, positive correlations were also observed between vitamin E levels and the number of positive DCH responses. Subjects with tocopherol levels greater than 135 mg/liter were found to have higher helper–inducer/cytotoxic–suppressor ratios. Blood vitamin E concentrations were negatively correlated with the number of infectious disease episodes in the three preceding years.

Table I. Effects of Vitamin E on Immune Responsiveness of 24-Month-Old Mice[a]

Parameters	Control	Dietary vitamin E[b] 30 ppm	500 ppm
Serum α-tocopherol	236 ± 3 μg/dl	71	194*
Delayed hypersensitivity	59.9 ± 13.8%	36*	75
T-cell lymphocyte proliferation	119,611 ± 35,491 cpm	5*	38
B-cell lymphocyte proliferation	25,074 ± 5,149 cpm	24*	85
Ex vivo splenic PGE_2 synthesis	2.60 ± 0.08 μg/g	123*	89
Interleukin 2	27 ± 4 unit/ml	44*	85

[a]Data adapted from Meydani *et al.* (1986a).
[b]All values expressed as percentage of 3-month-old control group (fed 30 ppm vitamin E). *, significantly different from control and other experimental group, $P \leq 0.05$.

Studies on the effect of vitamin E on immune function thus provide encouraging evidence that dietary tocopherol supplementation might be beneficial in enhancing the immune response in aged animal models and the elderly. However, well-controlled and long-term human studies that could provide less equivocal data are still lacking. Further research is also required to clarify the mechanism of the immunostimulatory effect of tocopherol.

3.5. Vitamin B_6

Humoral and cell-mediated immunity are affected by vitamin B_6 deficiency states. Vitamin-B_6-deficient animals have reduced DCH and antibody-forming cells (Axelrod, 1971), prolonged skin allograft survival time and diminished mitogen-induced lymphocyte proliferation (Robson and Schwarz, 1975). Inadequate vitamin B_6 intakes among the elderly and age-related declines in fasting plasma and serum pyridoxal phosphate levels and other indices of vitamin B_6 nutriture have been reported (Garry *et al.*, 1982; Rose *et al.*, 1976). In adults depleted of vitamin B_6, antibody production is decreased, and lymphocytopenia is produced (Hodges *et al.*, 1962; Cheslock and McCully, 1960). Talbott *et al.* (1987) examined the effect of 50 mg/day vitamin B_6 supplementation for 2 months on lymphocyte responsiveness of a group of 11 healthy individuals over 65 years of age. The vitamin-B_6-supplemented group showed a significant increase in lymphocyte proliferation in response to PHA, pokeweed mitogen, and *Staphylococcus aureus* (Cowain I) relative to a placebo control group of four elderly subjects. Percentages of helper but not suppressor cytotoxic T cells increased significantly in the pyridoxine-treated subjects. The supplementation was more effective in those subjects with the lowest initial plasma pyridoxal phosphate levels, indicating that low vitamin B_6 contributes to impaired immunocompetence in the elderly.

3.6. Glutathione

Glutathione (GSH) is the most abundant low-molecular-weight thiol-containing compound in living cells. In its reduced form, GSH protects cells against various oxidants, free radicals, and cytotoxic agents (Sies and Wendell, 1978). Furthermore, it maintains a variety of cellular molecules in their functionally active form (Flohe and Gunzler, 1976). Recent studies indicate that GSH plays a role in lymphocyte activation. The depletion of GSH lowers mitogenic response, and the addition of this tripeptide into culture medium reverses this effect (Noelle and Lawrence, 1981; Gougerst-Poidals *et al.*, 1985). Decreased GSH levels as a function of age have been reported to occur in liver, kidney, heart, and blood of mice and have been suggested to be responsible for progression of the aging process (Hazelton and Lang, 1980; Abraham *et al.*, 1978).

Furukawa *et al.* (1987) showed that 0.1% to 1.0% dietary GSH supplementation of a semipurified, nutritionally adequate diet significantly increased mitogenic response of aged mice to Con A and enhanced their *in vivo* T-cell-mediated immune response as measured by DCH compared to that of aged mice fed control diet. Furthermore, they found that spleen and livers from aged mice had a lower GSH content than those from younger mice; GSH supplementation reversed this age-related decrease. Lacombe *et al.* (1985) showed that the level of intracellular −SH declines during mitogenic stimulation with Con A. However, Furukawa *et al.* (1987) found that old mice supplemented with GSH showed a smaller decline in intracellular GSH than control mice, suggesting that splenocytes from the aged mice supplemented with GSH maintain a more vigorous cellular GSH metabolism and are more responsive to mitogenic stimulation.

Methionine, a precursor of GSH biosynthesis, has been reported not to have an immunostimulatory effect (Radix *et al.*, 1983). An immunostimulatory effect in experimental animals has been reported for another sulfhydryl-containing compound, 2-mercaptoethanolamine (Heindrick *et al.*, 1984); however, this antioxidant is not suitable for human use.

3.7. Zinc

Marginal deficiencies of zinc and chromium may occur with aging. Sandstead *et al.* (1982) showed that zinc intake declines with advancing age in parallel with many other nutrients. Abdulla *et al.* (1977) found that zinc content of self-selected diets of 37 65-year-old Swedes averaged 8.2 mg/day compared to a recommended dietary allowance (RDA) of 15 mg/day. Clinical symptoms associated with zinc deficiency such as decreased taste acuity, impaired wound healing, increased prevalence of cell-mediated immune disorders, and hypogonadism in males are not uncommon among the elderly. Although some studies have not shown an association between plasma zinc level and age (Sandstead, 1982), Linderman *et al.* (1971) found a decrease in plasma zinc level with age, and Stiedeman and Harrell (1980) showed a negative correlation between age and serum zinc level.

Zinc is essential for the maintenance of cell-mediated immune function (Fraker *et al.*, 1977; Frost *et al.*, 1977; Ruhl and Kirchner, 1978), particularly T-cell-mediated functions. Zinc deficiency has been shown to cause thymus involution and decreased antibody formation in SRBC (Fraker, 1977). Furthermore, thymic hormone levels necessary for T-cell maturation have been reported to be decreased in both zinc-deficient mice and humans (Iwata *et al.*, 1979). Several investigators have reported depressed mitogenic responses of lymphocytes in zinc-deficient animals (Alford, 1970; Fraker *et al.*, 1977; Ruhl and Kirchner, 1978; Meydani *et al.*, 1983). Conditions in humans that are associated with zinc deficiency, such as acrodermatitis enteropathica, Down's syndrome, protein–energy malnutrition, and those in hospitalized patients receiving zinc-free total parental nutrition, are associated with thymic atrophy, decreased thymic hormone level, and a decrease in certain T-cell populations. Zinc supplementation has been shown to increase thymic size and improve DCH response to *Candida* antigen in children with PEM (Golden *et al.*, 1977). In 12 patients with Down's syndrome, zinc supplementation increased serum zinc level, neutrophil chemotactic activity, lymphocyte reactivity, and DCH response to dinitrochlorbenzene (Bjorksten *et al.*, 1980). In children with acrodermatitis enteropathica, supplementation for 2 weeks with zinc sulfate increased serum zinc level and resulted in greater lymphocyte proliferation and improved DCH to a battery of recall antigens (Chandra, 1980).

More than 70 metalloenzymes are zinc dependent, among them thymidine kinase, DNA polymerase, and DNA-dependent RNA polymerase. In addition, thymic hormone is a zinc-containing metallopeptide produced by epithelial cells of the thymus. Changes in the thymic hormone level can result in an inability of immature T cells and prothymocytes to differentiate properly, resulting in decreased T-cell numbers as well as specific defects that cause loss of functional subpopulations dependent on the presence of circulating thymic hormones. Gross *et al.* (1979) showed that treatment of zinc-deficient rats with levamisole, which acts on precursor cells, significantly increased their depressed mitogenic response to PHA. This finding suggests that although stem cells in zinc-deficient rats are not altered, T-cell differentiation and maturation are affected through a defect in thymic hormones.

Zinc may also intervene in nonenzymic free-radical reactions, as superoxide dismutase is a zinc-containing enzyme. Bettger and O'Dell (1981) have suggested that zinc plays a role analogous to vitamin E in stabilizing membrane structures and reducing peroxidative damage to the cell. Zinc has also been indicated as affecting arachidonic acid metabolism (Bettger and O'Dell, 1981; Meydani *et al.*, 1983).

Wagner *et al.* (1983) studied 173 heterogeneous low-income elderly subjects aged 60–97 for zinc intake, plasma and hair zinc concentration, and DCH to four antigens. The average zinc intake of the study population was 7.3 mg/day, approximately 50% of the RDA, and average serum zinc level was 92 ± 20 mg/dl. Twenty-two percent of the subjects were anergic and had a serum zinc level of 83 ± 18 μg/dl compared to 94 ± 20 μg/dl in the nonanergic subjects. A significant improvement in DCH response was observed in five anergic subjects supplemented with 55 mg zinc sulfate/day for 4 weeks. Even though the study was not done in a double-blind fashion and lacked the placebo control group, it does suggest that inadequate zinc nutriture in the elderly might contribute to immune dysfunction.

Weindruch *et al.* (1984) looked at the effect of *in vitro* addition of $ZnCl_2$ on *in vitro* antibody formation by cells from spleens of young and old mice and found that 10^{-4} M $ZnCl_2$ in most old mice tested increased the number of PFC to SRBC; however, the effect was not specific to old mice, since the same concentration of $ZnCl_2$ increased PFC in younger mice as well. The stimulatory effect of zinc was not caused by increasing the lower zinc content of spleen in the old mice, since young and old mice had similar concentrations. Zinc supplementation was most effective when added 0–48 hr after initiation of the culture, indicating that zinc influences early events in antibody formation such as interaction between antigen-presenting cells and T cells or between T cells and the precursor forms of antibody-forming cells. Duchateau *et al.* (1981) examined the effect of oral zinc supplementation (440 mg/day for 1 month) on T-cell-mediated immune function of healthy institutionalized subjects over 70 years old compared to an age- and sex-matched untreated group. The zinc supplementation did not have an effect on *in vitro* lymphocyte proliferation, but it significantly increased the percentage of circulating T cells and the number of positive tests and mean diameter of positive reaction in DCH to *Candida,* streptokinase–streptodornase, and PPD antigens. The zinc supplementation also improved antibody formation against tetanus toxin. Whether the immunostimulatory effect of zinc resulted from the presence of a marginal zinc deficiency in these elderly subjects or from a nonspecific immunostimulatory effect is not clear. It should be noted that there is pronounced thymus atrophy with aging, accompanied by a decrease in the level of thymic hormone. Zinc has been shown to increase serum levels of thymic hormones (Iwata *et al.*, 1979), and thymic atrophy is observed in zinc deficiency. Therefore, the beneficial effect of supplemental zinc might result from increases in thymic hormone levels or from its antioxidant and membrane-stabilizing action. Confirmation of these mechanisms of action will require direct assessment of changes in thymic hormones and membrane characteristics.

4. Conclusion

Nutritional factors act at multiple sites within the immune system by modulating metabolic processes. These metabolic changes may include the activation or inhibition of key enzymes, immunoregulatory mediators, and/or products of the major histocompatibility gene complex. These nutritionally induced changes may result in altered cellular immune functions, particularly in cells of the T-lymphocyte lineage. The immunologic approach to the study of nutrition and aging (and its associated disease processes) appears useful, as certain immune functions, particularly those that are thymus-related, consistently decline in quantity and efficiency with aging. This decline has been linked to increased susceptibility to bacterial, fungal, and viral infection as well as to the development of cancer and autoimmune disease.

Despite the documented decline in immune responsiveness with age and the established changes in nutritional status in the elderly, little conclusive evidence is available about dietary interventions and immune function in the aged. As is evident from the discussion above, few studies with the exception of food restriction in animal models have addressed the role of nutrient deficiencies or supplementation in the immune response of the aged. Unfortunately, most relevant human investigations suffer from an inadequate number of study subjects, poorly defined or documented population cohorts, and the lack of placebo controls. Further, review of these studies reveals inadequate attention to diet composition other than to those single nutrients specifically being examined. The apparent difficulty in obtaining more than one pre- and posttreatment value for immune function makes extrapolation and practical recommendations to the general population almost impossible. The inability of most investigators to control carefully for pertinent environmental factors also limits the utility of the studies. Nevertheless, the results of these studies and the potential benefit to be derived from their practical application are sufficiently encouraging to warrant further and more expansive studies in this area.

Interestingly, several of the potential beneficial actions of nutrients on the immune system appear to involve dietary antioxidants. Age-related increases in free radical reactions and associated lipid peroxidation events could be contributing to the aging process via several mechanisms. Free radicals and the oxidative products of arachidonic acid have been shown to have a suppressive effect on most cell-mediated immune functions. Dietary antioxidants may act to increase immune responsiveness by altering macrophage events mediated by cyclooxygenase, e.g., generation of prostaglandins, and lipoxygenase, e.g., generation of hydroxyeicosatetraenoic acid and leukotrienes, or IL-1 production. The mechanism(s) of such action could be based on antioxidant dampening of enzyme activity, quenching of lipid peroxidation, and/or altering fatty acid precursor pools of splenocyte phospholipids, which dictate prostaglandin and leukotriene synthesis.

It seems reasonable to postulate that any factors that might delay, decrease, or reverse the rates of immunologic decline may also beneficially affect the development of age-related diseases. Cellular and molecular analyses have revealed that the function of the immunoregulatory network is in an intimate relationship with other important biological systems, including the brain and endocrine systems, which are also affected by nutritional status. Therefore, nutritional modulation of the aged immune system presents a practical approach to improving immunocompetence and may promote the realization of a more productive, full life span for the elderly.

5. *References*

Abdulla, M., Jagerstad, M., Norden, A., Orist, I., and Svensson, S., 1977, Dietary intake of electrolytes and trace elements in the elderly, *Nutr. Metab.* **21**[*Suppl.* 1]:41–44.

Abraham, C., Tal, Y., and Gershon, H., 1977, Reduced *in vitro* response to concanavalin A and lipopolysaccharide in senescent mice: A function of reduced number of responding cells, *Eur. J. Immunol.* **7**:301–304.

Abraham, E. C., Taylor, F. F., and Lang, C. A., 1978, Influence of mouse age and erythrocyte age on glutathione metabolism, *Biochem. J.* **174**:819–825.

Alford, R. M., 1970, Metal cation requirements for phytohemagglutinin-induced transformation of human peripheral blood leukocytes, *J. Immunol.* **104**:698–703.

Anderson, R., Oosthuigen, R., Maritz, R., Theron, A., and Van Rensburg, A., 1980, The effect of increasing weekly doses of ascorbate on certain cellular and humoral immune functions in normal volunteers, *Am. J. Clin. Nutr.* **33**:71–76.

Antel, J. P., Weinrich, M., and Aranson, B. G. W., 1978, Circulating suppressor cells in man as a function of age, *Clin. Immunol. Immunopathol.* **9**:134–141.

Atkinson, J., Kelly, J., Weiss, A., Wedner, H., and Parker, C., 1978, Enhanced intracellular cGMP concentrations and lectin-induced lymphocyte transformation, *J. Immunol.* **121**:2282–2291.

Axelrod, A. E., 1971, Immune processes in vitamin deficiency states, *Am. J. Clin. Nutr.* **24**:265–271.

Bach, M. A., 1979, Influence of aging on T-cell subpopulations involved in the *in vitro* generation of allogeneic cytotoxicity, *Immunol. Immunopathol.* **13**:220–230.

Barnes, K. J., and Chen, L. H., 1981, Vitamin E status of the elderly in central Kentucky, *J. Nutr. Elderly* **1**:41–49.

Barrett, D. J., Steinmark, S., and Wara, D. W., and Ammann, A. J., 1980, Immunoregulation in aged humans, *Clin. Immunol. Immunopathol.* **17**:203–211.
Bartocci, A., Maggi, F. M., Welker, R. D., and Veronese, F., 1982, Age-related immunosuppression: Putative role of prostaglandins, in: *Prostaglandins and Cancer* (T. J. Powles, R. S. Backman, K. V. Honn, and P. Ramwell, eds.), Alan R. Liss, New York, pp. 725–730.
Bash, J. A., 1983, Cellular immunosenescence in F344 rats; decline in responsiveness to phytohemagglutinin involves changes in both T cells and macrophages, *Mech. Ageing Dev.* **21**:323–333.
Beach, R. S., Gershwin, M. E., and Hurley, L. S., 1982, Nutritional factors and autoimmunity, III. Zinc deprivation versus restricted food intake in MRL/1 mice; the distinction between interacting dietary influences, *J. Immunol.* **129**:2686.
Becker, M. J., Farkas, R., Schneider, M., Drucker, L., and Klajman, A., 1979, Cell mediated cytotoxicity in humans: Age-related decline as measured by xenogeneic assay, *Immunol. Immunopathol.* **14**:204–210.
Beisel, W. R., 1982, Single nutrients and immunity, *Am. J. Clin. Nutr.* **35**:417–468.
Bendich, A., Gabriel, E., and Machlin, L. J., 1983, Effect of dietary level of vitamin E in the immune system of the spontaneously hypertensive (SHR) and mormotensive Wistar Kyoto (WKY) rats, *J. Nutr.* **113**:1920–1926.
Bendich, A., Gabriel, E., and Machlin, L. J., 1986, Dietary vitamin E requirement for optimum immune response in the rat, *J. Nutr.* **116**:675–681.
Bettger, W. J., and O'Dell, B. L., 1981, A critical physiological role in zinc in the structure and function of biomembranes, *Life Sci.* **28**:1425–1438.
Bjorksten, B., Back, O., Gustavson, K. H., Hallmans, G., Hagglof, B., and Tarnvik, A., 1980, Zinc and immune function in Down's syndrome, *Acta Paediatr. Scand.* **69**:183–187.
Blumberg, J. B., 1987, Vitamin E requirements during aging, in: *Clinical and Nutritional Aspects of Vitamin E* (O. Hayaishi and M. Mino, eds.), Elsevier, Amsterdam, pp. 53–61.
Blumberg, J. B., and Meydani, S. N., 1986, Role of dietary antioxidants in aging, in: *Nutrition and Aging*, Volume 5 (H. Munro and M. Hutchinson, eds.), Academic Press, New York, pp. 85–97.
Bowers, T. K., and Eckert, E., 1978, Leukopenia in anorexia nervosa, *Arch. Intern. Med.* **138**:1520–1523.
Brennan, P. C., and Jaroslow, B. N., 1975, Age-associated decline in theta antigen on spleen thymus-derived lymphocytes of B6CF1 mice, *Cell. Immunol.* **15**:51–56.
Burr, M. L., Elwood, P. C., Hole, D. J., Hurley, R. J., and Hughes, R. E., 1974, Plasma and leukocyte ascorbic acid levels in the elderly, *Am. J. Clin. Nutr.* **27**:144–151.
Burr, M. L., Hurley, R. J., and Sweetnam, P. M., 1975, Vitamin C supplementation of old people with low blood levels, *Gerontol. Clin.* **17**:236–243.
Callard, R. E., and Basten, A., 1978, Immune function in aged mice, IV. Loss of T cell and B cell function in thymus-dependent antibody responses, *Eur. J. Immunol.* **8**:552–558.
Ceuppens, J. L., and Goodwin, J. S., 1982, Regulation of immunoglobulin production in pokeweed mitogen-stimulated cultures of lymphocytes from young and old adults, *J. Immunol.* **128**:2429–2434.
Chandra, R. K., 1972, Immunocompetence in undernutrition, *J. Pediatr.* **81**:1194–1200.
Chandra, R. K., 1980, Acrodermatitis enteropathica: Zinc levels and cell-mediated immunity, *Pediatrics* **66**:789–791.
Chandra, R. K., 1985, Nutritional regulation of immunity and infection: From epidemiology to phenomenology and clinical practice, *J. Pediatr. Gastroenterol. Nutr.* **5**:844–852.
Chandra, R. K., and Puri, S., 1985, Nutritional support improves antibody response to influenza virus vaccine in the elderly, *Br. Med. J.* **291**:705–706.
Chandra, S., and Chandra, R. K., 1986, Nutrition, immune response, and outcome, *Prog. Food Nutr. Sci.* **10**:1–65.
Chang, M. P., Makinodan, T., Peterson, W. J., and Strehler, B. L., 1982, Role of T cells and adherent cells in age-related decline in murine interleukin 2 production, *J. Immunol.* **129**:2426–2430.
Chavance, M., Brubacher, G., Herberth, B., Vernes, G., Mistacki, T., Deti, F., Fournier, C., and Janot, C., 1985, Immunological and nutritional status among the elderly, in: *Nutrition, Immunity, and Illness in the Elderly* (R. K. Chandra, ed.), Pergamon Press, New York, pp. 137–142.
Chen, C. H., Hsu, S. J., Huang, P. C., and Chen, J. S., 1977, Vitamin E status of Chinese population in Taiwan, *Am. J. Clin. Nutr.* **30**:728–735.

Cheney, K. E., Liu, R. K., Smith, G. S., Leung, R. E., Mickey, M. R., and Walford, R. L., 1980, Survival and disease patterns in C57BL/6J mice subjected to undernutrition, *Exp. Gerontol.* **15:**237–258.

Cheslock, K. E., and McCulley, M. T., 1960, Response of human beings to a low vitamin B_6 diet, *J. Nutr.* **70:**507–513.

Cobleigh, M. A., Braun, D. P., and Harris, J. E., 1980, Age-dependent changes in human peripheral blood B cells and T cell subsets: Correlation with mitogen responsiveness, *Clin. Immunol. Immunopathol.* **15:**162–173.

Corman, L. C., 1985, The relationship between nutrition, infection, and immunity, *Med. Clin. North Am.* **69:**519–532.

Corwin, L. M., and Shloss, J., 1980a, Influence of vitamin E on the mitogenic response of murine lymphoid cells, *J. Nutr.* **110:**916–923.

Corwin, L. M., and Shloss, J., 1980b, Role of antioxidants on the stimulation of the mitogenic response, *J. Nutr.* **110:**2397–2505.

DeKruyff, R. H., Kim, Y. T., Siskind, G. W., and Weksler, M. E., 1980, Age related changes in the *in vitro* immune response: Increased suppressor activity in immature and aged mice, *J. Immunol.* **125:**142–147.

Delafuente, J. C., Dlesk, A., and Panush, R. S., 1981, Cellular immunity, in: *Principles of Rheumatic Diseases* (R. S. Panush, ed.), John Wiley & Sons, New York, pp. 89–102.

Delafuente, J. C., Eisenberg, J. D., Hoelzer, D. R., and Slavin, R. G., 1983, Tetanus toxoid as an antigen for delayed cutaneous hypersensitivity, *J.A.M.A.* **249:**3209–3211.

Delafuente, J. C., Prendergast, J. M., and Modigh, A., 1986, Immunological modulation by vitamin C in the elderly, *Int. J. Immunopharmacol.* **8:**205–211.

Delfraissy, J. F., Galanaud, P., Wallon, C., Balavoine, J. F., and Dormont, J., 1982, Abolished *in vitro* antibody response in elderly: Exclusive involvement of prostaglandin-induced T-suppressor cells, *Clin. Immunol. Immunopathol.* **24:**377–385.

Dowd, P. S., and Eckert, E., 1984, The influence of undernutrition on immunity, *Clin. Sci.* **66:**241–248.

Duchateau, J., Delepesse, G., Vrijens, R., and Collet, H., 1981, Beneficial effects of oral zinc supplementation on the immune response of old people, *Am. J. Med.* **70:**1001–1004.

Dworksky, R., Paganini-Hill, A., Arthur, M., and Parker, J., 1983, Immune response of healthy humans 83–104 years of age, *J. Natl. Cancer Inst.* **71:**265–268.

Effros, R. B., and Walford, R. L., 1983, Diminished T-cell response to influenza virus in aged mice, *Immunology* **49:**387–392.

Fernandes, G., 1984, Nutritional factors: Modulating effects on immune function and aging, *Pharmacol. Rev.* **36:**1235–1295.

Fernandes, G., and Gupta, S., 1981, Natural killing and antibody-dependent cytotoxicity by lymphocyte subpopulations in young and aging humans, *J. Clin. Immunol.* **1:**141–148.

Fernandes, G., Yunis, E., and Good, R., 1976, Suppression of adenocarcinoma by the immunological consequences of calorie restriction, *Nature* **263:**504–507.

Fernandes, G., Friend, P., Yunis, E. J., and Good, R. A., 1978, Influence of dietary restriction on immunologic function and renal disease in (NZB × NZW) F_1 mice, *Proc. Natl. Acad. Sci. U.S.A.* **75:**1500–1504.

Fernandez, L. A., and Macsween, J. M., 1980, Decreased autologous mixed lymphocyte reaction with aging, *Mech. Ageing Dev.* **12:**245–248.

Flohe, L., and Gunzler, W. A., 1976, Glutathione-dependent oxido-reduction reactions, in: *Glutathione: Metabolism and Function* (I. M. Arias and W. B. Jakoby, eds.), Raven Press, New York, pp. 17–34.

Fraker, P. J., Haas, S., and Luecke, R. W., 1977, Effect of zinc deficiency on the immune response of the young adult/Jax mouse, *J. Nutr.* **107:**1889–1895.

Frost, P., Chen, J. C., Rabbani, P., Smith, J., and Prasad, A. S., 1977, The effect of zinc deficiency on the immune response, in: *Zinc Metabolism: Current Aspects in Health and Disease* (G. J. Brewer and A. S. Prasad, eds.), Alan R. Liss, New York, pp. 143–150.

Furukawa, T., Meydani, S. N., and Blumberg, J. B., 1987, Reversal of age-associated decline in immune responsiveness, *Mech. Ageing Dev.* **38:**107–117.

Gardner, N. D., Lim, S. T., and Lawton, J. W. M., 1981, Monocyte function in aging humans, *Mech. Ageing Dev.* **16:**233–239.

Garry, P. J., Goodwin, J. S., Hunt, W. C., Hooper, E. M., and Leonard, A. G., 1982, Nutritional status in a healthy elderly population: dietary and supplemental intakes, *Am. J. Clin. Nutr.* **36:** 319–331.

Gebrase-DeLima, M., Liu, R. K., Cheney, K. E., Mickey, R., and Walford, R. L., 1975, Immune function and survival in a long-lived mouse strain subjected to undernutrition, *Gerontology* **21:**184–189.

Gershwin, M. E., Beach, R. S., and Hurley, L. S., 1985, *Nutrition and Immunity,* Academic Press, Orlando, FL.

Gilman, S., Woda, B., and Feldman, J., 1981, T lymphocytes of young and aged rats, I. Distribution, density and capping of T antigens, *J. Immunol.* **127:**149–153.

Gladstone, J. L., and Recco, R., 1976, Host function and infectious disease in elderly, *Med. Clin. North Am.* **60:**1225–1240.

Golden, M. H. N., Jackson, A. A., and Golden, B. E., 1977, Effect of zinc on thymus of recently malnourished children, *Lancet* **2:**1057–1059.

Golla, J. A., Larson, L. A., Anderson, C. F., Lucas, A. R., Wilson, W. R., and Tomasi, T. B., 1981, An immunological assessment of patients with anorexia nervosa, *Am. J. Clin. Nutr.* **34:**2756–2762.

Goodwin, J. S., and Garry, T. J., 1983, Relationship between megadose vitamin supplementation and immunological function in a healthy elderly population, *Clin. Exp. Immunol.* **51:**647–653.

Gougerst-Poidals, M. A., Fay, M., Roche, Y., Lacombe, P., and Marquetty, C., 1985, Immune oxidative injury in mice exposed to normabaric O_2: Effects of thiol compounds on the splenic cell sulfhdryl content and Con A proliferative response, *J. Immunol.* **135:**2045–2051.

Gross, R. L., Osdin, N., Fong, L., and Newberne, P. M., 1979, *In vitro* restoration by levamisole of mitogen responsiveness in zinc-deprived rats, *Am. J. Clin. Nutr.* **32:**1267–1271.

Gupta, S., and Good, R. A., 1979, Subpopulations of human T lymphocytes, X. Alterations in T, B. third population cells, and T cells with receptors for immunoglobulin M (T_m) or G (T_{gamma}) in aging humans, *J. Immunol.* **122:**1214–1219.

Haaijman, I., Berg, P., and Brinkhoff, J., 1977, Immunoglobulin class and subclass levels in the serum of CBA mice throughout life, *Immunology* **32:**923–927.

Haaijman, J. J., and Hijmans, W., 1978, Influence of age on immunological activity and capacity of the CBA mouse, *Mech. Ageing Dev.* **7:**375–398.

Haffer, K., Freeman, M. J., and Watson, R. R., 1979, Effects of age on cellular immune responses in BALB/C mice: Increase in antibody-dependent T lymphocyte mediated cytotoxicity, *Mech. Ageing Dev.* **11:**279–285.

Hallgren, H. M., and Yunis, E. J., 1977, Suppressor lymphocytes in young and aged humans, *J. Immunol.* **118:**2004–2008.

Hallgren, H. M., Buckley, C. E. III, Gilbertsen, V. A., and Yunis, E. J., 1973, Lymphocyte phytohemagglutinin responsiveness, immunoglobulins, and autoantibodies in aging humans, *J. Immunol.* **111:**1101–1107.

Hallgren, H. M., Jacola, D. R., and O'Leary, J. J., 1983, Unusual pattern of surface marker expression on peripheral lymphocytes from aged humans suggestive of a population of less differentiated cells, *J. Immunol.* **131:**191–194.

Hamm, M. W., Winick, M., and Schachter, D., 1985, Macrophage phagocytosis and membrane fluidity in mice: The effect of age and dietary protein, *Mech. Ageing Dev.* **32:**11–20.

Harman, D., 1980, Free radical theory of aging: Beneficial effect of antixoxidants on the lifespan of male NZB mice; role of free radical reactions in the deterioration of the immune system with age and in the pathogenesis of systemic lupus erythematosus, *Age* **3:**64–73.

Harman, D., 1982, The free-radical theory of aging, in: *Free Radicals in Biology,* Volume 5 (W. A. Pryor, ed.), Academic Press, New York, pp. 255–273.

Harman, D., and Miller, R. W., 1986, Effect of vitamin E on the immune response to influenza virus vaccine and incidence of infectious disease in man, *Age* **9:**21–23.

Hausman, P. B., and Weksler, M. E., 1985, Changes in the immune response with age, in: *Handbook of the Biology of Aging* (C. E. Finch and E. L. Schneider, eds.), Van Nostrand-Reinhold, New York, pp. 414–432.

Hazelton, G. A., and Lang, C. A., 1980, Glutathione contents of tissues in the aging mouse, *Biochem. J.* **188:**25–30.

Heindrick, M. L., Hendricks, L. C., and Cook, D. E., 1984, Effect of dietary 2-mercaptoethanol on the life span, immune system, tumor incidence and lipid peroxidation damage in spleen lymphocytes of aging $BC3F_1$ mice, *Mech. Ageing Dev.* **27**:341–358.

Hodges, R. E., Bean, W. B., Ohlson, M. A., and Bleiler, R. E., 1962, Factors affecting human antibody response, IV. Pyridoxine deficiency, *Am. J. Clin. Nutr.* **11**:180–186.

Hodkinson, H. M., and Exton-Smith, A. N., 1976, Factors predicting mortality in the elderly in the community, *Age Aging* **5**:110–115.

Horowitt, M. K., Harvey, C. C., Dahm, C. J., Jr., and Searey, M. T., 1972, Relationship between tocopherol and serum lipid levels for determination of nutritional adequacy, *Ann. N.Y. Acad. Sci.* **203**:223–236.

Indiveri, F., Perri, I., Viglione, D., Pende, D., Russo, C., Pelligrino, M. A., and Ferrone, S., 1983, Human T lymphocytes in aging and malignancy: Abnormalities in pha-induced ia antigen expression and in functional activity in autologous and allogeneic MLR, *Cell. Immunol.* **76**:224–231.

Iwata, T., Incefy, G., Tanaka, T., Fernandes, G., Menendez-Botet, C. J., Pih, K., and Good, R. A., 1979, Circulating thymic hormone levels in zinc deficiency, *Cell. Immunol.* **47**:100–105.

James, S. J., and Makinodan, T., 1984, Nutritional intervention during immunologic aging: Past and present, in: *Nutritional Intervention in the Aging Process* (H. J. Armbrecht, J. M. Prendergast, and R. M. Coe, eds.), Springer-Verlag, New York, pp. 209–229.

Joncourt, F., Wang, Y., Kristensen, F., and DeWeck, A. L., 1982, Aging and immunity: Decrease in interleukin-2 production and interleukin-2-dependent RNA synthesis in lectin-stimulated murine spleen cells, *Immunobiology* **163**:521–526.

Jose, D. G., and Good, R. A., 1971, Absence of enhancing antibody ion cell mediated immunity to tumor heterografts in protein deficient rats, *Nature* **231**:323–325.

Jose, D. G., and Good, R. A., 1973, Quantitative effects of nutritional protein and calorie deficiency upon immune responses to tumors in mice, *Cancer Res.* **33**:807–812.

Kagawa, Y., 1978, Impact of westernization on the nutrition of Japanaese: Changes in physique, cancer, longevity and centenarians, *Prev. Med.* **7**:205–217.

Kataria, M. S., Rao, D. B., and Curtis, R. C., 1965, Vitamin C levels in elderly, *Gerontol. Clin.* **7**:189–190.

Katz, S., Kierszenbaum, F., and Waksman, B., 1978, Mechanism of action of lymphocyte activating factor, III. Evidence that LAF acts on stimulated lymphocytes by raising cyclic GMP in G1, *J. Immunol.* **126**:2386–2391.

Kay, M. M. B., 1979, Effect of age on human immunological parameters including T and B cell colony formation, in: *Recent Advances in Gerontology* (H. Orimo, K. Shimada, M. Iriki, and D. Maeda, eds.), Excerpta Medica, Amsterdam, pp. 442–443.

Kay, M. M. B., 1985, Immunobiology of Aging, in: *Nutrition, Immunity and Illness in the Elderly* (R. K. Chandra, ed.), Pergamon Press, New York, pp. 97–119.

Kay, M. M. B., Mendoza, J., Diven, J., Denton, T., Union, N., and Lajiness, L., 1979, Age related changes in the immune system of mice of 8 medium and long-lived strains and hybrids, I. Organ, cellular, and activity changes, *Mech. Ageing Dev.* **211**:295–346.

Kay, M. M. B., Goodman, S., Sorensen, K., Whitfield, C., Wong, P., Zaki, L., and Rudoloff, U. V., 1983, The senescent cell antigen is immunologically related to band 3, *Proc. Natl. Acad. Sci. U.S.A.* **80**:1631–1635.

Kelleher, J., and Losowsky, M. S., 1978, Vitamin E in the elderly, in: *Tocopherol, Oxygen and Biomembranes* (C. DeDuve and O. Hayaishi, eds.), Elsevier/North Holland Biomedical Press, Amsterdam, pp. 311–327.

Kennes, B., Hubert, C., Brohee, D., and Neve, P., 1981, Early biochemical events associated with lymphocyte activation in ageing, I. Evidence that Ca^{2+} dependent processes induced by PHA are impaired, *Immunology* **42**:119–126.

Kennes, B., Dumont, I., Brohee, D., Hubert, C., and Neve, P., 1983, Effect of vitamin C supplementation on cell-mediated immunity in old people, *Gerontology* **29**:305–310.

Kessler, J. O., Jarvik, L. J., Fu, T. M., and Matsuyama, S., 1979, Thermotaxis, chemotaxis, and age, *Age* **2**:5–11.

Keusch, G. T., Wilson, C. S., and Waksal, S. D., 1983, Nutrition, host defenses, and the lymphoid system, in: *Advances in Host Defense Mechanisms,* Volume 2 (J. I. Gallin and A. S. Fauci, eds.) Raven Press, New York, pp. 275–359.

Keystone, E. L., Demerieux, P., Gladman, D., Poplonski, L., Piper, S., and Buchanan, R., 1980, Enhanced delayed hypersensitivity skin test reactivity with serial testing in healthy volunteers, *Clin. Exp. Immunol.* **40:**202–205.

Kishimoto, S., Tomino, S., Mitsuya, H., Fujiwara, H., and Tsuda, H., 1980, Age-related decline in the *in vitro* and *in vivo* synthesis of antitetanus toxoid antibody in humans, *J. Immunol.* **125:**2347–2352.

Knicker, W. T., Anderson, C. T., McBryde, J. L., Roumiantzeff, M., and Lesourd, B., 1984, Multitest, C.M.I. for standardized measurement of delayed cutaneous hypersensitivity and cell-mediated immunity: Normal values and proposed scoring system for healthy adults in the U.S.A., *Ann. Allergy* **52:**75–82.

Krogsrud, R. L., and Perkins, E. H., 1977, Age-related changes in T cell function, *J. Immunol.* **118:**1607–1611.

Kubo, C., Johnson, B. C., Day, K., and Good, R. A., 1984, Calorie source, calorie restriction, immunity and aging of (NZB/NZW)F_1 mice, *J. Nutr.* **114:**1884–1899.

Kubo, C., Johnson, B. C., Gajjar, A., and Good, R. A., 1987, Crucial dietary factors in maximizing life span and longevity in autoimmune prone mice, *J. Nutr.* **117:**1129–1135.

Lacombe, P., Kraus, L., Fay, M., and Pocidalo, J., 1985, Lymphocyte glutathione status in relation to their Con A proliferative response, *FEBS Lett.* **191:**227–230.

Langweiler, M., Schultz, R. D., and Sheffy, B. E., 1981, Effect of vitamin E deficiency on the proliferative response of canine lymphocytes, *Am. J. Vet. Res.* **42:**1681–1685.

Larsen, H. J., and Tollersrud, S., 1981, Effect of dietary vitamin E and selenium on the phytohaemagglutinin response of pig lymphocytes, *Am. J. Vet. Sci.* **31:**301–305.

Ledbetter, J. A., Rouse, R. V., Michlem, H. S., and Herzenberg, L. A., 1980, T cell subsets defined by expression of Lyt-1,2,3 and Thy-1 antigens: Two parameter immunofluorescence and cytotoxicity analysis with monoclonal antibodies modifies current views, *J. Exp. Med.* **152:**280–295.

Leibovitz, B. E., and Siegel, B. V., 1980, Aspects of free radical reactions in biological systems, *Aging J. Gerontol.* **7:**45–56.

Leichter, J., Angel, J. F., and Lee, M., 1978, Nutritional status of a select groups of free-living elderly people in Vancouver, *Can. Med. Assoc. J.* **118:**40–43.

Licastro, F., Tabacchi, P. L., Chiricolo, R., Parente, R., Cenci, M., Barboni, F., and Franceschi, C., 1983, Defective self-recognition in subjects of far advanced age, *Gerontology* **29:**64–72.

Linderman, R. D., Clark, M. L., and Colemore, J. P., 1971, Influence of age and sex on plasma and red cell zinc concentrations, *J. Gerontol.* **26:**358–363.

Linn, B. S., and Jensen, J., 1984, Malnutrition and immunocompetence in older and younger outpatients, *South. Med. J.* **77:**1098–1102.

Lipschitz, D. A., and Udupa, K. B., 1986, Influence of aging and protein deficiency on neutrophil function, *J. Gerontol.* **41:**690–694.

Makinodan, T., 1976, Immunobiology of aging, *J. Am. Geriatr. Assoc.* **24:**249–252.

McGandy, R. B., Russell, R. M., Hartz, S. C., Jacob, R. A., Tannenbaum, S., Peters, H., Sahyoun, N., and Otradovec, C. L., 1986, Nutritional status survey of healthy noninstitutionalized elderly: energy and nutrient intakes from three-day diet records and nutrient supplements, *Nutr. Res.* **6:**785–798.

McLaughlin, B., O'Malley, K., and Cotton, T. G., 1986, Age-related differences in granulocyte chemotaxis and degranulation, *Clin. Sci.* **70:**59–62.

McMurray, D. N., Rey, H., Casazza, C. J., and Watson, R. R., 1977, Effect of moderate malnutrition on concentrations of immunoglobulins and enzymes in tears and saliva of young Colombian children, *Am. J. Clin. Nutr.* **30:**1944–1948.

Meydani, S. N., and Dupont, J., 1982, Effect of zinc efficiency on prostaglandin levels in different organs of the rat, *J. Nutr.* **112:**1098–1104.

Meydani, S. N., Meydani, M., and Dupont, J., 1983, Effect of prostaglandin modifiers and zinc deficiency on possibly related functions in rats, *J. Nutr.* **133:**494–500.

Meydani, S. N., Meydani, M., Verdon, C. P., Shapiro, A. C., Blumberg, J. B., and Hayes, K. C., 1986a, Vitamin E supplementation suppresses prostaglandin E_2 synthesis and enhances the immune response in aged mice, *Mech. Ageing Dev.* **34:**191–201.

Meydani, S. N., Cathcart, E. S., Hopkins, R. E., Meydani, M., Hayes, K. C., and Blumberg, J. B., 1986b, Antioxidants in experimental amyloidosis of young and old mice, in: *Fourth International Symposium of Amyloidosis* (G. G. Glenner, E. P. Asserman, E. Benditt, E. Calkins, A. S. Cohen, and D. Zucker-Franklin, eds.), Plenum Press, New York, pp. 683–692.

Meydani, S. N., Yogeeswaran, G., Liu, S., Baskar, S., and Meydani, M., 1988, Fish oil and tocopherol induced changes in natural killer cell mediated cytotoxicity and PGE_2 synthesis in young and old mice, *J. Nutr.* (in press).

Miller, A. E., 1980, Selective decline in cellular immune response to varicella–zoster in the elderly, *Neurology (Minneap.)* **30:**582–587.

Miller, R. A., 1983, Age-associated decline in precursor frequency for different T-cell mediated reactions, with preservation of helper or cytotoxic effect per precursor cell, *J. Immunol.* **132:**63–68.

Moldawer, L. L., Nauss, K., Bistrian, B. R., and Blackburn, G. L., 1979, Cellular immunity in protein malnutrition: Differences in *in vivo* and *in vitro* responses, *Surg. Forum* **30:**138–140.

Moody, C. E., Innes, J. B., Staiano-Coico, L., Incefy, G. S., Thaler, H. T., and Weksler, M. E., 1981, Lymphocyte transformation induced by autologous cells, XI. The effect of age on the autologous mixed lymphocyte reaction, *Immunology* **44:**431–438.

Munro, H. N., Suter, P. M., and Russell, R. M., 1987, Nutritional requirements of the elderly, *Annu. Rev. Nutr.* **7:**23–49.

Murray, J., and Murray, A., 1981, Toward a nutritional concept of lost resistance to malignancy and intracellular infection, *Perspect. Biol. Med.* **24:**290–301.

Nagel, J. E., Chrest, F. J., and Adler, W. H., 1981, Enumeration of T-lymphocyte subsets by monoclonal antibodies in young and aged humans, *J. Immunol.* **127:**2086.

Nagel, J. E., Pyle, R. S., Chrest, F. J., and Adler, W. H., 1982, Oxidative metabolism and bactericidal capacity of polymorphonuclear leukocyte from young and aged adults, *J. Gerontol.* **37:**529–534.

Nagel, J. E., Chrest, F. J., Pyle, R. S., and Adler, W. H., 1983, Monoclonal antibody analysis of T-lymphocyte subsets in young and aged adults, *Immunol. Commun.* **12:**223–237.

Nakayama, E., Dippold, W., Shiku, H., Oettgen, H. F., and Old, L. J., 1980, Alloantigen-induced T-cell proliferation: Lyt phenotype of responding cells and blocking of proliferation by Lyt antisera, *Proc. Natl. Acad. Sci. U.S.A.* **77:**2890–2894.

Nerenberg, S. T., and Prasad, R., 1975, Radioimmunoassays for Ig Classes G, A, M, D, and E in spinal fluids: Normal values for different age groups, *J. Lab. Clin. Med.* **86:**887–893.

Noelle, R. J., and Lawrence, D. A., 1981, Determination of glutathione in lymphocyte and possible association of redox state and proliferative capacity of lymphocytes, *Biochem. J.* **198:**571–579.

Otte, R. G., Wormsley, S., and Hollingsworth, J. W., 1983, Cytofluorographic analysis of pokeweed mitogen-stimulated human peripheral blood cells in culture; age-related characteristics, *J. Am. Geriatr. Soc.* **31:**49–56.

Palmblad, J., 1976, Fasting (acute energy deprivation) in man: Effect on polymorphonuclear granulocyte functions, plasma iron and serum transferrin, *Scand. J. Haematol.* **17:**217–226.

Palmblad, J., Cantell, K., Holm, G., Nordberg, R., Stranders, H., and Sunblad, I., 1977, Acute energy deprivation in man: Effect on serum immunoglobulins antibody response, complement factors 3 and 4, acute phase reactants and interferon-producing capacity of blood lymphocytes, *Clin. Exp. Immunol.* **30:**50–55.

Penschow, J., and Mackay, I. R., 1980, NK and K cell activity of human blood: Differences according to sex, age, and disease, *Ann. Rheum. Dis.* **39:**82–86.

Popp, D. M., and Francis, M., 1979, Age-associated changes T–B cell cooperation demonstrated by the allogeneic effect, *Mech. Ageing Dev.* **10:**341–353.

Price, G. B., and Makinodan, T., 1972a, Immunologic deficiencies in senescence, I. Characterization of intrinsic deficiencies, *J. Immunol.* **108:**403–412.

Price, G. B., and Makinodan, T., 1972b, Immunologic deficiencies in senescence, II. Characterization of extrinsic deficiencies, *J. Immunol.* **108:**413–417.

Radix, P. M., Walters, C. S., and Adkins, J. A., 1983, The influence of ethionine-supplemented soy protein diet on cell-mediated and humoral immunity, *J. Nutr.* **113:**159–164.

Radl, J., Sepers, J. M., Skvaril, F., Morell, A., and Hijmans, W., 1975, Immunological patterns in humans over 95 years of age, *Clin. Exp. Immunol.* **22:**84–90.

Robson, S., and Schwarz, M. R., 1975, Vitamin B_6 deficiency and the lymphoid system. I. Effects on cellular immunity and in vitro incorporation of 3H-uridine by small lymphocytes. *Cell. Immunol.* **16:**135–144.

Roghmann, K. J., Tabloshki, P. A., Bentley, D. W., and Schiffman, G., 1987, Immune response of elderly adults to pneumococcus: Variation by age, sex, and functional impairment, *J. Gerontol.* **42:**265–270.

Rose, C. S., Gyorgy, P., Butler, M., Andres, R., Norris, A. H., Shock, N. W., Tobin, J., Brin, M., and Spiegel, H., 1976, Age differences in vitamin B_6 status of 617 men, *Am. J. Clin. Nutr.* **29:**847–853.

Rosenberg, J. S., Gilman, S. C., and Feldman, J. D., 1983, Effect of aging on cell cooperation and lymphocyte responsiveness to cytokines, *J. Immunol.* **130:**1754–1758.

Rosenkoetter, C. M., Antel, J. P., and Oger, J. J. F., 1983, Modulation of T lymphocyte differentiation antigens: Influence of aging, *Cell. Immunol.* **77:**395–401.

Rosenstein, M. M., and Strauser, H. R., 1980, Macrophage induced T-cell mitogen suppression with age, *J. Reticuloendothel. Soc.* **27:**159–166.

Ruhl, H., and Kirchner, H., 1978, Monocyte-dependent stimulation of human T cells by zinc, *Clin. Exp. Immunol.* **32:**484–488.

Sandstead, H. H., Henriksen, L. K., Greger, J. L., Parsad, A. S., and Good, R. A., 1982, Zinc nutriture in the elderly in relation to taste acuity, immune response, and wound healing, *Am. J. Clin. Nutr.* **26:**1046–1059.

Satoh, K., 1978, Serum lipid peroxides in cerebrovascular disorders determined by a new caloremetric method, *Clin. Chim. Acta* **90:**37–43.

Shofield, J. D., and Davies, I., 1978, Theories of aging, in: *Geriatric Medicine and Gerontology* (J. C. Brocklehurst, ed.), Churchill Livingstone, Edinburgh, pp. 37–70.

Schulof, R. S., Garofalo, J. A., Good, R. A., and Gupta, S., 1980, Concanavalin A-induced suppressor cell activity for T-cell proliferative responses: Autologous and allogeneic suppression in aging humans, *Cell. Immunol.* **56:**80–88.

Scrimshaw, N. S., 1964, Protein deficiency and infective disease, in: *Mammalian Protein Metabolism,* Volume 2 (H. N. Munro and J. B. Allison, eds.), Academic Press, New York, pp. 569–592.

Scrimshaw, N. S., Taylor, C. E., and Gordon, J. E., 1959, Interactions of nutrition and infection, *Am. J. Med. Sci.* **237:**367–403.

Segal, J., 1986, Studies on the age-related decline in the response of lymphoid cells to mitogens: Measurement of concanavalin A binding and stimulation of calcium and sugar uptake in thymocytes from rats of varying ages, *Mech. Ageing Dev.* **33:**295–303.

Sies, H., and Wendel, A. (eds.), 1978, *Functions of Glutathione in Liver and Kidney,* Springer-Verlag, New York.

Smythe, P. M., Schonland, M., and Breneton-Stiles, C. C., 1971, Thymolymphatic deficiency and depression of cell-mediated immunity in protein–calorie malnutrition, *Lancet* **2:**939–943.

Stiedeman, M., and Harrell, I., 1980, Relation of immunocompetence to selected nutrients in elderly women, *Nutr. Rep. Int.* **21:**931–940.

Stinnett, J. D., 1983, Historical perspectives of malnutrition and disease, in: *Nutrition and the Immune Response,* (J. D. Stinnett, ed.) CRC Press, Boca Raton, FL, pp. 1–5.

Suzuki, K., Swenson, C., Sasagawa, S., Sakatani, T., Watanabe, M., Kobayashi, M., and Fujikura, T., 1982, Age-related decline in lysosomal enzyme release from polymorphonuclear leukocytes after N-formyl-methionylleucyl-phenylalanine stimulation, *Exp. Hematol.* **11:**1005–1013.

Svematsu, T., Kamada, T., Abe, H., Kikudzi, S., and Yagi, K., 1977, Serum lipoperoxide level in patients suffering from liver disease, *Clin. Chim. Acta* **79:**267–271.

Talbott, M. C., Miller, L. T., and Kerkvliet, N., 1987, Pyridoxine supplementation: Effect of lymphocyte response in elderly persons, *Am. J. Clin. Nutr.* **46:**659–664.

Tam, C. F., and Walford, R. L., 1978, Cyclic nucleotide levels in resting and mitogen-stimulated spleen cell suspensions from young and old mice, *Mech. Ageing Dev.* **7:**309–320.

Tanka, J., Fuyiwara, H., and Torisu, M., 1979, Vitamin E and immune response: Enhancement of helper T cell activity by dietary supplementation of vitamin E in mice, *Immunology* **38:**727–734.

Taylor, G., 1966, Diet of elderly women, *Lancet* **1:**926.

Tengerdy, P., and Brown, J. C., 1977, Effect of vitamin E and A on humoral immunity and phagocytosis in *E. coli* infected chickens, *Poultry Sci.* **56:**957–963.

Tengerdy, R. P., 1980, Effect of vitamin E on immune responses, *Basic Clin. Nutr.* **1:**429–445.

Thoman, M. L., and Weigle, W. O., 1982, Lymphokines and aging: Interleukin-2 production and activity in aged animals, *J. Immunol.* **127:**2102–2106.

Twomey, J. J., Luchi, R. J., and Kouttab, N. M., 1982, Null cell senescence and its potential significance to the immunobiology of aging, *J. Clin. Invest.* **70:**201–204.

Underwood, B. A., Sigel, H., Dolinski, M., and Weisell, R. C., 1970, Liver stores of alpha-tocopherol in a normal population dying suddenly and rapidly from unnatural causes in New York City, *Am. J. Clin. Nutr.* **23:**1314–1321.

Vatassery, G. T., Johnson, G. J., and Krezowski, A. M., 1983, Changes in vitamin E concentrations in human plasma and platelets with age, *J. Am. Coll. Nutr.* **4:**369–375.

Vie, H., and Miller, R. A., 1986, Decline, with age, in the proportions of mouse T cells that express IL-2 receptors after mitogen stimulation, *Mech. Ageing Dev.* **33:**313–322.

Wagner, P. A., Jernigan, J. A., Baily, L. B., Nickens, C., and Brazzi, G. A., 1983, Zinc nutriture and cell mediated immunity in the aged, *Int. J. Vitam. Nutr. Res.* **53:**94–101.

Walford, R. L., 1982, Studies in immunogerontology. *J. Am. Geriatr. Soc.* **30:**617–622.

Walford, R. L., Liu, R. K., Gebrase-DeLima, M., Mathies, M., and Smith, G. S., 1973, Longterm dietary restriction and immune function in mice: Response to sheep red blood cells and to mitogenic agents, *Mech. Ageing Dev.* **2:**447–454.

Walford, R. L., Gottesman, S. R. S., and Weindruch, R. H., 1981, Immunopathology of aging, *Annu. Rev. Gerontol. Geriatr.* **2:**3–15.

Wartanowicz, M., Panczenko-Kresowska, B., Ziemlanski, S., Kowalska, M., and Okolska, G., 1984, The effect of alpha-tocopherol and ascorbic acid on the serum lipid peroxide level in elderly people, *Am. Nutr. Metab.* **28:**186–191.

Weindruch, R. H., and Suffin, S. L., 1980, Quantitative histologic effects on mouse thymus of controlled dietary restriction, *J. Gerontol.* **4:**525–531.

Weindruch, R. H., and Walford, R. L., 1982, Dietary restriction in mice beginning at 1 year of age: Effect on lifespan and spontaneous cancer incidence, *Science* **215:**1415–1418.

Weindruch, R. H., Kristie, J. A., Cheney, K. E., and Walford, R. L., 1979, Influence of controlled dietary restriction on immunologic function and aging, *Fed. Proc.* **38**(6):2007–2016.

Weindruch, R. H., Gottesman, S. R. S., and Walford, R. L., 1982a, Modification of age-related immune decline in mice dietarily restricted from or after midadulthood, *Proc. Natl. Acad. Sci. U.S.A.* **79:**898–902.

Weindruch, R. H., Kristie, J. A., Noeim, F., Mullen, B. G., and Walford, R. L., 1982b, Influence of weaning-initiated dietary restriction on responses to T cell mitogens and on splenic T cell levels in a long-lived F_1-hybrid mouse strain, *Exp. Gerontol.* **17:**49–64.

Weindruch, R. H., Devens, B. H., Raff, H. V., and Walford, R. L., 1983, Influence of dietary restriction and aging on natural killer cell activity in mice, *J. Immunol.* **130:**993–996.

Weindruch, R. A., Thomas, D. J., Adler, W. H., and Lindsay, T. J., 1984, Supplemental zinc restores antibody formation in cultures of aged spleen cells, *J. Immunol.* **133:**569–571.

Weindruch, R., Walford, R. L., Fligiel, S., and Guthrie, D., 1986, The retardation of aging in mice by dietary restriction: Longevity, cancer, immunity and lifetime energy intake, *J. Nutr.* **116:**641–654.

Weitekamp, M. R., and Aber, R. C., 1984, Nonbacterial and unusual pneumonias in the elderly, *Geriatrics* **39:**87–100.

Wei Wo, C. K., and Draper, H. H., 1975, Vitamin E status of Alaskan Eskimos, *Am. J. Clin. Nutr.* **28:**808–813.

Weksler, M. E., 1981, The senescence of the immune system, *Hosp. Pract.* **16:**53–64.

Weksler, M. E., 1983, Senescence of the immune system, *Med. Clin. North Am.* **67:**263–272.

Williams, G. O., 1980, Vaccines in older patients: Combating the risk of mortality, *Geriatrics* **35:**55–64.

Wilson, T. S., Weeks, M. M., Mukheyee, S. K., Murrell, J. S.. and Andrews, C. T., 1972, A study of vitamin C levels in the aged and subsequent mortality, *Gerontol. Clin.* **14:**17–24.

Wilson, T. S., Datta, S. B., Murrell, J. S., and Andrews, C. T., 1973, Relationship of vitamin C to mortality in a geriatric hospital: A study of the effect of vitamin C administration, *Age Aging* **2:**163–171.

Yu, B. F., Masoro, E. J., Murata, I., Bertrand, H. A., and Lynd, F. T., 1982, Life span study of SPF Fischer 344 male rats fed *ad libitum* on restricted diets: Longevity, growth, lean body mass and disease, *J. Gerontol.* **37:**130–141.

Ziemlanski, S., Wartanowicz, M., Kios, A., Raczka, A., and Kios, M., 1986, The effects of ascorbic acid and alpha-tocopherol supplementation on serum proteins and immunoglobulin concentrations in the elderly, *Nutr. Internatl.* **2:**1–5.

5

Exercise and Nutrition in the Elderly

William J. Evans and Carol N. Meredith

1. Introduction

Old age has traditionally been considered a time for reducing activity and accepting a decline in health and vigor that eventually leads to death. Images of old people in literature and art show them involved in a sedentary existence that was the reward for a lifetime of hard work; indeed, places that house and care for the aged have been called "rest homes." The large and increasing number of people aged over 65 (more than 22% of the U.S. population by the year 2050) and their better health have pushed back the limits of old age. One hundred years ago, at the age of 58 a man could be considered used up. Five hundred years ago, Christopher Columbus at 51 was dangerously old for embarking on his fourth voyage to America, and Emperor Charles V of Spain at age 55 was ready to abdicate and retire to a monastery, to prepare for death by prayer and meditation (Braudel, 1979). Today, only 3 to 4% of those aged 55 to 64 are too disabled to walk half a mile or climb stairs, although by age 75 to 84 more than 15% have difficulties in walking and more than half cannot lift or move large objects, as shown in Fig. 1 (Jette and Branch, 1981).

The biological length of human life has not changed. Only 0.01% of the population in developed countries can expect to live beyond 100 years, and life expectancy at age 75 has increased by only 3 years in this century (Fries, 1980). The great achievement of medicine and public health has been to increase life expectancy at birth (Fries, 1980), mainly through better hygiene and nutrition, to improve active life expectancy, defined as the age after which people need help in order to eat, move about, dress, or bathe, and to reduce the mortality rate of chronic degenerative diseases such as ischemic heart disease and stroke (Manton and Soldo, 1985). At present, people aged 65–70 can expect another 10 years of life, whereas active life expectancy for those over 85 is only 2.9 years (Katz *et al.*, 1983). Many of the changes that lead to loss of function result from biological effects of age. However, the similarity between changes found

William J. Evans and Carol N. Meredith • USDA Human Nutrition Research Center on Aging, Tufts University, Boston, Massachusetts 02111.

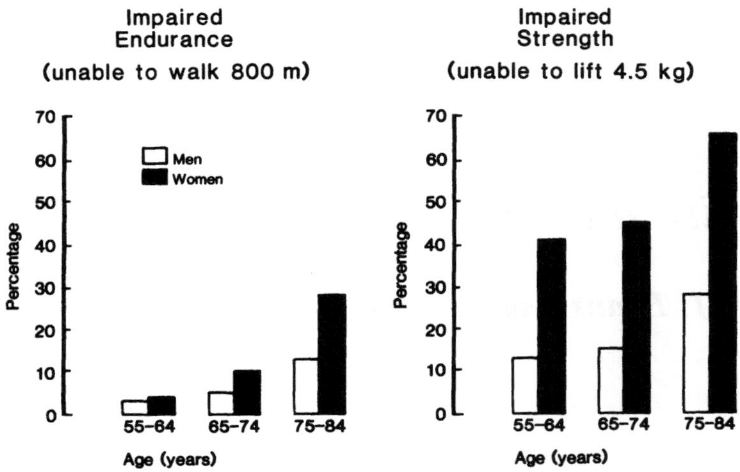

Fig. 1. Prevalence of impaired endurance or impaired strength among aging men and women, from the Framingham Study. Functional impairment was greatest in elderly women. (Drawn from data of Jette and Branch, 1981.)

with age and the loss of function induced by physical inactivity has suggested that disuse may result in so called "age-related changes" (Bortz, 1982).

The amount of daily activity and of regular physical exercise undertaken by children and adults living in a prosperous country today is mainly a matter of personal choice. This unprecedented change is recent. Up to the first decades of this century, most people lived on farms and spent long days doing moderately hard physical labor. Only a fraction of the U.S. population today can be described as working in moderate to hard occupations such as mining or lumberjacking. Until the industrial age, holidays also were celebrated not only by eating and drinking but by exuberant activities involving dancing and the types of round games now relegated to small children (Aries, 1962). Today, time not used earning wages is spent doing less exercise than ever before. Recreation tends to involve hours in front of the television set (Dietz and Gortmaker, 1985). Vigorous play is socially acceptable mainly as organized team sports for children and young men, with few activities considered proper for women or for men beyond middle-age. At the same time, the cost of food in proportion to earnings has declined, and the variety and palatability of the diet have increased. In 17th century Europe, 80% of the dietary calories consumed by all except the richest people were provided by carbohydrates, mainly as bread and gruel (Braudel, 1979). Although dietary abundance and variety have led to the virtual disappearance of specific nutrient deficiencies in the United States, it has also encouraged overeating.

As people eat more and exercise less, at their discretion, by the onset of middle-age about 20% of men and 40% of women are obese (Ten-State Nutrition Survey, 1968). Obesity, which is most prevalent in persons aged 40 to 60, is in itself a health hazard and further discourages exercise because of the effort of breathing and moving (Whipp and Davis, 1984). Among the "oldest old" (those aged over 85), exercise is often limited by physical or mental disability: 24% of men and 35% of women of this age cannot independently perform activities of daily living, and about 20% have Alzheimer's disease (Manton and Soldo, 1985). There is little information about how the impaired mobility of very old people could be prevented or treated with exercise rehabilitation, yet there is an increasing need for strategies to prevent old people from becoming "frail elderly." In 1980, there were about 2 million people over the age of 85 in the United States, but by 2050 this group will have grown to 16 million (Suzman and White-Riley, 1985).

Changing exercise habits in a sedentary population is already a challenge, but it is probably more difficult in the aging because there seems to be a natural reduction in voluntary activity with age. In rodents, voluntary activity increases during development and then gradually declines after 3 or 4 months of age (Mondon *et al.*, 1985; Smith and Dugal, 1965; Mark *et al.*, 1986). Activity in rodents is greater in females throughout life (Tokuyama *et al.*, 1982), in underfed males (Yu *et al.*, 1985), and in males subjected to intermittent fasting and also shows marked individual variability (Mondon *et al.*, 1985). In humans, the decline in voluntary activity with age can be judged from questionnaires and estimated from functional tests that measure physical fitness. Table I shows the aerobic capacity of men at different ages in different societies, reflecting their habitual activity and exercise levels.

In young men chosen from the general urban population, aerobic capacity or Vo_2-max tends to be low; it is slightly higher in men from rural areas of developed countries, such as Israeli kibbutzim. Modern Canadian wheat farmers (average age 42 years) have an average Vo_2max of 37.5 ml/kg per min during the harvesting season, higher than for the general population but still suggestive of a sedentary life (Cumming and Bailey, 1974; Bailey *et al.*, 1974). The Vo_2max is higher in athletes or men from rural, primitive societies. In unmechanized farming or manual work, where wages are earned from physical labor, physical fitness contributes directly to income, as productivity is a linear function of Vo_2max (Spurr, 1984). The capacity to carry out hard and prolonged physical activity has become less important in prosperous, highly mechanized societies. In the Masai, Vo_2max does not decline until after age 40 (Mann *et al.*,

Table I. Vo_2max and Age in Different Populations of Men[a]

	Vo_2max (ml/kg per min)			
Subjects	Age 21–30	Age 31–40	Age 51–60	Age 61–70
(1) Masai	58	58	40	—
(2) Israeli kibbutz	41	39	—	—
Israeli urban	36	33	—	—
(3) Canadian, 1974	36	32	26	—
(4) U.S., 1938	48	42	40	30
(5) U.S., 1986	36	28	—	—
(6) Czechoslovakian urban	42	—	—	18
(7) Swedish laborers	—	43	34	29

[a]From: (1) Mann *et al.*, 1965; (2) Epstein *et al.*, 1982; (3) Bailey *et al.*, 1974; (4) Robinson, 1983; (5) Higginbotham *et al.*, 1986; (6) Parizkova *et al.*, 1971; (7) Astrand, 1967.

Table II. Daily Activity and Body Composition of Iranian Rural Men at Different Ages[a]

Age	Body mass index (kg/m^2)	Energy expenditure (kcal/kg per day)
21–30	21.3 ± 0.8	58.4 ± 6.4
31–40	21.8 ± 1.6	56.8 ± 9.5
41–50	21.0 ± 1.1	53.4 ± 10.9

[a]Results are mean ± S.D. for a cross-sectional study. Calculated from Brun *et al.* (1979).

1965), whereas in developed countries the decline in activity and physical fitness occurs soon after adolescence or early adult life. In rural Iran (Table II), energy expenditure among men in their 20s is about 27% higher than for U.S. college students and declines only 9% over two decades of aging (Brun *et al.*, 1979; Scrimshaw *et al.*, 1972); Iranian farmers also maintain low body fat as they age. In Holland, a linear decline in energy output occurs throughout adolescence, from age 12 to 18, because less time is spent walking, cycling, and participating in sports (Verschuur and Kemper, 1985).

Few studies have accurately examined exercise habits and phyical fitness of the elderly in less-developed countries, although they are believed to be exceptionally vigorous (Leaf, 1973). Isolated ethnic groups may have developed over many generations a genetically different pattern of aging. This may explain the low prevalence of osteoporosis among elderly blacks in the United States or the 50% prevalence of diabetes mellitus among Pima Indians over the age of 50 (Bourliere, 1978). Nonetheless, differences in aging between populations, ethnic groups, and social classes mostly reflect life-long habits and adaptation to ecological factors. Old people living in an unmechanized, rugged environment appear more active, but the intensity of daily exercise may be insufficient to produce a marked effect on functional capacity. In Nepalese elderly men, only 5 to 30% of those aged over 60 engaged in strenuous activity (determined by heart rate monitor) for more than 20 min a day. Although they were smaller and leaner than average for 63-year-old U.S. workers, they showed a similar heart rate during exercise at a workload of 74 watts suggesting similar physical fitness (Beall *et al.*, 1985). A study of 50 men and women aged 60 to 69 in southern China showed a large daily energy intake of about 44 kcal/kg per day: 48% worked in the fields for a few hours every day, 36% did heavy work at home, and 16 % were unable to do more than light work (Ho, 1982). Habitual low-intensity activity in rural environments may have a greater effect on food intake and body fat than on functional capacity.

Elderly Americans today have led a more sedentary and well-fed existence than ever before in history. Among Harvard graduates of all ages, not more than 20% spend more than 2 hr a week playing sports (Paffenbarger *et al.*, 1986). A study in California showed that only 8% of men and 2% of women aged 50 to 64 reported regular vigorous exercise during the previous year (Sallis *et al.*, 1985). Many older people are obese, unable to tolerate intense or prolonged physical activity, and susceptible to cardiovascular disease, hypertension, and diabetes. Measures to prevent obesity and to increase physical activity, both light and vigorous, are needed to improve the health and longevity of the aging.

In rodents, physical activity increases longevity (Mark *et al.*, 1986; Goodrick, 1980), although dietary restriction has a greater effect (Ross, 1977). There is an inverse correlation between body weight and longevity: exercised rats grow more slowly, which may account for the life-prolonging effects of exercise. In humans it has been difficult to establish the effects of exercise on health and longevity independently from associated changes in fatness. With or without considering hypertension, cigarette smoking, weight gain, or early parental death as factors, mortality is significantly lower among physically active men (Paffenbarger *et al.*, 1986). Maintaining physical activity throughout life is more important than early athletic prowess: former international rugby players show the same survival curve as the general population (Beaglehole and Stewart, 1983), and the death rate among aging, sedentary men who had been college athletes in the United States is only slightly lower than for men who had never been physically active (Paffenbarger *et al.*, 1986). Even in men with familial hypercholesterolemia and at high risk for early coronary heart disease, a physically active life style seems to delay the expression of this lethal trait (William *et al.*, 1986).

The term "exercise" can be used for a variety of voluntary contractions of the skeletal muscles. Physical training is achieved by performing a certain type of exercise with a given intensity, duration, and frequency. The improvement in health and physical function depends on the type of training. Endurance exercise has been defined as any activity that uses large muscle groups, is rhythmical in nature, and can be sustained for a long time, such as walking, jogging, bicycling, rowing, or skiing. Strength exercise involves exerting force against an immovable object (static strength) or exerting force in order to lift or lower a weight (dynamic strength). The capacity to perform

Table III. Endurance Training and Strength Training: Typical Exercise Programs and Results

Exercise prescription	Endurance	Strength
Type	Many rhythmical contractions of large muscle groups	A few repeated contractions of muscle groups
Intensity	60 to 75% of $\dot{V}O_2$max[a]	Over 60% of 1 RM[a]
Duration	15 to 20 min/session	15 to 21 repetitions/session
Frequency	3 to 5 days/week	3 days/week
Training effects	Increased $\dot{V}O_2$max Improved cardiovascular function Increased oxidative capacity of muscle fibers Increased capillarization of muscle	Increased strength Increased muscle mass Increased muscle fiber size

[a] $\dot{V}O_2$max is maximum oxygen consumption during graded exercise and determines the maximum intensity of aerobic exercise. One RM is one repetition maximum, i.e., the maximum weight that can be lifted once through a complete range of motion. This determines maximum dynamic strength.

low-intensity endurance exercise or weight-lifting exercise is impaired in a substantial part of the elderly population, especially in women, as shown in Fig. 1. Typical exercise prescriptions for these two types of training and some of their effects are summarized in Table III.

The evidence that leaner, more active people live longer and healthier lives is giving rise to new questions. In a sedentary population of old people, what type and intensity of exercise will benefit health and functional capacity? In preventing and treating the increased adiposity of middle age, what is the role of diet and of exercise? How do diet and exercise affect the appearance, progress, and treatment of age-related diseases? What age-related changes are inevitable, and which may be caused in part or entirely by changes in activity? How are the nutritional needs of the elderly affected by extremes of inactivity or activity? What difference is there in metabolic adaptation to exercise and training in the elderly compared to the young?

In this chapter, information from the scientific literature is brought together to address these questions.

2. *Energy Metabolism*

Daily energy expenditure declines progressively throughout adult life in all societies (McGandy *et al.*, 1966; Ho, 1982). Under sedentary conditions, the main determinant of energy expenditure is fat-free mass (Ravussin *et al.*, 1986), which declines about 15% between the ages 20–29 and 70–79, contributing to a lower basal metabolic rate in the elderly (Cohn *et al.*, 1980). Exercise training has no effect on basal energy expenditure of the elderly: in highly active old men, basal metabolic rate was not higher than for sedentary controls (Lundholm *et al.*, 1986).

A minor component of daily energy output is the thermogenic effect of food (TEF). The increase in energy output after a meal depends on the diet and the physical characteristics of the person consuming the meal. A larger energy intake and higher protein content of meals increase TEF in young subjects (Belko *et al.*, 1986). As people become older and fatter, there is a reduction in TEF (Schutz *et al.*, 1984; Golay *et al.*, 1983). The inverse correlation found between TEF and age (Golay *et al.*, 1983) could result from age itself or from lower physical training, decreased glucose tolerance, or increased adiposity among older subjects, but the biochemical mechanisms for these effects are not known. It has been suggested that insulin resistance, which reduces glucose uptake and glucose storage as glycogen in muscles, is responsible for decreasing the thermic effect of food (Ravussin *et al.*, 1985). Physical exercise increases TEF. In lean, young persons, aerobic training increased TEF in proportion to the improvement in Vo_2max (Davis *et al.*, 1983), and the effects of a single bout of exercise depend on the time elapsed between the end of exercise and the test meal. Immediately after an exercise bout, TEF increases (Segal *et al.*, 1985; Young *et al.*, 1986), partly because of the cost of storing glucose as glycogen (Devlin and Horton, 1986), but by 16 hr after exercise TEF is lower than initial values (Tremblay *et al.*, 1985). In ten highly trained old men (69 ± 2 years old) studied at least 2 days after their last exercise bout, the thermic effects of a 500-kcal mixed meal were about 36% higher than for sedentary men of similar weight, height, and age (Lundholm *et al.*,

1986); the authors suggest that enhanced sensitivity to catecholamines in the trained men could account for their higher TEF.

Energy needs of the general population in developed countries are low and decline from an early age. Male high school students in Holland or college students in the United States need about 46 kcal/kg per day to maintain body weight (Verschuur and Kemper, 1985; Scrimshaw *et al.*, 1972). Female high school students in Holland need about 41 kcal/kg per day (Verschuur and Kemper, 1985), and English women aged 31 ± 7 years and working in clerical jobs or as housewives have an average energy expenditure of 31 kcal/kg per day, only 35% more than basal metabolic rate (Prentice *et al.*, 1985). In the elderly, energy intake is remarkably low, as shown by nutrition surveys of persons aged over 65 in the United States: about 1400 kcal/day (23 kcal/kg per day) for women and about 1870 kcal/day (27 kcal/kg per day) for men (Brown *et al.*, 1977; McGandy *et al.*, 1966; Dibble *et al.*, 1967; Ten-State Survey, 1972). Although surveys may underestimate food intake (Hallfrisch *et al.*, 1982), weighed intake methods used to study the food consumption of elderly men and women living in institutions or at home also show energy intakes that tend to be below the U.S. recommended dietary allowance (Table IV). Metabolic ward studies of noninstitutionalized elderly men and women in which energy intakes for maintenance of body weight were exactly measured show a tendency for energy needs to decrease with age (Table V). The remarkably low energy intakes shown by Stiedemann *et al.* (1978) may be because 48% of the people studied were between 85 and 98 years of age. Declining physical activity partly accounts for low energy intake. A cross-sectional study of elderly French women has shown that energy intakes are lower and decline at an earlier age in urban areas, where everyday living and work demand less physical effort than in rural areas (Debry *et al.*, 1977).

There are few studies available on the exact energy needs of the "oldest old," although it is likely that increasing disability in this group further reduces physical movement and leads to very low energy expenditure (Minaker and Rowe, 1985). Because the intake of most nutrients depends on total energy intake, elderly people

Table IV. Energy Consumption (Mean ± S.E.M.) of Elderly Men and Women, Measured by Weighing Food Intake

Group[a]	Men	Women
(1) U.S., aged 62–98	1720 ± 310	1330 ± 270
(2) Spain, average age 82	1830 ± 120	1690 ± 140
(3) France, rural and urban		
age 65–77	—	1950
age > 78	—	1730
(4) England, aged 70–86	2200	1650
RDA	2400	1800

[a]From: (1) Stiedmann *et al.*, 1978; (2) Moreiras-Varela *et al.*, 1986; (3) Debry and Bleyer, 1969; (4) Bunker *et al.*, 1984.

Table V. Energy Needs of Elderly Subjects Studied in a Metabolic Ward[a]

Ref.[b]	Sex	N	Age (years)	Energy requirements (kcal/kg per day)
(1)	M	5	64 ± 2	34.1 ± 1.8
(4)	M	6	68 ± 5	30.2 ± 1.4
(2)	M	7	71 ± 2	31.5 ± 4.1
(3)	M	5	75 ± 5	32.7 ± 3.2
(1)	F	5	65 ± 2	39.7 ± 2.3
(2)	F	7	74 ± 2	27.6 ± 6.1
(3)	F	5	79 ± 12	31.4 ± 3.3

[a]Daily energy intake (mean ± S.D.) for maintenance of body weight for 10 to 30 days. Data selected for subjects whose weight varied less than 0.6 kg over each study period.

[b]From: (1) C. N. Meredith and W. J. Evans, unpublished observations; (2) Uauy *et al.*, 1978; (3) Gersovitz *et al.*, 1982; (4) Calloway and Zanni, 1980.

who maintain body weight with a small intake of food may be consuming undesirably low amounts of proteins, minerals, and vitamins. An increase in activity leading to greater food intake could be the best strategy for reducing the risk of malnutrition in ambulatory elderly people.

Activity accounts for most of the difference in the energy needs of people throughout life. Even in the absence of conscious physical exercise, a large part of the variability in energy expenditure depends on minor movements or fidgeting (Ravussin *et al.*, 1986). An increase in physical activity has different effects depending on its nature, intensity, and frequency. Physiological adaptations to training in young subjects occur with aerobic exercise performed at least three times a week for sessions of more than 30 min, preferably at intensities greater than 70% Vo_2max, although in elderly subjects whose initial physical fitness may be very low, moderate exercise at 57% of Vo_2max is a conditioning stimulus and can substantially increase weekly energy expenditure (Badenhop *et al.*, 1983).

It is important to point out that exercise of any intensity will increase energy expenditure even if it fails to increase endurance or strength. However, as a treatment for middle-aged obesity, exercise with no dietary restriction is not consistently effective, and the weight loss is slight, as shown in Table VI, although it tends to be greater as the duration of the exercise program increases. In middle-aged subjects, exercise combined with dietary restriction has sometimes been shown to produce weight loss similar to diet treatment alone. Improved fat loss with a combination of diet and exercise was shown in 72 obese middle-aged men, who lost 10.1 kg of fat and 0.11 kg of protein compared to a 5.3-kg fat loss and 0.64-kg protein loss with diet alone (Pavlou *et al.*, 1985). However, in a younger and smaller group of seven women and one man, the 8-kg fat loss obtained when exercise was incorporated into the restricted diet program was not significantly higher than the 7-kg fat loss obtained with diet alone (Bogardus *et al.*, 1984).

In contrast to endurance training, strength training to achieve an increase in energy expenditure has not been extensively studied. In young men and women, 10

Table VI. Changes in Energy Reserves with Exercise and No Dietary Restriction in Men and Women of Different Ages

N^a	Age (years)	Exercise program	Weight change	Changes in subcutaneous fat (mm skinfolds)
(1) 55 M	17–59	10 weeks, aerobic	−1%	−7%
(2) 13 M, 25 F	65	14 weeks, aerobic	NS	−8%
(3) 36 M	60–79	14 weeks, aerobic	−2%	−4%
(4) 7 M	48	25 weeks, aerobic	−2%	—
(4) 8 M	58	25 weeks, aerobic	−2%	—
(5) 169 M,F	35–50	68 weeks, aerobic	−5%	—
(6) 7 M	39–59	96 weeks, aerobic	−6%	−20%
(7) 6 M	60–69	12 weeks, strength	NS	NS

[a]From: (1) Wilmore *et al.*, 1974; (2) Sidney *et al.*, 1977; (3) Buccola and Stone, 1975; (4) Tzankoff *et al.*, 1972; (5) Kukkonen *et al.*, 1982; (6) Carter and Phillips, 1969; (7) Frontera *et al.*, 1988.

weeks of strength training for muscles of the upper and lower body with no dietary restriction did not affect body weight but increased lean mass by 2% and decreased fat mass by 8–9% (Wilmore, 1974). However, in six men aged 64 ± 2 years, a 12-week strength-training program of only extensors and flexors of the legs, while eating their usual diet, did not alter body weight or body fat (Frontera, 1986). There are no studies available on the effects of weight training in older women.

For the elderly, an increase in energy expenditure with the purpose of improving appetite and nutrient intake can best be achieved by prolonging the time spent in light to moderate activities such as walking, cycling, playing golf, doing calisthenics, or dancing. These types of exercises allow the expenditure of about 4 to 5 kcal/min (Passmore and Durnin, 1955; Calloway and Zanni, 1980) and are least likely to produce injury. Elderly people enrolled in a training program tend to drop out after an episode of illness or disability (Kriska *et al.*, 1986), so it is particularly important for them to avoid strain, pain, or injury.

Although middle-aged runners develop an energy intake that is 40 to 60% greater than sedentary men and women of the same age (Blair *et al.*, 1981), there is no information available on the change in food intake produced by an active life style or an exercise program in elderly subjects. However, the prevalence of extremely low energy intake is less among elderly people who are physically active. In elderly women, energy intakes below 1500 kcal/day were found in 33% of those classified as "inactive," in 12% of "moderately active," and only 9% of the "very active" women (Debry *et al.*, 1977). In endurance-trained middle-aged men, energy needs were a linear function of hours spent exercising per week in the same way as for young men (Meredith *et al.*, 1987). This suggests that better nutrition may be achieved in sedentary middle-aged or old people by increasing activity, together with an improvement in physical endurance and strength.

In conclusion, increased physical activity in the elderly is associated with a larger food intake together with a reduction in body energy stores, and these changes have a favorable effect on health

3. Carbohydrate Metabolism

3.1. Effects of Age

Increasing age is associated with major changes in whole-body carbohydrate metabolism. The two-hour plasma glucose level during an oral glucose tolerance test increases by an average 5.3 mg/dl per decade, and fasting plasma glucose increases by an average of 1 mg/dl per decade (Davidson, 1979). These age-related changes in glucose tolerance can result in non-insulin-dependent diabetes mellitus (NIDDM). A large survey in the United States that used the oral glucose tolerance test showed that 13% of men and women between the ages of 60 and 74 had impaired glucose tolerance and an additional 17% had NIDDM (Harris, 1982).

Chronically elevated insulin levels may have a role in the development of atherosclerosis, as exogenous insulin enhances the synthesis of cholesterol, triglyceride, and fatty acids in the aorta (Stout, 1981). It has been speculated that even the mild hyperinsulinemia seen in the elderly may play a role in the atherogenic process (Fink *et al.*, 1984). High insulin levels have been shown to be an independent risk factor for the development and subsequent complications of coronary artery disease (Ducimetiere *et al.*, 1980; Jarret *et al.*, 1982). Impaired glucose tolerance is also associated with an increased risk of developing atherosclerotic disease and cataracts and a greatly increased risk of developing NIDDM (Holloszy *et al.*, 1986); NIDDM increases the risk of intermittent claudication, microvascular disease leading to retinopathy and nephropathy, neuropathy, cataracts, and increased risk of infections.

The relationship between aging, body composition, activity, and glucose tolerance was examined in 270 female and 462 male factory workers aged 22 to 73 years, none of whom were retired (Zavaroni *et al.*, 1986). Plasma glucose levels, both fasting and after a glucose load, increased with age, but the correlation between age and total integrated glucose response following a glucose load was weak: in women, only 3% of the variance could be attributed to age. When activity levels and drug use were factored in, age accounted for only 1% of the variance in women and 6.25% in men. The response to meals is different from the response to oral glucose. In elderly (aged 60–83 years) and young (aged 23–58 years) subjects, the glucose and insulin response were studied following an oral glucose tolerance test and a mixed liquid meal (Fink *et al.*, 1984). The total glucose response following oral glucose was 24% higher in the older subjects but only 11% higher after the meal tolerance test. Similarly, insulin levels were 127% greater in the old subjects following the OGTT but only 40% greater following the meal tolerance test compared to the young subjects.

Older persons, who are generally less physically active than young people, have more fat and less lean tissue, as can be observed in Fig. 2. Reaven and Reaven (1980) have stated that "Age itself, as differentiated from the effects of obesity, diabetes, etc., has a relatively trivial effect on glucose tolerance, and even this effect is largely confined to patients over 60. The effect of age, *per se,* on glucose tolerance is quantitatively minor in magnitude."

The rate of glucose disposal and the sensitivity of tissues to insulin have been studied by the euglycemic glucose clamp technique described by DeFronzo *et al.* (1979). Insulin is infused into a subject at a constant rate while plasma glucose

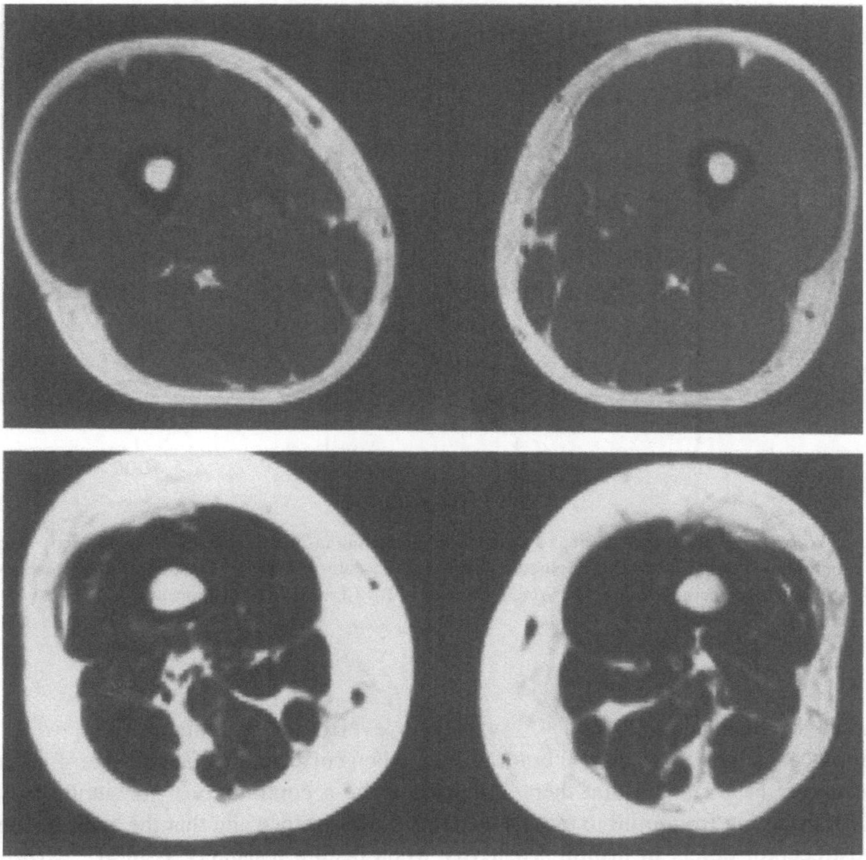

Fig. 2. Magnetic resonance images of the thigh, showing differences in total muscle, intramuscular fat, subcutaneous fat, and bone between a young woman athlete (age 20, BMI 22.6) and an old sedentary woman (age 64, BMI 30.7). BMI, body mass index (wt/ht^2).

concentration is monitored and kept constant by adjusting the rate of infusion of glucose. In this way, the rate of whole-body glucose disposal at different plasma insulin levels can be accurately assessed. The euglycemic glucose clamp has been used to determine if insulin resistance is the mechanism responsible for the demonstrated glucose intolerance of aging, as shown in Fig. 3 (Rowe *et al.*, 1983). A study by Fink *et al.* (1983) showed that fasting serum glucose levels were not different between young and elderly subjects, but fasting serum insulin levels were greater in the elderly (13 ± 1 versus 9 ± 1 μU/ml). There was a negative correlation between glucose disposal rate and age ($r = -0.53$, $P < 0.01$). Insulin resistance was only observed in the subjects aged over 60 years, and there was no decrease in *in vivo* insulin action to promote glucose uptake in the middle-aged group. This contrasts with the findings of DeFronzo (1979), who demonstrated that the decline in insulin sensitivity was most

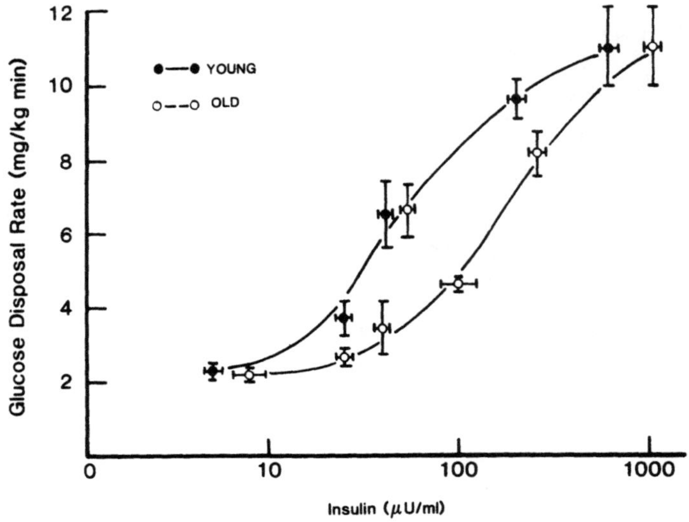

Fig. 3. Whole-body glucose disposal as a function of circulating insulin in young and old subjects. Normal old people show a shift towards lower glucose disposal at physiological levels of insulin. (From Rowe *et al.*, 1983, by copyright permission of The American Society for Clinical Investigation.)

marked between ages 20 and 45 years and leveled off thereafter. There were no differences in adipocyte insulin binding even when corrected for fat cell size. Fink and co-workers (1983) state that there "appears to be a continuum of metabolic abnormalities ranging from mild to more severe insulin resistance and that the basic lesion is a postreceptor defect in insulin sensitivity when insulin resistance is mild." Rowe *et al.* (1983) have described a need for greater insulin levels in the elderly to achieve a similar uptake of glucose; the age-related decline in insulin sensitivity has been attributed to a postreceptor defect in insulin action, shown by a lower response to very high doses of insulin during a glucose clamp.

Although the effects of aging on glucose tolerance appear to be unequivocal, many studies have not taken into consideration diet, nutritional status, or age-related changes in activity. Impaired glucose utilization has been linked to fat accumulation in growing and mature rats (Narimiya *et al.*, 1984). Insulin-stimulated glucose utilization *in vivo* and body composition were examined in 1.5-, 4-, and 12-month-old rats, and the greatest increase in insulin resistance was found between the ages of 1.5 and 4 months, when the animals accumulated the greatest amount of fat. Furthermore, *in vivo* insulin resistance does not develop in rats if obesity is prevented by using a hypocaloric diet (Reaven *et al.*, 1983). Thus, *in vivo* insulin resistance of older rats "is due in large measure to the obesity that develops in these animals and is primarily due to environmental factors and is not an inevitable consequence of the aging process."

Obese humans have a reduced insulin sensitivity and demonstrate an increased risk of developing non-insulin-dependent diabetes that is proportional to their degree of obesity (Hartz *et al.*, 1984). Increased body fat has been associated with reduced rates of insulin-mediated glucose disposal (Rabinovitz and Zierler, 1962; Kolterman *et al.*,

1980). For this reason, the increasing obesity of advancing age is thought to be causally related to age-related decreases in glucose tolerance, especially if body fat is accumulated in the upper body, i.e., "android" obesity versus "gynoid" obesity. Upper body fat accumulation is associated with insulin resistance, hyperinsulinemia, diminished glucose tolerance, lower sensitivity to insulin in skeletal muscle, and a reduced rate of hepatic insulin extraction (Peiris *et al.*, 1986; Evans *et al.*, 1984; Kissebah *et al.*, 1982). The influence of body composition in humans has not been accurately studied since anthropometric measurements have been routinely used to estimate body fat, and these do not reflect the intraabdominal and intramuscular accumulation of fat that occurs with aging (Borkan *et al.*, 1983).

3.2. *Effects of Diet*

Changes in the diet can affect carbohydrate metabolism. Simple overnutrition can reduce glucose disposal; a 65% increase in calorie consumption without changing diet composition reduced rates of glucose disposal during a euglycemic glucose clamp mainly by decreasing the rate of glucose storage as glycogen (Mott *et al.*, 1986). The composition of the diet also affects glucose disposal. An increased consumption of fat alone leads to whole-body insulin resistance and lowers thermogenesis (Storelien *et al.*, 1986); in individual muscles, insulin-stimulated glucose utilization decreases, primarily in muscles with a high percentage of type I, oxidative fibers.

In contrast to the deleterious effects of excess dietary fat, increasing the percentage of calories from carbohydrate and an increase in the intake of fiber improve insulin sensitivity and glucose tolerance. Studies by Anderson and his group have demonstrated that a high-carbohydrate, high-fiber diet can lower fasting serum insulin levels and lower the insulin response to an oral glucose load in both NIDDM and nondiabetics (Anderson *et al.*, 1976). These changes have been associated with a twofold increase in insulin sensitivity, an increased number of insulin receptors, and lower serum cholesterol and triglycerides (Kiehm *et al.*, 1976; Anderson *et al.*, 1976; Anderson and Gustafsson, 1986). No effect is found if for 4 weeks the fiber content of the diet is increased from 11 to only 27 g/100 kcal without changing the carbohydrate or fat composition (Hollenbeck *et al.*, 1986). Reaven (1986) has stated that the beneficial effects of high-carbohydrate, high-fiber diets on glucose metabolism and plasma cholesterol depend primarily on fiber content. If these diets are not greatly fiber enriched, the "beneficial effect on plasma glucose and LDL cholesterol is dissipated, and deleterious effects on plasma VLDL-TG and HDL cholesterol concentrations are seen."

Significant effects on fasting blood glucose levels by dietary chromium supplementation have been demonstrated. In slightly glucose-intolerant persons, a 3-month supplementation with chromium (200 μg/day) reduced fasting blood glucose levels and the blood glucose response to a glucose challenge (Anderson *et al.*, 1983). In elderly subjects, a daily chromium supplement for 8 weeks, in the form of chromium-rich brewer's yeast, improved glucose tolerance, reduced insulin output, and decreased total plasma lipids and cholesterol levels in diabetic and nondiabetic subjects (Offenbacher and Pi-Sunyer, 1980). Chromium supplementation improves glucose utilization in older (age 66 ± 4 years), glucose-intolerant subjects through higher circulating insulin levels (Potter *et al.*, 1985). This effect may be caused by an increased β-cell sensitivity to glucose or a decreased insulin clearance.

3.3. Effects of Inactivity and Exercise

Carbohydrate utilization changes with a reduction or an increase in physical activity. The detrimental effects of reduced activity have long been recognized. Hippocrates (Chadwick and Mann, 1950) stated, "For if the whole body is rested much more than is usual, there is no immediate increase in strength. In fact, should a long period of inactivity be followed by a sudden return to exercise, there will be an obvious deterioration. The same is true of each separate part of the body." Lower physical activity has been linked to age-related decreases in glucose tolerance and increases in blood pressure (Cederholm and Wibell, 1986).

It is well known that immobilization rapidly decreases glucose tolerance. In 1959, Lutwak and Whedon (1959) reported that intravenous glucose tolerance is significantly decreased after 1 to 3 weeks of bed rest in normal subjects. After only 3 days of complete bed rest in young healthy men, forearm glucose uptake during intravenous glucose infusion was significantly reduced (Lipman *et al.*, 1972). In mice, there is a decrease in the insulin responsiveness of the soleus muscle after only 1 day of immobilization with the limb fixed so that the length of the soleus was less than its normal resting length. The increase in insulin resistance in muscle occurred independently of plasma insulin levels and led to decreased glucose uptake and a diminished capacity to synthesize glycogen. It has been suggested that bed rest may, in fact, lead to a false-positive glucose tolerance test and a diagnosis of diabetes (Steinke and Soeldner, 1977). Sieder *et al.* (1982) suggest that responsiveness of the muscle to insulin is directly related to its immediate history of usage.

The decreased capacity of insulin to stimulate glucose uptake after only 24 hr of immobilization is suggestive of a postreceptor defect, since there is no change in insulin binding to muscle (Nicholson *et al.*, 1984). The same mechanism has been suggested for denervation atrophy and for age-related glucose intolerance (Burant *et al.*, 1984). When muscle contractile activity is greatly reduced, there is a downward regulation of skeletal muscle insulin binding, perhaps as a result of a decreased number of receptor sites and a reduced capacity for glucose disposal (Donaldson *et al.*, 1986). There is a reduced capacity for glycogen synthesis, which is most likely a result of a postreceptor defect.

Increased physical activity has the opposite effect on glucose metabolism. When individuals with normal glucose tolerance engage in endurance exercise training, insulin sensitivity increases, and glucose tolerance is improved (Bjorntorp *et al.*, 1972; Seals *et al.*, 1984b; Holloszy *et al.*, 1986). In middle-aged men who are endurance-trained, fat mass is lower, $V\text{O}_2\text{max}$ is higher, and there is a greater oral glucose tolerance and intravenous lipid tolerance compared to sedentary age-matched controls (Bjorntorp *et al.*, 1972). However, it is difficult to differentiate between the effects of body composition and of diet. Glucose tolerance and insulin resistance were studied in older untrained men, lean older men, endurance-trained young and older athletes, and young untrained men in an attempt to assess the separate effects of age, physical activity, and body composition (Seals *et al.*, 1984a). The response of these groups to an oral glucose load is shown in Fig. 4. The older and young athletes as well as the young untrained men had similar glucose tolerance, whereas the two groups of older untrained men had an almost twofold greater total area under the glucose curve. The

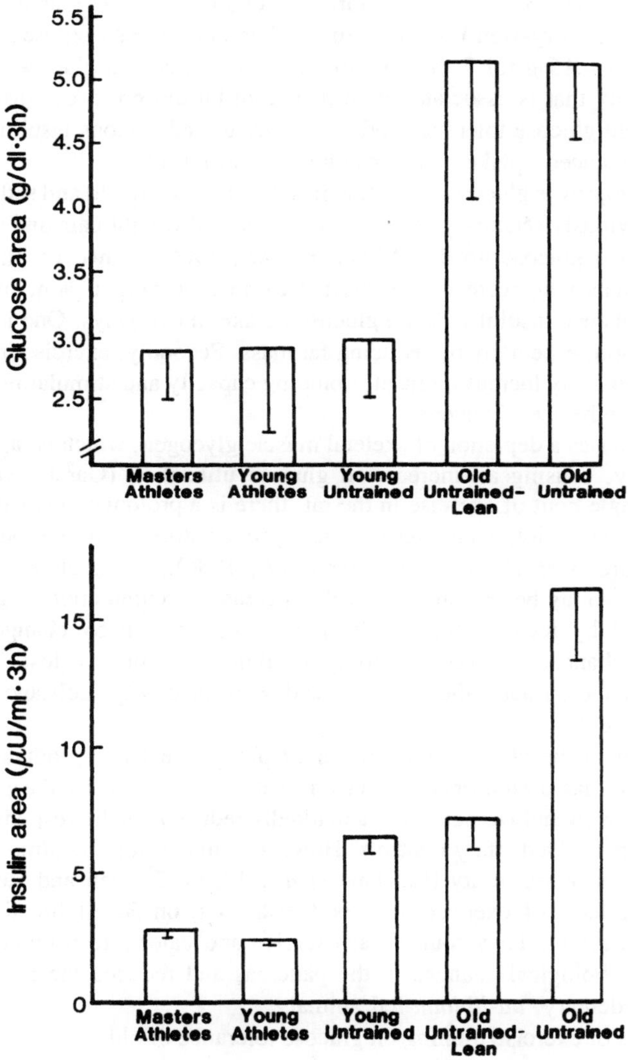

Fig. 4. Glucose and insulin response (mean ± S.E.M.) to a 100-g load of glucose in young and old, trained and untrained men. Athletes showed the lowest increase in glucose or insulin ($P < 0.05$) irrespective of age. (From Seals *et al.*, 1984a, by copyright permission of The American Physiological Society.)

older and young athletes had similar plasma insulin responses, the lean older men had an intermediate response, and the older untrained group demonstrated the greatest insulin response. This study indicates that habitual exercise can prevent the typical age-related changes in glucose tolerance and insulin sensitivity. Rosenthal *et al.* (1983) found a significant correlation between $V\text{O}_2$max and *in vivo* insulin-stimulated glucose utilization that was independent of age and obesity.

Other types of exercise also improve glucose utilization. Swim training increased insulin-stimulated glucose disposal in normal (Berger *et al.*, 1979) as well as severely diabetic rats (Walleberg-Henriksson, 1986). In 1-month-old rats exposed to continuous centrifugation at 4.15 *g* for 7 months, the normal decrease in glucose tolerance and insulin sensitivity that is associated with increased fat did not occur (Mondon *et al.*, 1981). Increased glucose tolerance and sensitivity to endogenous insulin resulted primarily from enhanced uptake of glucose by skeletal muscle.

Exercise improves glucose utilization in subjects who are old and sedentary. Daily exercise in previously sedentary year-old rats prevented weight gain and the decline of insulin-stimulated glucose uptake (Mondon *et al.*, 1986). However, this effect was greater in animals who were food-restricted to prevent weight gain, indicating that exercise can enhance insulin-induced glucose uptake in two ways. One is by affecting body composition, especially by reducing fat mass. Secondly, exercise increases rates of glucose disposal by increasing insulin-binding capacity and stimulating the capacity of muscle to synthesize glycogen.

Exercise causes a depletion of skeletal muscle glycogen, which is rapidly repleted during recovery, causing an increase in glucose utilization (Garetto *et al.*, 1984). Following a single bout of exercise in the rat, there is a prolonged increase in skeletal muscle insulin sensitivity, even after muscle glycogen stores have returned to preexercise values (Garetto *et al.*, 1984; Richter *et al.*, 1984). The prolonged increase in insulin sensitivity may be responsible for the increased accumulation of glycogen and is likely caused by local factors in the muscle rather than by changes in insulin metabolism. Enhanced insulin sensitivity is almost completely lost, however, in trained animals and humans after only a few days of inactivity (LeBlanc *et al.*, 1981; Heath *et al.*, 1983).

In addition to the changes that increased physical activity produces in skeletal muscle, exercise has a significant effect on insulin production by the pancreas. Endurance-trained men and women show a markedly reduced insulin response to injected glucose compared to sedentary controls. However, this disappears almost completely after only 3 days of inactivity (LeBlanc *et al.*, 1981). Reaven and Reaven (1981) examined the effects of exercise and food restriction on β-cell function and morphology in aging rats. They found that exercise and caloric restriction prevented a number of morphological changes in the pancreas and reduced the need for insulin compared to sedentary, *ad-libitum*-fed animals.

The effects of exercise training on glucose tolerance of older men and women has been examined by a number of investigators with mixed results. Seals *et al.* (1984a) examined the effects of 1 year of low-intensity and high-intensity endurance exercise training in older (63 ± 1 years) subjects with normal glucose tolerance. Although the insulin response to an oral glucose load was reduced by both training intensities, glucose tolerance was unchanged after 1 year. In elderly, sedentary men and women, skeletal muscle glycogen stores are lower than for sedentary young men and women but are more responsive to 12 weeks of endurance training (Meredith *et al.*, in press). Only small improvements in glucose tolerance have been seen in response to aerobic exercise training in subjects with NIDDM (Ruderman *et al.*, 1979; Saltin *et al.*, 1979; Schneider *et al.*, 1984). However, when exercise training is of sufficient intensity, there are marked improvements in insulin sensitivity and glucose tolerance in subjects with impaired glucose tolerance or NIDDM (Holloszy *et al.*, 1986). The beneficial effects of exercise training on glucose metabolism are lost within a few days following the cessation of training (Heath *et al.*, 1983).

Changes in diet and levels of physical activity apparently have a synergistic effect. Although decreased amounts of exercise and increased dietary fat can decrease glucose tolerance and insulin sensitivity, exercise coupled with a hypocaloric diet or reduced-fat diet can improve carbohydrate and lipid metabolism (O'Dea, 1984). In rats a combination of increased dietary sucrose and exercise training had synergistic effects (Vallerand *et al.*, 1986). Increased dietary sucrose in sedentary animals led to a marked hyperinsulinemia but did not improve glucose tolerance, but exercise training with a normal diet improved glucose tolerance by increasing muscle sensitivity to insulin. The synergistic action was caused by higher insulinemia and enhanced sensitivity to insulin.

In middle-aged men and women, the effects of 12 weeks of endurance training plus a hypocaloric diet were compared to the effects of the diet alone (Bogardus *et al.*, 1984). Only the exercise-trained group showed an increased rate of glucose disposal. Diet therapy alone improved glucose tolerance, mainly by reducing basal endogenous glucose production and improving hepatic sensitivity to insulin. Exercise training, on the other hand, increased carbohydrate storage rates, and, therefore, "diet therapy plus physical training produced a more significant approach toward normal."

3.4. Conclusions

An improvement in glucose tolerance in the elderly can be obtained through fat loss or endurance training. The increased sensitivity to insulin found after exercise is not caused by an enhanced antilipolytic effect on fat cells (Krotkiewski, 1983) but rather by an enhanced capacity of the muscles to take up and store glucose. The effects of exercise on carbohydrate metabolism are transient, disappearing after a few days of inactivity.

4. Protein Metabolism

4.1. Protein Reserves

The protein content of the body declines with age: in elderly men and women, total body protein is about 1.8 kg lower than for young adults, as shown in Table VII. Skeletal muscle, which in a young man makes up about 45% of body weight, accounts for most of the decrease in protein reserves with age (Cohn *et al.*, 1980).

Loss of muscle mass with age in humans has been demonstrated both indirectly and directly. The excretion of urinary creatinine, reflecting muscle creatine content and total muscle mass, decreases by nearly 50% between the ages of 20 and 90 (Tzankoff and Norris, 1978). This reduction in muscle mass is closely associated with age-related reductions in basal metabolic rate. About 60% of the body's potassium is found in skeletal muscle, and the ratio of potassium to nitrogen is higher in muscle than in nonmuscle lean tissue; muscle and nonmuscle mass can be calculated from total potassium and nitrogen (Cohn *et al.*, 1980). Loss of muscle protein with age has thus

Table VII. Total Body Protein (kg) in a Cross-Sectional Study of Men and Women[a]

	Young (20–29 years)	Middle-aged (40–49 years)	Elderly (70–79 years)
Men			
Muscle protein	4.54	3.80	2.50
Nonmuscle protein	8.32	8.20	8.60
Total protein	12.86	12.00	11.10
Women			
Muscle protein	1.85	1.94	1.11
Nonmuscle protein	7.23	6.53	6.10
Total protein	9.08	8.47	7.21

[a]From Cohn *et al.* (1980).

been calculated from the different decline in the whole-body content of potassium, measured from endogenous ^{40}K, and in nitrogen, measured by prompt γ radiation (Table VII).

Computed tomography of individual muscles shows that after age 30, there is a decrease in cross-sectional areas of the thigh along with decreased muscle density associated with increased intramuscular fat. Images obtained by magnetic resonance show a dramatic decrease in muscle size with age together with increased intramuscular and subcutaneous fat, as illustrated in the MR cross sections of the thigh in Fig. 2. These changes were most pronounced in women (Imamura *et al.*, 1983). Muscle atrophy may result from a gradual and selective loss of muscle fibers. The number of muscle fibers in the midsection of the vastus lateralis of autopsy specimens is lower by about 110,000 in elderly men (age 70–73) than in young men (age 19–37), a 23% difference (Lexel *et al.*, 1983). The decline is more marked in those muscles involved in high-intensity "sprinting" type movement (type II fibers), while those muscles necessary for posture and most low-intensity movement (type I fibers) are preserved. The proportion of type II fibers falls from about 60% in sedentary young men to below 30% after the age of 80 (Larsson, 1983). The atrophy of type II fibers is significantly related to age-related decreases in strength ($r = 0.54$, $P < 0.001$) (Larsson, 1983).

It has not been shown that the decline in muscle mass with age is affected by endurance training, which involves prolonged, rhythmical exercise using large muscle groups. Young subjects who exercise aerobically do not increase their muscle mass (Edstrom and Grimby, 1986). The effects of endurance training on lean body mass are related to the lowering of body fat. In elderly men who have trained hard throughout their lives, potassium per unit of body weight is 12% higher than for sedentary men of the same age and weight, but it is likely that these results reflect lower body fat rather than increased muscle mass (Lundholm *et al.*, 1986). Age-related reduction in oxidative capacity per gram of skeletal muscle of rats can be prevented by endurance exercise; however, it cannot prevent the typical atrophy associated with aging (Farrar *et al.*, 1981). A comparison of the body composition and exercise habits of young and middle-aged endurance-trained men showed that although body mass index in the two groups was identical, fat was greater in the older men (Meredith *et al.*, 1987). However, fat mass and Vo_2max were closely related to the amount of time spent exercising every week and were not a function of age.

Strength training, which involves resisting, lifting, or lowering heavy weights, can increase lean body mass in young subjects (Fahey *et al.*, 1975). Strength training in the elderly has been shown to result in significant gains in strength with small increases in the size of type II fibers (Aniansson and Gustaffsson, 1981) and no muscle hypertrophy detected by anthropometric measurements (Moritani and DeVries, 1980). However, 12 weeks of progressive resistance training of the leg extensors and flexors in elderly men resulted in substantial increases in muscle strength and size measured by computerized tomography (Frontera, 1986). The CT scan showed a 10% increase in the cross-sectional area of the muscles of both thighs, which is greater than has been reported for similarly trained young men (Larsson, 1982). Increased leg muscle mass in the elderly men was associated with hypertrophy of type I and type II muscle fibers. It is likely that strength training of large groups of muscles in the elderly would significantly increase muscle protein reserves.

4.2. Protein Requirements

Because of the decreased active cell mass of the elderly, dietary protein needs might be similar or lower than for young persons. In the 1950s, protein requirements were estimated from the amount of nitrogen lost from the body while consuming a protein-free diet, assuming that a diet had to provide at least that amount of protein nitrogen to prevent negative balance. Table VIII summarizes obligatory urinary nitrogen losses in young and old men and women, showing that these are only slightly decreased by age. Although this suggests that protein requirements are unchanged as people age, the utilization of dietary protein at various intake levels seems to be lower in the elderly. This has been shown by nitrogen balance studies at protein intakes between 0.5 and 0.85 g/kg per day (Table IX) to test the adequacy of levels considered safe by FAO/WHO or by the National Research Council of the United States. The results are variable but suggest that the elderly have increased protein requirements, as

Table VIII. Obligatory Urinary Nitrogen Loss (Mean ± S.D.) in Young and Old Men and Women in Response to a Protein-Free Diet[a]

	Protein loss (mg N/kg per day)	
	Men	Women
Young	37 ± 6	28 ± 4
Old	35 ± 10	24 ± 5

[a]From Bodwell *et al.* (1979).

Table IX. Protein Needs of Sedentary Elderly Men (M) and Women (W)

Ref.[a]	*N*	Age (yrs)	Protein intake (g/kg per day)	Diet duration (days)	Mean N balance (g/day)	Number in negative balance	Comments
(1)	7M	60–73	0.8	11	0.03	3/7	High energy intake (40 kcal/kg per day)
(2)	6M	63–77	1.3 to 1.8 × endogenous losses	15	−0.5	5/6	Slightly obese subjects; protein-free diet for previous 17 days
(3)	7M	68–74	0.57, 0.70, 0.85	10 each	—	5/7 at 0.85 g/kg per day	Variable data did not allow calculation of N requirement High fecal losses in three men with partial gastrectomy
(4)	7M	70–82	0.8	30	+0.4	2/7	Most had one or more chronic diseases
(3)	7W	70–84	0.52, 0.65, 0.80	10 each	—	5/7 at 0.80 g/kg per day	Mean requirement was 0.83 g/kg per day; most had one or more chronic diseases
(4)	8W	71–99	0.8	30	−2.3	3/8	Most had one or more chronic diseases

[a]From: (1) Cheng *et al.*, 1978; (2) Zanni *et al.*, 1979; (3) Uauy *et al.*, 1978; (4) Gersovitz *et al.*, 1982.

Table X. Habitual Protein Intake (Mean ± S.E.M.) in Elderly Men and Women, Measured by Weighing Food Intake

		Men		Women	
Ref.[a]	Subjects	Weight (kg)	Protein (g/day)	Weight (kg)	Protein (g/day)
(1)	U.S., nursing home, ages 62–98	63 ± 9	67 ± 14	58 ± 14	48 ± 14
(2)	Spain, nursing home, average age 82	—	66 ± 6	—	62 ± 6
(3)	France, free-living, ages 65–80				
	Urban	—	—	—	57 ± 13
	Rural	—	—	—	69 ± 17
(4)	England, free-living, ages 70–86	—	69	—	60

[a]From: (1) Stiedman *et al.*, 1978; (2) Moreiras-Varela *et al.*, 1986; (3) Debry *et al.*, 1977; (4) Bunker *et al.*, 1984.

discussed in Chapter 7. Even when better protein utilization was favored by a large energy intake (Cheng *et al.*, 1978) or the consumption of a protein-free diet for the previous 14 days (Zanni *et al.*, 1979), many of the elderly men were in negative nitrogen balance with protein intakes of 0.57 or 0.85 g/kg per day. When 0.80 g/kg per day was consumed for 30 days, protein utilization improved over time, but in the final 10-day period 36% of the elderly men and women remained in negative nitrogen balance (Gersovitz *et al.*, 1982). In elderly women, a mean protein requirement of 0.83 g/kg per day was calculated; in a similar study in elderly men, nitrogen balance results did not permit the calculation of protein requirements (Uauy *et al.*, 1978).

Under everyday circumstances, it is likely that in the elderly the high incidence of illness and consequent bed rest, fever, or surgery would further increase dietary protein needs. Protein utilization is also markedly affected by energy intake (Munro, 1951). Low energy intakes in sedentary elderly plus episodes of anorexia induced by illness or immobilization would diminish protein retention.

If the protein requirement of the elderly is at least 0.8 g/kg per day, it is apparent from food intake measurements that a substantial number of old people may not consume enough protein, as shown in Table X. The consequences for the elderly of consuming marginally low protein are not known, but it has been suggested that immunocompetence and recovery from illness or surgery could be compromised (Chandra, 1985; Symreng *et al.*, 1983). In active elderly people who have a higher food intake, protein requirements are covered with an average American diet. The protein density of a diet would probably have to be higher than 12 to 14% during convalescence from illness or for the very old whose total intake is low.

The effects of increased physical activity on protein needs have been studied mainly in young people, as shown in Table XI. At the onset of endurance or isometric training, nitrogen balance in young men is achieved if more than 0.85 g protein/kg per day is consumed. In young and middle-aged men who are already endurance-trained,

Table XI. Protein Intake and Nitrogen Balance during Exercise Training in Men Receiving an Adequate Energy Intake

Ref.[a]	*N*	Age (years)	Exercise	Protein intake (g/kg per day)	Results and comments
			Untrained men		
(1)	7	18–21	Isometric, 2 hr/day for 28–49 days	0.5	Approx. N balance −0.2 g/day
				1.0	Approx. N balance +1.1 g/day
(2)	8	20–23	Aerobic, to expend 450–500 kcal/day for 40 days	1.39	N balance +0.26 g/day
(3)	12	21–29	Aerobic, 2 hr/day for 21 days	1.0	N balance −2.0 g/day (day 4) N balance −0.3 g/day (day 20)
(4)	12	23–35	Aerobic, 1 hr/day for 18 days	0.57	N balance −0.19 g/day
				0.85	N balance +0.82 g/day
			Trained men		
(5)	6	22–30	Aerobic, 8–18 hr/week	0.6, 0.9, 1.2	Protein requirement 0.92 ± 0.13 (S.D.)
(5)	6	48–59	Aerobic, 4–14 hr/week	0.6, 0.9, 1.2	Protein requirement 0.96 ± 0.19 (S.D.)

[a]From: (1) Torun *et al.*, 1977; (2) Consolazio *et al.*, 1975; (3) Gontzea *et al.*, 1975; (4) Todd *et al.*, 1984; (5) Meredith *et al.*, 1988.

protein requirements are close to 1 g/kg per day for both age groups (Meredith *et al.*, in press). There is evidence that during an exercise bout there is a net breakdown of body proteins: leucine oxidation increases severalfold, lysine oxidation increases by about 40% (Wolfe, 1984), there is a net release of amino acids and ammonia from muscles (Felig, 1975), and urinary nitrogen increases immediately after exercise (Millward *et al.*, 1982). On the other hand, nitrogen balance studies have shown that moderate endurance exercise has an anabolic effect as long as energy needs are covered (Todd *et al.*, 1984; Butterfield and Calloway, 1984). The effect of exercise on individual amino acid requirements is not known. However, the oxidation of leucine and probably of the other branched-chain amino acids increases during exercise in proportion to its intensity (Millward *et al.*, 1982). These limited studies have led to the suggestion that endurance athletes may have an increased need for some or all of the indispensable amino acids (Evans *et al.*, 1983). It is not known how a physical training program affects the protein or amino acid needs of the elderly.

4.3. Protein Turnover

In experimental animals, the rate of protein synthesis in the whole body, and especially in skeletal muscles, gradually declines throughout adult life (Kelly *et al.*, 1984; Goldspink and Kelly, 1984). It is reported that aging decreases the rate of mRNA translation (Richardson and Birchenall-Sparks, 1983). The changes in muscle protein turnover with age, discussed in Chapter 7, may also be the result of decreased physical activity. Inactive muscles atrophy as protein synthesis decreases and breakdown increases (Goldspink *et al.*, 1986). Conversely, increased activity alters the synthesis of specific muscle proteins and total protein turnover rate in a way that is specific to the type of training. Endurance training increases the levels of mitochondrial proteins, and weight training increases myofibrillar proteins, sarcoplasmic proteins, and collagen in exercised muscles. Studies on the turnover of total muscle proteins in rats have shown that aerobic training does not alter muscle protein turnover (Tapscott *et al.*, 1982), whereas weight training leads to muscle hypertrophy by markedly increasing protein synthesis and slightly increasing protein breakdown (Laurent *et al.*, 1978).

In humans, studies of whole-body protein turnover using [^{15}N]glycine as a tracer for exchangeable nitrogen have not shown that aging or physical activity have any effect on the rate of whole-body protein synthesis or breakdown per unit body weight, as shown in Table XII (Young *et al.*, 1982; Meredith *et al.*, 1988). Rates obtained with other tracers are similar, as discussed in Chapter 7.

The turnover rate of specific proteins has also been studied in the elderly. The breakdown rate of actomyosin, estimated from urinary excretion of 3-methylhistidine, has been studied in young and old men who are sedentary, endurance trained, or weight trained (Table XIII). Actomyosin is found mainly in skeletal muscles, although it has a higher turnover rate in smaller tissues such as smooth muscle (Rennie and Millward, 1983). Thus, 3-methylhistidine excretion is a measure of contractile protein breakdown but not exclusively of skeletal muscle protein breakdown. In sedentary men, the rate of 3-methylhistidine excretion per day or per unit of creatinine (i.e., per unit of muscle mass) was lower in the oldest subjects. Endurance training had no apparent effect on daily 3-methylhistidine excretion, although in the middle-aged men there was a tendency for increased actomyosin turnover per unit muscle mass. Strength training, which is known to increase myofibrillar protein content, had the most marked effect on actomyosin turnover. The high daily excretion of 3-methylhistidine in young weight lifters could reflect a large muscle mass. In elderly men after 12 weeks of strength training, actomyosin turnover per gram creatinine unit (i.e., per unit muscle mass) was similar to that of young weight lifters and greater ($P < 0.05$) than values obtained before training (Frontera, 1986). Despite the variability of 3-methylhistidine

Table XII. Whole-Body Protein Synthesis and Breakdown in Young and Old Sedentary or Endurance-Trained Men[a]

	Sedentary		Endurance-trained	
	Young	Old	Young	Middle-aged
N	5	6	6	6
Age (years)	21 ± 1	72 ± 2	27 ± 1	52 ± 1
Protein synthesis (g/kg per day)	3.1 ± 0.2	3.3 ± 0.3	3.5 ± 0.2	4.0 ± 0.2
Protein breakdown (g/kg per day)	3.0 ± 0.2	2.7 ± 0.2	3.1 ± 0.2	3.7 ± 0.3

[a]Rates (mean ± S.E.M.) were calculated from urinary urea ^{15}N enrichment following 60 hr of oral [^{15}N]glycine. From Young *et al.*, 1982; Meredith *et al.*, 1988.

Table XIII. Actomyosin Breakdown in Young and Old Men: Effects of Physical Training[a]

Ref.[b]	Subjects	Age (years)	Weight (kg)	3-Methylhistidine excretion (μmole/day)	3-Methylhistidine excretion (μmole/g creatinine)
			Sedentary		
(1)	5 Young	21 ± 1	77 ± 5	287 ± 33	137 ± 6
(2)	14 Young	25 ± 1	74 ± 2	224 ± 11	132 ± 3
(3)	12 Old	66 ± 1	78 ± 2	212 ± 16	144 ± 10
(1)	6 Old	72 ± 2	69 ± 4	151 ± 9	118 ± 6
			Endurance-trained		
(4)	6 Young	27 ± 1	71 ± 5	238 ± 34	136 ± 11
(4)	6 Middle-aged	52 ± 1	72 ± 3	260 ± 15	167 ± 4
			Strength-trained		
(5)	4 Young	23 ± 2	77 ± 9	408 ± 27	187 ± 13
(3)	12 Old	66 ± 1	78 ± 2	279 ± 31	184 ± 21

[a]Results are mean ± S.E.M.
[b]From: (1) Young *et al.*, 1982; (2) Lukaski *et al.*, 1981; (3) Frontera, 1986; (4) Meredith *et al.*, 1988; (5) Hickson and Hinkelman, 1985.

excretion, the results suggest that weight training but not endurance training increases actomyosin turnover, similar to the effects of these types of training on muscle protein synthesis and breakdown rates in animals. In addition, actomyosin turnover per unit of muscle mass in active men is not markedly affected by age.

The mediators for exercise-induced changes in the synthesis of total proteins or specific proteins in muscles are not known. Hormonal changes during and immediately after exercise may favor a net anabolic effect. Following endurance exercise, there is an enhancement of insulin-stimulated amino acid uptake by skeletal muscles, especially slow twitch muscles (Zorzano *et al.*, 1985). Other hormonal changes that could enhance protein synthesis include increased growth hormone levels with exercise (Schalch, 1967), increased testosterone after weight-lifting (Weiss *et al.*, 1983; Hakkinen *et al.*, 1985), and increased prostaglandins after muscle contraction (Young and Sparks, 1980; Smith *et al.*, 1983). In mice, exhaustive exercise causes a delayed increase in the activities of skeletal muscle acid hydrolases (Salminen and Kihlstrom, 1985), which may be indicative of increased muscle protein turnover. These increases following exercise are much greater in young than in old animals (Salminen and Vihko, 1981). However, there is at present no complete biochemical explanation for the effects of exercise on muscle protein metabolism or for how these are affected by age.

5. *Fat Metabolism*

Aging affects body fat content and fat mobilization, and endurance exercise has effects that oppose those of aging. Fat content tends to be greatest among the middle-aged, especially in women. The distribution of body fat also changes with age, with marked accumulation of abdominal fat, especially in men (Haffner *et al.*, 1987). This type of "android" obesity is associated with a greater risk for diabetes, hypertension, coronary heart disease, and hypertension and with a greater proportion of highly glycolytic fast twitch fibers (type II fibers) in skeletal muscle (Krotkiewski, 1983). In aging women, fat tends to be more evenly distributed between central and subcutaneous deposits and appears to be less hazardous (Bjorntorp, 1985). The mobilization of fat through dieting and exercise is more rapid in the abdominal area (Smith *et al.*, 1979). Exercise alone, with no dietary restriction, has a minimal effect on fat loss in short-term studies, as shown in Table VI, but in trained men who exercise habitually, body fat is inversely related to weekly hours of training (Meredith *et al.*, 1987).

The levels of circulating triglycerides increase with age by an average 16 mg/dl per decade (Greenfield *et al.*, 1980). Circulating cholesterol also increases with age and is associated with an increased risk for atherosclerosis and coronary heart disease (Chapman *et al.*, 1964; Bjorntorp and Malmcrowa, 1960). However, the various cholesterol-containing lipoprotein fractions are more important than total cholesterol in predicting the risk of coronary heart disease (Miller and Miller, 1975). Populations with higher HDL-cholesterol levels have a lower incidence of coronary heart disease (Castelli *et al.*, 1977; Gordon *et al.*, 1977). Increasing endurance exercise in middle-aged men has been shown to increase HDL-cholesterol and decrease LDL-cholesterol (Wood *et al.*, 1983). The amount of endurance exercise determines the extent of the increase in HDL-cholesterol; below 8 miles run per week, plasma HDL-cholesterol in previously sedentary middle-aged men did not change, but above that threshold of activity, changes in plasma HDL-cholesterol were related to weekly distance run. The LDL-cholesterol showed a negative correlation with weekly distance run. Exercise reduces plasma triglyceride levels even if the diet is high in fat (Mann *et al.*, 1955) or provides the usual amount of energy (Holloszy *et al.*, 1964).

Increased physical activity also affects plasma lipoprotein levels by reducing body fat content. In post-myocardial-infarct patients undergoing cardiac rehabilitation, exercise without weight loss appeared to have no effect on lipoprotein profile (LaRosa *et al.*, 1982; Allison *et al.*, 1981). However, in healthy young and middle-aged subjects there is an increase in HDL-cholesterol and a decrease in LDL-cholesterol with exercise alone, with or without weight reduction (Kiens *et al.*, 1980). It is possible that the intensity and duration of training sessions were greater in the healthy men compared to the myocardial infarct patients, and this might explain the difference in HDL response.

A survey of 95 studies carried out between 1955 and 1983 on the effects of exercise on serum lipids and lipoproteins showed that exercise combined with weight reduction led to the greatest reduction in cholesterol, LDL-cholesterol, and triglycerides (Tran and Weltman, 1985). Exercise with no weight loss had similar but less marked effects, but in subjects who increased in weight during an exercise program the changes in serum lipids and lipoproteins were in the opposite direction. Thus, exercise cannot counteract the effects of weight gain but increases the beneficial effects of weight loss.

6. Minerals and Vitamins

6.1. Calcium

Calcium stores in bone decline throughout adult life at a rate of about 1% per year (Hansson and Roos, 1986; Riggs *et al.*, 1982). In advanced old age, especially in women of Caucasian or Oriental race, this leads to osteoporosis, i.e., bone fractures, which is a major cause of disability and death among the elderly. Both diet and exercise have been shown to affect bone mineral content during growth and old age (see Chapter 8). Epidemiologic studies have shown that in populations that consume more calcium in the form of dairy products, the elderly have a lower incidence of bone fracture (Matkovic *et al.*, 1979). This may be the result of high calcium intake during childhood and adolescence, leading to a larger bone mass in early adult life (Sandler *et al.*, 1985).

Physical activity in young people is also associated with a larger bone mass. Young men and women marathon runners have a greater bone mass (Aloia *et al.*, 1978; Lane *et al.*, 1986). Mechanical strain increases bone mass, and the stress on the skeleton during running may increase the bone calcium stores of runners (Rubin and Lanyon, 1985). On the other hand, in some women whose energy expenditure in exercise is apparently not compensated by an adequate food intake, low estrogen levels associated with amenorrhea have been associated with lower lumbar bone mass (Nelson *et al.*, 1986). Other factors influence bone health and can be affected by exercise, as shown in Table XIV: of most concern to the elderly are the effects of low estrogen in women, low weight, and immobilization during bed rest.

In old persons, especially postmenopausal women, the effects of dietary calcium intake and the influence of exercise have recently received a lot of attention. The benefits of dietary calcium supplements in persons who are already elderly are not well established. The current recommended dietary allowance for calcium is 800 mg/day for adults. Based on the negative calcium balance of pre- and postmenopausal women consuming between 600 and 700 mg/day, a new RDA of 1500 mg/day has been proposed for older persons (Heaney *et al.*, 1977). However, there is little evidence that 1500 mg/day or more would decrease the rate of bone loss in elderly women (Riis *et al.*, 1987). On the other hand, the rate of lumbar bone mineral loss is greater in postmenopausal women consuming less than 405 mg/day compared to the rate in women consuming more than 777 mg/day (Dawson-Hughes *et al.*, 1987). A weak but significant relationship has been found between the milk consumption of elderly Japanese-Americans and their bone mineral content; average dietary calcium intake was 497 mg/day for men and 429 mg/day for women (Yano *et al.*, 1985). These studies suggest that low calcium intake in the elderly may be linked to a rapid rate of bone loss, but very high calcium intakes in persons who are already old do not have a protective effect.

In the United States, calcium intake declines with age, and many elderly persons consume very little calcium. In addition, calcium absorption declines with age and is lower in women with osteoporosis (Gallagher *et al.*, 1979) and in elderly persons with lactase deficiency (Pacifici *et al.*, 1985) or gastric atrophy (Russell, 1986). In 43% of the elderly women living in a nursing home, calcium intake was less than 530 mg/day

Table XIV. Some Nonhereditary Factors Other Than Calcium Intake That Can Affect Bone Health

Factor	Effect of exercise[a]
	Improve bone status
Estrogen	Amenorrhea (low estrogens) is prevalent in young runners, gymnasts, dancers (1)
	Athletic women have later puberty and earlier menopause, suggesting lower lifetime exposure to estrogen (2)
	Athletic women with anorexia and amenorrhea have normal bone density, suggesting that exercise has a protective effect (3)
	Bone density in post-menopausal athletic women is similar to that of sedentary women, despite lower body weight (4)
Obesity	Weight-bearing exercise places a greater stress on bones of obese persons
Vitamin D	Active people may get more exposure to sun; vitamin D + Ca and exercise is not more effective than exercise alone in preventing bone loss from the radius (4)
Fluoride	Exercise effect not known
	Impair bone status
Smoking	Smoking is less prevalent among athletes (5)
Caffeine, other drugs	Exercise effect not known
Bed rest	Calcium loss during bed rest is not prevented by exercise that does not involve weight bearing (6)

[a]From: (1) Sanborn *et al.*, 1982; (2) Frisch *et al.*, 1987; (3) Rigotti *et al.*, 1984; (4) Nelson *et al.*, 1988; (5) Morgan *et al.*, 1976; (6) Issekutz *et al.*, 1966.

(Stiedemann *et al.*, 1978). Low calcium intakes result from a decreased intake of all foods, which is associated with declining physical activity, and from a tendency for old people to avoid milk and other dairy products (Sellery, 1984).

The rate of bone mineral loss increases about 50-fold during prolonged bed rest (Krolner and Toft, 1983). This is a major problem for the elderly, in whom illness and disability can lead to more frequent periods of bed rest. In persons aged 18 to 60, normal reambulation following prolonged bed rest restores bone mineral in about 4 months (Krolner *et al.*, 1983). It is not known whether increased exercise and calcium during convalescence can accelerate the rate of bone mineral gain in the elderly.

Exercise in the ambulatory elderly has been shown to reduce the rate of bone loss. Training programs of 8 to 24 months in postmenopausal women have produced an increase in total body calcium (Aloia *et al.*, 1978), in lumbar spine mineral content (Krolner *et al.*, 1983), and in the bone density of the forearm (Smith *et al.*, 1981). A significant correlation between physical fitness ($V\text{O}_2$max) and bone mineral of the trunk and femur has been found in women aged 50 to 59 years (Chow *et al.*, 1986). Moderate exercise combined with calcium and vitamin D supplementation in postmenopausal women was not more effective in preventing bone loss from the radius than exercise alone over a 3-year period (Smith *et al.*, 1981).

6.2. Other Minerals and Vitamins

Little is known about how physical activity in the elderly changes the metabolism or requirements of minerals and vitamins. Age may alter the need for some vitamins and minerals, especially in persons with gastric atrophy or osteoporosis (Suter and Russell, 1987). Poverty and a decreased consumption of all foods have been related to low intake of micronutrients; conversely, among prosperous elderly Americans, 95% take vitamin and/or mineral supplements, and 31% take daily multivitamin preparations (Garry and Hunt, 1986).

Despite the widespread use of vitamin and mineral supplements in young athletes, there is little evidence to suggest that their needs are increased beyond the capacity of a normal diet to cover requirements (Williams, 1984). In older people, it is likely that the increased food intake promoted by physical activity would tend to decrease the need for vitamin and mineral supplements.

7. Water

Thermoregulation in the heat and during exercise occurs primarily as a result of the evaporative cooling of sweat. The maintenance of normal body temperature during exercise and/or heat exposure depends on adequate cutaneous blood flow and continued sweating. Dehydration and heat-related injuries are much more common among the elderly (Levine, 1969; Lye, 1977). Sweating can result in dehydration, which compromises cardiac output. After loss of only 2% of body weight through dehydration as a result of exercise in the heat, the heart rate response to exercise increases compared to the hydrated state (Costill *et al.*, 1976). During exercise in the heat (35°C), older subjects have a lower heart rate response and smaller stroke volume than younger subjects (Irion *et al.*, 1984). This reduced cardiac output, which impairs skin blood flow and limits evaporative heat loss in the older subjects, may result from lower physical fitness. It has been suggested that a decrease in aerobic power rather than an impaired thermoregulatory system is the limiting factor when older men (Dill and Consolazio, 1962; Robinson *et al.*, 1965) and women (Drinkwater *et al.*, 1982) exercise in a hot environment.

Dehydration in the elderly may also result from reduced renal function (Rowe *et al.*, 1976) and an impaired ability to concentrate urine in addition to a reduced sensation of thirst (Philips *et al.*, 1984). Healthy elderly men have been shown to have a significantly reduced thirst and water intake following 24 hr of no fluid intake compared to weight-matched young men (Philips *et al.*, 1984). This occurred despite an increase in plasma sodium and osmolality in the older men.

Reduced water intake, reduced ability to concentrate urine, lower total body water levels, and lower fitness all work together to decrease the ability of the elderly to maintain body temperature during exercise in hot or humid environments. Older men and women should pay particular attention to fluid intake during and following exercise. Strenuous exercise by the unacclimatized elderly during very hot and humid environmental conditions should be discouraged.

8. Conclusions

Increased physical activity in the elderly has been shown to increase life expectancy even into advanced old age (Kaplan *et al.*, 1987). Normal age-related changes in body composition that include increased fat mass and decreased muscle and bone mass may result in part from decreasing physical activity. By improving the utilization of glucose and fats, endurance exercise may reverse these trends and lead to a lower, more youthful metabolism and body composition as well as delay the onset of debilitating diseases. Loss of excess fat in middle-aged and elderly persons can be achieved with a hypocaloric diet alone, but an endurance exercise program can reduce the loss of lean tissue during dieting. Endurance exercise and weight training can significantly improve the low functional capacity in the elderly even after a lifetime of sedentary living. Age-related chronic diseases such as diabetes, hypertension, and cardiovascular disease are less prevalent among elderly athletes. In sedentary persons favorable changes in fat metabolism and glucose metabolism occur in response to individual bouts of endurance exercise in addition to improvements in cardiovascular health that result from progressive training. In the sedentary elderly whose daily food intake is too low to ensure adequate consumption of proteins, minerals, vitamins, and water, a program of exercise may improve nutritional status by simply increasing appetite. The interaction between exercise and nutrient metabolism is not well studied in the "oldest old," and this rapidly increasing population may benefit the most from strategies for improving both physical fitness and nutritional status.

9. References

Allison, T. G., Iammarino, R. M., and Metz, K. F., 1981, Failure of exercise to increase high-density lipoprotein cholesterol, *J. Card. Rehab.* **1**:257–265.

Aloia, J. F., Cohn, S. H., Babu, T., Abemasis, C., Kalici, N., and Ellis, K., 1978, Skeletal mass and body composition in marathon runners, *Metabolism* **27**:1793–1796.

Anderson, J. W., and Gustafsson, N. J., 1986, Type II diabetes: Current nutrition management concepts, *Geriatrics* **41**:28–38.

Anderson, J. W., Story, L., and Sieling, B., 1976, Hypocholesterolemic effects of oat-bran or bean intake for hypercholesterolemic men, *Am. J. Clin. Nutr.* **40**:1146–1155.

Anderson, R. A., Polansky, M. M., Bryden, N. A., Roginski, E. E., Mertz, W., and Glinsmann, W., 1983, Chromium supplementation of human subjects: Effects on glucose, insulin, and lipid variables, *Metabolism* **32**:894–899.

Aniansson, A., and Gustafsson, N. J., 1981, Physical training in elderly men with special reference to quadriceps muscle strength and morphology, *Clin. Physiol.* **1**:87–98.

Aries, P., 1962, *Centuries of Childhood,* Alfred A. Knopf, New York.

Astrand, I., 1967, Degree of strain during building work related to individual aerobic work capacity, *Ergonomics* **10**:293–303.

Badenhop, D. T., Cleary, P. A., Schaal, S. F., Fox, E. L., and Bartels, R. L., 1983, Physiological adjustments to higher or lower intensity exercise in elders, *Med. Sci. Sports Exercise* **15**:496–502.

Bailey, D. A., Shephard, R. J., Mirwald, R. L., and MacBride, G. A., 1974, Current levels of Canadian cardio-respiratory fitness, *Can. Med. Assoc. J.* **111**:25–30.

Beaglehole, R., and Stewart, A., 1983, Longevity of international rugby players, *N.Z. Med. J.* **96**:513–515.

Beall, C. M., Goldstein, M. C., and Feldman, E. S., 1985, The physical fitness of elderly Nepalese farmers residing in rugged mountain and flat terrain, *J. Gerotol.* **40**:529–535.

Belko, A. Z., Barbieri, T. F., and Wong, E. C., 1986, Effect of energy and protein intake and exercise intensity on the thermic effect of food, *Am. J. Clin. Nutr.* **43:**863–869.

Berger, M. F., Kemmer, W., Becker, K., Hergerg, L., Schwenen, M., Gjinavci, A., and Berchtold, P., 1979, Effect of physical training on glucose tolerance and on glucose metabolism of skeletal muscle in anaesthetized normal rats, *Diabetologia* **16:**179–184.

Bjorntorp, P., 1985, Regional patterns of fat distribution, *Ann. Intern. Med.* **103:**994–995.

Bjorntorp, P., and Malmcrona, R., 1960, Serum cholesterol in patients with myocardial infarction in younger ages, *Acta Med. Scand.* **168:**151–160.

Bjorntorp, P., Fahlen, M., Grimby, G., Gustafson, A., Holm, J., Renstrom, P., and Schersten, T., 1972, Carbohydrate and lipid metabolism in middle-aged physically well-trained men, *Metabolism* **21:**1037–1044.

Blair, S. N., Ellsworth, N. M., Haskell, W. L., Stern, M. P., Farquhar, J. W., and Wood, P. D., 1981, Comparison of nutrient intake in middle-aged men and women runners and controls, *Med. Sci. Sports Exercise* **13:**310–315.

Bodwell, C. E., Schuster, E. M., Kyle, E., Brooks, B., Womack, M., Steele, P., and Ahrens, R., 1979, Obligatory urinary and fecal nitrogen losses in young women, older men, and young men and the factorial estimation of adult human protein requirements, *Am. J. Clin. Nutr.* **32:**2450–2459.

Bogardus, C., Ravussin, E., Robbins, D. C., Wolfe, R. R., Horton, E. S., and Sims, E. A. H., 1984, Effects of physical training and diet therapy on carbohydrate metabolism in patients with glucose intolerance and non-insulin-dependent diabetes mellitus, *Diabetes* **33:**311–318.

Borkan, G., Hults, D. E., Gerzof, S. G., Robbins, A. H., and Silbert, C. K., 1983, Age changes in body composition revealed by computed tomography, *J. Gerontol.* **38:**673–677.

Bortz, W. M., 1982, Disuse and aging, *J.A.M.A.* **248:**1203–1208.

Bourliere, F., 1978, Ecology of human senescence, in: *Textbook of Geriatric Medicine and Gerontology* (J. C. Brocklehurst, ed.), Churchill-Livingston, New York, pp. 71–85.

Braudel, F., 1979, *The Structures of Everyday Life,* Harper & Row, New York, pp. 104–182.

Brown, P. T., Bergan, J. G., Parsons, E. P., and Krol, I., 1977, Dietary status of elderly people, *J. Am. Diet. Assoc.* **71:**41–45.

Brun, T. A., Geissler, C. A., Mirbagheri, I., Hormozdiary, H., Bastani, J., and Hedayat, H., 1979, The energy expenditure of Iranian agricultural workers, *Am. J. Clin. Nutr.* **32:**2154–2161.

Buccola, V. A., and Stone, W. J., 1975, Effects of jogging and cycling programs on physiological and personality variables in aged men, *Res. Q.* **46:**134–139.

Bunker, V. W., Hinks, L. J., Lawson, M. S., and Clayton, B. E., 1984, Assessment of zinc and copper status of healthy elderly people using metabolic balance studies and measurement of leukocyte concentrations, *Am. J. Clin. Nutr.* **40:**1096–1102.

Burant, C. F., Lemmon, S. K., Treutelaar, M. K., and Buse, M. G., 1984, Insulin resistance of denervated rat muscle: A model for impaired receptor function coupling, *Am. J. Physiol.* **247:**E647–E666.

Butterfield, G. E., and Calloway, D. H., 1984, Physical activity improves protein utilization in young men, *Br. J. Nutr.* **51:**171–184.

Calloway, D. H., and Zanni, E., 1980, Energy requirements and energy expenditure of elderly men, *Am. J. Clin. Nutr.* **33:**2088–2092.

Carter, J. E. L., and Phillpis, W. H., 1969, Structural changes in exercising middle-aged males during a 2-year period, *J. Appl. Physiol.* **27:**787–794.

Castelli, W. P., Doyle, J. T., Gorden, T., Hames, C. G., Hjortland, M. C., Hully, S. B., Kagan, A., and Zukel, W. J., 1977, HDL-cholesterol and other lipids in coronary heart disease: The cooperative lipoprotein phenotyping study, *Circulation* **55:**767–772.

Cederholm, J., and Wibell, L., 1986, The relationship of blood pressure to blood glucose and physical leisure time activity, *Acta Med. Scand.* **219:**37–46.

Chadwick, J., and Mann, W. M., 1950, *The Medical Works of Hippocrates,* Blackwell, Oxford, p. 140.

Chandra, R. K., 1985, Nutrition–immunity–infection interactions in old age, in: *Nutrition, Immunity and Illness in the Elderly* (R. K. Chandra, ed.), Pergamon Press, New York, pp. 87–96.

Chapman, J. M., and Massey, F. J., 1964, The interrelationship of serum cholesterol, hypertension, body weight, and risk of coronary artery disease, *J. Chron. Dis.* **17:**933–940.

Cheng, A. H. R., Gomez, A., Bergan, J. G., Lee, F. C., Monckeberg, F., and Chichester, C. O., 1978,

Comparative nitrogen balance study between young and aged adults using three levels of protein intake from a combination wheat–soy-milk mixture, *Am. J. Clin. Nutr.* **31**:12–22.

Chow, R. K., Harrison, J. E., Brown, C. E., and Hajek, V., 1986, Physical fitness effect on bone mass in postmenopausal women, *Arch. Phys. Med. Rehab.* **67**:231–234.

Cohn, S. H., Vartsky, D., Yasumura, S., Savitsky, A., Zanzi, I., Vaswani, A., and Ellis, K. J., 1980, Compartmental body composition based on total-body nitrogen, potassium, and calcium, *Am. J. Physiol.* **239**:E524–E530.

Consolazio, C. F., and Johnson, H. L., 1975, Protein metabolism during intensive physical training in young adults, *Am. J. Clin. Nutr.* **28**:29–35.

Costill, D. L., Cote, R., and Fink, W., 1976, Muscle water and electrolytes following varied levels of dehydration in man, *J. Appl. Physiol.* **40**:6–11.

Cumming, G. R., and Bailey, G. J., 1974, Seasonal variation of cardiorespiratory fitness of grain farmers, *J. Occup. Med.* **16**:91–93.

Davis, J. R., Tagliaferro, A. R., Kertzer, R., Gerardo, T., Nichols, J., and Wheeler, J., 1983, Variations in dietary-induced thermogenesis and body fatness with aerobic capacity, *Eur. J. Appl. Physiol.* **50**:319–329.

Dawson-Hughes, B., Jacques, P., and Shipp, C., 1987, Dietary calcium and bone loss from the spine in healthy postmenopausal women, *Am. J. Clin. Nutr.* **46**:685–687.

Debry, G., and Bleyer, R., 1969, Habitudes alimentaires et risques de carence chez le vieillard, *Rev. Fr. Gerontol.* **15**:393–399.

Debry, G., Bleyer, R., and Martin, J. M., 1977, Nutrition of the elderly, *J. Hum. Nutr.* **31**:195–203.

DeFronzo, R. A., 1979, Glucose tolerance and aging: Evidence for tissue insensitivity to insulin, *Diabetes* **28**:1095–1101.

DeFronzo, R. A., Tobin, J. D., and Andres, R., 1979, Glucose clamp technique: A method for quantifying insulin secretion and resistance, *Am. J. Physiol.* **237**:E214–E223.

Devlin, J. T., and Horton, E. S., 1986, Potentiation of the thermic effect of insulin by exercise: Differences between lean, obese, and non-insulin-dependent diabetic men, *Am. J. Clin. Nutr.* **43**:884–890.

Dibble, M. V., Brin, M., Thiele, V. F., Peel, A., Chen, N., and McMullen, E., 1967, Evaluation of the nutritional status of elderly subjects, with a comparison between fall and spring, *J. Am. Geriatr. Soc.* **15**:1031–1061.

Dietz, W. H., and Gortmaker, S. L., 1985, Do we fatten our children at the TV set? *Pediatrics* **75**:807–812.

Dill, D. B., Consolazio, C. F., 1962, Responses to exercise as related to age and environmental temperature, *J. Appl. Physiol.* **17**:647–658.

Donaldson, D., Evans, O. B., and Harrison, R. W., 1986, Insulin binding in denervated muscle, *Muscle Nerve* **9**:211–215.

Drinkwater, B. I., Bedi, J. F., Loucks, A. B., Roche, S., and Horvath, S. M., 1982, Sweating sensitivity and capacity of women in relation to age, *J. Appl. Physiol.* **53**:671–676.

Ducimetiere, P., Eschwege, L., Papoz, J., Richard, J. L., Claude, J. R., and Rosselin, G., 1980, Relationship of plasma insulin levels to the incidence of myocardial infarction and coronary heart disease mortality in a middle-aged population, *Diabetologia* **19**:205–210.

Edstrom, L., and Grimby, G., 1986, Effect of exercise on the motor unit, *Muscle Nerve* **9**:104–126.

Epstein, Y., Keren, G., Udassin, R., and Shapiro, Y., 1981, Way of life as a determinant of physical fitness, *Eur. J. Appl. Physiol.* **47**:1–5.

Evans, D. J., Hoffmann, R. G., Kalfhoff, R. K., and Kissebah, A. H., 1984, Relationship of body fat topography to insulin sensitivity and metabolic profiles in premenopausal women, *Metab. Clin. Exp.* **33**:68–75.

Evans, W. J., Fisher, E. C., and Hoerr, R. A., and Young, V. R., 1983, Protein metabolism and endurance exercise, *Physician Sports Med.* **11**:63–72.

Fahey, T. D., Akka, L., and Rolph, R., 1975, Body composition and $V\text{O}_2$max of exceptional weight-trained athletes, *J. Appl. Physiol.* **39**:559–561.

Farrar, R. P., Martin, T. P., and Ardies, C., 1981, The interaction of aging and endurance exercise upon the mitochondrial function of skeletal muscle, *J. Gerontol.* **36**:642–647.

Felig, P., 1975, Amino acid metabolism in man, *Annu. Rev. Biochem.* **44**:933–955.

Fink, R. I., Kolterman, O. G., Griffin, J., and Olefsky, J. M., 1983, Mechanism of insulin resistance in aging, *J. Clin. Invest.* **71**:1523–1535.

Fink, R. I., Kolterman, O. G., and Olefsky, J. M., 1984, The physiological significance of the glucose intolerance of aging, *J. Gerontol.* **39:**273–278.

Fries, J. F., 1980, Aging, natural death, and the compression of morbidity, *N. Engl. J. Med.* **303:**130–135.

Frisch, R. E., Wyshak, G., Albright, N. L., Albright, T. E., Schiff, I., Witschi, J., and Marguglio, M., 1987, Lower lifetime occurrence of breast cancer and cancers of the reproductive system among former college athletes, *Am. J. Clin. Nutr.* **45:**328–335.

Frontera, W. R., 1986, *Strength Training and Diet: Effects on Skeletal Muscle in Older Men,* Ph.D. Thesis, Boston University, Boston.

Gallagher, J. C., Riggs, B. L., Eisman, J., Hamstra, A., Arnaud, S. B., and DeLuca, H. F., 1979, Intestinal calcium absorption and serum vitamin D. metabolites in normal subjects and osteoporotic patients, *J. Clin. Invest.* **64:**729–736.

Garetto, L. P., Richter, E. A., Goodman, M. N., and Ruderman, N. B., 1984, Enhanced muscle glucose metabolism after exercise in the rat: The two phases, *Am. J. Physiol.* **246:**E471–E475.

Garry, P. J., and Hunt, W. C., 1986, Vitamin status of healthy elderly, in: *Nutrition and Aging* (M. L. Hutchinson and H. N. Munro, eds.), Academic Press, New York, pp. 117–137.

Gersovitz, M., Motil, K., Munro, H. N., Scrimshaw, N. S., and Young, V. R., 1982, Human protein requirements: Assessment of the adequacy of the current recommended dietary allowance for dietary protein in elderly men and women, *Am. J. Clin. Nutr.* **35:**6–14.

Golay, A., Schutz, Y., Broguet, C., Moeri, R., Felber, J. P., and Jequier, E., 1983, Decreased thermogenic response to an oral glucose load in older subjects, *J. Am. Geriatr. Soc.* **31:**144–148.

Goldspink, D. F., and Kelly, F. J., 1984, Protein turnover and growth in the whole body, liver and kidney of the rat from the fetus to senility, *Biochem. J.* **217:**507–516.

Goldspink, D. F., Morton, A. J., Loughna, P., and Goldspink, G., 1986, The effect of hypokinesia and hypodynamia on protein turnover and the growth of four skeletal muscles of the rat, *Pflugers Arch.* **407:**333–340.

Gontzea, I., Sutzescu, P., and Dumitrache, S., 1975, The influence of adaptation to physical effort on nitrogen balance in man, *Nutr. Rep. Int.* **11:**233–236.

Goodrick, C. L., 1980, Effects of long-term voluntary wheel exercise on male and female rats. I. Longevity, body weight, and metabolic rate, *Gerontology* **26:**22–33.

Gordon, T. W., Castelli, W. P., Hjortland, M. J., Kannel, W. B., and Dawbe, T. R., 1977, HDL as a protective factor against CHD: The Framingham study, *Am. J. Med.* **62:**707–712.

Greenfield, M. S., Kraemer, F., Tobey, T., and Reaven, G., 1980, Effect of age on plasma triglyceride concentrations in man, *Metabolism* **29:**1095–1099.

Haffner, S. M., Stern, M. P., Hazuda, H. P., Pugh, J., and Patterson, J. K., 1987, Do upper-body and centralized adiposity measure different aspects of regional body-fat distribution? *Diabetes* **36:**43–51.

Hakkinen, K., Pakarinen, A., Alen, M., and Komi, P. V., 1985, Serum hormones during prolonged training of neuromuscular performance, *Eur. J. Appl. Physiol.* **53:**287–293.

Hallfrisch, J., Steele, P., and Cohen, L., 1982, Comparison of a seven-day diet record with measured food intake of twenty-four subjects, *Nutr. Res.* **2:**263–273.

Hansson, T., and Roos, B., 1986, Age changes in the bone mineral of the lumbar spine in normal women, *Calcif. Tissue Int.* **38:**249–251.

Harris, M., 1982, The prevalence of diabetes, undiagnosed diabetes and impaired glucose tolerance in the United States, in: *Genetic Environmental Interaction in Diabetes Mellitus* (H. S. Melish, J. Hanna, and S. Baba, eds.), Exerpta Medica, Amsterdam, pp. 70–76.

Hartz, A. J., Rupley, D. C., and Rimm, A. A., 1984, The association of girth measurements with disease in 32,856 women, *Am. J. Epidemiol.* **119:**71–80.

Heaney, R. P., Recker, R. R., and Saville, P. D., 1977, Calcium balance and calcium requirements in middle-aged women, *Am. J. Clin. Nutr.* **30:**1603–1611.

Heath, G. W., Gavin, J. R. III, Hinderliter, J. M., Hagberg, J. M., Bloomfield, S. A., and Holloszy, J. O., 1983, Effects of exercise and lack of exercise on glucose tolerance and insulin sensitivity, *J. Appl. Physiol.* **55:**512–517.

Hickson, J. F., and Hinkelman, K., 1985, Exercise and protein intake effects on urinary 3-methylhistidine excretion, *Am. J. Clin. Nutr.* **41:**246–253.

Higginbotham, M. B., Morris, K. G., Williams, R. S., Coleman, E., and Cobb, F. R., 1986, Physiologic basis for the age-related decline in aerobic work capacity, *Am. J. Cardiol.* **57:**1374–1379.

Ho, Z. C., 1982, A study of longevity and protein requirements of individuals 90 to 112 years old in southern China, *J. Appl. Nutr.* **34:**12–23.

Hollenbeck, C. B., Coulston, A. M., and Reaven, G. M., 1986, To what extent does increased dietary fiber improve glucose and lipid metabolism in patients with noninsulin-dependent diabetes mellitus (NIDDM)? *Am. J. Clin. Nutr.* **43:**16–24.

Holloszy, J. O., Skinner, S., Toro, G., and Cureton, T. K., 1964, Effects of a six-month program of endurance exercise on the serum lipids of middle-aged men, *Am. J. Cardiol.* **14:**753–760.

Holloszy, J. D., Schultz, J., Kusnierkiewicz, J., Hagberg, J. M., and Ehsani, A. A., 1986, Effects of exercise on glucose tolerance and insulin resistance, *Acta Med. Scand. [Suppl.]* **711:**55–65.

Imamura, K., Ashida, H., Ishikawa, T., and Fujii, M., 1983, Human major psoas muscle and sacrospinalis muscle in relation to age: A study by computed tomography, *J. Gerontol.* **38:**678–681.

Irion, G., Wailgum, T. D., Stevens, C., Kendrick, Z. V., and Paolone, A. M., 1984, The effect of age on the hemodynamic responses to thermal stress during exercise, in: *Modern Aging Research,* Volume 6 (V. J. Cristofalo, G. T. Blaker, R. C. Adelman, and J. Roberts, eds.), Alan R. Liss, New York.

Issekutz, B., Blizzard, J. J., Birkhead, N. C., and Rodahl, K., 1966, Effect of prolonged bed rest on urinary calcium output, *J. Appl. Physiol.* **21:**1013–1020.

Jarret, R. J., McCartney, P., and Keen, J., 1982, The Bedford survey: Ten year mortality rates in newly diagnosed diabetics, borderline diabetics and normoglycemic controls and risk indices for coronary heart disease in borderline diabetics, *Diabetologia* **22:**79–84.

Jette, A. M., and Branch, L. G., 1981, The Framingham disability study: II. Physical disability among the aging, *Am. J. Public Health* **71:**1211–1216.

Kaplan, G. A., Seeman, T. E., Cohen, R. D., Knudsen, L. P., and Guralnik, J., 1987, Mortality among the elderly in the Alameda County study: Behavioral and demographic risk factors, *Am. J. Public Health* **x7:**307–312.

Katz, S., Branch, L. G., Branson, M. H., Papsidero, J. A., Beck, J. C., and Greer, D. S., 1983, Active life expectancy, *N. Engl. J. Med.* **309:**1218–1224.

Kelly, F. J., Lewis, S. E., Anderson, P., and Goldspink, D. F., 1984, Pre and postnatal growth and protein turnover in four muscles of the rat, *Muscle Nerve* **7:**235–242.

Kiehm, T. G., Anderson, J. W., and Ward, K., 1976, Beneficial effects of a high carbohydrate high fiber diet on hyperglycemic diabetic men, *Am. J. Clin. Nutr.* **29:**895–899.

Kiens, B., Jorgensen, I., Lewis, S., Jensen, G., Lithell, H., Vessby, B., Hoe, S., and Schnohr, P., 1980, Increased plasma HDL-cholesterol and apoA-1 in sedentary middle-aged men after physical conditioning, *Eur. J. Clin. Invest.* **10:**203–209.

Kissebah, A. N., Vydelingum, N., Murry, R., Evans, D. J., Hartz, A. J., Kalkhoff, R. K., and Adams, P. N., 1982, Relation of body fat distribution to metabolic complications of obesity, *J. Clin. Endorinol. Metab.* **54:**254–260.

Kolterman, O. G., Insel, J., Saekow, M., and Olefsky, J. M., 1980, Mechanisms of insulin resistance in human obesity. Evidence for receptor and postreceptor defects, *J. Clin. Invest* **65:**1272–1284.

Kriska, A. M., Bayles, C., Cauley, J. A., Laporte, R. E., Black, R., and Pambianco, G., 1986, A randomized exercise trial in older women: Increased activity over two years and the factors associated with complicance, *Med. Sci. Sports Exercise* **18:**557–562.

Krolner, B., and Toft, B., 1983, Vertebral bone loss: An unheeded side effect of therapeutic bed rest, *Clin. Sci.* **64:**537–540.

Krolner, B., Toft, B., Nielsen, S. P., and Tondevold, E., 1983, Physical exercise as prophylaxis against involutional vertebral bone loss: A controlled trial, *Clin. Sci.* **64:**541–546.

Krotkiewski, M., 1983, Physical training in the prophylaxis and treatment of obesity, hypertension and diabetes, *Scand. J. Rehab. [Suppl.]* **9:**55–70.

Kukkonen, K., Rauramaa, R., Siitonen, O., and Hanninen, O., 1982, Physical training of obese middle-aged persons, *Ann. Clin. Res.* **14:**80–85.

Lane, N. E., Bloch, D. A., Jones, H. H., Marshall, W. H., Wood, P. D., and Fries, J. F., 1986, Long-distance running, bone density and osteoarthritis, *J.A.M.A.* **255:**1147–1151.

LaRosa, J. C., Cleary, P., Muesing, R. A., Gorman, P., Hellerstein, H. K., and Naughton, T., 1982, Effect of long-term moderate physical exercise on plasma lipoproteins: The National Exercise and Heart Disease Project, *Arch. Intern. Med.* **142:**2269–2274.

Larsson, L., 1982, Physical training effects on muscle morphology in sedentary males at different ages, *Med. Sci. Sports Exercise* **14:**203–206.

Larsson, L., 1983, Histochemical characteristics of human skeletal muscle during aging, *Acta Physiol. Scand.* **117**:469–471.

Laurent, G. J., Sparrow, M. P., and Millward, D. J., 1978, Turnover of muscle protein in the fowl, *Biochem. J.* **176**:407–417.

Leaf, A., 1973, Unusual longevity: The common demoninators, *Hosp. Pract.* **8**(10):75–86.

LeBlanc, J., Nadeau, A., Richard, D., and Tremblay, A., 1981, Studies on the sparing effect of exercise on insulin requirements in human subjects, *Metabolism* **30**:1119–1124.

Levine, J. A., 1969, Heat stroke in the aged, *Am. J. Med.* **47**:251–256.

Lexell, J., Henriksson-Larsen, K., Wimblod, B., and Sjostrom, M., 1983, Distribution of different fiber types in human skeletal muscles: Effects of aging studied in whole muscle cross sections, *Muscle Nerve* **6**:588–595.

Lipman, R. L., Raskin, P., Love, T., Triebwasser, J., Lecocq, F. R., and Schnure, J. J., 1972, Glucose intolerance during decreased physical activity in man, *Diabetes* **21**(2):101–107.

Lukaski, H. C., Mendez, J., Buskirk, E. R., and Cohn, S. H., 1981, Relationship between endogenous 3-methyl-histidine excretion and body composition, *Am. J. Physiol.* **240**:E302–E307.

Lundholm, K., Holm, G., Lindmark, L., Larsson, B., Sjostrom, L., and Bjorntorp, P., 1986, Thermogenic effect of food in physically well-trained elderly men, *Eur. J. Appl. Physiol.* **55**:486–492.

Lutwak, L., and Whedon, G. J., 1959, The effect of physical conditioning on glucose tolerance, *Clin. Res.* **7**:143–144.

Lye, M., 1977, Effects of a heatwave on mortality-rates in elderly inpatients, *Lancet* **1**:529–531.

Mann, G. V., Teel, K., Hayes, O., McNally, A., and Bruno, D., 1955, Exercise in the disposition of dietary calories: Regulation of serum lipoprotein and cholesterol levels in human subjects, *N. Engl. J. Med.* **253**:349–355.

Mann, G. V., Shaffer, R. D., and Rich, A., 1965, Physical fitness and immunity to heart-disease in Masai, *Lancet* **2**:1308–1310.

Manton, K. G., and Soldo, B. J., 1985, Dynamics of health changes in the oldest old: New perspectives and evidence, *Milbank Mem. Fund Q.* **63**:206–285.

Mark, D. A., Borbjerg, D., Katzeff, H., Rivlin, R. S., and Weksler, M. E., 1986, Effects of voluntary exercise and caloric restriction on murine lymphocyte responses, thyroid hormone levels, and life span, in: *Nutrition, Immunity and Illness in the Elderly* (R. K. Chandra, ed.), Pergamon Press, New York, pp. 192–199.

Matkovic, V., Kostial, K., Simonovic, I., Buzina, R., Brodarec, A., and Nordin, B. E., 1979, Bone status and fracture rates in two regions of Yugoslavia, *Am. J. Clin. Nutr.* **32**:540–549.

McGandy, R. B., Barrows, C. H., Spanias, A., Meredith, A., Stone, J. L., and Norris, A. H., 1966, Nutrient intake and energy expenditure in men of different ages, *J. Gerontol.* **21**:581–587.

Meredith, C. N., Zackin, M. J., Frontera, W. R., and Evans, W. J., 1988, Protein metabolism in young and middle-aged endurance-trained men, *Am. J. Physiol.* (in press).

Meredith, C. N., Zackin, M. J., Frontera, W. R., and Evans, W. J., 1987, Body composition and aerobic capacity in endurance-trained men: Effects of age and habitual exercise, *Med. Sci. Sports Exercise* **19**:557–563.

Meredith, C. N., Frontera, W. J., Fisher, E. C., Hughes, V. A., Herland, J. S., Edwards, J., and Evans, W. J., Endurance training in young and old men and women: effects on body composition, VO_2 max and muscle metabolism, *J. Appl. Physiol.* (in press).

Miller, G. J., and Miller, N. E., 1975, Plasma high density lipoprotein concentration and the development of ischaemic heart disease, *Lancet* **1**:16–19.

Millward, D. J., Davies, C. T. M., Halliday, D., Wolman, S., Matthews, D., and Rennie, M., 1982, Effect of exercise on protein metabolism in humans as explored by stable isotopes, *Fed. Proc.* **41**:2686–2691.

Minaker, K. L., and Rowe, J., 1985, Health and disease among the oldest old: A clinical perspective, *Millbank Mem. Fund Q.* **63**:324–349.

Mondon, C. E., Dolkas, C. B., and Oyama, J., 1981, Enhanced skeletal muscle insulin sensitivity in year-old rats adapted to hypergravity, *Am. J. Physiol.* **240**:E482–E488.

Mondon, C. E., Dolkas, C. B., Sims, C., and Reaven, G. M., 1985, Spontaneous running activity in male rats: Effect of age, *J. Appl. Physiol.* **58**:1553–1557.

Mondon, C. E., Sims, C., Dolkas, C. B., Reaven, E. P., and Reaven, G. M., 1986, The effect of exercise training on insulin resistance in sedentary year old rats, *J. Gerontol.* **41**:605–610.

Moreiras-Varela, O., Ortega, R. M., Ruiz, B., and Varela, G., 1986, Nutritional status of an institutionalized elderly group in Segovia, Spain, *Int. J. Vitam. Nutr. Res.* **56:**109–117.

Morgan, P., Gildiner, M., and Wright, G. R., 1976, Smoking reduction in adults who take up exercise: A survey of a running club for adults, *CAHPER J.* **42:**39–43.

Moritani, T., and DeVries, H. A., 1980, Potential for gross muscle hypertrophy in older men, *J. Gerontol.* **35:**672–682.

Mott, D. M., Lillioja, S., and Bogardus, C., 1986, Overnutrition induced decrease in insulin action for glucose storage *in vivo in vitro* in man, *Metabolism* **35:**160–165.

Munro, H. N., 1951, Carbohydrate and fat as factors in protein utilization and metabolism, *Physiol. Rev.* **31:**449–488.

Narimiya, M., Azhar, S., Dolkas, C. B., Mondon, C. E., Sims, C., Wright, D. W., and Reaven, G. M., 1984, Insulin resistance in older rats, *Am. J. Physiol.* **246:**E397–E404.

Nelson, M. E., Meredith, C. N., Dawson-Hughes, B., and Evans, W. J., 1988, Hormone and bone mineral status in endurance-trained and sedentary postmenopausal women, *J. Clin. Endocrinol. Metab.* **66:**927–933.

Nelson, M. E., Fisher, E. C., Catsos, P. D., Meredith, C. N., Turksoy, R. N., and Evans, W. J., 1986, Diet and bone status in amenorrheic athletes, *Am. J. Clin. Nutr.* **43:**910–916.

Nicholson, W. F., Watson, P. A., and Booth, F. W., 1984, Glucose uptake and glycogen synthesis in muscles from immobilized limbs, *J. Appl. Physiol.* **56:**431–435.

O'Dea, K., 1984, Marked improvement in carbohydrate and lipid metabolism in diabetic Australian aborigines after temporary reversion to traditional lifestyle, *Diabetes* **33:**596–603.

Offenbacher, E. G., and Pi-Sunyer, F. X., 1980, Beneficial effect of chromium-rich yeast on glucose tolerance and blood lipids in elderly subjects, *Diabetes* **29:**919–925.

Pacifici, R., Droke, D., and Avioli, L. V., 1985, Intestinal lactase activity and calcium absorption in the aging female with osteoporosis, *Calcif. Tissue Int.* **37:**101–102.

Paffenbarger, R. S., Hyde, R. T., Wing, A. L., and Hsieh, C. C., 1986, Physical activity, all-cause mortality, and longevity of college alumni, *N. Engl. J. Med.* **314:**605–613.

Parizkova, J., Eiselt, E., Sprynarova, S., and Wachtlova, M., 1971, Body composition, aerobic capacity, and density of muscle capillaries in young and old men, *J. Appl. Physiol.* **31:**323–325.

Passmore, R., and Durnin, J. V., 1955, Human energy expenditure, *Physiol. Rev.* **35:**801–840.

Pavlou, K. N., Steffee, W. P., Lerman, R. H., and Burrows, B. A., 1985, Effects of dieting and exercise on lean body mass, oxygen uptake, and strength, *Med. Sci. Sports Exercise* **17:**466–471.

Peiris, A. N., Mueller, R. A., Smith, G. A., Struve, M. F., and Kissebah, A. H., 1986, Splanchnic insulin metabolism in obesity: Influence of body fat distribution, *J. Clin. Invest.* **78:**1648–1657.

Philips, P. A., Rolls, B. J., Ledingham, J. G. G., Forsling, M. L., Morton, J. J., Crowe, M. J., and Wollner, L., 1984, Reduced thirst after water deprivation in healthy elderly men, *N. Engl. J. Med.* **311:**753–759.

Potter, J. F., Levin, P., Anderson, R. A., Freiberg, J. M., Andres, R., and Elahi, D., 1985, Glucose metabolism in glucose-intolerant older people during chromium supplementation, *Metabolism* 34:199–204.

Prentice, A. M., Coward, W. A., Davies, H. L., Murgatroyd, P. R., Black, A. E., Goldberg, G. R., Ashford, J., Sawyer, M., and Whitehead, R. G., 1985, Unexpectedly low levels of energy expenditure in healthy women, *Lancet* **1:**1419–1422.

Rabinovitz, D., and Zierler, K. L., 1962, Forearm metabolism in obesity and its response to intra-arterial insulin: Characterization of insulin resistance and evidence for adaptive hyperinsulinism, *J. Clin. Invest.* **41:**2173–2182.

Ravussin, E., Acheson, K. J., Vernet, O., Danforth, E., and Jequier, E., 1985, Evidence that insulin resistance is responsible for the decreased thermic effect of glucose in human obesity, *J. Clin. Invest.* **76:**1268–1273.

Ravussin, E., Lillioja, S., Anderson, T. E., Cristin, L., and Bogardus, C., 1986, Determinants of 24-hour energy expenditure in man, *J. Clin. Invest.* **78:**1568–1578.

Reaven, E. P., and Reaven, G. M., 1981, Structure and function changes in the endocrine pancreas of aging rats with reference to the modulating effects of exercise and caloric restriction, *J. Clin. Invest.* **68:**75–84.

Reaven, E., Wright, D., Mondon, E. E., Solomon, R., Ho, H., and Reaven, G. M., 1983, Effect of age and diet on insulin secretion and insulin action in the rat, *Diabetes* **32:**175–180.

Reaven, G. M., 1986, Effect of dietary carbohydrate on the metabolism of patients with non-insulin dependent diabetes mellitus, *Nutr. Rev.* **44:**65–73.

Reaven, G. M., and Reaven, E. P., 1980, Effects of age on various aspects of glucose and insulin metabolism, *Mol. Cell. Biochem.* **31:**37–47.

Rennie, M. J., and Millward, D. J., 1983, 3-Methylhistidine excretion and the 3-methylhistidine/creatinine ratio are poor indicators of skeletal muscle protein breakdown, *Clin. Sci.* **65:**217–225.

Richter, E. A., Garetto, L. P., Goodman, M. N., and Ruderman, N. B., 1984, Enhanced muscle glucose metabolism after exercise: Modulation by local factors, *Am. J. Physiol.* **246:**E476–E482.

Riggs, B. L., Wahner, H. W., Seeman, E., Offord, K. P., Dunn, W. L., Mazess, R. B., Johnson, K. A., and Melton, L. J., 1982, Changes in bone mineral density of the proximal femur and spine with aging, *J. Clin. Invest.* **70:**716–723.

Rigotti, N. A., Nussbaum, S. R., Herzog, D. B., and Neer, R. M., 1984, Osteoporosis in women with anorexia nervosa, *N. Engl. J. Med.* **311:**1601–1606.

Riis, B., Thomsen, K., and Christiansen, C., 1987, Does calcium supplementation prevent postmenopausal bone loss? *N. Engl. J. Med.* **316:**173–177.

Robinson, S., 1938, Experimental studies of physical fitness in relation to age, *Arbeitsphysiologie* **10:**251–323.

Robinson, S., Belding, H. S., Consolazio, F. C., Horvath, S. M., and Turrell, E. S., 1965, Acclimatization of older men to work in heat, *J. Appl. Physiol.* **20:**583–586.

Rosenthal, M., Haskell, W. L., Solomon, R., Widstrom, A., and Reaven, G. M., 1983, Demonstration of a relationship between level of physical training and insulin-stimulated glucose utilization in normal humans, *Diabetes* **32:**408–411.

Ross, M. H., 1977, Dietary behavior and longevity, *Nutr. Rev.* **35:**257–265.

Rowe, J. W., Shock, N. W., and DeFronzo, R. A., 1976, The influence of age on the renal response to water deprivation in man, *Nephron* **17:**270–278.

Rowe, J. W., Minaker, K. L., Pallotta, J. A., and Flier, J. S., 1983, Characterization of the insulin resistance of aging, *J. Clin. Invest.* **71:**1581–1587.

Rubin, C. T., and Lanyon, L. E., 1985, Regulation of bone mass by mechanical strain magnitude, *Calcif. Tissue Int.* **37:**411–417.

Ruderman, N. B., Ganda, O. B., and Johansen, K., 1979, The effect of physical training on glucose tolerance and plasma lipids in maturity onset diabetes, *Diabetes* **28**(Suppl. 1)**:**89–92.

Russell, R. M., 1986, Implications of gastric atrophy for vitamin and mineral nutrition, in: *Nutrition and Aging* (M. L. Hutchinson and H. N. Munro, eds.), Academic Press, New York, pp. 59–69.

Sallis, J. F., Haskell, W. L., Wood, P. D., and Fortman, S. P., 1985, Physical activity assessment methodology in the Five City project, *Am. J. Epidemiol.* **121:**91–106.

Salminen, A., and Kihlstrom, M., 1985, Lysosomal changes in mouse skeletal muscle during the repari of exercise injuries, *Muscle & Nerve* **8:**269–279.

Salminen, A., and Vihko, V., 1981, Acid hydrolase activities in mouse cardiac and skeletal muscle following exhaustive exercise, *Eur. J. Appl. Physiol.* **47:**57–64.

Saltin, B., Lindgarde, F., Houston, M., Horlin, R., Nygaard, E., and Gad, P., 1979, Physical training and glucose tolerance in middle-aged men with chemical diabetes, *Diabetes* **28**(Suppl. 1)**:**30–32.

Sanborn, C. F., Martin, B. J., and Wagner, W. W., 1982, Is athletic amenorrhea specific to runners? *Am. J. Obstet. Gynecol.* **143:**859–861.

Sandler, R. B., Slemenda, C. W., LaPorte, R. E., Cauley, J. A., Schramm, M. M., Barresi, M. L., and Kriska, A. M., 1985, Postmenopausal bone density and milk consumption in childhood and adolescence, *Am. J. Clin. Nutr.* **42:**270–274.

Schalch, D., 1967. The influence of physical stress and exercise on growth hormone and insulin secretion in men. *J. Lab. Clin. Med.* **69:**256–260.

Schneider, S. H., Amorosa, L. F., Kachadurinan, A. K., and Ruderman, N. B., 1984, Studies on the mechanisms of improved glucose control during regular exercise in type 2 (non-insulin dependent) diabetics, *Diabetologia* **26:**355–360.

Schutz, Y., Bessard, T., and Jequier, E., 1984, Diet-induced thermogenesis measured over a whole day in obese and non-obese women, *Am. J. Clin. Nutr.* **40:**542–552.

Scrimshaw, M. S., Hussein, M. A., Murray, E., Rand, W. M., and Young, V. R., 1972, Protein requirements of man: Variations in obligatory urinary and fecal nitrogen losses in young men, *J. Nutr.* **102:**1595–1604.

Seals, D. R., Hagberg, J. M., and Allen, W. K., 1984a, Glucose tolerance in young and older athletes and sedentary men, *J. Appl. Physiol.: Respirat. Environ. Exercise Physiol.* **56:**1521–1525.

Seals, D. R., Hagberg, J. M., Hurley, B. F., Ehsani, A. A., and Holloszy, J. O., 1984b, Effects of endurance training on glucose tolerance and plasma lipid levels in older men and women, *J.A.M.A.* **252:**645–649.

Segal, K. R., Gutin, B., Nyman, A. M., and Pi-Sunyer, F. X., 1985, Thermic effect of food at rest, during exercise, and after exercise in lean and obese men of similar body weight, *J. Clin. Invest.* **76:**1107–1112.

Sellery, S. B., 1984, New product opportunities: diet food for older Americans, *J. Nutr. Elderly* **4:**31–41.

Sidney, K. H., Shephard, R. J., and Harrison, J. E., 1977, Endurance training and body composition of the elderly, *Am. J. Clin. Nutr.* **30:**326–333.

Sieder, M. J., Nicholson, W. F., and Booth, F. W., 1982, Insulin resistance for glucose metabolism in disused soleus muscle of mice, *Am. J. Physiol.* **242:**E121–E128.

Siegel, C., Blomquist, A., and Mitchell, J. H., 1970, Effects of a quantitated physical training program on middle-aged sedentary men, *Circulation* **41:**19–25.

Smith, E. L., Reddan, W., and Smith, P. E., 1981, Physical activity and calcium modalities for bone mineral increase in aged women, *Med. Sci. Sports Exercise* **13:**60–64.

Smith, L. C., and Dugal, L. P., 1965, Age and spontaneous activity of male rats, *Can. J. Physiol. Pharmacol.* **43:**852–856.

Smith, R. H., Palmer, R. M., and Reeds, P. J., 1983, Protein synthesis in isolated rabbit forelimb muscles, *Biochem. J.* **214:**153–161.

Smith, U., Hammarsten, J., Bjorntorp, P., and Kral, J., 1979, Regional differences and effect of weight reduction on human fat cell metabolism, *Eur. J. Clin. Invest.* **9:**327–332.

Spurr, G. B., 1984, Physical activity, nutritional status, and physical work in relation to agricultural productivity, in: *Energy Intake and Activity* (E. Pollitt and P. Amante, eds.), Alan R. Liss, New York, pp. 207–261.

Steinke, J., and Soeldner, J. S., 1977, Diabetes mellitus, in: *Harrison's Principles of Internal Medicine*, 8th ed. (G. W. Thorn, R. D. Adams, E. Braunwald, K. J. Isselbacher, and R. G. Petersdorf, eds.), McGraw-Hill, New York, p. 569.

Stiedemann, M., Jansen, C., and Harrill, J., 1978, Nutritional status of elderly men and women, *J. Am. Diet. Assoc.* **73:**132–139.

Storlien, L. H., James, D. E., Burleigh, K. M., Chisolm, D. J., and Kraegen, E. W., 1986, Fat feeding causes widespread *in vivo* insulin resistance, decreased energy expenditure, and obesity in rats, *Am. J. Physiol.* **251:**E576–E583.

Suter, P. M., and Russell, R. M., 1987, Vitamin requirements of the elderly: A review, *Am. J. Clin. Nutr.* **45:**501–512.

Suzman, R., and White-Riley, M., 1985, Introducing the "oldest old," *Milbank Mem. Fund Q.* **63:**177–186.

Symreng, T., Anderberg, B., Kagedal, B., Norr, A., Schildt, B., and Sjodahl, R., 1983, Nutritional assessment and clinical course in 112 elective surgical patients, *Acta Chir. Scand.* **149:**657–662.

Tapscott, E. B., Kasperek, G. J., and Dohm, G. L., 1982, Effect of training on muscle protein turnover in male and female rats, *Biochem. Med.* **27:**254–259.

Ten-State Nutrition Survey, 1968–1970, 1972, Highlights, DHEW Pub. No. (HSM) 72-8134, Government Printing Office, Washington.

Todd, K. S., Butterfield, G. E., and Calloway, D. H., 1984, Nitrogen balance in men with adequate and deficient energy intake at three levels of work, *J. Nutr.* **114:**2107–2118.

Tokuyama, K., Saito, M., and Okuda, H., 1982, Effects of wheel running on food intake and weight gain of male and female rats, *Physiol. Behav.* **28:**899–903.

Torun, B., Scrimshaw, N. S., and Young, V.R., 1977, Effect of isometric exercises on body potassium and dietary protein requirements of young men, *Am. J. Clin. Nutr.* **30:**1983–1993.

Tran, Z. V., and Weltman, A., 1985, Differential effects of exercise on serum lipid and lipoprotein levels seen with changes in body weight: A meta-analysis, *J.A.M.A.* **254:**919–924.

Tremblay, A., Fontaine, E., and Nadeau, A., 1985, Contribution of post-exercise increment in glucose storage to variations in glucose-induced thermogenesis in endurance athletes, *Can. J. Physiol. Pharmacol.* **63:**1165–1169.

Tzankoff, S. P., and Norris, A. H., 1978, Longitudinal changes in basal metabolic rate in man, *J. Appl. Physiol.* **45:**536–539.

Tzankoff, S. P., Robinson, S., Pyke, F. S., and Brawn, C. A., 1972, Physiological adjustments to work in older men as affected by physical training, *J. Appl. Physiol.* **33:**346–350.

Uauy, R., Scrimshaw, M. S., and Young, V. R., 1978, Human protein requirements: Nitrogen balance response to graded levels of egg protein in elderly men and women, *Am. J. Clin. Nutr.* **31:**779–785.

Vallerand, A. L., Lupien, J., and Bukowiecki, J., 1986, Synergistic improvement of glucose tolerance by sucrose feeding and exercise training, *Am. J. Physiol.* **250:**E607–E614.

Verschuur, R., and Kemper, H. C. G., 1985, The pattern of daily physical activity, *Med. Sport Sci.* **20:**169–186.

Wallenberg-Henriksson, H., 1986, Repeated exercise regulates glucose transport capacity in skeletal muscle, *Acta Physiol. Scand.* **127:**39–43.

Weiss, L. W., Cureton, K. J., and Thompson, F. N., 1983, Comparison of serum testosterone and androstenedione responses to weight lifting in men and women, *Eur. J. Appl. Physiol.* **50:**413–419.

Whipp, B. J., and Davis, J. A., 1984, The ventrilatory stress of exercise in obesity, *Am. Rev. Respir. Dis.* **129:**S90–S92.

Williams, M. H., 1984, Vitamin and mineral supplements to athletes: Do they help? *Clin. Sports Med.* **3:**623–637.

Williams, R. R., Hasstedt, S. J., Wilson, D. E., Ash, K. O., Yanowitz, F. F., Reiber, G. E., and Kuida, H., 1986, Evidence that men with familial hypercholesterolemia can avoid early coronary death, *J.A.M.A.* **255:**219–224.

Wilmore, J., Royce, J., Girandola, R. N., Katch, F. I., and Katch, V. L., 1970, Body composition changes with a 10-week program of jogging, *Med. Sci. Sports* **2:**113–117.

Wilmore, J., 1974, Alterations in strength body composition and anthropometric measurements consequent to a 10-week training program, *Med. Sci. Sports* **6:**133–138.

Wolfe, R. R., 1984, Whole body protein turnover, in: *Tracers in Metabolic Research* Alan R. Liss, New York, pp. 157–173.

Wood, P. D., Haskell, W. L., Blair, S. N., Williams, P. T., Krauss, R. M., Lindgren, F. T., Albers, J. J., Ho, P. H., and Farquhar, J. W., 1983, Increased exercise level and plasma lipoprotein concentrations: A one year, randomized, controlled study in sedentary middle-aged men, *Metabolism* **32:**31–39.

Yano, K., Heilbrun, L. K., Wasnich, R. D., Hankin, J. H., and Vogel, J. M., 1985, The relationship between diet and bone mineral content of multiple skeletal sites in elderly Japanese-American men and women living in Hawaii, *Am. J. Clin. Nutr.* **42:**877–888.

Young, E. W., and Sparks, H. V., 1980, Prostaglandins and exercise hyperemia of dog skeletal muscle, *Am. J. Physiol.* **238:**H190–H195.

Young, J. C., Treadway, J. L., Balon, T. W., Gavras, H. P., and Ruderman, N. B., 1986, Prior exercise potentiates the thermic effect of a carbohydrate load, *Metabolism* **35:**1048–1053.

Young, V. R., Gersovitz, M., and Munro, H. N., 1982, Human aging: Protein and amino acid metabolism and implications for protein and amino acid requirements, in: *Nutritional Approaches to Aging Research* (G. B. Moment, ed.), CRC Press, Boca Raton, FL, pp. 47–81.

Yu, B. P., Basoro, E. J., and McMahan, C. A., 1985, Nutritional influences on aging of Fischer 344 rats: I. Physical, metabolic, and longevity characteristics, *J. Gerontol.* **40:**657–670.

Zackin, M. J., 1986, *Protein Requirements and Metabolism in Middle-Aged and Young Endurance-Trained Men*, Ph.D. Thesis, Tufts University, Boston.

Zanni, E., Calloway, D. H., and Zezulka, A. Y., 1979, Protein requirements of elderly men, *J. Nutr.* **109:**513–524.

Zavaroni, I., Dall'Aglio, E., Bruschi, F., Bonora, E., Alpi, O., Pezzarossa, A., and Butturini, U., 1986, Effect of age and environmental factors on glucose tolerance and insulin secretion in a worker population, *J. Am. Gerontol. Soc.* **34:**271–275.

Zorzano, A., Balon, T., Garetto, L. P., Goodman, M. N., and Ruderman, N. B., 1985, Muscle alpha-aminoisobutyric acid transport after exercise: Enhanced stimulation by insulin, *Am. J. Physiol.* **248:**E546–E552.

II

Nutrient Needs of the Elderly

6

Energy Needs of the Elderly

A New Approach

W. P. T. James, Ann Ralph, and Anna Ferro-Luzzi

1. Introduction

A discussion of human energy needs in the elderly as well as in other age groups raises the issue of what we mean by the term "needs." A recent international report on energy and protein requirements (FAO/WHO/UNU, 1985) has dealt in some detail with this question, but the analysis warrants further emphasis because the question of needs is particularly relevant to the elderly. Indeed, most of the literature that purports to assess the adequacy of diets in the elderly ignores the principles of energy requirements. This chapter sets out a collection of some of the literature on energy requirements, supplemented where there are deficiencies by unpublished data collected as part of a current study of the nutritional status of elderly men and women in Italy (A. Ferro-Luzzi, unpublished data). The implications of these studies are then considered and set in the context of the new approach to assessing energy needs embodied in the recent FAO/WHO/UNU (1985) report.

2. Studies on Energy Intake for Specific Needs

The term "need" in energy terms implies that there is a requirement for dietary energy to meet the demands of a variety of components of energy expenditure. The focus must therefore be on energy expenditure and not on intake. To monitor energy intake as a method of assessing energy needs is inappropriate unless only a very crude analysis is required in a group of individuals who are specified on other grounds as being healthy and having access to unlimited food supplies. Intake data then only help in specifying whether requirements are being met. This conclusion has important implications for the way in which one assesses nutritional data. For example, energy

---

W. P. T. James and Ann Ralph • Rowett Research Institute, Bucksburn, Aberdeen AB2 9SB, Scotland, United Kingdom *Anna Ferro-Luzzi* • National Institute on Nutrition, 00179 Rome, Italy.

intake may be low in a group of people who appear at the time to be reasonably healthy; this low intake may, however, reflect a behavioral response to the investigation, methodological errors, or a state of apathy with limited activity that is not conducive to the individual's long-term health or to the welfare of the family or community.

A behavioral response to dietary surveys is well recognized, with adults altering their behavior either consciously or unconsciously in order to impress the investigator or to conform to some idealized goal. Dietary surveys are notoriously unreliable, a feature that many epidemiologists and nutritionists find hard to countenance because this makes even general statements about dietary intake difficult. Thus, for example, old people asked to respond to a request for a dietary history may have poor recall of what they have eaten. They may also find the technical details of the survey too difficult, particularly if they have to undertake the documentation of intake themselves. An unconscious reduction in the number of foods specified in a history of food intake or a reduction in the variety of foods eaten may occur if food recording is required. This simplifies the monitoring process for the subject but leads to substantial errors.

The problems of dietary survey methodology have been dealt with elsewhere (James *et al.*, 1981; Bingham, 1987; see also Chapter 1). Where systematic errors do occur, the trend is usually to underestimate energy intakes (e.g., in a 24-hr recall approach). Social reasons can be important. Thus, women in developing countries often seem to consider themselves as "needing" less than the men and children of their families (James and Shetty, 1982). It is therefore important when assessing energy intakes to ensure that some validation of the dietary survey is included as well as a check on whether individuals are in a phase of energy imbalance for medical or social reasons. Changes in the seasonal availability of food may be important, as are religious effects on eating, e.g., fasting during Ramadan or overeating at times of Thanksgiving in the United States and Christmas in that and other communities.

In the context of cross-sectional studies of food intake at different ages, it may be noted that a longitudinal study of nutritional intake of men of all ages undertaken over a 15-year period by Elahi *et al.* (1983) confirmed earlier cross-sectional evidence on the same group (McGandy *et al.*, 1966) that total caloric intake per subject declined with age in parallel with a fall in basal metabolic rate and physical activity. However, although the data of Elahi *et al.* (1983), expressed as calories per kilogram body weight, also show an aging-related decline over the whole adult age range, the slope for subgroups of elderly does not attain significance. These older subgroups are represented by few subjects, making it difficult to draw conclusions.

3. Assessing Energy Expenditure

The true energy needs of an individual or population should therefore be considered in a new light; the requirement is the amount of dietary energy that should be eaten to match the appropriate energy expenditure of the individual. Idealized energy needs refer to the dietary energy necessary to match the requirements of a healthy, active individual of normal size and body composition. As will become clear, the choice of a single value such as 2500 kcal/day for the energy requirement of all men is far too crude an approach and should be abandoned for medical, nutritional, and planning purposes. Many investigators have misinterpreted the use of the recommended dietary allowance (National Academy of Sciences, 1980) figure. This is only relevant when planning the likely requirements of a group of men of presumed age, size, and physical activity. To disregard the importance of age, body size, and activity has led to major errors in nutritional understanding; the emphasis on these factors is an important feature of the new FAO/WHO/UNU (1985) approach.

4. *Components of Energy Expenditure*

First, energy is needed to maintain normal body functions. This energy includes that for the maintenance of the usual organ size, i.e., of body composition and the maintenance of each organ's contribution to the body's function. In addition, dietary energy has to be provided to meet the necessary costs of metabolizing and storing the food that is ingested (thermogenesis). These are physiological needs, so we can expect that both the processes of body function and those of assimilating ingested food will show the normal intraindividual biological variation. Additional energy has to be provided for people who are engaged in different activities, and these additions therefore add a social as well as a biological dimension to the variability that we can expect to find between the energy needs of different individuals. People expend energy not only on physical activity that relates to their essential needs, i.e., for work, but also to their wish to engage in recreation and social interactions. Thus, there are biological and social needs for individuals. An individual or societal view of energy requirements is therefore complex, and only by recognizing the different components can one make an appropriate set of judgments on need. To these biological and social needs we then may have to add a medical or public health perspective, since in many affluent societies physical inactivity on a long-term basis may be disadvantageous. This then leads to a "prescriptive" as well as a descriptive approach to energy expenditure. Thus, the biological, social, and medical components of "need" have to be collated (Table I) and aggregated before being converted to a single value of prescribed dietary energy. This single value is classically specified as the recommended energy allowance or requirement of the individual or group of similar individuals. The implications of this for predicting energy requirements are dealt with later.

Figure 1 illustrates the relative sizes of the different components of energy expenditure in a young man in his 20s engaged in moderate activity compared with the same components of an elderly man's expenditure. Several of these components have already been specified in the preceeding analysis of "needs," but if one wishes to specify all factors that lead to an increase in energy expenditure, e.g., caffeine drinking and smoking, then one must clearly build up a much more complicated picture. In theory, one can then simply sum all the different components illustrated in Fig. 1. However, a number of components interact so that a combination of factors can either amplify energy expenditure by synergism or reduce the total because the interaction of two components induces less expenditure than the sum of the individual effects. Thus,

Table I. Components of Energy Expenditure[a]

	Biological
1.	Maintaining normal organ function, i.e., basal metabolic rate
2.	Maintaining normal body composition
3.	Processing food after ingestion
	Physical activity
4.	Economic, i.e., "survival" purposes
5.	Socially desirable: (a) housework; (b) recreational
	Medically desirable
6.	High-intensity exercise for cardiovascular conditioning

[a]These distinctions are somewhat arbitrary. For example, medically desirable energy expenditure could be defined more widely to include component 2, i.e., the prevention of wasting or obesity; component 5(a) includes housework, which is also essential for cooking and maintaining hygenic conditions. Components based on concepts specified in the FAO/WHO/UNU report (1985).

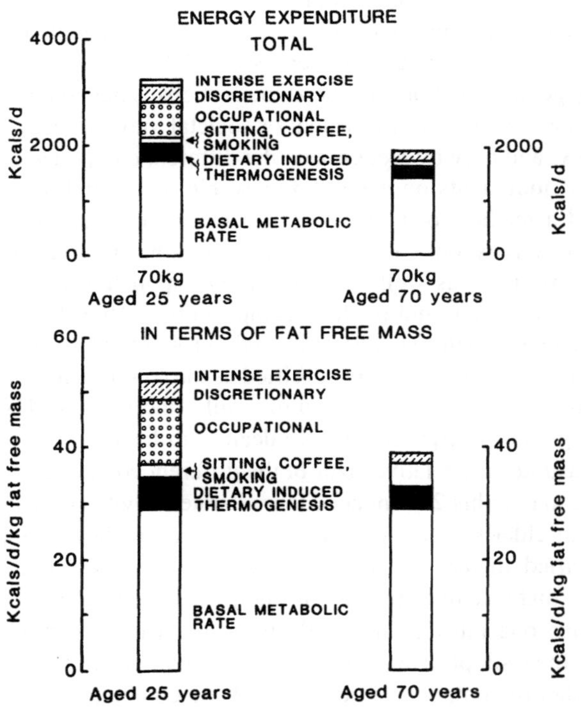

Fig. 1. Distribution of components of energy expenditure at age 25 years and at 70 years. Upper diagram, total energy output per day. Lower diagram, daily energy output expressed per kilogram fat-free mass.

smoking tends to amplify diet-induced thermogenesis (Robinson and York, 1986), but cold-induced thermogenesis may only occur in cooler environments when behavioral changes, e.g., putting on thicker clothes, are not made. When cold-induced thermogenesis does occur, it may also only be relevant long after a meal, when dietary thermogenesis can no longer provide the heat required to satisfy the need for cold-induced thermogenesis (Dauncey, 1981). In this case, therefore, there are subtle interactions that may depend on the precise interplay of the environmental effects during the day. Similarly, there are now several reports of an interaction of physical activity and diet-induced thermogenesis (Segal *et al.*, 1985; Tagliaferro *et al.*, 1986; Davis *et al.*, 1983; Samueloff *et al.*, 1982). Physical activity may amplify dietary thermogenesis only if exercise is intense; if exercise is taken some time after the meal, then the interaction is lost.

Given all these components of energy expenditure, with their supposed marked variation, it is little wonder that most physiologists, physicians, and nutritionists have considered the problem of energy requirements, whether of young adults or of the elderly, as too complicated to warrant any serious analysis. Not only do individuals differ one from another, but within any one individual, alterations in energy output occur from day to day or even from hour to hour in response to coexistent stimuli of, for example food, cold, caffeine drinking, and smoking. In practice, however, these conclusions prove to be too pessimistic, since they neglect our increasing recognition that the impact of many of the interactions is very small. Indeed, one of the major conclusions of the last decade of research is that the metabolic rate of an individual, whether in the basal or fed state, is far less flexible than previously imagined. Thus, if physical activity is kept constant, the 24-hr energy expenditure of individuals in energy balance is remarkably constant from day to day and week to week, with a coefficient of variation of only about 1.3%. Some of this variation relates to the technical error of measurement (Dallosso *et al.*, 1982). A similar conclusion was made for BMR recently by Bogardus *et al.* (1986).

The interactions of cold- and diet-induced thermogenesis (Dauncey, 1981) are also very small, as are the interactions between exercise and diet (Segal *et al.*, 1985), amounting to a change of only 1–2% of total daily energy turnover. Similarly, the effects of caffeine and smoking on daily energy expenditure amount to about 3% of the daily total expended for caffeine and up to 10% for smoking (Acheson *et al.*, 1980; Jung *et al.*, 1981; Dallosso and James, 1984; Hofstetter *et al.*, 1986). Thus, the interactions are interesting but small in magnitude and require specialized facilities and standardized conditions for their display. Even when overfeeding occurs, the effects are subtle, amounting to an increase in 24-hr energy expenditure of only about 10% when there is a 50% increase in energy intake (Ravussin *et al.*, 1985). Thus, the stability of metabolism is a major feature of adults, and changes in energy expenditure are mainly derived from alterations in the amount of physical activity taken. Differences between people also depend on the biological differences in the basal metabolic rate (BMR), which reflect differences in both body composition and metabolic efficiency. Given this perspective on energy requirements, we need to examine the components to see if, with aging, there is a differential effect on the basal metabolic rate, on physical activity, or on the other components of energy expenditure.

Table II. Equations for Predicting the Basal Metabolic Rate of Adults[a]

Subjects	Basal metabolic rate (kcal/day)	
	Based on weight (W)[b]	Based on weight (W) and height (H)[b]
Men		
18–29	$15.3W + 679$	$15.4W - 27H + 717$
30–59	$11.6W + 879$	$11.3W + 16H + 901$
60 and over	$13.5W + 487$	$8.8W + 1128H - 1071$
Women		
18–29	$14.7W + 496$	$13.3W + 334H + 35$
30–59	$8.7W + 829$	$8.7W - 25H + 865$
60 and over	$10.5W + 596$	$9.2W + 637H - 302$

[a]Tables taken from the FAO/WHO/UNU (1985) report, not from Schofield *et al.* (1985), who produced slightly different equations from an expanded data base.
[b]Weight is expressed in kilograms, and height in meters.

4.1. Basal Metabolic Rate in the Elderly

A number of studies have suggested that with aging the basal metabolic rate diminishes when expressed in absolute terms, e.g., as kilocalories per day. However, it has been recognized for many years that the basal metabolic rate of an individual depends on body size, and many equations have been developed to predict the BMR from body weight, from weight and height, or from some index derived from these two measures such as surface area. The latest collation of equations was constructed by Schofield *et al.* (1985). This incorporated an analysis of the BMR of most of the published data in the world's literature, including individual data on 7549 people. Similar equations have been used in the latest FAO/WHO/UNU (1985) report on protein and energy needs and are summarized in Table II for adults of various ages. These equations are based only on age, sex, and body weight. Adding a value for height makes a small difference in the elderly not sufficient to justify its routine use.

Tables III and IV provide a collation of the published studies on the BMR of the elderly. The BMR values of a group of young men and women are given for comparison. These studies are cross sectional, and on this basis it would be wrong to presume that aging results in a decline in BMR. For example, a secular trend for increasing height, weight, and lean body mass, well recognized in many countries and pronounced in Japan and some developing countries, would result in a secular increase in absolute basal metabolic rate of the different cohorts. Cross-sectional studies could therefore show a marked difference in the BMR of 20- and 80-year-olds because of the greater stature of those aged 20. The BMRs could in theory then simply reflect the different heights and weights of each cohort if there were no other explanation for the decline in the BMR. Clearly, it is important to understand the basis for the decline in BMR with age. Without an analysis of changes in body size and composition, even repeated longitudinal studies on individuals over decades would not allow a reasonable analysis to be made.

Tables III and IV provide a very much larger data base for the over-60s than that

Table III. The Basal Metabolic Rate of Men in Different Studies

Number	Age (years)	Weight (kg)	Height (cm)	Basal metabolic rate kcal/day	Basal metabolic rate kcal/kg per day	Reference
172	60	78.0	176	1541	19.8	Baltimore[a]
6	68 ± 5	82.2 ± 5.2	174 ± 4	1627 ± 187	19.6 ± 1.2	Calloway and Zanni (1980)
162	70	76.5	174	1472	19.2	Baltimore[a]
87	71.4 ± 2.7	75.9 ± 108	176.6 ± 6	1519 ± 229	20.0 ± 2.8	Keys (1973)
163	74.7 ± 9.1	68.2 ± 177	162 ± 77	1426 ± 173	20.9	A. Ferro-Luzzi (unpublished data)
103	79	73.1	175	1369	18.7	Baltimore[a]
12	90	—	—	1286	—	Baltimore[a]
		Previously collated data by Schofield *et al.* (1985)				
2879	22.5 ± 7.4	63.0 ± 8.7	170 ± 0.1	1642	26.1	
50	72.4 ± 10.5	62.3 ± 12.8	165 ± 0.1	1336	21.4	

[a]The Baltimore survey data have been calculated by reading data on oxygen consumption from a graph by Tzankoff and Norris (1978) and then relating this to age and the anthropometric data given in Shock *et al.* (1984).

used in generating the equations shown in Table II because in the Baltimore study individual values were not published. A substantial amount of unpublished information on Italian men and women has also been added. By using averaged data on large groups and the new Italian work, it becomes apparent that appreciable reductions in absolute BMR (kcal/day) occur between the ages of 20 and 60 years and that thereafter a further decline in BMR per day is also apparent, since Tables III and IV are set out in order of increasing age. If a comparison based on kilocalories per body weight is then made between the data of Schofield *et al.* (1985) for young men and women and the 60-year-old men (Table III, Baltimore) and women (Table IV; Miller *et al.*, 1957; Durnin *et al.*, 1961), it seems that there is still a 24% decline in the case of men (26.1 versus 19.8 kcal/kg) and a 15% decline in the case of women (24.1 versus 20.4 kcal/kg) when both are expressed on a body weight basis.

However, the apparent effect of age is less clear because the comparisons are being made between the world-wide data collated by Schofield on young men of smaller average stature and those from older Baltimore men, where the North American males are both taller and heavier. Since on a per-kilogram basis it has been established that heavier adults have a lower BMR than lighter adults, this in theory could explain the male data. However, recalculating the Schofield data for young men to a weight appropriate for the Baltimore 60-year-olds suggests that at an equivalent weight there would still have been an 18% decline in BMR per kilogram between young and old. This underestimates the change, because Schofield showed that the BMR of North American adults is on average about 5% above the world-wide average at equivalent weights. Accordingly, it seems reasonable to conclude that there is a reduction of 20–25% in BMR from the third to the seventh decade of life in men. Similar arguments applied to women in Table IV do not change this picture, but it

Table IV. Basal Metabolic Rate of Elderly Women in Different Studies[a]

Number	Age (years)	Weight (kg)	Height (cm)	BMR		Reference
				kcal/day	kcal/kg per day	
2	60–61	53.5 ± 6.1	148 ± 3.5	1081 ± 116	20.2 ± 0.1	Miller *et al.* (1957)
21	60 ± 3.7	60.4 ± 9.6	155 ± 6.4	1253	20.7	Durnin *et al.* (1961)
1	61	50.5	159	1166	23.1	Chambers and Lewis (1969)
6	66–68	53.6 ± 9.9	146 ± 4.9	1089 ± 121	20.7 ± 3.0	Miller *et al.* (1957)
5	70–74	51.1 ± 6.9	146 ± 2.6	1121 ± 65	22.2 ± 3.0	Miller *et al.* (1957)
152	73.4 ± 9.3	63.2 ± 19.0	151 ± 6.5	1267	20.0	A. Ferro-Luzzi (unpublished)
3	75–79	47.9 ± 4.5	143 ± 8.9	1000 ± 109	20.9 ± 1.6	Miller *et al.* (1957)
			Previous data collated by Schofield *et al.* (1985)			
829	22.3 ± 7.8	52.9 ± 8.4	160 ± 0.07	1274	24.1	
38	66.4 ± 5.3	55.5 ± 10.9	153 ± 0.09	1159	20.9	

[a]Chambers and Lewis' subject was from Tristan da Cunha. Miller *et al.*'s subjects were Japanese in Hawaii. Durnin's subjects were Scottish. The unpublished data of Ferro-Luzzi relate to Italians.

seems that men do tend to show a greater fall in BMR than women from young adult life to the time they consider retiring at the age of 60 years. Further changes beyond 60 years are examined in the next section.

4.1.1. *Changes in Basal Metabolic Rate with Aging in the Elderly*

Table III suggests that there is a further appreciable fall in the total calorie cost of basal metabolism per day as men age from 60 to 90 years. However, on a weight basis there is little difference in the BMR between the different aged men in Table III. Thus, the dominant effect relates to size. There is less of an age range in the female studies shown in Table IV, with little change in the total energy cost of the BMR. Again, there is no evidence of a difference between women at 60 years of age and those in their mid-70s when the BMR is expressed on a body weight basis.

In the cross-sectional Italian study (A. Ferro-Luzzi, unpublished*), detailed analysis shows that there is a decline in basal metabolic rate that amounts in absolute terms in men to 3% (130 kcal/day) for each decade of age from age 60 years; in the women there is also a clear but smaller decline, namely, 86 kcal per 24 hr for each decade from 60 years, amounting to a fall of 6% in each decade. Thus, older men do seem to show a greater absolute fall in BMR during the elderly years with little evidence of any change in metabolic efficiency (BMR in kcal/kg).

4.1.2. *Sex Differences in Basal Metabolic Rate in the Elderly*

The data in Tables III and IV illustrate the well-recognized point that although the absolute BMR of women is lower than that of men, most of this effect depends on the lower body weight of women. Nevertheless, if the BMRs of young adult men and women are compared on a body-weight basis, men still have a slightly higher BMR per kilogram than women, but the difference amounts to only about 8%. The data on the BMR of the elderly collated from the literature and published by Schofield *et al.* (1985) suggest that the difference between elderly men and women in their BMRs expressed per kilogram body weight is negligible (Tables III and IV).

The Italian study (A. Ferro-Luzzi, unpublished) provides a better opportunity to make these comparisons, since the techniques were comparable and a large number (200 subjects) were studied in each sex group by the same investigators. In this large study, any difference between the sexes observable in younger adults had disappeared, both men and women having a BMR of about 20 kcal/kg per day (compare Tables III and IV). Detailed analysis within the group of elderly men and women shows, as expected, that body weight affected the value of BMR per kilogram, that of lighter individuals being higher than that of heavier subjects in both sexes. The BMR per kilogram for a 50-kg Italian man is about 24 kcal/kg per day, whereas that for a 75-kg man is about 20 kcal/kg per day. Similarly, 50-kg and 75-kg elderly Italian women have BMRs of approximately 22.5 kcal/kg per day and 18 kcal/kg per day, respectively. On this basis, elderly men may still have a slightly higher BMR per kilogram

*Frequent references in the text to A. Ferro-Luzzi (unpublished data) are to a comprehensive study of Italian men and women by A. Ferro-Luzzi, C. Scattini, A. D'Aminisis, and S. Selte.

than women of equivalent weight, but any such effect is small. Since these data may reflect differences in the composition of the men and women of different weights, this now needs to be considered in greater detail.

4.1.3. Body Compositional Changes and Basal Metabolic Rate

It is now well recognized that basal metabolism is best related to the fat-free mass (FFM) of the body and that the quantity of fat has little effect in itself on the BMR. This is not surprising, since the FFM of the body includes the enzymatic and other cellular proteins of adipose tissue; the FFM of individuals increases in obesity at least in part because the protein mass of adipose tissue increases as fat is deposited. The triacylglycerol in adipose tissue cannot be expected to have metabolic activity, since it is deposited as an inert mass for later mobilization as substrate for metabolism. Therefore, any analysis of BMR should ideally be assessed in terms of the total FFM of the body.

Table V presents cross-sectional BMR data that have all been put on a comparable basis and expressed in terms of fat-free mass. Once any loss of active tissue mass (FFM) is taken into account, there seems to be little indication of any loss of metabolic activity in the fat-free mass itself with age. In the Baltimore study, the men with an average age of 79 had only a 2% lower BMR than men with an average age of 60 years. When the total sample of Italian men was assessed separately to see whether there was any decline in BMR per kilogram FFM with age, only a small effect was observed, amounting to 1.6 kcal/kg FFM (5%) per decade from the age of 60 to 90 years ($P > 0.05$). In the women, however, no discernible decrement was observed. These data

Table V. Basal Metabolic Rate and Fat-Free Mass of the Elderly[a]

Number	Age (years)	Height (cm)	Fat-free mass (kg)	BMR/kg FFM (kcal/kg per day)	Reference
Men					
172	60	176	57.7	26.7	Baltimore
6	68	174	52.7	30.9	Calloway and Zanni (1980)
162	70	174	54.5	27.0	Baltimore
163	75	162	48.7	23.9	A. Ferro-Luzzo (unpublished data, Italy)
103	79	175	52.3	26.2	Baltimore
Women					
152	73	151	36.5	34.7	A. Ferro-Luzzi (unpublished data, Italy)

[a]For the Baltimore survey, data have been calculated by obtaining the oxygen consumption from a graph presented by Tzankoff and Norris (1978) and relating these values, converted to kcal per day, to data on body composition. This was estimated from measurements of total body water and reported by Borkan and Norris (1977). Unpublished Italian data rely on estimating body fat from skinfold measurement by the use of the predictive equations developed by Durnin and Womersley (1974), based on measurements of body density.

suggest that there is no intrinsic biological effect of aging on the metabolic activity of lean tissue.

No simple explanation for the higher BMR per kilogram body weight of lighter individuals has yet been forthcoming. One possibility is that heavier adults have a greater proportion of body fat with therefore a lower proportion of metabolically active lean tissue (Ferro-Luzzi, 1985). This theory would not explain the persistence of the phenomenon in groups with a similar physique but of different stature. One explanation may lie in the components of the fat-free mass, since it is recognized that the visceral organs and the brain are metabolically very active compared with muscle. When the Italian data are expressed in terms of total FFM, then there is a statistically significant decline in metabolic rate per kilogram FFM with the increasing size of the fat-free mass of the individual. Table V also shows that the Italian elderly women appear to have a higher BMR per kilogram FFM than the men, the difference amounting to about 17%. This could readily be explained if the men had a larger muscle mass than women and therefore a greater mass of a tissue that is metabolically relatively inactive at rest.

In practice only a few longitudinal studies of BMR have been conducted. These are only in men enrolled in the Baltimore study and are included in Tables III and V. They lend validity to the suggestion that the decline in BMR depends essentially on the loss of lean, metabolically active tissue; once an adjustment is made for this (kcal/FFM in Table V), there is no evidence of an intrinsic decline in the energy turnover of the active tissue itself.

4.1.4. Metabolic Adaptation to Low Energy Intakes

It is well recognized that within a few days of starting on a low energy intake, the BMR falls, part of this decline being in the metabolic activity of the tissue itself; subsequently a further fall occurs as lean tissue is lost. Keys and his colleagues, in the classic Minnesota semistarvation experiments (Keys *et al.*, 1950), observed that young, initially normal-weight male volunteers reduce their BMR expressed in absolute terms, i.e., kilocalories/day, by 40% over a period of 6 months. However, the maximum decline in the metabolic activity of the residual lean tissue (BMR/kg FFM) amounted to only 15%, the other 25% of the fall depending on the loss of lean tissue itself. Other studies have shown that changes in metabolic efficiency start about 4 days after the onset of semistarvation and reach their maximum within 2 weeks. Thereafter, further lowering of the BMR occurs only as lean tissue is lost. The early change in metabolic efficiency is in part dependent on a fall in the concentration of the circulating thyroid hormone triiodothyronine (Jung *et al.*, 1980a). Theoretically, therefore, the lower BMR per kilogram body weight in the 60-year-olds could reflect a metabolic adaptation to their low energy intakes. However, when BMR is related to fat-free mass, there is no evidence of a change in metabolic efficiency during early adult life. Furthermore, the failure to find any substantial decline in BMR in men and women from 60 years onwards, once the BMR is expressed on a weight or fat-free mass basis (Table V), again argues against any metabolic adaptation in response to low energy intakes by the elderly.

It would seem best, therefore, to conclude that any changes that occur in the BMR of the elderly relate primarily to the consequences of a change in the fat-free mass of the body and not to an aging effect or to an intake-mediated effect on metabolic efficiency.

4.2. Thermogenic Responses in the Elderly

In response to a meal, there is an increase in caloric expenditure; i.e., thermogenesis occurs. Many stimuli can induce thermogenesis, but the most important is that occurring in response to food. Numerous studies have shown that the magnitude of the response varies according to the source of energy, with protein inducing the largest response, carbohydrate having a modest effect, and fat very little. Reduced thermogenic responses to a meal by the elderly have been reported by Morgan and York (1983) and by Golay *et al.* (1983). The effect depends on the size and composition of the meal. The response was found to be 20–30% lower than in younger adults.

This topic has reemerged as a possible variable determining whether individuals remain slim throughout life or are prone to obesity (James, 1983). Since most of the energy dissipated as thermogenesis following a meal can be accounted for by the additional energy needed to process and store the ingested nutrients, any difference between the young and old is likely to reflect the use of different metabolic routes for storing dietary nutrients. Some of the enhanced thermogenic energy output has, however, been ascribed to the activation of metabolites, e.g., by the sympathetic nervous system, since a component of the thermogenic response to glucose can be blocked by the use of a β-adrenergic blocking drug such as propranolol (Jung *et al.*, 1980b). The extent to which the response to a normal meal can be blocked by propranolol is, however, debatable (Zed and James, 1986a), and furthermore, if individuals are overfed with a mixed diet for several days, it is by no means clear that any general stimulus to metabolism occurs (Zed and James, 1986b). Nevertheless, should there be a decline in the response to sympathetic nervous activity with age, it is possible that a small component of energy expenditure amounting to perhaps 2–5% at most of total energy expenditure would be affected. However, most studies show an enhanced output of norepinephrine to a variety of physiological stimuli in the elderly (Young *et al.*, 1980), but the overall metabolic effect is uncertain.

4.3. Physical Activity

4.3.1. Mechanical Efficiency in the Elderly

The elderly often develop a different gait when walking, and this may alter the energy cost of walking. In addition, there could be a change in the energy cost of muscular contraction. Although the elderly lose muscular mass and tend to have a selective loss of type II fibers (see Chapter 5), there is little evidence that the actual cost of a standardized activity such as that on a bicycle ergometer changes. Table VI displays a selection of data on the cost of a variety of activities in elderly Italian men (A. Ferro-Luzzi, unpublished data). The data have been compared with those obtained in young and middle-aged adults (E. C. Schofield, H. M. Dallosso, and W. P. T. James, unpublished data). The data for the elderly have been expressed in relation to

Table VI. Activity Factors for Elderly Men and Women: Comparison with Younger Adults[a]

Activity	Elderly men	Younger adult men	Elderly women	Younger adult women
Resting metabolic rate	1.16 (35)	1.05 (229)	1.19 (35)	1.05 (229)
Sitting inactive	1.23 (103)	1.19 (122)	1.19 (98)	1.19 (172)
Standing inactive	1.46 (91)	1.26 (156)	1.41 (68)	1.26 (156)
Walking 3–4 km/hr	3.38 (37)	2.87 (30)	3.44 (66)	2.87 (30)
Cooking	2.34 (2)	1.80 (15)	2.02 (12)	1.80 (15)

[a]The number of individuals measured to obtain each rate is given in parentheses. They are unpublished data from a large survey of elderly Italian men and women over the age of 60 years. The energy expenditure in each activity is expressed as a ratio of the measured basal metabolic rate of each individual. A comparison is made with data on individual young and middle-aged adults in the literature, the data being recalculated as the ratio to their predicted basal metabolic rate. This BMR was predicted from the sex, age, and weight of the subjects using the FAO/WHO/UNU (1985) equations (E. C. Schofield, H. M. Dallosso, and W. P. T. James, unpublished data).

the measured BMR of the individual being studied, whereas the BMR data on the younger adults had to be predicted from their sex, age, and body weight, making use of the FAO/WHO/UNU (1985) equations. It is apparent that, when measuring very sedentary activities such as those at rest or when sitting inactive, there is no evidence that these elderly Italian men and women have a more "efficient" metabolism than that of younger adults. Since these measurements were made in the fed state, they will have included the thermic effect of food. Thus, it is unlikely that their diet-induced thermogenesis is markedly different.

More active tasks in the elderly seem to be associated with a greater level of energy expenditure than that in the young. Thus, simple activities such as inactive standing, walking briskly, or even cooking seem, if anything, to incur higher costs in the elderly. This feature probably relates to the greater efforts that older subjects have to exert, given their somewhat arthritic state and changed gait. Certainly, there is no evidence of an enhanced mechanical efficiency of work with a reduced energy cost for specific tasks. It therefore appears that any decrease in the total level of energy expended on physical activity in old age must come from a reduction in the time spent on different activities rather than from a fall in the energy cost of the activities.

4.3.2. Physical Activity Patterns in the Elderly

There is a surprising paucity of data on the physical activity patterns of the elderly despite increasing evidence of its importance for preventing muscle atrophy and for maintaining bone mass (see Chapter 5 for a review). The overall level of physical activity also affects food intake, since there has to be a concordance between intake and expenditure if weight changes are not to occur. The higher the physical activity, therefore, the greater will be the food intake, and the greater the likelihood of individuals meeting their requirements for vitamins, minerals, and other nutrients. On this basis it could be argued that the maintenance of physical activity into old age is of major importance for the well-being of the elderly.

The most comprehensive data on the overall effect of age on physical activity are

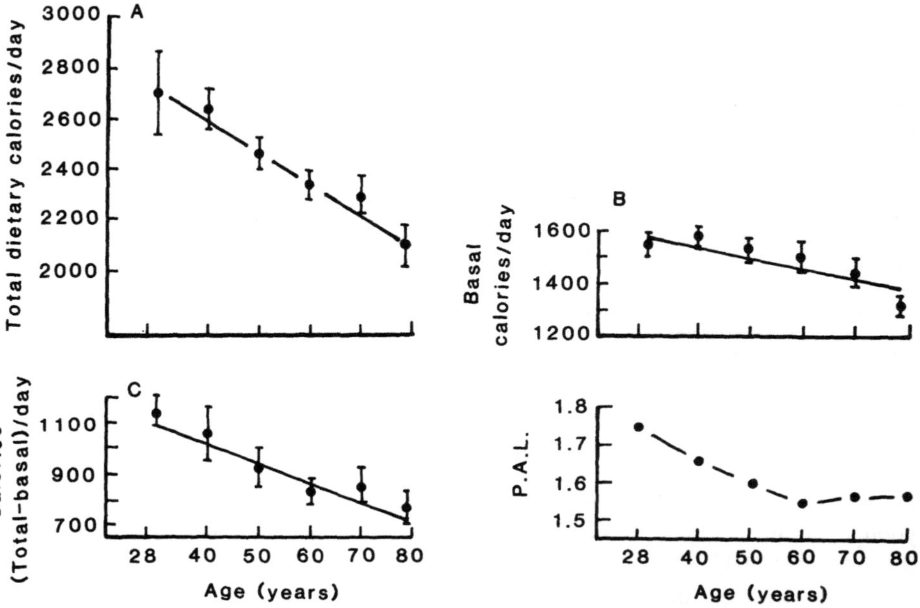

Fig. 2. The effect of age on the total daily energy intake of men (A), on their basal metabolism (B), and on the caloric expenditure not accounted for by basal metabolism (C) (From McGandy *et al.*, 1966). A fourth diagram has been added (lower right) to provide physical activity level (P.A.L.) by expressing the total daily energy expenditure as a multiple of the observed basal metabolic rate.

those given by McGandy *et al.* (1966), whose data are redrawn in Fig. 2. It is apparent that the energy expended on processes other than basal metabolic rate falls progressively from young adult life to old age in this study conducted in Baltimore. When expressed per kilogram body weight, this seems to leave only about 11 kcal/kg body weight per day out of 30 kcal/kg total energy (Table VII) in the elderly for diet-induced thermogenesis, for the enhanced muscle tone in the nonbasal state, and for overt physical activity. If diet-induced thermogenesis accounts for perhaps 10% of energy intake, this amounts to about 3 kcal/kg per day in the elderly men studied, leaving only 8 kcal/kg per day for activity *per se*.

Another approach to assessing the overall effect of physical activity is to assess the total energy turnover as a multiple of the BMR. This then allows the pattern to be compared with the new estimates of energy requirements produced in 1985 by the FAO/WHO/UNU Commission. Table VII presents data for the elderly collected from the United States, Sweden, and Scotland. It is clear that the data collected by McGandy *et al.* (1966) are not unusual, with the energy intake amounting to about 30 kcal/kg, yielding a ratio of about 1.5 times the BMR. The intake/BMR ratio provides an index of the physical activity level of the subjects. The data are reasonably comparable except for the Swedish women, who either underestimated their total energy intake or were extraordinarily inactive.

The most detailed studies of activity patterns shown in Table VI have been conducted in Italy (A. Ferro-Luzzi, unpublished data), and a more extensive account

Table VII. Daily Energy Intakes in Groups of Elderly People

	McGandy *et al.* (1966), U.S.A.		Borgström *et al.* (1979), Sweden		Uauy *et al.* (1978), U.S.A.		Calloway and Zanni (1980), U.S.A.	Durnin *et al.* (1961), Scotland
Sex	M	M	M	F	M	F	M	F
N	50	37	17	20	6	6	6	17
Age	67–74	77–79	67–73	67–73	68–74	70–84	63–77	60–69
Height (mean)	1.74	1.72	1.68	1.60	1.70	1.59	1.74	1.55
Weight (mean)	77.7	70.9	76.4	68.8	73.7	68.9	82.2	60.7
Energy intake (kcal)	2297	2093	2050	1600	2325	1904	2554	1894
Energy intake kcal/kg wt.	29.6	29.5	26.8	23.3	31.5	27.6	31.1	31.2
Intake/estimated BMR[a]	1.53	1.47	1.38	1.25	1.62	1.49	1.58	1.57

[a]Basal metabolic rate (BMR) was estimated from body weight from the equations in Table III and taken to indicate the physical activity level of the subjects.

will be published elsewhere. For these measurements, indirect calorimetric monitoring was undertaken in the homes of the elderly subjects, with account taken of the full range of the individual's activities. In addition, the basal metabolic rate was measured so that, once the time allocated to each task and its energy cost had been collated, it was then possible to assess the total energy expenditure as a multiple of the individual's measured BMR. The overall change in total energy expenditure from 60 to 90 years was substantial, amounting to a decline of 675 kcal for men and 459 kcal for women. When activity is expressed as physical activity ratios (i.e., the ratio of total expenditure to BMR), men show a fall from 1.45 in the seventh decade of life to 1.34 in the ninth decade, with women also becoming more inactive; their ratios fell from 1.41 to 1.32. Since there is little evidence of any intrinsic change in the metabolic cost of physical activity measured in the fed state (Table VI), these findings must reflect the progressive decline in spontaneous physical activity in the elderly. The nonbasal energy expenditure, i.e., that involved in the thermic response to food and in physical activity, declined faster in absolute terms than the BMR. Thus, on a daily kilocalorie basis, the total energy expenditure of men declined by 10% per decade from the age of 60 years, and that of women by 8%, but the corresponding data on the BMR changes were −8% and −6% per decade. In Fig. 1, we have included our estimate of the change in total energy expenditure from young adulthood to old age. It is apparent that the decline in physical activity and the fall in body weight dominate the picture and provide the explanation for the dramatic decline in energy turnover in the course of adult life.

5. *Defining the Energy Requirements of the Elderly*

Table VIII reproduces an example of how the FAO/WHO/UNU expert group approached the issue of energy requirements in the elderly. As with other age groups,

Table VIII. Specifying Energy Requirements of Elderly Men[a]

	Hours	Energy (kcal)	Energy (kJ)
In bed at 1.0 × BMR	8	430	1810
Occupational activities	0	0	0
Discretionary activities:			
Socially desirable at 3.3 × BMR[b]	2	355	1490
Household tasks at 2.7 × BMR	1	145	610
Cardiovascular and muscular maintenance at 4 × BMR	20 min	70	300
For residual time, energy needs at 1.4 × BMR	12 hr 40 min	960	4020
Total (1.51 × BMR)		1960	8220

[a]Age 75 years, weight 60 kg, height 1.6 m, BMI 23.5. Estimated basal metabolic rate: 54 kcal (225 kJ) per hour.
[b]Because the elderly man has no occupational demands on his time, an extra hour has been allocated for walking and other similar activities.

Table IX. A Simple Guide to the Energy Cost of Various Occupational Tasks in Which the Elderly Might Be Engaged[a]

	Cost as a ratio of BMR	
	Male	Female
1. Professional, technical, and related workers	1.7	1.7
2. Administrative and managerial	1.7	1.7
3. Clerical and related workers	1.7	1.7
4. Sales workers	2.3	2.0
5. Service workers	2.3	2.0
6. Agricultural, animal husbandry, forestry, fishing, and hunting	2.7	2.2
7. Production and related transport equipment operators and laborers	2.7	2.2
8. Subsistence farmers	2.7	2.2
9. Domestic helpers	2.7	2.2

[a]Many of these categories are those specified by the International Labor Organization, but they have been amplified to include work that is not considered by ILO as gainful employment such as numbers 8 and 9. The values chosen are necessarily very approximate and relate to the type of work expected in rather more affluent countries.

the approach simply involves specifying the time allocated to different activities throughout the 24 hr and then assigning an energy cost to each activity. Thus, in Table VIII, the time spent in bed is taken as costing in energy terms the equivalent of the estimated BMR of the individual. This value can be estimated from Table II, which provides the value for the 24-hr energy cost of the BMR estimated from body weight. Then activity values are provided for any work undertaken before the energy cost of housework and other discretionary activities is considered. Clearly, there are several approaches of increasing complexity, the most detailed being that which requires a time and motion study of the individuals and a measurement of the energy cost of each activity. This approach was used in the Italian studies already mentioned (A. Ferro-Luzzi, unpublished data). Nevertheless, for simplicity, one can make a reasonable estimate of the different forms of activity and collate them. This approach was used in developing Table VIII. Although the table specifies that no work was being undertaken, many elderly men and women in different countries do continue with their employment beyond the age of 60. If so, the energy cost of their work can be readily specified by reference to the FAO/WHO/UNU (1985) report, which provides values for the activity cost of many jobs. A crude classification, analogous to those provided by the International Labor Organization's classification of work, may be used to simplify the process even further. This classification, developed from the 1985 FAO/WHO/UNU report, is displayed in Table IX. These are crude figures that specify the likely energy cost as an overall figure for the whole time that the elderly are considered to work and include the rests and pauses while engaged in employment. The work time is averaged over a 7-day week and may amount to perhaps only 3 hr a day if the employment is part time. Once the BMR is calculated on an hourly basis from Table II and multiplied by the work activity factor shown in Table IX, it can then be multiplied by the hours spent on the activity and inserted in Table VIII.

5.1. Socially Desirable Activities

This term was developed in the FAO/WHO/UNU (1985) report to indicate the prescriptive nature of the approach being adopted. Nevertheless, one can distinguish some of the different components as specified in Table VIII. Housework is readily dealt with. Here it is expected that a man may contribute an hour to helping about the house, but it was considered that women usually spend 2 hr a day engaged in these tasks. The actual cost obviously varies with the task, but an overall average figure amounts to an integrated value of 2.7 times the BMR. This level of activity is quite high and does not include many other household tasks such as sewing or knitting, ironing, or some food preparation that are undertaken at a much lower rate of energy expenditure and can be included under the residual light activity specified in Table VIII as having a maintenance cost of 1.4 × BMR for the hours out of bed.

In addition to these household duties, the 1985 report suggested two new approaches to providing what in effect is an extra energy allowance for the elderly. These allowances are summarized in Tables X and XI. First, it is suggested that an allowance should be made for the type of activity that is behaviorally important—walking out to meet friends, going for a walk, taking part in social events with various activities involved, e.g., dancing or playing cards. The emphasis was on activity as well as community interactions, so a figure of 3.3 × BMR was chosen, and the elderly were considered to be benefiting if they engaged in this for 2 hr rather than 1 hr daily as recommended for younger adults. This activity might also be expected to maintain neuromuscular coordination, muscle tone, and perhaps muscle mass. In addition, a further, more intense exercise period was suggested for the elderly, which involved activity for about 20 min each day at a ratio equivalent to four times the BMR.

The overall effect of these inclusions shown in Table VIII may be assessed by calculating the contribution each factor makes to the overall daily rate of energy expenditure. These calculations are provided in Table XI. Bed-bound elderly people can be expected to need about 1.2 times their BMR. This allows for the thermogenic response to meals and for the mild physical exertion involved in sitting up in bed. If, however, they spend only 8 hr a day in bed and the rest out of bed sitting up in a chair with a little exertion involved in washing and dressing and with the occasional short walk to the table to eat, then their BMR ratio will increase to about 1.27. Further

Table X. Characteristics of the Prescriptive Approach to Specifying Energy Requirements in the Elderly and the Effect on 24-hr Energy Expenditure

1. Allow for any occupational activity
2. Include a total of 2 hr rather than the single hour for adults for socially desirable activity at a cost of 3.3 times estimated BMR
3. Maintain 1 hr allocated for household tasks at 2.7 times estimated BMR for men and 2 hr for women
4. Maintain 20 min daily high-intensity exercise but reduce intensity from 6 × BMR for younger adults to 4 × BMR

Table XI. Effect on Ratio of 24-hr Activity to BMR for Different Degrees of Activity in the Elderly[a]

		Men	Women
1.	No occupation	1.51	1.56
2.	No cardiovascular work	1.49	1.55
3.	No additional social activity, i.e., 1 hr only	1.42	1.47
4.	No social activity at all	1.34	1.39
5.	No housework	1.27	1.27
6.	In bed all day	1.20	1.20

[a]This table is based on the assumption that there is a sequential reduction in each of the activities specified in Table VIII with women doing 2 hr rather than 1 hr of housework.

increases can be estimated as in Table XI. From these calculations, it can be seen that the prescriptive approach to energy allowances makes an appreciable difference in the final value. In practice, in Italy for example, 60-year-old men have an expenditure ratio of about 1.45, implying that they are on their feet and active for about 3–4 hr a day, but by the age of 90 they exercise very little, spending most of their time sitting, with a 24-hr energy ratio of only 1.34 (A. Ferro-Luzzi, unpublished data). The data on elderly Italian women also implies that, even at 60 years of age, they are only active and on their feet and working at energetic household tasks for 2–3 hr daily, with a total energy expenditure ratio to BMR of 1.41, and that they undertake very little housework or external activity by the time they are in their late 80s. Thus, the prescriptive approach in the elderly allows for much more exercise than they take in practice.

More direct evidence of this picture comes from monitoring the time spent on

Table XII. Time Allocation (as Percentage of 24 hr) of Elderly Men and Women Living in Italy[a]

	Women			Men		
Activity	60–69	70–79	>79	60–69	70–79	>79
Sleep	31	33	34	31	33	35
Rest in bed	8	10	13	8	8	12
Sitting						
Inactive	22	24	27	25	27	28
Active	8	9	8	7	7	7
Standing						
Inactive	4	3	3	6	5	3
Active	4	3	1	9	8	5
Walk, stairs	3	3	2	5	4	3
Moving about	19	15	11	9	8	7
Other activity	<1	<1	<1	<1	<1	<1
Total	100	100	100	100	100	100

[a]From A. Ferro-Luzzi (unpublished data).

different activities by different age groups of the Italian elderly. This is illustrated in Table XII, which shows a progressive increase as age advances in the time spent in bed and inactive sitting as well as a decline in the amount of time walking and exercising. Similar data have been collated by Shepherd (1978).

These detailed monitoring studies may in part be replaced by the advent of the $D_2{}^{18}O$ method of measuring the total energy expenditure. This method depends on the turnover of deuterium in body water being compared with that of ^{18}O, which has additional turnover by exchange with the bicarbonate pool. It is therefore possible to calculate CO_2 production rates and from this to derive an estimate for oxygen uptakes measured over a 2 to 3-week period. The technique has many attractions since it involves giving a dose of nonradioactive isotopically labeled water and then monitoring the rate of dilution of the labels in samples of urine collected at the beginning and end of the period or, preferably, throughout the time of study. This method is still being developed, and there is a need to validate some of the assumptions (James *et al.*, 1988). Nevertheless, it could be useful in future studies in the elderly and would allow an activity ratio to be derived once the BMR has been measured.

5.2. *Variability in Energy Expenditure*

It is well recognized that individuals differ in their energy requirement. Nevertheless, it has too often been assumed that the wide range of apparent energy intakes measured by standard techniques in the community reflect an equally large variation in energy needs. This is not true, since the variability in intake is much greater than the variability in expenditure. Intake, even in affluent conditions where social patterns affect eating, is still under physiological control, and adjustments are made within 3–6 days of there being an energy imbalance (James, 1985). The sensitivity of the control mechanism is unknown in either adults generally or the elderly specifically, but the effect of these adjustments will be to increase the range of intraindividual variability and therefore of the apparent interindividual variability in intakes measured over a short time scale.

Detailed analyses of a large body of information on the variability of energy expenditure are given elsewhere (Ferro-Luzzi, 1985). Even if expenditure is expressed in absolute terms, thereby discounting the importance of relating the data to body weight, the mean interindividual variation still amounts to only 14% when each study from less-developed and developed countries is considered separately. Standardizing for activity and weight reduces the interindividual variation to about 6–8%. If 24-hr energy expenditure is expressed as a multiple of the BMR, then the variability for individuals classified into the three categories of light, moderate, or heavy activity remains below 10%.

Finally, when dealing with individual elderly subjects, it may not always be possible to measure their BMR. Nevertheless, the BMR can still be estimated from the equations in Table II. If the appropriate BMR factors from Tables X and XI are then applied, an estimate of the individual's energy needs to within an error of 10% will be obtained. This error is readily acceptable for anything other than basic research purposes.

6. Concluding Remarks

The two dominating changes in the energy requirements of the elderly are the decline in physical activity and the fall in energy needs as the lean body mass declines. It is tempting to link these two phenomena, since bed rest certainly leads to marked muscle wasting, and exercise is a recognized way of maintaining muscular strength and coordination. Isometric exercise also maintains or even increases muscle mass, although the degree to which this is possible in the elderly seems uncertain (see Chapter 5).

The last 5 years have seen renewed interest in studies on energy metabolism in man, and further information is beginning to emerge on the elderly. We still, however, have a paucity of data and must rely on judgments about the likely impact of changes in body composition and physical activity. Nevertheless, we now have a much more coherent strategy for the analysis of energy needs in old people, and, with the approach set out in this chapter, it should be possible to judge the needs of the elderly, whether inactive and bedridden or mobile and engaged in a variety of activities.

7. References

Acheson, K. J., Zahorska-Markiewicz, B., Pittet, P., Anantharaman, K., and Jequier, E., 1980, Caffeine and coffee: Their influence on metabolic rate and substrate utilization in normal weight and obese individuals, *Am. J. Clin. Nutr.* **33**:989–997.

Bingham, S. A., 1987, The dietary assessment of individuals; methods, accuracy, new techniques and recommendations, *Nutr. Abstr. Rev.* **57**:705–742.

Bogardus, C., Lillioja, S., Ravussin, E., Abbot, W., Zawadzki, J. K., Young, A., Knowler, W. C., Jacobowitz, R., and Moli, P. P., 1986, Familial dependence of the resting metabolic rate, *N. Engl. J. Med.* **315**:96–100.

Borgström, B., Norden, A., Åkesson, B., Abdulla, M., and Jagerstad, M., 1979, Nutrition in old age. Chemical analyses of what old people eat and their states of health during 6 years follow-up, *Scand. J. Gastroenterol. [Suppl.]* **52**:1–299.

Borkan, G. A., and Norris, A. H., 1977, Fat redistribution and the changing body dimensions of the adult male, *Human Biol.* **49**:495–514.

Calloway, D. H., and Zanni, E., 1980, Energy requirements and energy expenditure of elderly men, *Am. J. Clin. Nutr.* **33**:2088–2092.

Chambers, M. A., and Lewis, H. E., 1969, Nutritional study of the islanders on Tristan da Cunha 1966. 2. The energy expenditure and food intake of Tristan islanders, *Br. J. Nutr.* **23**:237–247.

Dallosso, H. M., and James, W. P. T., 1984, The role of smoking in the regulation of energy balance, *Int. J. Obesity* **8**:365–375.

Dallosso, H. M., Murgatroyd, P. R., and James, W. P. T., 1982, Feeding frequency and energy balance in adult males, *Human Nutr. Clin. Nutr.* **36C**:25–39.

Dauncey, M. J., 1981, Influence of mild cold on 24 h energy expenditure, resting metabolism and diet-induced thermogenesis, *Br. J. Nutr.* **45**:257–267.

Davis, J. R., Tagliaferro, A. R., Kertzer, R., Gerrardo, T., Nichols, J., and Wheeler, J., 1983, Variations of dietary-induced thermogenesis and body fatness with aerobic capacity, *Eur. J. Appl. Physiol.* **50**:319–329.

Durnin, J. V. G. A., and Womersley, J., 1974, Body fat assessed from total body density and its estimation from skinfold thickness: Measurements on 481 men and women aged from 16–72 years, *Br. J. Nutr.* **32**:77–97.

Durnin, J. V. G. A., Blake, E. C., Brockway, J. M., and Drury, E. A., 1961, The food intake and energy expenditure of elderly women living alone, *Br. J. Nutr.* **15**:499–506.

Elahi, V. K., Elahi, D., Andres, R., Tobin, J. D., Butler, M. G., and Norris, A. H., 1983, A longitudinal study of nutritional intake in men, *J. Gerontol.* **38:**162–180.

FAO/WHO/UNU, 1985, *Energy and Protein Requirements,* Technical Report Series 724, WHO, Geneva.

Ferro-Luzzi, A., 1985, Range of variation in energy expenditure and scope for regulation, in: *Proceedings XIII International Conference on Nutrition* (T. G. Taylor and N. K. Jenkins, eds.), John Libbey, London, pp. 393–399.

Golay, A., Schutz, Y., Broquet, C., Moeri, R., Selber, J. P., and Jéquier, E., 1983, Decreased thermogenic response to an oral glucose load in older subjects, *J. Am. Geriatr. Soc.* **31:**144–148.

Hofstetter, A., Schutz, Y., Jequier, E., and Wahren, J., 1986, Increased energy expenditure in cigarette smokers, *N. Engl. J. Med.* **314:**79–82.

James, W. P. T., 1983, Energy requirements and obesity, *Lancet* **2:**386–389.

James, W. P. T., 1985, Appetite control and other mechanisms of weight homeostasis, in: *Nutritional Adaptation in Man* (K. Blaxter and J. C. Waterlow, eds.), John Libbey, London, pp. 141–154.

James, W. P. T., and Shetty, P., 1982, Metabolic adaptation and energy requirements in developing countries, *Hum. Nutr. Clin. Nutr.* **36C:**331–336.

James, W. P. T., Bingham, S. A., and Cole, T. J., 1981, Epidemiological assessment of dietary intake, *Nutr. Cancer* **2:**203–212.

James, W. P. T., Haggarty, P., and McGaw, B. A., 1988, Recent progress in studies on energy expenditure; are the new methods providing answers to the old questions? *Proc. Nutr. Soc.* (in press).

Jung, R. T., Shetty, P. S., and James, W. P. T., 1980a, Nutritional effects on thyroidal and catecholamine metabolism, *Clin. Sci.* **58:**183–191.

Jung, R. T., Shetty, P. S., and James, W. P. T., 1980b, The effect of beta-adrenergic blockade on metabolic rate and peripheral thyroid metabolism in obesity, *Eur. J. Clin. Invest.* **10:**179–182.

Jung, R. T., Shetty, P. S., James, W. P. T., Barrand, M. A., and Callingham, B. A., 1981, Caffeine: Its effect on catecholamines and metabolism in lean and obese humans, *Clin. Sci.* **60:**527–535.

Keys, A., Brozek, J., Henschel, A., Mickelson, O., and Taylor, H. L., 1950, *The Biology of Human Starvation,* University of Minnesota, Minneapolis, and Oxford University Press, London.

Keys, A., Taylor, H. L., and Grande, F., 1973, Basal metabolism and age of adult man, *Metabolism* **22:**579–587.

McGandy, R. B., Barrows, C. H., Spanias, A., Meredith, A., Stone, J. L., and Norris, A. H., 1966, Nutrient intakes and energy expenditure in men of different ages, *J. Gerontol.* **21:**581–587.

Miller, C. D., Wenkam, N. S., and Kimura, A. M., 1957, Basal metabolism in the elderly, *J. Am. Diet. Assoc.* **33:**1259–1265.

Morgan, J. B., and York, C. A., 1983, Thermic effects of food in relation to energy balance in elderly men, *Ann. Nutr. Metab.* **27:**71–77.

National Academy of Sciences, 1980, *Recommended Dietary Allowances,* 9th rev. ed., National Academy Press, Washington.

Ravussin, E., Schutz, Y., Acheson, K. J., Dusmet, M., Bourquin, L., and Jéquier, E., 1985, Short-term, mixed-diet overfeeding in man: No evidence for "luxuskonsumption," *Am. J. Physiol.* **249:**E470–E477.

Robinson, S., and York, D. A., 1986, The effect of cigarette smoking on the thermic response to feeding, *Int. J. Obesity* **10:**407–417.

Samueloff, S., Beer, G., and Blondheim, S. H., 1982, Influence of physical activity on the thermic effect of food in young men, *Israel. J. Med. Sci.* **18:**193–196.

Schofield, W. N., Schofield, C., and James, W. P. T., 1985, Basal metabolic rate. Review and prediction, together with an annotated bibliography of source material, *Hum. Nutr. Clin. Nutr.***39c** (Suppl. 1):1–96.

Segal, K. R., Gutin, B., Nyman, A. M., and Pi-Sunyer F. X., 1985, Thermic effect of food at rest, during exercise and after exercise in lean and obese men of similar body weight, *J. Clin. Invest.* **76:**1107–1112.

Shepherd, R. J., 1978, *Physical Activity and Aging,* Croom Helm, London.

Shock, N. W., Greulich, R., Andres, R., Arenberg, D., Costa, P. T., Lakatta, E. G., and Tobin, J. D. (eds.), 1984, *Normal Human Aging: The Baltimore Longitudinal Study of Aging,* NIH Publication 84/2450, DHHS, Washington.

Tagliaferro, A. R., Kertzer, R., Davis, J. R., Janson, C., and Tse, S. K., 1986, Effects of exercise-training on the thermic effect of food and body fatness of adult women, *Physiol. Behav.* **38:**703–710.

Tzankoff, S. P., and Norris, A. H., 1978, Longitudinal changes in basal metabolism in man, *J. Appl. Physiol.* **45:**536– 539.

Uauy, R. B., Scrimshaw, N. S., and Young, V., 1978, Human protein requirements: Nitrogen balance response to graded levels of egg protein in elderly men and women, *Am. J. Clin. Nutr.* **31:**779–785.

Young, J. B., Rowe, J. W., Pallotta, J. A., Sparrow, D., and Landsberg, L., 1980, Enhanced plasma norepinephrine response to upright posture and oral glucose administration in elderly human subjects, *Metabolism* **29:**532–539.

Zed, C., and James, W. P. T., 1986a, Dietary thermogenesis in obesity. Response to carbohydrate and protein meals: The effect of β-adrenergic blockade and semi-starvation, *Int. J. Obesity* 10:391–405.

Zed, C., and James, W. P. T., 1986b, Dietary thermogenesis in obesity. Fat feeding at different energy intakes, *Int. J. Obesity* **10:**375–390.

7

Protein Nutriture and Requirements of the Elderly

Hamish N. Munro

1. Introduction

Protein requirements of populations have been estimated for more than a century (see Munro, 1964a, 1985, for the historical references in the paragraph). In 1853 and again in 1865, Playfair reported the protein intakes of different classes of the population of Britain and concluded that the requirements of adults ranged from 57 g protein per day in the case of a subsistence diet to 184 g for laborers doing heavy work. Later in the same century, Voit and Atwater both supported generous allowances of protein for the average working man, but several subsequent investigators publishing just before World War I concluded that 30 to 50 g protein daily was not only adequate to maintain nitrogen balance but even improved the general health and vigor of young adults. Following the first global war, the League of Nations was formed, and in 1936 a health committee reported that the safe protein intake for adults was 1 g per kilogram body weight and that some of the protein should come from animal sources.

Following World War II, the Food and Agricultural Organization (FAO) in Rome and the World Health Organization (WHO) in Geneva and recently the United Nations University (UNU) in Tokyo have taken responsibility for periodic reports on protein and energy requirements (FAO, 1957; FAO/WHO, 1965, 1973; FAO/WHO/UNU, 1985) and have in general agreed to a level of 0.8 g protein per kilogram body weight as being safe for almost all adults in a population, irrespective of age and sex. In the most recent report (FAO/WHO/UNU, 1985), the protein requirement of an individual is defined as

> the lowest level of dietary protein intake that will balance the losses of nitrogen from the body in persons maintaining energy balance at modest levels of physical activity. In children and pregnant or lactating women, the protein requirement is taken to include the needs associated with the deposition of tissues or the secretion of milk at rates consistent with good health (p. 12).

Hamish N. Munro • USDA Human Nutrition Research Center on Aging, Tufts University, Boston, Massachusetts 02111.

Also from the same report, there is a statement that "for adults the protein requirement per kilogram body weight is considered to be the same for both sexes at all ages and body weights. The values accepted for the safe level of intake is 0.75 g per kg per day, in terms of proteins with the digestibility of milk or egg" (p. 132). They conclude (p. 84) that "the safe intake of protein should not be lower than 0.75 g/kg per day for older adults and the elderly. This figure is higher than that for younger adults in relation to lean body mass because it is an accepted fact that protein utilization is less efficient in the elderly."

The stage is thus set for asking three questions. Is nitrogen balance an adequate criterion for setting intakes of protein appropriate for different stages of the aging process? Are there better ways of evaluating protein needs? Is it adequate to conclude from present evidence that protein needs do not deviate from 0.75 g per kg during the whole adult life span? In order to answer these questions, we consider, first, the effect of the aging process on body protein content and body protein metabolism. Second, this chapter analyzes studies on the protein requirements of elderly people that have appeared in publications since World War II. Third, surveys of the protein nutriture of elderly populations will be reviewed for evidence of protein–calorie malnutrition. Finally, some conclusions about the current state of our knowledge and potential directions for future research will be summarized.

2. Body Protein Content and Metabolism in Relation to Age

In order to understand how the protein needs of the aging and the elderly can be approached in a basic fashion, it is necessary to review what we know about the effect of aging on the protein content of the body and its organs and how aging affects protein metabolism.

2.1. Age-Related Changes in Body Protein Content

The aging adult undergoes continuous change in body composition, which is not confined to old age. During the course of adult life, body protein in the form of lean tissues (lean body mass) diminishes progressively while body fat increases, so that overall weight does not necessarily diminish during most of the adult years. The loss of lean body mass has been demonstrated most directly by several cross-sectional and a few longitudinal studies of populations at different ages by measuring ^{40}K radiation from the subjects in a whole-body counter. Since body potassium is mainly concentrated in lean (active) tissues and is naturally radioactive, reduction in the amount of radiation from ^{40}K with advancing age is equated with loss of the lean tissues of the body in which most of the body protein resides. An excellent survey on age-related changes in ^{40}K content of the adult has been assembled by Forbes (1976). He demonstrates a continuous decrease in lean body mass as age advances, with a hint of acceleration in the rate of loss when old age is attained. This increasing rate of loss among the elderly may also be evident in data published by Steen *et al.* (1979). In their longitudinal study of Swedish subjects between the ages of 70 and 75 years, an average loss of 1 kg of lean body mass was observed over the 5-year period, a rate that could hardly be sustained if it also applied to the earlier years of adult life.

Table I. Age-Related Changes in Body Composition of Adult Men[a]

Age group (years)	Body weight (kg)	Body fat (kg)	Nonmuscle mass (kg)	Muscle mass (kg)
20–29	80	15	37	24
40–49	81	19	38	20
60–69	79	23	37	17
70–79	80	24	38	18

[a]Abstracted from data of Cohn *et al.* (1980).

Not only is aging associated with the overall loss of lean body mass, it is also selective for different tissues and organs. Korenchevsky (1961) used autopsy findings to show that people over the age of 70 years have internal organs that weight 9 to 18% less than the same visceral organs in young adults, whereas skeletal muscle has lost 40% of its weight. In consequence, the muscle of elderly people represents about 27% of body weight, whereas the slim young man has 45% muscle in his body. Evidence from alternative measurements of muscle mass support this selective erosion with age and demonstrate that it is a progressive process throughout adult life. Thus, Cohn *et al.* (1980) report studies on men and women varying in age from 20 to 80 years whose total body nitrogen was measured using prompt-γ neutron activation and in addition whose total body potassium was obtained by counting ^{40}K. They found that ^{40}K, which is more concentrated in muscle cells, is lost more extensively as age advances than is total body nitrogen, which is more uniformly distributed among the lean tissues. With differential equations, it was possible to demonstrate from these data that muscle is extensively lost during the aging process, whereas nonmuscular lean tissues do not undergo detectable loss over the adult life span (Table I). Borkan *et al.* (1983) have applied computed tomography scans (CAT scans) to compare the muscle content of the upper arms and legs of elderly men with that of middle-aged men. Aging not only caused a 12% loss of muscle mass over an average age difference of 23 years but also resulted in infiltration of the muscle with fat, thus reducing the lean tissue even further. In contrast, the tissues of the chest and abdomen lost 3% of their lean mass as measured by CAT scans.

The large change in muscle mass during aging can also be inferred from measurement of two urinary metabolites of muscle origin, namely, creatinine and 3-methylhistidine. Urinary creatinine is derived from creatine and its high-energy form, creatine phosphate, which are present in largest amount in muscle. Creatinine is made from these precursors by a nonenzymic chemical reaction that occurs at a constant rate of 1.5% per day. In consequence, the urinary output of creatinine becomes a measure of the body creatine pool and, if we assume a constant concentration in muscle, provides an approximate index of muscle mass. Table II shows that the output of creatinine by a group of old men was only 60% of its output by young men (Uauy *et al.*, 1978a). This is confirmed by an extensive cross-sectional study of creatinine output reported by Tzankoff and Norris (1977) for men in the Baltimore Longitudinal Study of Aging. From the age of 20 years to 90 years, output decreased progressively

Table II. Whole-Body Protein Breakdown and Muscle Protein Breakdown in Young and Old Adults[a]

Group	Mean age (yr)	Whole-body protein breakdown (g/day per kg body weight)	Creatinine output (mg/kg body weight)	Muscle protein breakdown (g/day)[b]		
				Per kg body weight	Per g creatinine	Percentage whole-body protein breakdown
Males						
Young	22	2.94	26	0.76	30	26%
Old	70	2.64	16	0.53	32	20%
Difference		0.30 (−10%)		0.23 (−41%)		
Females						
Young	20	2.35	23	0.64	28	27%
Old	76	1.94	13	0.31	26	16%
Difference		0.41 (−17%)		0.33 (−51%)		

[a]Abstracted from data of Uauy *et al.* (1978a).
[b]Computed from output of 3-methylhistidine.

with age, the mean value at 90 years being only 50% of that at 20 years of age. These findings are also seen in aging rats. Neumaster and Ring (1965) report studies on male and female rats at about 200 days and 800 days of age. The mass of selected muscles per 100 g body weight was 17–29% less in the older males and females, whereas the liver did not lose weight and the spleen increased markedly. Urinary output of creatinine decreased in males by 18% and in females by 8%.

The second metabolite of muscle origin, 3-methylhistidine, is released during breakdown (turnover) of the myofibrillar proteins of muscle, namely, actin and myosin (Young and Munro, 1978; Munro and Young, 1978). When these proteins break down, they release 3-methylhistidine, which is not reutilized or metabolized but is quantitatively and rapidly excreted in the urine of man and the rat. Muscle proteins provide the major pool of 3-methylhistidine in the body, but some other tissues (e.g., intestine, skin) may contribute in aggregate up to 25% of the urinary output of this metabolite in the rat but probably a lesser proportion in man, for whom intestine and skin provide a lower percentage of body weight. Measurements of urinary output of 3-methylhistidine in young and elderly subjects by Uauy *et al.* (1978a) show (Table II) that output declines with age in parallel with creatinine output, indicating that the greatly reduced excretion by the older men and women is related to the smaller muscle mass and not to a reduction in turnover rate per unit of muscle protein. The same table also shows that whole-body protein turnover is only slightly reduced by old age, a change that can be accounted for by the large change in muscle protein.

From the point of view of nutrition in relation to aging, the question arises whether this extensive and selective loss of muscle with aging can be influenced by nutrition. This topic is part of another section of this volume (Chapter 5), but it may be remarked here that Ståhlberg and Fawcett (1982) have concluded that the reduction in muscle mass results from a progressive loss of motor units within the spinal cord as the subject ages. This conclusion makes the relationship to nutrition, if any, a matter of effects on the nervous system.

2.2. Age-Related Changes in Protein Metabolism

One feature of aging is the continuous reduction in the capacity to adapt to environmental factors. Thus, it is well known that tolerance for carbohydrate diminishes as the subject grows older (Silverberg, 1984). Changes in the regulation of protein metabolism can also be identified. Here, we look for clues to the impact of such changes in relation to protein and amino acid utilization and requirements as age advances. This covers whole-body protein turnover, the synthesis of individual proteins, and the metabolism of selected amino acids. Some of these age-related changes may be related to the reduction in muscle mass in the elderly.

2.2.1. Whole-Body Protein Turnover

The greater availability in recent years of amino acids labeled with stable isotopes has encouraged investigators to explore the turnover and metabolism of protein in human subjects. A short account of the principles and limitations of these studies now follows. More detailed accounts can be found in the comprehensive volume written by

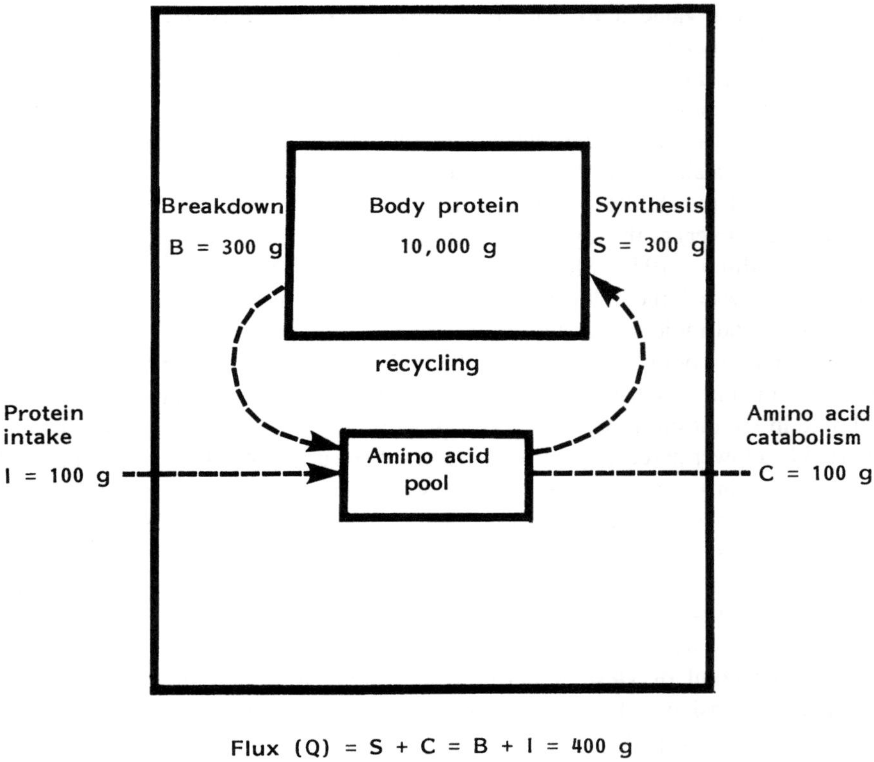

Fig. 1. Components of daily whole-body protein turnover for an adult man of 70 kg body weight. The relationships are expressed by the equation $Q = B + I = S + C$, where Q is total amino acid flux, I is amino acid intake, usually as dietary protein, B is body protein breakdown, S is body protein synthesis, and C is amino acid catabolism.

Waterlow *et al.* (1978) and in a recent symposium volume (Garrow and Halliday, 1985) and are the basis of the following theoretical description.

Turnover of protein is sometimes taken to be equivalent to breakdown but is more correctly used to mean the combination of synthesis (S) and breakdown (B) that results in continuous replacement of the proteins of different organs at different rates (Fig. 1). When synthesis and breakdown of body protein or organ proteins are equal in magnitude ($S = B$), the protein content of the body or organ remains constant even although turnover is often extensive. If synthesis is less than breakdown ($S < B$), there will be loss of protein from the body or organ, whereas there is a gain in protein when synthesis exceeds breakdown ($S > B$). In order to explore body protein turnover, two additional measurements need to be made, namely, protein (or amino acid) intake and amino acid catabolism. This allows the investigator to calculate the amount of amino acids entering the free amino acid pool from dietary protein intake (I) as well as from protein breakdown (B), while the pool loses amino acids through protein synthesis (S) and amino acid catabolism (C). This traffic through the free amino acid pool of the body is known as flux (Q) and is illustrated in Fig. 1. In the equilibrium state shown in the diagram, flux Q thus consists of I (100 g per day) plus amino acids coming from body protein breakdown B (300 g per day), total 400 g. This has to be balanced by removal of amino acids from the pool in the form of protein synthesis, S (300 g), and amino acid catabolism, C (100 g). Thus, the equation becomes:

$$Q = S + C = B + I = 400 \text{ g}$$

Figure 1 represents protein metabolic dynamics typical of a 70-kg man and shows that most of the amino acids for synthesis of new body protein comes from reutilization (recycling) of amino acids entering the pool as a result of protein breakdown. Indeed, it is three times larger than the intake from the diet. What advantage justifies the extensive and energy-costly process of turnover on this scale? It seems probable that this lability of body protein allows rapid adaptation to stress circumstances such as starvation (maintaining gluconeogenesis from amino acids released from muscle protein) and sepsis and injury (corticosteroid action on muscle protein to supply amino acids for other tissues). Thus, a large turnover of body protein is compatible with considerable flexibility, allowing diversion of amino acids and their metabolites without depending on dietary protein as an amino acid source in emergencies.

Elderly humans display partial loss of one major component of recycling, namely, extensive reduction of muscle protein. This is emphasized in a study of the changing pattern of whole-body protein metabolism in aging humans (Uauy *et al.*, 1978a). Rate of breakdown of body protein was measured on healthy young adults and elderly men and women who were administered [^{15}N[glycine over a 60-hr period during which urine was collected over 3-hr periods and the rate of body protein breakdown was computed at plateau output levels of ^{15}N according to the formula of Picou and Taylor-Roberts (1969). Table II shows that rate of whole-body protein breakdown per kilogram body weight diminishes about 10% in elderly men and about 15% in old women. Three-quarters of the reduction can be accounted for by reduced breakdown of muscle protein, as measured by urinary excretion of 3-methylhistidine (Table II). This preferential reduction in muscle protein turnover with age results in the contribution of muscle to whole body turnover shrinking from 26% in young men and 27% in young women to 20% and 16%, respectively, in their elderly counterparts.

Other data in the literature support these data but provide a less comprehensive picture (Table III). Thus, Golden and Waterlow (1977) measured rate of protein synthesis in elderly subjects using both [^{15}N]glycine, whose end product (C) is urinary N, and [1-^{14}C]leucine, for which C is measured as $^{14}CO_2$ in the breath. Thus, they had two independent measures of protein metabolic dynamics. Six patients over 65 years of age and free of metabolic diseases were studied. They computed the rate of whole-body protein synthesis of these old people in several different ways and concluded that the values were lower than those reported in the literature for middle-aged or young adults measured in the same way. Robert *et al.* (1984) measured protein synthesis and breakdown using infusions of [1-^{14}C]leucine (Table III). In agreement with Uauy *et al.* (1978a; Table II), their data display a larger difference in rates of both synthesis and breakdown for old women than for old men when compared with young women and men. M. K. Gersovitz, H. N. Munro, and V. R. Young (unpublished data) confirm with [^{15}N]glycine that the effect of aging on protein turnover in men is small. Then

Table III. Whole-Body Protein Synthesis and Breakdown in Young and Old Men and Women

Authors	Labeled amino acid	Sex of subjects	Protein synthesis[a] (g/kg per day)			Protein breakdown[a] (g/kg per day)		
			Young	Old	Difference	Young	Old	Difference
Golden and Waterlow (1977)	[1-^{14}C]Leucine	M + F	4.0[b]	2.7 (6)	−32%	—	—	—
	[^{15}N]Glycine	M + F	3.8[c]	3.3 (6)	−13%	—	—	—
Robert *et al.* (1984)	[1-^{13}C]Leucine[d]	M	3.1 (10)	2.8 (6)	−10%	4.0 (10)	3.6 (6)	−5%
	[1-^{13}C]Leucine	F	3.9 (5)	2.7 (4)	−31%	4.8 (5)	3.3 (4)	−31%
M. Gersovitz, H. N. Munro, and V. R. Young (unpublished)	[^{15}N]Glycine	M	3.1 (5)	3.1 (6)	± 0%	3.0 (5)	2.7 (6)	−10%

[a]Number of subjects in parentheses.
[b]Data of O'Keefe *et al.* (1974) on young subjects used for comparison.
[c]Data of Crane *et al.* (1977) on young subjects used for comparison.
[d]Computed from Robert *et al.* (1984) using the data showing micromoles leucine incorporated per kilogram per hour and expressing it as grams protein per kilogram per day assuming 8% body protein to be leucine.

corrected for the smaller lean body mass of older subjects, the small diminution in male subjects disappears in their data and those of Robert *et al.* (1984).

It can be cautiously concluded from Tables II and III that the elderly, especially women, have a smaller protein turnover because of a smaller muscle mass. With these small differences in whole-body protein turnover during adult aging, it seems unlikely that further studies of this parameter will improve the data. Since meals affect rates of protein synthesis and breakdown in individual organs, it may, however, be profitable to determine whether this phase of the daily metabolic cycle is less efficient in older people. If further studies of this kind are to be pursued, it will be necessary to reconcile the different absolute values for protein turnover that have been reported using various labeled amino acids (Garlick and Fern, 1985).

2.2.2. *Effect of Aging on Specific Proteins*

The most accessible proteins for study are those in the plasma, which have been used extensively to monitor malnutrition (e.g., Shetty *et al.*, 1979). The literature contains a number of observations showing depressed levels of albumin and other plasma proteins in older people, but the effect of chronic disease and malnutrition must be excluded. Our studies (Gersovitz *et al.*, 1980a) on ostensibly healthy young and elderly men show about 10% less albumin in the plasma as age advances (Table IV). In the case of a recent survey (Munro *et al.*, 1987) of healthy elderly people aged 60–75 years and 76 years onwards, the latter group showed a further significant reduction of about 3%; the relevance of nutritional status to this continuing reduction in old age is discussed in Section 4 of this chapter.

The effect of aging on the rate of albumin synthesis and degradation has been studied on both rats and human subjects. Old rats show evidence of accelerated albumin synthesis (Beauchene *et al.*, 1970; Chen *et al.*, 1973; Obenrader *et al.*, 1975; Van Bezooijen *et al.*, 1976, 1977). However, aged rats tend to lose albumin through albuminuria, which may be the reason for the accelerated synthesis with aging. In human elderly, two groups of investigators have studied the rate of degradation of

Table IV. Albumin Metabolism in Young and Elderly Men Studied with [^{15}N]Glycine at Two Dietary Protein Levels[a]

Measurement	Young men: Low protein	Young men: Adequate protein	Old men: Low protein	Old men: Adequate protein
Serum albumin (g/dl)	4.58	4.52	4.22[b]	4.12[c]
Albumin synthesis (mg/kg per day)	140	186[b]	147	149
Percentage whole-body protein synthesis	4.6	6.2[b]	5.6	4.8

[a]Data abstracted from Gersovitz *et al.* (1980a).
[b]Significantly different from young men on low protein.
[c]Significantly different from young men on adequate protein diet.

injected plasma albumin labeled with ^{131}I or ^{125}I. In comparison with published data from young adults, Yan and Franks (1968) found decreased intravascular and extravascular albumin pools in elderly people but no change in fractional degradation rate. In contrast, Misra *et al.* (1975) report increased fractional and absolute rates of albumin catabolism in elderly men and women, some of whom had severe hypoalbuminemia. Neither Yan and Franks (1969) nor Misra *et al.* (1975) report the nutritional status of their subjects.

We (Gersovitz *et al.*, 1980a) have studied albumin synthesis by young and elderly human subjects receiving different levels of protein intake. Albumin synthesis was measured by using a new stable isotope procedure in which we fed [^{15}N]glycine every 3 hr throughout a 60-hr period. The labeled ^{15}N was incorporated through glutamate into the pool of liver arginine via the ornithine–arginine cycle and was thus available for both [^{15}N]urea labeling and also for incorporation of [^{15}N]arginine into plasma albumin. The specific activity of the precursor free arginine could be inferred from the labeling of the body pool of [^{15}N]urea and used to correct the incorporation of [^{14}C]arginine into albumin. Fractional synthetic rates were calculated and converted to absolute synthesis rates as milligrams per kilogram body weight per day. The study was carried out with young and old adult subjects receiving a formula diet containing either a high level of protein (1.5 g/kg) for 7 days or a low level of protein (0.4 g/kg) for 14 days. Table IV shows that albumin concentration was about 10% less in the elderly irrespective of the diet. In the young subjects, the absolute synthesis rate rose significantly from 140 mg/kg per day on the inadequate protein intake to 186 mg/kg per day on the high protein intake, whereas the synthesis rate of the elderly subjects remained unaffected (147 mg/kg to 149 mg/kg). The rate of synthesis of albumin by the young adults on an adequate intake of protein (186 mg/kg per day) is in good agreement with the catabolic rate measured with radioiodinated albumin, namely, 180 mg/kg per day (McFarlane, 1964).

The differing responses of young and old subjects to raising the level of protein intake is important. It implies that the elderly respond differently to dietary protein level because in older people there is a cap limiting the response of albumin synthesis to a level lower than in the young. This limitation is also seen in a rat. Ove *et al.* (1972) demonstrated that young rats increase their albumin synthesis rate by 40% in response to bleeding, but old rats do not show this response. In both studies, the regulating factor could reside in a reduced capacity of the older animal to transcribe more albumin mRNA in response to the stimulus of protein intake or of hypoalbuminemia. In support of this interpretation, Pain *et al.* (1978) have demonstrated that protein-depleted young rats have less available mRNA for albumin in their cell cytoplasm, and we (Zähringer *et al.*, 1976) have found more albumin mRNA when young rats develop hypoalbuminemia following puromycin nephrosis. It would be interesting to extend these observations on the age-related change in responsiveness of albumin synthesis to dietary protein to other plasma proteins. Since most plasma proteins other than albumin are glycoproteins, it is worth commenting that a new procedure for measuring the specific activity in the liver of precursor sugars for synthesis of the carbohydrate component of plasma glycoproteins is available (Hellerstein and Munro, 1987). In this procedure, acetaminophen is administered, causing excretion in the urine of acetaminophen glucuronide made from glucose via UDP-glucose, which is also a precursor of galactose incorporated into plasma glycoprotein synthesized in the liver (Hellerstein *et al.*,

1987). Thus, when labeled glucose is administered, the labeling of acetaminophen-glucuronide provides the specific activity of precursor liver galactose used for glycoprotein synthesis.

2.2.3. *Aging and Amino Acid Metabolism*

Amino acid metabolism involves extensive interactions between organs (Munro, 1982), and it might be thought that plasma free amino acid levels would reflect age-related losses of function, notably the extensive reduction in muscle mass. Indeed, the levels of free amino acids in the plasma of elderly subjects have been reported by several investigators, often without restricting their observations to healthy elderly of good nutritional status or on similar diets as young controls. The findings show little uniformity. Thus, Ackerman and Kheim (1964) observed lower levels of most free amino acids in the plasma of the elderly, whereas Wehr and Lewis (1966) found two-thirds of plasma amino acids to be raised in the elderly, and Armstrong and Stave (1973) report elevations in levels of alanine, citrulline, tyrosine, and cystine but depression in serine level. Similarly, in a comparison of young and elderly men and women, Robert *et al.* (1984) report consistent depressions in plasma serine and threonine levels of the elderly of both sexes. A study of glycine metabolism discussed below (Gersovitz *et al.*, 1980b) did not indicate any age-related reduction in conversion of glycine to serine.

One might expect the extensive loss of muscle mass in old people to have an important effect on amino acid metabolism, notably on the branched-chain amino acids (Munro, 1982), but there is little in the literature to support this. In a comparison of levels of free amino acids in plasma and muscle, Möller *et al.* (1979) found elevations of most essential and some nonessential amino acids. Young *et al.* (1982) report unpublished studies (W. D. A. Perera and V. R. Young, unpublished data) in which a diet with protein replaced by amino acids could be varied. They found that as leucine intake was lowered, plasma levels of this amino acid decreased with a similar pattern in both young and old adults, whereas valine concentration rose to similar levels in both age-groups. These patterns of similar levels and responses in the plasma amino acids of the young and the elderly have also been recorded for subjects fed graded doses of tryptophan (Young *et al.*, 1971; Tontisirin *et al.*, 1973a) or of valine (Young *et al.*, 1972). Such findings indicate that the plasma free amino acid levels can reflect the patterns of amino acid intakes.

It might be thought that plasma amino acid levels are sometimes elevated in the elderly because of the well-known insulin resistance of older people. However, release of insulin by infusion of glucose into young and old adults produced the same reduction in plasma leucine level and in plasma flux measured with [1-^{13}C]leucine (Robert *et al.*, 1984). The action of insulin in depressing plasma amino acids has been examined in young and elderly men by Fukagawa *et al.* (1988) using the insulin-clamp procedure. They find that the dose of insulin needed to half-maximally depress glucose in young subjects was the same as the dose needed for depressing most plasma amino acids to this extent. In contrast, the elderly needed about twice the level of insulin to achieve half-maximal reduction in glucose, but the dose needed for depression of amino acids to a similar extent remained essentially the same as in the young men. Thus, insulin

Table V. Glycine Flux and Its Components in Young and Elderly Subjects Receiving Adequate (1.5 g/kg) and Low (0.4 g/kg) Intakes of Protein[a]

Group and protein intake	Total glycine flux (μmole/kg per hr)	Components of glycine flux[b] (μmole/kg per hr): Glycine intake	Glycine release from protein	Glycine synthesis
Young adults				
Adequate protein	458	27 (6%)	80 (18%)	351 (78%)
Low protein	301[c]	7 (2%)	87[d] (29%)	206[c] (68%)
Elderly				
Adequate protein	409	27 (7%)	74 (19%)	308 (75%)
Low protein	291[c]	7 (2%)	81[d] (28%)	204[c] (70%)

[a]From data of Gersovitz *et al.* (1980b).
[b]Figures in parentheses are percentages of total glycine flux.
[c]Significant reduction on low-protein diet ($P < 0.01$).
[d]Significant increase on low-protein diet ($P < 0.05$).

resistance for glucose disposal by the elderly is not shared by amino acids. An insulin-clamp study of leucine flux by the same investigators led to the conclusion that the lowered plasma levels caused by insulin administration were caused by reduced protein breakdown, which diminished leucine flux. Thus, there appears to be no support for a change in leucine metabolism in the elderly because of diminishing muscle mass.

Finally, the metabolism of individual amino acids in the young and the elderly has occasionally been examined following administration of labeled amino acids. A detailed study has been made of glycine metabolism in young and elderly subjects using continuous administration of [^{15}N]glycine fed orally over 60 hr (Gersovitz *et al.*, 1980b). Endogenous glycine synthesis was estimated from the dilution of oral [^{15}N]glycine in the plasma glycine in excess of glycine entering the pool from protein breakdown (Fig. 1). The diets fed the young and elderly subjects contained either 1.5 or 0.4 g protein/kg. Table V shows that glycine flux and its components at the two levels of protein intake. Glycine flux did not differ between young and elderly subjects at the same level of protein intake but was extensively reduced at the lower intake of protein. The contribution of dietary glycine to the flux was small (2–7%), that of protein breakdown was 18–29%, and that of glycine synthesis was 68–75%. Age had no significant effect on glycine synthesis or its percentage contribution to whole-body glycine flux, although the absolute rate of glycine synthesis fell extensively at the lower level of protein intake. The lack of a difference between young and old may reflect the finding that the major site of glycine metabolism lies in the viscera (Yoshida and Kikuchi, 1973), so that the age-related loss of muscle will have a minimal influence on glycine synthesis.

3. *Requirements for Protein and for Essential Amino Acids*

Energy intake usually declines progressively throughout adult life. In the Baltimore Longitudinal Study of Aging, cross-sectional measurement of the food intake of

Table VI. Protein and Energy Intakes of Groups of Adults in Scotland[a]

Group	Number in group	Mean age (yr)	Mean energy intake per day (kcal)	Mean protein intake per day: Total (g)	As percentage of total energy intake	Intake per kilogram body weight (with range) (g/kg)
Younger men						
Students	9	22	3060	91	11.9	1.28 (1.05–1.46)
Clerks	10	28	3040	96	12.6	1.49 —
Coal miners	19	36	4030	121	12.0	1.84 —
Older men						
Older clerks	8	56	2440	83	13.6	1.24 (1.04–1.52)
Older workers (heavy work)	26	60	3430	113	13.2	1.48 (1.24–1.86)
Older workers (moderate work)	24	61	2910	90	12.4	1.31 (0.85–1.80)
Retired men (living alone)	9	73	2050	72	14.0	1.03 (0.78–1.24)
Younger women						
Technicians	18	19	2200	64	11.6	1.18 (0.89–1.65)
Young shop assistants	12	21	2220	70	12.3	1.21 (0.99–1.63)
Older women						
Older housewives	21	60	1940	62	12.7	1.02 (0.69–1.39)
Elderly women (living alone)	17	66	1890	62	13.2	1.03 (0.69–1.59)

[a]From Munro (1964c), with permission.

this cohort of men (McGandy *et al.*, 1966) showed that their energy intake fell from 2700 kcal at age 30 years to 2100 kcal at 80 years, the reduction being partly related to diminished lean body mass but mostly to reduced physical activity. As energy intake falls, so do intakes of other nutrients contained in the dietary sources of energy. Thus, Table VI, taken from studies performed in Scotland in 1958, shows that young men had a daily intake of 3000–4000 kcal energy, depending on physical work demands, whereas retired men living alone could survive on 2050 kcal.These different caloric intakes were paralleled by proportional intakes of protein, so that the protein–calorie ratio deviated little from 12–14% despite large changes in caloric intake. We can, therefore, ask whether the reduction in protein intake, coupled with a lower intake of energy, contributes to the age-related reduction in lean body mass noted earlier. One objective should thus be to identify a level of protein intake that would result in the least erosion of lean body mass.

3.1. Protein Requirements of the Elderly

The protein requirements of adults have traditionally been based on nitrogen (N) balance in which intake of N is compared with N output (Munro, 1985). The amount of protein required to achieve equilibrium and thus prevent loss of body protein N has been approached in two ways (see FAO/WHO/UNU, 1985, for detailed discussion). In the "factorial" method, loss of body protein by subjects on a protein-free diet is measured as N lost in the urine, feces, from the skin, and by other minor routes, the so-called "obligatory N losses" when no protein is available from the diet (FAO/WHO, 1973). In this approach, the protein requirement of the subject is the amount of dietary protein equivalent to these losses with additions representing the upper limit of variability of individuals (2 standard deviations, usually +25% or +30% above the mean) and a further correction for incomplete utilization of protein because of the nonlinear (diminishing) response to increasing protein intake, for which a further 30% is added to the estimate. Thus, a typical young man weighing 70 kg and receiving a protein-free diet for 10 days would have a urinary excretion at plateau of 37 mg N daily per kilogram body weight, to which is added 12 mg N for fecal N, and 5 mg N for cutaneous and miscellaneous N losses. The total daily obligatory (endogenous) N loss thus amounts to 54 mg N, equivalent to consuming 0.34 g protein/kg daily. When corrected for individual variability of subjects (+30%) and for curvilinear response increments in protein intakes (+30%), this becomes 0.57 g protein/kg. When corrected for the alleged biological utilization of the average dietary protein by adults on Western diets (75%), this becomes 0.8 g protein/kg (FAO/WHO, 1973).

A limited number of investigators have studied elderly subjects on protein-free diets by measuring their obligatory N losses via the urine and feces, to which can be added estimated losses by minor routes, to add up to total obligatory N losses on a protein-free diet. In two cases, published data allow us to compare the findings for young and elderly subjects studied by the same investigators. In the first case, the total obligatory losses were 51 mg N/kg body weight for young men (Scrimshaw *et al.*, 1972) and 52 mg N for old men (Uauy *et al.*, 1978b). In contrast, Calloway and Margen (1971) obtained an obligatory output of 57 mg N/kg body weight in young men, but the same laboratory (Zanni *et al.*, 1979) assessed the obligatory N losses of old men to be only 42 mg N/kg. Finally, comparison of women at two different laboratories shows almost identical obligatory N losses of 38 mg N/kg by young women (Bricker and Smith, 1951) and 39 mg N/kg by old women (Scrimshaw *et al.*, 1976). In general, therefore, calculated requirements based on endogenous N output corrected for the various factors described above predict a need not exceeding 0.8 g protein/kg body weight by both young and elderly adults. It should be emphasized that the obligatory N losses only allow us to estimate the protein needs of young and old on the assumption that efficiency of dietary protein utilization is the same at both ages and that variability in protein requirements is similar in the two populations. If we accept this, the obligatory N loss approach does not suggest greater needs by the elderly.

The second procedure for determining protein requirements involves finding the minimum amount of dietary protein required to maintain the subject in N equilibrium (zero N balance). The subject is fed several levels of dietary protein below and above the amount needed to achieve equilibrium, and the point of N equilibrium can be identified by interpolation (Fig. 2). To this is added an amount representing individual variations (+2 standard deviations, usually 25–30%). There are several features of N balance determinations that limit the precision of this approach (Munro and Young, 1981). (1) Minor routes of N excretion are usually not directly measured but are

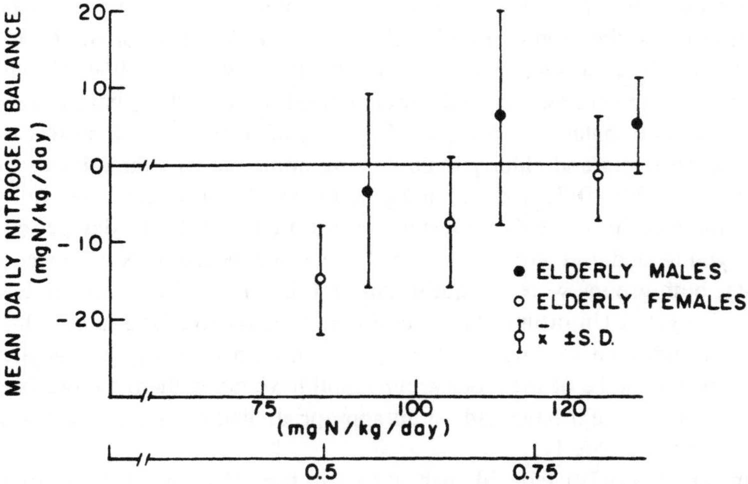

Fig. 2. Nitrogen balance data for seven elderly men and seven elderly women receiving graded amounts of whole-egg protein from submaintenance to maintenance levels. (From Uauy *et al.*, 1978c, with permission.)

estimated from the literature. (2) The previous nutritional status of the subject can affect the level of protein intake at which N equilibrium is achieved; subjects who have been depleted of protein reach this level on less protein. (3) Energy intake affects N balance, even when the amount of energy is well above requirements (Cuthbertson and Munro, 1937; Munro, 1964b). Kishi *et al.* (1978) provide a good illustration (Table VII) of how increasing the energy intake of young men can alter the amount of dietary protein needed to achieve N equilibrium and also the recommended requirement, which includes two standard deviations above this average value, covering 97.5% of the population's needs.

Table VII. Effect of Energy Intake on the Amount of Dietary Protein Required by Adult Men to Achieve Zero Nitrogen Balance and on the Corresponding Safe Allowance of Dietary Protein[a]

Energy (kcal/kg body weight)	Mean requirement of dietary protein for zero N balance (g protein/kg body weight)	Safe allowance of protein (mean requirement + 2 standard deviations) Grams protein/kg body weight	Grams protein/70-kg man
40	0.78	1.02	72
45	0.56	0.74	52
48	0.51	0.62	44
57	0.42	0.50	35
Recommended dietary allowance[b]		0.80	56

[a]Data computed from Kishi *et al.* (1978).
[b]National Academy of Sciences (1980).

As reviewed by Munro (1983), studies of protein requirements in the 1950s led to the conclusion that the protein needs of the elderly are less than or similar to those of young adults (Albanese *et al.*, 1952; Horwitt, 1953; Watkin, 1964; Kountz *et al.*, 1951). Four more recent reports on the protein needs of the elderly have benefited from improvements in N balance techniques. Cheng *et al.* (1978), working in Chile, gave young male prisoners and elderly male nursing home patients three levels of protein intake, namely, 0.4, 0.8, and 1.6 g/kg body weight, a wheat–soy–milk mixture providing the protein of the diet. During the last 5 days of the 11-day period on each diet, the young and old groups averaged the same negative N balance on 0.4 g protein/kg; both groups were in equilibrium at 0.8 g/kg and were in similar positive balance at 1.6 g/kg. Unfortunately, men of both ages received the same caloric intake (40 kcal/kg), although we know that old people need less energy. Consequently, the excessive energy intake of the older group could have given them a more favorable N balance than they would have had on an appropriate energy intake, thus obscuring a greater need by the elderly.

Zanni *et al.* (1979) fed old men a protein-free diet for 17 days, followed by addition of two levels of egg-white protein to the diet. From N balance determinations made while these diets were consumed, the authors were able to apply regression analysis to predict that N equilibrium would be reached by these old men on a diet containing 0.59 g protein/kg, an estimate that includes two standard deviations above the mean. This value is almost identical to the FAO/WHO (1973) estimate for the amount of egg protein needed for N equilibrium by young men. Although the elderly men in the study received an appropriate energy intake (31 kcal/kg), it can be criticized on the grounds that the preliminary feeding of a protein-free diet could promote more efficient use of the dietary protein fed immediately afterwards. The study also suffers from basing regression analysis on two levels of protein intake that were rather close together.

Uauy *et al.* (1978c) report a study of seven elderly men and seven elderly women over 68 years of age who were given graded amounts of whole-egg protein between 0.52 and 0.85 g/kg body weight and an appropriate caloric intake (32 kcal/kg). Five of the women were still in negative N balance at 0.8 g protein/kg, whereas only two men remained in slightly negative N balance at 0.85 g protein/kg (Fig. 2). Finally, Gersovitz *et al.* (1982) describe a much longer study on seven men and seven women over the age of 70 years who were given 0.8 g whole egg protein along with about 30 kcal/kg throughout a 30-day experiment. The study was divided into three 10-day periods, during the last 5 days of which N balances were determined. Table VIII shows that the men were all in negative balance in the first period but averaged a positive balance during the last two periods, although at the end of the study three of the seven still were in negative balance. The women showed an average negative balance throughout, four out of eight being in negative balance. This study and the one reported by Uauy *et al.* (1978c) agree in showing that 0.8 g protein/kg is only marginal in maintaining zero N balance in older people. In addition, both reports suggest that old women have a greater need than old men for dietary protein.

It is apparent from these four recent studies that nitrogen balance is a difficult technique with which to achieve precision. In one laboratory with extensive experience in this field, values for the protein requirements of young men have been estimated at

Table VIII. Nitrogen Balance of Elderly Men and Women Fed 0.8 G Egg Protein per Kilogram Body Weight for 30 Days[a]

Group	Period of 10 days on diet	N intake (mg N/kg)	N balance (mg N/kg)	Number in negative balance
Men	I	129	−7.4	7/7
	II	130	+1.6	4/7
	III	130	+0.4	3/7
Women	I	128	−0.8	4/8
	II	129	−7.8	7/8
	III	129	−2.3	4/8

[a]Adapted from Gersovitz *et al.* (1982).

different times to be either 0.43 g protein/kg (Calloway and Margen, 1971) or 0.56 g protein/kg (Calloway, 1975), a 25% difference. This contrasts with the need for a technique that can detect differences in rate of loss of lean body mass at different levels of protein intake. For example, Steen *et al.* (1979) found that elderly people lost about 1 kg lean body mass between the ages of 70 and 75 years, which represents 40 g protein per year, equivalent to a daily negative N balance of 20 mg N for a 70-kg man. It is likely that N balance is not more precise than several hundred milligrams N per day. In consequence, this technique is unlikely to detect subtle but important differences in rate of loss of protein from whole-body mass as a result of changes in protein intake. It may be noted, however, that Steen and others study changes of lean body mass of adult populations consuming twice the recommended protein level of 0.8 g/kg body weight and, nevertheless, still observe loss of lean body mass. High intakes of protein are thus unlikely to eliminate this loss.

Of some interest is a study of the effect of level of protein intake on the synthesis and breakdown of body protein in young and elderly subjects (M. Gersovitz, H. N. Munro, and V. R. Young, unpublished data). Table IX summarizes the findings of an experiment in which young and old men were given a formula diet containing either 1.5 g, 0.8 g, or 0.4 g protein/kg body weight. [^{15}N]Glycine was administered orally for 60 hr, and urinary urea isotopic enrichment was employed to compute protein synthesis and breakdown over a 24-hr period (see Section 2.2.1). Protein synthesis was not significantly affected by level of dietary protein over the whole range, but breakdown was accelerated by decreasing intake from 1.5 to 0.4 g/kg but not by changing it from 1.5 to 0.8 g/kg. This lends support to a requirement not exceeding 0.8 g/kg as the safe level for old men. The most recent Recommended Dietary Allowances (National Academy of Sciences, 1980) prescribe 56 gm protein for a 70-kg adult male and 44 gm for a 56-kg woman, irrespective of age, i.e., 0.8 gm protein per kg of body weight.

3.2. Requirements for Essential Amino Acids

The requirement for protein represents a need for both essential amino acids and for total nitrogen. The requirements for the eight essential amino acids not synthesized

Table IX. Protein Synthesis and Breakdown in Young and Elderly Subjects at Different Levels of Protein Intake[a]

Components	Young males			Elderly males			Elderly males		
	1.5 g protein	0.4 g protein	Difference	1.5 g protein	0.4 g protein	Difference	1.5 g protein	0.8 g protein	Difference
Protein synthesis	3.13	3.15	−0.02	3.08	2.96	+0.12	3.58	3.49	+0.09
Protein breakdown	2.96	3.22	−0.26*	2.74	2.98	−0.24	3.44	3.43	+0.01
Difference	+0.17	−0.07	+0.24*	+0.34	−0.02	+0.36*	+0.14	+0.06	+0.08

[a]From M. K. Gersovitz, H. N. Munro, and V. R. Young (unpublished). Data are expressed as grams of protein per kilogram body weight.
*Difference between levels in diet significant ($P < 0.05$).

by man have been studied by feeding human subjects with complete amino acid mixtures in place of protein and varying the intake of one essential amino acid at a time, thus establishing the least amount compatible with N equilibrium (Rose, 1957). This approach has led to different results at different ages (see review by Munro, 1972). In infancy, about 43% of the total dietary nitrogen has to be provided by the proper proportions of the essential amino acids in order to achieve optimal N retention and growth. At 10–12 years of age, the percentage is 36%, whereas in young adults it need only be 19%, this last finding recently being confirmed by Inoue *et al.* (1983). This implies that most mixed proteins in diets will contain more than enough of each essential amino acid to meet the small requirements of the adult. In the most recent FAO/WHO/UNU (1985) report it was recognized that, because of this low essential amino acid requirement for adults, most dietary proteins have 100% quality and thus do not need a correction for this factor. The authors of the FAO/WHO/UNU (1985) report do, however, add a small factor for lack of complete digestibility of dietary protein, about 5% loss on Western diets and more for the diets of some other countries.

Few studies of essential amino acid requirements have been made on elderly subjects. In an experiment on men between the ages of 52 and 68 years of age fed on amino acid mixtures in place of protein, Tuttle *et al.* (1957) found that N balance remained negative at levels of intake at which N equilibrium could be achieved in young adults. They therefore suspected that the requirement for one or more of the essential amino acids is increased in the elderly. They followed this by another study (Tuttle *et al.*, 1959) on adults over 50 years of age in which they brought the subjects into N equilibrium on a diet providing 7 g nitrogen as essential and nonessential amino acids. When N intake was raised to 15 g by addition of glycine and diammonium citrate, seven of the eight older men went into negative N balance. This suggested that the source of nonessential N can affect utilization of the amino acid mixture, a conclusion confirmed by replacing glycine with a mixture of nonessential N and obtaining better N balance (Tuttle *et al.*, 1965a).

Finally, requirements for two essential amino acids have been directly evaluated by Tuttle *et al.* (1965b) using a synthetic L-amino acid mixture patterned after whole-egg protein fed to their older subjects in place of dietary protein. Based on the amount needed to achieve N equilibrium, the requirement for the sulfur amino acids methionine plus cystine was 46 mg/kg, and that for lysine was 30 mg/kg, compared with 13 mg and 11 mg/kg, respectively, in young adults (Munro, 1972). In contrast, Watts *et al.* (1964) report that the requirements of old black men for the sulfur amino acids in order to achieve N equilibrium is less than that of young men. However, it should be noted that Mertz *et al.* (1952) found that old women on self-selected diets were in negative N balance, which they attributed to intakes of methionine below the recommended level, whereas Albanese *et al.* (1957) concluded that elderly women in a nursing home were in negative N balance because of inadequate intakes of lysine and could be restored to zero N balance by adding extra lysine to the diet.

Another approach has been used to determine essential amino acid requirements, namely, by increasing the intake of one amino acid in a mixture and observing the response of plasma amino acid levels of that amino acid. When intake of an essential amino acid exceeds requirement the plasma level starts to rise sharply in some cases, less acutely in the case of some other amino acids. In the former case, the point of

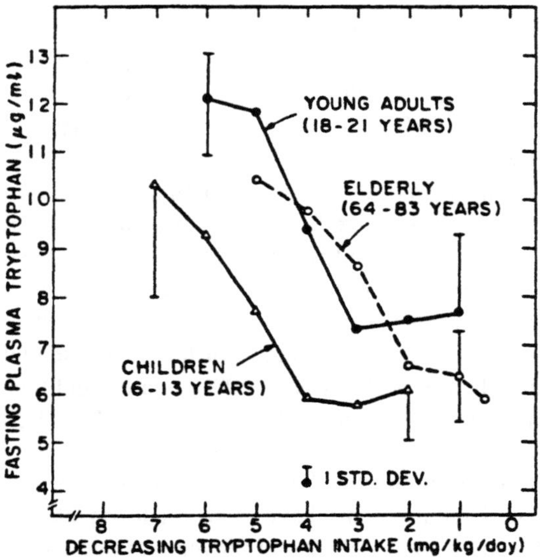

Fig. 3. Changes in plasma tryptophan at various levels of tryptophan intake by children, young adult men, and elderly men. (From Young *et al.*, 1976, with permission.)

inflection has been found to coincide with the requirement for that amino acid. Thus, in a study by Young and Munro (1973), progressively increasing the intake of tryptophan of the growing rat resulted in a sharp inflection at 0.11% tryptophan in the diet, whereas the adult rat showed a less acute inflection at 0.04%; these inflection points correspond reasonably well with the needs of the rat for maximal growth (0.14% of total diet) compared with the tryptophan need for maintenance (0.04%). Animal studies of this kind using other essential amino acids gave similar correlations between the point of inflection and the requirements.

In the case of human subjects, Fig. 3 shows that variations in tryptophan content of the diet result in a sharp increase in plasma tryptophan level above intakes of 4 mg/kg body weight for infants, 3 mg/kg for young adults, and 2 mg/kg for the elderly (Young *et al.*, 1976; Tontisirin *et al.*, 1973). The inflection points agree reasonably well with the tryptophan requirements determined by N balance for the child and the young adult (Munro, 1972), but we have no corresponding data for the elderly. The same approach has been applied to the threonine needs of the elderly (Tontisirin *et al.*, 1974). In this case, both young and elderly adults showed an inflection in plasma level when more than 7 mg threonine/kg body weight was fed, thus agreeing with the need of young men assessed by N balance to be 6 mg/kg (Munro, 1972). Since lean body mass is a smaller proportion of the body weight of elderly people, the requirements for tryptophan and threonine may indeed be somewhat greater for the elderly relative to active tissue than these data suggest when expressed in relation to total body weight.

3.3. *Effects of High Intakes of Protein*

Protein can affect the utilization of other dietary nutrients. The best-authenticated example is the increased loss of body calcium caused by raising the intake of protein. With young adults, Anand and Linksweiler (1974) showed that raising protein intake increases urinary output of calcium which continues for many weeks (Allen *et al.*, 1979). Even when the diet contains little or no calcium (Margen *et al.*, 1974), this effect of protein still occurs, indicating that the protein of the diet does not affect calcium absorption but probably reduces renal reabsorption of calcium. This is compatible with the observation (Bengoa *et al.*, 1983) that level of parenteral infusion of an amino acid mixture affects calcium excretion in the urine. These findings imply that high intakes of dietary protein can contribute to loss of skeletal calcium in osteoporosis. However, Spencer *et al.* (1978) found that addition to the diet of meat as the form of extra protein produced only a transient increase in urinary calcium output, which they ascribe to the beneficial effect of phosphorus in the meat. In contrast, Heaney and Recker (1982) conclude from a study of the calcium balances of women on self-selected diets that the usual amount of dietary phosphorus is insufficient to counteract the effect of large intakes of dietary protein.

Brenner *et al.* (1982) have assembled evidence suggesting that a high intake of protein in the diet may increase the age-related loss of kidney function. However, the Baltimore Longitudinal Study of Aging failed to show such a relationship (Tobin, 1986). In aging rats, however, the lowering of protein intake reduces the incidence of renal pathology (see Masoro, Chapter 2).

Finally, a high intake of protein increases the need for vitamin B_6, which is extensively involved in amino acid metabolism (National Academy of Sciences, 1980). Examination of a population of elderly in Boston (Munro *et al.*, 1987) showed a strong positive correlation between their protein intakes and their dietary vitamin B_6 intakes, making it improbable that high intakes of protein will not be accompanied by increased intakes of this vitamin from the diet.

4. *Protein Nutriture of the Elderly*

If the safe level of daily protein intake for elderly people is 0.8 g/kg or even higher, we can determine by population studies whether there are a significant number of malnourished people in such a cohort, and particularly whether it includes cases of protein malnutrition or protein–calorie malnutrition. This involves taking a dietary history, measuring biochemical indices such as plasma protein levels, and carrying out a clinical examination including measurement of muscle mass and skinfold thickness.

In Britain, government surveys have used these approaches to determine the nutritional status of the elderly (Department of Health and Social Security, 1979). A representative group of 365 men and women 70 years of age and older were examined for nutrient intake and for nutritional status as judged by biochemical tests and clinical evaluation. This resulted in the identification of 26 individuals with malnutrition, the incidence between 70 and 79 years being 6% for men and 5% for women. From 80 years on, the incidence rose to 12% for men and 8% for women. Caloric and protein intakes by the malnourished subjects were less than by their age-matched controls, and there was a tendency for plasma albumin to be lower. Indeed, protein–calorie malnutrition was the primary deficiency diagnosed in one-quarter of the total malnourished elderly. The report provides a brief clinical history for each subject, from which it is apparent that all but one of the 26 malnourished subjects had an underlying disease

Table X. Protein and Energy Intakes, Concentrations of Plasma Constituents, and Body Composition of Old Men and Women[a]

	Males		Females		Statistics		
Measurement	60–75 yr	76+ yr	60–75 yr	76+ yr	Age	Sex	Interaction
Diet							
Protein (g/day)	83	74	65	64	x	xx	x
Protein (g/kg body wt.)	1.06	1.05	1.02	1.06			
Energy (kcal/day)	1941	1778	1503	1479	x	xx	x
Plasma (per 100 ml)							
Total protein (g)	7.01	7.03	7.00	6.86			
Albumin (g)	4.23	4.11	4.20	4.05	xx		
Prealbumin (mg)	33.8	29.3	21.0	28.7			xx
Transferrin (mg)	298	296	303	292	x		
Ceruloplasmin (mg)	32.1	34.8	36.4	35.8		xx	xx
Retinol-binding protein (mg)	6.00	6.23	5.88	5.79			
Blood urea (mg)	19.1	23.3	17.1	19.9	xx	xx	
Creatinine (mg)	1.24	1.35	1.01	1.11	xx	xx	
Uric acid (mg)	7.32	6.99	5.89	6.27		xx	
Body composition							
Skin thickness (mm)	18.4	16.4	29.5	24.5	xx	xx	x
Arm muscle (cm^2)	44.7	37.1	31.2	28.9	xx	xx	x

[a]Adapted from Munro *et al.* (1987). x, significant, $P < 0.05$; xx, significant, $P < 0.01$.

process. These consisted of chronic bronchitis (nine cases), emphysema (seven), postgastrectomy malnutrition (five), mental depression (nine), dementia (six), alcoholism (three), and some other causes (four). (Note that these numbers add up to more than 26, since many subjects had more than one cause.) Thus, malnutrition was secondary to chronic disease in essentially all of this group.

This picture contrasts with a nutritional status study in Boston of 239 men and 452 women between 60 and 98 years of age who were ambulatory and free from overt chronic disease likely to cause malnutrition (Munro *et al.*, 1987). The subjects were divided into men and women of 60–75 years and those aged 76 years and older. For each of these four groups, Table X shows protein and energy intakes together with plasma protein and other blood concentrations, and Table XI presents the relationship of these to protein intakes by individuals. The older group of men had significantly smaller total caloric and protein intakes than the group of men aged 60–75 years, whereas the women in the two age categories showed no difference (Table X). However, when expressed per kilogram of body weight, mean intakes of protein were essentially similar for both sexes and both ages, ranging from 1.02 to 1.06 g protein/kg, averaging well above the recommended safe intake of 0.8 g/kg. Within each of the four age–sex categories, some 12–15% of individuals recorded intakes less than 0.8 g/kg, some of them probably because of deviations in reporting of their 3-day intakes compared with their true long-term eating habits. As in other studies (Table

Table XI. Correlations of Body Components with Protein Intake[a]

Blood or body component	Men[b] 60–75 yr	Men[b] 76+ yr	Women[b] 60–75 yr	Women[b] 76+ yr
Total protein (g/dl)	−0.27*	+0.02	+0.03	−0.25*
Albumin (g/dl)	−0.02	+0.22	+0.08	−0.14
Prealbumin (mg/dl)	0.00	−0.02	−0.02	−0.26**
Transferrin (mg/dl)	+0.04	−0.10	−0.16**	−0.12
Ceruloplasmin (mg/dl)	−0.09	−0.07	−0.12*	−0.08
Retinol-binding protein (mg/dl)	+0.13	−0.04	−0.17**	−0.15*
Blood urea N (mg/dl)	+0.14*	+0.27*	+0.01	−0.06
Creatinine (mg/dl)	−0.18**	−0.18	−0.05	+0.04
Uric acid (mg/dl)	−0.33**	−0.03	−0.07	−0.14
Triceps skinfold (mm)	−0.22**	−0.21*	−0.34*	−0.31**
Arm muscle (cm^2)	−0.24**	+0.05	−0.21**	−0.21**

[a]Adapted from Munro *et al.* (1987). Protein intake in g/kg body weight.
[b]*, significant correlation ($P < 0.05$); **, significant correlation ($P < 0.01$).

VI), energy intake and protein intake were closely correlated within each group. The correlation coefficients between caloric intake (total kcal/day) and protein intake (g/day) were +0.74 for men aged 60–75 years, +0.63 for men over 75 years, and for the two age groups of women they were +0.66 and +0.54, respectively, all coefficients being highly significant ($P < 0.01$).

The concentrations of several plasma proteins have been used to identify protein–calorie malnutrition (Ingenbleek *et al.*, 1975; Shetty *et al.*, 1979). As Table X shows, concentrations of several plasma proteins were measured by us as indices of protein–calorie malnutrition. Levels of albumin, prealbumin, and transferrin were significantly lower in the plasma of men and women over 75 years of age, but within each group the only significant correlations of individual values with protein intake were in a negative direction (Table XI), implying that some factor associated with higher intakes of protein was related to slight reductions in the levels of certain plasma proteins. Thus, insufficiency of dietary protein is not a factor in the age-related decline in the levels of some plasma proteins.

Other parameters were also examined in the four groups of elderly. Blood urea levels of men and women rose significantly with age (Table X), being higher in men at both ages, and individual levels were positively correlated with the protein intake of the men (Table XI). However, this is unlikely to reflect renal damage from the higher intake of protein (Brenner *et al.*, 1982), since blood creatinine and uric acid levels were not positively correlated with protein intake (Table XI). The elevated blood urea levels in elderly men on higher protein intakes must therefore be accepted as direct consequences of the higher protein load.

Finally, body composition changed with the advance of aging. In both age groups, skinfold thickness was greater in women, while muscle mass was less, and both components of body composition decreased with aging (Table X), observations that are in agreement with expectation. However, these changes could not be linked to low intakes of protein within each age–sex group (Table XI).

In order to coordinate the evidence suggesting that protein malnutrition is not present in an overtly healthy elderly population, a formula used to identify malnutrition in patients (Mullen *et al.*, 1979) was applied in slightly modified form to the data:

$$\text{Nutritional index} = 150 - 16.6 \times Alb - 0.78 \times TSF - 20 \times TFN,$$

where *Alb* is plasma albumin (g/100 ml plasma), *TSF* is triceps skinfold thickness (mm), and *TFN* is plasma transferrin level (mg/100 ml plasma) (delayed hypersensitivity was not done on our elderly subjects but contributes little to the nutritional index). The nutritional indices so generated were low (indicating little tendency to malnutrition) and within each age and sex group showed no correlation with the protein intake of individuals that would suggest higher indices with lower intakes of protein. Thus, the exclusion of subjects with chronic debilitating illnesses allows one to conclude that, despite the continued reduction in food intake with aging, healthy old age can be maintained on diets providing an average daily intake of 1 g protein/kg body weight or perhaps less. The occurrence of malnutrition in elderly people is discussed in detail by Exton-Smith (1980), who also emphasizes its association with chronic physical and mental disease.

5. *Conclusions*

The protein requirements of the elderly are difficult to identify with precision. A first step is to decide what criteria are the most appropriate. The achievement of zero nitrogen balance has been used in adults as the endpoint for many years but cannot provide accurate estimates of small but physiologically important daily losses of body protein as, for example, occur in the age-related reduction of lean body mass. Measurements of lean body mass have been confined to Western countries and, despite the high protein intakes in these countries, still continue to show progressive reductions in lean tissue with aging. Thus, high protein intakes are unlikely to suppress this phenomenon.

Other criteria would also be valuable in monitoring protein needs during the adult life span. In this connection, the somatomedin (IGFs, insulinlike growth factors) family may provide criteria of suffiency of protein intake. During pregnancy, inadequacy of dietary protein can cause lowering of plasma levels of IGF-I and II because of insufficient release of lactogen from the placenta (Pilistine and Munro, 1984; Pilistine *et al.*, 1984), and in the aging adult it has been reported (Florini *et al.*, 1985) that IGF-I levels decline. There is good evidence that inadequacy of both protein and energy intake reduce the IGF-I plasma levels in human subjects (Isley *et al.*, 1983; Unterman *et al.*, 1985; Clemmons *et al.*, 1985) and in rats (Prewitt *et al.*, 1982). These findings suggest that levels of protein intake sustaining optimal levels of plasma somatomedins could be used as endpoints for requirements of protein and energy. This might be combined with plasma levels of prealbumin and of retinol-binding proteins, which are also sensitive to adequacy of protein and energy intakes (Shetty *et al.*, 1979; Sachs and Bernstein, 1986).

Finally, the protein and energy intakes of elderly people with chronic diseases are often inadequate to prevent malnutrition (Department of Health and Social Security, 1979). This results from a lower level of intake than would suffice for a healthy old person and also from losses of body protein caused by the illness. Such cases, which become significant as old age advances, require special consideration from their physician.

6. References

Ackerman, P. G., and Kheim, T., 1964, Plasma amino acids in young and older adult human subjects, *Clin. Chem.* **10**:32–40.

Albanese, A. A., Higgens, R. A., Vestal, B., Stephanson, L., and Malsch, M., 1952, Protein requirements of old age, *Geriatrics* **7**:109–118.

Albanese, A. A., Higgens, R. A., Orto, L. A., and Zwattoro, D. N., 1957, Protein and amino needs in the aged in health and convalescence, *Geriatrics* **12**:443–452.

Allen, L. H., Oddoye, E. A., and Margen, S. (1979). Protein-induced hypercalciuria: a longer term study. *Am. J. Clin. Nutr.* **32**:741–749.

Anand, C. R., and Linksweiler, H. M., 1974, Effect of protein intake on calcium balance of young men given 500 mg calcium daily, *J. Nutr.* **104**:695–700.

Armstrong, M. D., and Stave, U., 1973, A study of plasma free amino acid levels. III. Variations during growth and aging, *Metabolism* **22**:571–578.

Beauchene, R. D., Roeder, L. M., and Barrows, C. H., 1970, The interrelationships of age, tissue protein synthesis and proteinuria, *J. Gerontol.* **25**:359–363.

Bengoa, J. M., Sitrin, M. D., Wood, R. J., and Rosenberg, I. H., 1983, Amino acid induced hypercalciuria in patients on total parenteral nutrition, *Am. J. Clin. Nutr.* **38**:264–269.

Borkan, G. A., Hults, D. E., Gerzof, S. G., Robbins, A. H., and Silbert, C. K., 1983, Age changes in body composition revealed by computed tomography, *J. Gerontol.* **38**:673–677.

Brenner, B. M., Meyer, T. W., and Hostetter, T. H., 1982, Dietary protein and the progressive nature of kidney disease, *N. Engl. J. Med.* **307**:652–659.

Bricker, M. L., and Smith, J. M., 1951, A study of the endogenous nitrogen output of college women with particular reference to the use of creatinine output in the calculation of the biological values of the protein of egg and sunflower seed flour, *J. Nutr.* **44**:553–573.

Calloway, D. H., 1975, Nitrogen balance of men with marginal intakes of protein and energy, *J. Nutr.* **105**:914–923.

Calloway, D. H., and Margen, S., 1971, Variation in endogenous nitrogen utilization as determinants of human protein requirement, *J. Nutr.* **101**:205–216.

Chen, J. C., Ove, P., and Lansing, A. I., 1973, *In vitro* synthesis of microsomal protein and albumin in young and old rats, *Biochim. Biophys. Acta* **312**:598–607.

Cheng, A. H. R., Gomez, A., Gergan, J. G., Lee, T. C., Monckeberg, F., and Chichester, C. O., 1978, Comparative nitrogen balance study between young and aged adults using three levels of protein intake from a combination of wheat–soy–milk-mixture, *Am. J. Clin. Nutr.* **31**:779–785.

Clemmons, D. R., Seek, M. M., and Underwood, L. E., 1985, Supplemental essential amino acids augment the somatomedin-C/insulin-like growth factor I response to refeeding after fasting, *Metabolism* **34**:391–394.

Cohn, S. H., Vartsky, D., Yasumura, S., Savintsky, A., Zanzi, I., Vaswani, A., and Ellis, K. J., 1980, Compartmental body composition based on total body nitrogen, potassium and calcium, *Am. J. Physiol.* **239**:E524–530.

Crane, C. W., Picou, D., Smith, R., and Waterlow, J. C., 1977, Protein turnover in patients before and after elective orthopaedic operations, *Br. J. Surg.* **64**:129–133.

Cuthbertson, D. P., and Munro, H. N., 1937, A study of the effect of overfeeding on the protein metabolism of man. III. The protein saving effect of carbohydrate and fat when superimposed on a diet adequate for maintenance, *Biochem. J.* **31**:694–705.

Department of Health and Social Security, 1979, *Nutrition and Health in Old Age, Report on Health and Social Subjects,* No. 16, Her Majesty's Stationery Office, London.

Exton-Smith, A. N., 1980, Nutritional status: Diagnosis and prevention of malnutrition, in: *Metabolic and Nutritional Disorders in the Elderly* (A. N. Exton-Smith and F. I. Caird, eds.), Wright, Bristol, pp. 66–76.

FAO, 1957, *Protein Requirements, FAO Nutritional Studies,* No. 16, FAO, Rome.

FAO/WHO, 1965, *Protein Requirements, FAO Nutrition Meetings Report Series,* No. 30, FAO, Rome.

FAO/WHO, 1973, *Energy and Protein Requirements, FAO Nutrition Meetings Report Series,* No. 52, FAO, Rome.

FAO/WHO/UNU, 1985, *Energy and Protein Requirements, WHO Technical Report Series,* No. 724, WHO, Geneva.

Florini, J. R., Prinz, P. N., Vitiello, M. V., and Hintz, R. L., 1985, Somatomedin-C levels in healthy young and old men: Relationship to peak and 24-hour integrated levels of growth hormone, *J. Gerontol.* **40:**2–7.

Forbes, G. B., 1976, The adult decline in lean body mass, *Hum. Biol.* **48:**161–173.

Fukagawa, N. K., Minaker, K., Rowe, J. W., Matthews, D. E., Bier, D. M., and Young, V. R., 1988, Differential insulin sensitivity of glucose and amino acid metabolism in aging man, *Metabolism* **37:**371–377.

Garlick, P. J., and Fern, E. B., 1985, Whole body protein turnover: Theoretical considerations: in: *Substrate and Energy Metabolism in Man* (J. S. Garrow and D. Halliday, eds.), John Libbey, London, pp. 7–14.

Garrow, J. S., and Halliday, D. (eds.), 1985, *Substrate and Energy Metabolism in Man,* John Libbey, London.

Gersovitz, M., Munro, H. N., Udall, J., and Young, V. R., 1980a, Albumin synthesis in young and elderly subjects using a new stable isotope methodology: Response to level of protein intake, *Metabolism* **29:**1075–1086.

Gersovitz, M., Bier, D., Matthews, D., Udall, J., Munro, H. N., and Young, V. R., 1980b, Dynamic aspects of whole body glycine metabolism: Influence of protein intake in young adult and elderly males, *Metabolism* **29:**1087–1094.

Gersovitz, M., Motil, K., Munro, H. N., Scrimshaw, N. S., and Young, V. R., 1982, Human protein requirements: Assessment of the adequacy of the current recommended dietary allowance for dietary protein in elderly men and women, *Am. J. Clin. Nutr.* **35:**6–14.

Golden, M. H. N., and Waterlow, J. C., 1977, Total protein synthesis in elderly people: A comparison of results with ^{15}N-glycine and [^{14}C]leucine, *Clin. Sci. Mol. Med.* **53:**277–288.

Heaney, R. P., and Recker, R. R., 1982, Effects of nitrogen, phosphorus and caffeine on calcium balance in women, *J. Lab. Clin. Med.* **99:**46–55.

Hellerstein, M. K., and Munro, H. N., 1987, Glycoconjugates as noninvasive probes of intrahepatic metabolism, II. Application to measurement of plasma alpha 1-acid glycoprotein turnover during experimental inflammation, *Metabolism* **36:**995–1000.

Hellerstein, M. K., Greenblatt, D. J., and Munro, H. N., 1987, Glycoconjugates as non-invasive probes of intrahepatic metabolism. I. Kinetics of labelling of urinary acetaminophen-glucuronide from carbohydrate precursors and absence of compartmentalized hepatic UDP-glucose pools for secreted glucuronyl- and galactosyl-conjugates, *Metabolism* **36:**988–994.

Horwitt, M. K., 1953, Dietary requirements of the aged, *J. Am. Diet. Assoc.* **29:**443–448.

Ingenbleek, Y., Van der Schrieck, H. G., De Nayer, P., and De Visscher, M., 1975, Albumin, transferrin and the thyroxine-binding prealbumin/retinol-binding protein (TBPA-RBP) complex in assessment of malnutrition. *Clin. Chim. Acta* **28:**9–19.

Inoue, G., Komatsu, T., Kishi, K., and Fujita, Y., 1983, Amino acid requirements of Japanese young men, in: *Amino Acids: Metabolism and Medical Applications* (G. L. Blackburn, J. P. Grant, and V. R. Young, eds.), Wright, Bristol, pp. 55–62.

Isley, W. L., Underwood, L. E., and Clemmons, D. R., 1983, Dietary components that regulate serum somatomedin-C concentrations in humans, *J. Clin. Invest.* **71:**175–182.

Kishi, K., Miyatani, S., and Inoue, G., 1978, Requirement and utilization of egg protein by Japanese young men with marginal intakes of energy, *J. Nutr.* **109:**658–669.

Korenchevsky, V., 1961, *Physiological and Pathological Aging,* Hafner, New York.

Kountz, W. B., Hofstatter, L., and Ackerman, P. G., 1951, Nitrogen balance studies in four elderly men, *J. Gerontol.* **6:**20–33.

Margen, S., Chu, J.-Y., Kaufman, N. A., and Calloway, D. H., 1974, Studies in calcium metabolism, I: The calciuretic effect of dietary protein, *Am. J. Clin. Nutr.* **27**:584–589.

McFarlane, A. S., 1964, Metabolism of plasma proteins, in: *Mammalian Protein Metabolism,* Volume 1 (H. N. Munro and J. B. Allison, eds.), Academic Press, New York, pp. 297–341.

McGandy, R. B., Barrows, C. H., Spanias, A., Meredith, A., Stone, J. L., and Norris, A. H., 1966, Nutrient intakes and energy expenditure in men of different ages, *J. Gerontol.* **21**:581–587.

Mertz, E. T., Baxter, E. J., Jackson, L. E., Roderuck, C. E., and Weis, A., 1952, Essential amino acids in self-selected diets of older women, *J. Nutr.* **46**:313–322.

Misra, D. P., Loudon, J. M., and Staddon, G. E., 1975, Albumin metabolism in elderly patients, *J. Gerontol.* **30**:304–306.

Möller, P., Bergström, J., Erickson, S., Fürst, P., and Hellerström, K., 1979, Effect of aging on free amino acids and electrolytes in leg muscle, *Clin. Sci.* **56**:427–432.

Mullen, J. L., Buzby, G. P., and Waldman, M. T., 1979, Prediction of operative morbidity and mortality by preoperative nutritional assessment, *Surg. Forum* **30**:80–82.

Munro, H. N., 1964a, Historical introduction: The origin and growth of our present concepts of protein metabolism, in: *Mammalian Protein Metabolism,* Volume I (H. N. Munro and J. B. Allison, eds.), Academic Press, New York, pp. 1–29.

Munro, H. N., 1964b, General aspects of the regulation of protein metabolism by diet and by hormones, in: *Mammalian Protein Metabolism,* Volume I (H. N. Munro and J. B. Allison, eds.), Academic Press, New York, pp. 381–481.

Munro, H. N., 1964c, An introduction to nutritional aspects of protein metabolism, in: *Mammalian Protein Metabolism,* Volume II (H. N. Munro and J. B. Allison, eds.), Academic Press, New York, pp. 3–39.

Munro, H. N., 1972, Amino acid requirements and metabolism and their relevance to parenteral nutrition, in: *Parenteral Nutrition* (A. W. Wilkinson, ed.), Churchill Livingstone, Edinburgh, pp. 34–67.

Munro, H. N., 1982, Interaction of liver and muscle in the regulation of metabolism in response to nutritional and other factors, in: *The Liver: Biology and Pathobiology* (I. Arias, H. Popper, D. Schachter, and D. A. Shafritz, eds.), Raven Press, New York, pp. 677–691.

Munro, H. N., 1983, Protein nutriture and requirement in elderly people, in: *Bibliotheca Nutritio et Dieta,* No. 33, (J. C. Somogyi, ed.), S. Karger, Basel, pp. 61–74.

Munro, H. N., 1985, Historical perspective on protein requirements: Objectives for the future, in: *Nutritional Adaptation in Man* (K. Blaxter and J. C. Waterlow, eds.), John Libby, London, pp. 155–166.

Munro, H. N., and Young, V. R., 1978, Urinary excretion of N^t-methylhistidine (3-methyl-histidine): A tool to study metabolic responses in relation to nutrient and hormonal status in health and disease in man, *Am. J. Clin. Nutr.* **31**:1608–1614.

Munro, H. N., and Young, V. R., 1981, New approaches to the assessment of protein status in man, in: *Recent Advances in Clinical Nutrition* (A. N. Howard and I. M. Baird, eds.), Libby, London, pp. 33–41.

Munro, H. N., McGandy, R. B., Hartz, S. C., Russell, R. M., Jacob, R. A., and Otradovec, C. L., 1987, Protein nutriture of a group of free-living elderly, *Am. J. Clin. Nutr.* **46**:586–592.

National Academy of Sciences, 1980, *Recommended Dietary Allowances,* 9th rev. ed., National Academy Press, Washington.

Neumaster, T. D., and Ring, G. C., 1965, Creatinine excretion and its relation to whole body potassium and muscle mass in inbred rats, *J. Gerontol.* **20**:379–382.

Obenrader, M. F., Lansing, A. I., and Ove, P., 1975, Evidence relating the amount of albumin mRNA to the increase albumin synthetic activity in old rats, *Adv. Exp. Med. Biol.* **61**:289–290.

O'Keefe, S. J. D., Sender, P. M., and James, W. P. T., 1974, 'Catabolic' loss of body nitrogen in response to surgery, *Lancet* **2**:1035–1038.

Ove, P., Obenrader, M., and Lansing, A., 1972, Synthesis and degradation of liver proteins in young and old rats, *Biochim. Biophys. Acta* **277**:211–221.

Pain, V. M., Clemens, M. J., and Garlick, P. J., 1978, The effect of dietary protein deficiency on albumin synthesis and the concentration of active albumin messenger ribonucleic acid in the rat liver, *Biochem. J.* **172**:129–135.

Picou, D., and Taylor-Roberts, T., 1969, The measurement of total protein synthesis and catabolism and nitrogen turnover in infants in different nutritional states and receiving different amounts of dietary protein, *Clin. Sci.* **36**:283–296.

Pilistine, S. J., and Munro, H. N., 1984, Protein deficiency in pregnant rats causes decreased levels of

plasma somatomedin and its carrier protein associated with reduced plasma levels of placental lactogen and hepatic lactogenic receptor number, *J. Nutr.* **114:**638–642.
Pilistine, S. H., Moses, A. C., and Munro, H. N., 1984, Placental lactogen administration reverses the effect of low protein diet on maternal and fetal serum somatomedin levels in the pregnant rat, *Proc. Natl. Acad. Sci. U.S.A.* **81:**5853–5857.
Prewitt, T. E., D'Ercole, A. J., Switzer, B. R., and Van Wyk, J. J., 1982, Relationship of serum immunoreactive somatomedin-C to dietary protein and energy in growing rats, *J. Nutr.* **112:**144–150.
Robert, J., Bier, D., Schoeller, D., Wolfe, R., Matthews, D., Munro, H. N., and Young, V. R., 1984, Effects of intravenous glucose on whole body leucine dynamics, studied with 1-^{13}C-leucine in healthy young and elderly adults, *J. Gerontol.* **39:**673–681.
Rose, W. C., 1957, The amino acid requirements of adult man, *Nutr. Abstr. Rev.* **27:**631–647.
Sachs, E., and Bernstein, L. H., 1986, Protein markers of nutrition status as related to sex and age, *Clin. Chem.* **32:**339–341.
Scrimshaw, N. S., Hussein, M. A., Murray, E., Rand, W. M., and Young, V. R., 1972, Protein requirements of man, *J. Nutr.* **102:**1595–1604.
Scrimshaw, N. S., Perera, W. D. A., and Young, V. R., 1976, Protein requirements of man: Obligatory urinary and fecal nitrogen losses in elderly women, *J. Nutr.* **106:**665–670.
Shetty, P. S., Watrasiewicz, K. E., Jung, R. T., and James, W. P. T., 1979, Rapid turnover transport proteins: An index of subclinical protein–energy malnutrition, *Lancet* **2:**230–232.
Silverberg, A. B., 1984, Carbohydrate metabolism and diabetes in the aged, in: *Nutritional Intervention in the Aging Process* (H. J. Ambrecht, J. M. Prendergast, and R. M. Coe, eds.), Springer, New York, pp. 191–208.
Spencer, H., Kramer, L., Osis, D., and Norris, C., 1978, Effect of a high protein (meat) intake on calcium metabolism in man, *Am. J. Clin. Nutr.* **36:**2167–2180.
Stålberg, E., and Fawcett, P. R., 1982, Macro EMG in healthy subjects of different ages, *J. Neurol. Neurosurg. Psychiatry* **45:**870–878.
Steen, G. B., Isaksson, B., and Svanberg, A., 1979, Body composition at 70 and 75 years of age: Longitudinal population study, *J. Clin. Exp. Gerontol.* **1:**185–200.
Tobin, J., 1986, Nutrition and organ function in a cohort of aging men, in: *Nutrition and Aging* (M. L. Hutchinson and H. N. Munro, eds.), Academic Press, New York, pp. 23–34.
Tontisirin, K., Young, V. R., Miller, M., and Scrimshaw, N. S., 1973, Plasma tryptophan response curve and tryptophan requirements of elderly people, *J. Nutr.* **103:**1220–1228.
Tontisirin, K., Young, V. R., Rand, W. M., and Scrimshaw, N. S., 1974, Plasma threonine response curve and threonine requirements of young men and elderly women, *J. Nutr.* **104:**495–505.
Tuttle, S. G., Swendseid, M. E., Mulcare, D., Griffith, W. H., and Basset, S. H., 1957, Study of the essential amino acid requirements of men over fifty, *Metabolism* **6:**564–573.
Tuttle, S. G., Swendseid, M. E., Mulcare, D., Griffith, W. H., and Basset, S. H., 1959, Essential amino acid requirements of older men in relation to nitrogen intake, *Metabolism* **8:**61–70.
Tuttle, S. G., Basset, S. H., Griffith, W. H., Mulcare, D. G., and Swendseid, M. E., 1965a, Further observations on the amino acid of older men. I. Effects of nonessential nitrogen supplements fed with different amounts of essential amino acids, *Am. J. Clin. Nutr.* **16:**225–228.
Tuttle, S. G., Bassett, S. H., Griffith, W. H., Mulcare, D. B., and Swendseid, M. E., 1965b, Further observations on amino acid requirements of older men. II. Methionine and lysine, *Am. J. Clin. Nutr.* **16:**229–231.
Tzankoff, S. P., and Norris, A. H., 1977, Effect of muscle mass decrease on age-related BMR changes, *J. Appl. Physiol.* **43:**1001–1006.
Uauy, R., Winterer, J. C., Bilmazes, C., Haverberg, L. N., Scrimshaw, N. S., Munro, H. N., and Young, V. R., 1978a, The changing pattern of whole body protein metabolism in aging humans, *J. Gerontol.* **33:**663–671.
Uauy, R., Scrimshaw, N. S., Rand, W. M., and Young, V. R., 1978b, Human protein requirements: Obligatory urinary and fecal nitrogen losses and the factorial estimation of protein needs in elderly men, *J. Nutr.* **108:**97–103.
Uauy, R., Scrimshaw, N. S., and Young, V. R., 1978c, Human protein requirements: Nitrogen balance response to graded levels of egg protein in elderly men and women, *Am. J. Clin. Nutr.* **31:**779–785.
Unterman, T. G., Vazquez, R. M., Slas, A. J., Martyn, P. A., and Phillips, L. S., 1985, Nutrition and somatomedin. XIII. Usefulness of somatomedin-C in nutritional assessment, *Am. J. Med.* **78:**228–234.

Van Bezooijen, C. F. A., Grell, R., and Knook, D. L., 1976, Albumin synthesis by liver parenchymal cells from young and old rats, *Biochem. Biophys. Res. Commun.* **71**:513–519.

Van Bezooijen, C. F. A., Grell, R., and Knook, D. L., 1977, The effect age on protein synthesis by isolated liver parenchymal cells, *Mech. Ageing Dev.* **6**:293–304.

Waterlow, J. C., Garlick, P. J., and Millward, D. C., 1978, *Protein Turnover in Mammalian Tissues and in the Whole Body,* North Holland, New York.

Watkin, D., 1964, Protein metabolism and requirements in the elderly, in: *Mammalian Protein Metabolism,* Volume 2 (H. N. Munro and J. B. Allison, eds.), Academic Press, New York, pp. 247–263.

Watts, J. H., Mann, A. N., Bradley, L., and Thompson, D. J., 1964, Nitrogen balances of men over 65 fed the FAO and milk patterns of essential amino acids, *J. Gerontol.* **19**:370–374.

Wehr, R. F., and Lewis, G. T., 1966, Amino acids in blood plasma of young and aged adults, *Proc. Soc. Exp. Biol. Med.* **121**:349–351.

Yan, S. H., and Franks, J. J., 1968, Albumin metabolism in elderly men and women, *J. Lab. Clin. Med.* **72**:449–454.

Yoshida, T., and Kikuchi, G., 1973, Major pathways of serine and glycine catabolism in various organs of the rat and cock, *J. Biochem. (Tokyo)* **73**:1013–1022.

Young, V. R., and Munro, H. N., 1973, Plasma and tissue tryptophan levels in relation to tryptophan requirements of weanling and adult rats, *J. Nutr.* **103**:1756–1763.

Young, V. R., and Munro, H. N., 1978, N^{τ}-methylhistidine (3-methylhistidine) and muscle protein turnover, *Fed. Proc.* **37**:2291–2300.

Young, V. R., Hussein, M. A., Murray, E., and Scrimshaw, N. S., 1971, Plasma tryptophan response curve in relation to tryptophan requirements in young men, *J. Nutr.* **101**:45–60.

Young, V. R., Uauy, R., Winterer, J. C., and Scrimshaw, N. S., 1976, Protein metabolism and needs in elderly people, in: *Nutrition, Longevity, and Aging* (M. Rockstein and M. L. Sussman, eds.), Academic Press, New York, pp. 67–102.

Young, V. R., Gersovitz, M., and Munro, H. N., 1982, Human aging: Protein and amino acid metabolism and implications for protein and amino acid requirements, in: *Nutritional Approaches to Aging Research,* (G. B. Moment, ed.), CRC Press, Boca Raton, FL, pp. 47–81.

Young, V. R., Tontisirin, K., Ozalp, I., Lakshamana, F., and Scrimshaw, N. S., 1972, Plasma amino acid response curve and amino acid requirements in young men: valine and lysine, *J. Nutr.* **102**:1159–1169.

Zähringer, J., Baliga, B. S., and Munro, H. N., 1976, Increased levels of microsomal albumin-mRNA in the liver of nephrotic rats, *FEBS Lett.* **62**:322.

Zanni, E., Calloway, D. H., and Zezulka, A. H., 1979, Protein requirements of elderly men, *J. Nutr.* **109**:513–524.

8

Calcium Nutrition and Its Relationship to Bone Health

Robert R. Recker and Robert P. Heaney

1. Introduction

In a sense, it is odd that there should be any doubt about this issue, since all of one's calcium must come from the diet aside from the rather small contribution made by the mother during pregnancy. Nevertheless, calcium nutrition and utilization vary so greatly from individual to individual, other factors affect bone health so profoundly, and measurement tools are so imprecise that the relationship has been difficult to document and characterize.

2. Confusing Reports

Careful studies done in the 1960s (Smith and Rizek, 1966; Smith and Frame, 1965) were unable to demonstrate a relationship between current bone mass and current calcium intake. Methods available for measuring bone mass were not very precise (estimating vertebral density on lateral spine films or measurement of metacarpel cortical thickness), yet the studies were carefully done, and the populations were very large. Later studies by Garn *et al.* (1981) demonstrated no more than a weak correlation between current calcium intake and metacarpal cortical thickness in elderly persons, and Pacifici *et al.* (1985) could find no correlation between vertebral density by quantitative computed tomography and calcium intake in healthy perimenopausal women, nor could Laval-Jeantet *et al.* (1984).

On the other hand, Kanders *et al.* (1984) reported a positive correlation between calcium intake and midshaft radial bone mineral content (BMC) in young women, and Anderson and Tylavsky (1984) were able to show that elderly women with high lifelong calcium intakes had greater BMC and bone density (BD) of the midradius that those with low lifelong calcium intakes.

Robert R. Recker • Creighton University School of Medicine, Omaha, Nebraska 68178. ***Robert P. Heaney*** • Creighton University, Omaha, Nebraska 68178.

Nordin (1961) and others (Riggs *et al.*, 1967; Hurxthal and Vose, 1969; Vinter-Paulsen, 1953) have demonstrated that patients with osteoporosis generally have lower calcium intakes than controls, but the differences are not great. In Riggs' (1967) study, for example, intake was 617 mg/day in patients versus 721 mg/day in controls, and others have not found such differences. Nordin *et al.* (1979a), in fact, could not find this difference in a more recent study in which intakes of patients and controls were 885 and 835 mg/day, respectively.

Two scientific reports have had major influence on current notions linking diet calcium and bone mass; these were by Heaney *et al.* (1978) and Matkovic *et al.* (1979). The former described transmenopausal changes in the efficiency of utilization of diet calcium, and the latter described lifelong intake effects on bone mass and fracture frequency.

In the report by Heaney *et al.* (1978), healthy perimenopausal women were studied under strict metabolic balance conditions on a diet carefully prepared to match their usual intakes of all nutrients including calcium. The usual intakes were carefully estimated by 7-day diaries and interview by a specially trained dietitian. There were 274 studies performed on 168 women. (Repeat studies were separated by an interval of 5 years.) Figure 1 summarizes the results of a plot of calcium balance as a function of dietary calcium intake. There were 233 studies on women who were estrogen-replete (premenopausal or postmenopausal and estrogen-treated) and 41 on women who were estrogen-deprived (postmenopausal, untreated). Calcium balance was more positive in both groups at higher calcium intakes, but at any given intake the estrogen-replete individuals had about 0.024 g/day more positive calcium balance. The mean zero

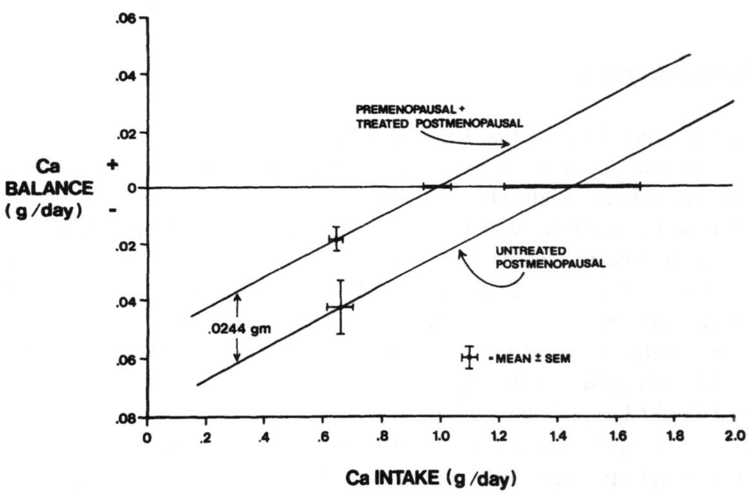

Fig. 1. Plot of the regression lines of calcium balance on calcium intake in two estrogen-status groups. The broad horizontal bands on the zero-balance line depict the 95% confidence range for the estimates of calcium intake predicted from these data to result in zero calcium balance for the two groups of women. The ranges for the calcium intake data used to compute these lines are as follows: For the combined premenopausal and treated postmenopausal group, 0.159 to 2.273; for the untreated postmenopausal group, 0.205 to 1.142. (Adapted from Heaney *et al.*, 1978.)

balance point for the estrogen-replete group was 0.990 g/day, and for the estrogen-deprived group was 1.504 g/day.

This study matched current calcium intake with current calcium balance performance and provided evidence in favor of a link between dietary calcium and bone health. It also demonstrated an estrogen effect on calcium utilization manifest as an interaction between hormone status and dietary calcium levels.

Matkovic's study (1979) was cross sectional. Two Yugoslavian communities were examined, one with an average lifelong calcium intake of about 0.950 g/day and the other about 0.424 g/day. In the high-calcium district both men and women had higher bone mass (by metacarpal radiogrammetry) at all ages than those in the low-calcium district, and the incidence of hip fracture was 34 times higher in the low-calcium district. The most important feature of this study was that bone mass was higher at ages 30–35 in the high-calcium district, the earliest age studied, suggesting that calcium nutrition is important early in life in achieving maximum peak skeletal mass. Reduction in bone mass was parallel in later ages in both communities, but the high-calcium district maintained an advantage in greater bone mass throughout the elderly years.

3. *Prospective Studies*

Another method of examining the link between calcium nutrition and bone health is through prospective studies of calcium supplementation, and several have been reported. Recker *et al.* (1977) demonstrated that calcium carbonate supplements will improve calcium balance and eliminate age-related bone loss (measured by metacarpal radiogrammetry) in healthy postmenopausal women compared to untreated controls. Calcium intake averaged 0.579 g/day in the controls and 1.482 g/day in the subjects. These findings were corroborated in a more recent study by these investigators (Recker *et al.*, 1985) in which the calcium supplement was from dairy products. Similar results have been published by others (Albanese *et al.*, 1973, 1975; Horsman *et al.*, 1977; Lee *et al.*, 1981), and Aloia and co-workers (1983) found that the rate of bone loss in postmenopausal women as measured by total body calcium was inversely correlated with levels of diet calcium and calcium absorption.

These studies suggest that calcium supplements or increased calcium intake from food sources can slow bone loss and, further, that calcium nutrition is important in childhood and young adult life in attaining peak skeletal mass.

On the other hand, careful studies by Nilas *et al.* (1984), Garsdal *et al.* (1984), and Sowers *et al.* (1985) could not demonstrate that calcium intake influences age-related bone loss in healthy postmenopausal women. In each of these studies, bone mass was measured at the distal radius, with other skeletal sites excluded from analysis. The Nilas and Garsdal studies were controlled and consisted of longitudinal observation during calcium supplementation, and the Sowers study examined two Iowa communities that differed in calcium intake largely because of markedly different calcium content of the community water supply.

A more recent study has added to the uncertainty about whether calcium nutrition has any impact on age-related bone loss in postmenopausal women. Riis *et al.* (1987)

examined the effect of estrogen replacement or calcium supplementation on the bone loss that occurs in the period immediately after menopause. The subjects entered study during the first 3 years after menopause, a time when the loss of bone associated with estrogen deprivation is greatest. Not surprisingly, the calcium supplements did not prevent bone loss at the distal radius. However, even during this period of exponential bone loss from estrogen deprivation, the calcium supplements did have an effect intermediate between estrogen replacement and placebo at the proximal radius and as evaluated by total body calcium measurements. This study has been cited as evidence against a favorable calcium nutrition effect on bone loss, but the data actually support such an effect, and the authors acknowledge this.

4. Resolving the Conflicts

The currently available data leave some uncertainty about the validity of a link between diet calcium and bone health, with some reports contradicting others. However, some progress has been made in resolving these contradictions.

Heaney, in a recent review of this topic, has pointed out (Heaney, 1986) that bone mass is the result of three general groups of forces: genetic endowment, mechanical loading, and endocrine/nutritional factors. The first two are causal and the third permissive, and this is the critical point. There are numerous examples of low bone mass caused by endocrine and nutritional (calcium) deficiencies but few examples (except perhaps acromegaly) of increased bone mass from nutritional or endocrine excess. An optimal endocrine and nutritional status permits realization of the full genetic potential of skeletal mass as modulated by mechanical loading, but neither endocrine nor nutritional factors are capable of causing appreciable increase in bone mass.

Thus, whenever a variable (diet calcium) exerts a permissive effect on another variable (bone mass), a threshold emerges below which the two variables are related and above which they are not. Figure 2 is a schematic illustration of this principle. Any population of subjects that might be examined for a relationship between diet calcium and bone mass will likely contain members above and below the threshold; further, the threshold cannot be expected to be the same in all members. Thus, the relationship may be very difficult to detect even though it is real.

Another problem in studying this relationship is that the variable, "diet calcium" should not really be defined as current diet calcium but rather as the diet calcium integrated over an individual's entire life history to date. Manifestly, this is very difficult to estimate with very much precision.

One can list a whole array of factors that may cause variation in the threshold level from individual to individual, obscuring the relationship between calcium intake and bone mass. For example, calcium absorption efficiency varies greatly from person to person (Heaney, 1986), and there is a decline in absorption efficiency with age (Nordin *et al.*, 1976, 1979b; Gallagher *et al.*, 1979; Lawson *et al.*, 1979). There is also variation in absorption efficiency because of digestive factors (Allen, 1982) and nutrient interactions such as found with dietary fiber (Godara, 1981). It should be remembered that these confounding factors do not indicate that a relationship does not exist, but they do make one difficult to detect in population studies.

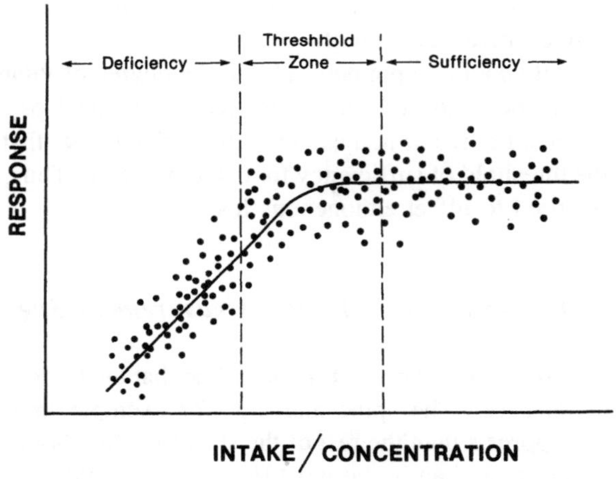

Fig. 2. Schematic representation of the observational relationship of two variables when the independent variable is permissive. The solid line represents the mean relationship, and the points, observational data. In the deficiency region, the permissive variable is limiting, and variations in its availability are observably related to the values of the outcome variable. In the sufficiency region, there is no discernable relationship between the two, either observationally or in reality. In the threshold zone, there is a real relationship, but it is often difficult to observe. (Adapted from Heaney, 1986.)

5. *Vitamin D*

Most students of this subject are now very familiar with the role of vitamin D in calcium absorption: sun exposure (UV light) to the skin provides the energy required to convert a precursor, 7-dehydrocholesterol, to cholecalciferol. Dietary sources of vitamin D are handled in the same manner as the skin sources except that the vitamin D precursor is fed. This is converted in the liver to another precursor, 25-hydroxyvitamin D, which in turn is converted to the active metabolite, 1,25-dihydroxyvitamin D, by the kidney. This compound regulates calcium absorption efficiency. Comprehensive reviews of this area of physiology are available (Parfitt, 1982), and this review touches only on one area that is important to the discussion of diet calcium, calcium absorption and the abovementioned thresholds.

Vitamin D status has been evaluated by measurement of serum 25-hydroxyvitamin D levels, and the lower end of the normal range has been found to be in the neighborhood of between 15 and 30 ng/ml based on studies of apparently healthy subjects (Heaney, 1986). However, studies of asymptomatic subjects may not be the best method of finding the optimal lower limit for serum 25-hydroxyvitamin D. The production rate of 1,25-dihydroxyvitamin D is substrate dependent, and Francis *et al.* (1983) have shown that when oral 25-hydroxyvitamin D is given to healthy subjects, the circulating 1,25-dihydroxyvitamin D levels will increase unless the pretreatment 25-hydroxyvitamin D levels are above about 30 ng/ml. The magnitude of the 1,25-dihydroxyvitamin D response is inversely related to the pretreatment serum 25-hydroxyvitamin D levels below this 30 ng/ml. These provocative findings suggest that our criteria for adequate vitamin D status should be reevaluated. It is interesting that serum 25-hydroxyvitamin D levels decline with age coincident with declining calcium absorption efficiency (Heaney, 1986). Vitamin D may then have a significant influence on the set point of the threshold phenomenon for diet calcium and its relationship to bone mass. Since serum 25-hydroxyvitamin D levels are generally below 30 ng/ml after age 30, this may account for some of the variation in the threshold in the relationship between diet calcium and bone mass described above. This is an area of active interest at present.

It should be pointed out that the degree of vitamin D deficiency described above would be mild and would not lead to clinical osteomalacia. However, it could be expected to result in a calcium absorptive defect that would account for an increase in the threshold of sufficiency for calcium intake. Thus, a higher calcium intake would be required to offset endogenous losses.

6. Problems with Skeletal Measurement Site

It has been known for some time that the skeleton does not behave uniformly in all of its parts. The spine and hip, for example, more frequently fracture because of osteoporosis than the rest of the skeleton. And bone loss after oophorectomy is greater in the spine than in the wrist (Riggs *et al.*, 1981). The wrist is a common site used to measure bone mass and the response to treatment or prophylactic interventions, and data from measurements at this site are used to extrapolate to other areas of the skeleton or the entire skeleton.

There are problems with the distal forearm site for measurement of bone mass in nutrition studies. To begin with, the fracture itself behaves differently. Colles' fractures occur at earlier ages than spine and hip fractures (Melton and Riggs, 1983), they do not tend to happen in the patients with spine or hip fractures as often as expected (Melton and Riggs, 1983; Nordin *et al.*, 1980), the rise in incidence begins well before menopause (Melton and Riggs, 1983), and there does not seem to be a clear association between bone mass of the forearm and fracture risk (Heaney, 1986). These data suggest that reduced bone mass may not be the principal factor in this fracture. It ought not to be surprising, then, that the forearm may respond differently to factors that affect the rest of the skeleton, such as diet calcium.

The three studies mentioned above by Nilas *et al.* (1984), Sowers *et al.* (1985), and Garsdal *et al.* (1984) all failed to demonstrate that higher calcium intake protects the skeleton from age-related bone loss during postmenopausal years. They had in common the fact that bone mass was measured at the distal radius. The calcium carbonate study of Recker *et al.* (1977) also failed to demonstrate an effect on the distal radius but did demonstrate an effect on metacarpal cortical thickness and on calcium balance. Most reports relating calcium intake to distal forearm BMC have been negative, as have studies of calcium supplements in preventing bone loss at this site. Thus, although one must conclude that BMC at this site is not related to calcium intake, it is not safe to extrapolate from this site to other skeletal regions. It is important to point out, however, that this site does respond to other agents, such as estrogen (Recker *et al.*, 1977; Horsman *et al.*, 1977; Nilsson and Westlin, 1975).

The Yugoslav study by Matkovic *et al.* (1979) supports the idea of a lack of responsiveness of the distal forearm to diet calcium. In that study, calcium intake influenced bone mass in the metacarpal region and reduced the incidence of hip fracture as well. On the other hand, there was no protection against Colles' fractures in the same subjects. Thus, one cannot relate bone mass and fracture susceptibility to each other at this site or to calcium intake or to events at other skeletal sites.

7. *Other Risk Factors*

It is important to note that much of the difficulty in relating calcium nutrition and bone health resides in the fact that numerous other factors, both nutritional and nonnutritional, affect bone mass and risk of fracture at any site. Nutritional factors include protein intake (Allen, 1982), caffeine intake (Heaney and Recker, 1982), and fiber content of food. Increases in each of these can result in loss of calcium from the body and can obscure the calcium/bone health relationship. Important nonnutritional factors include physical activity, susceptibility to falls, chronic disease of almost any kind, genetic or ethnic influences, smoking, number of pregnancies, degree of obesity, early menopause, treatment with steroids or anticonvulsants, and others. Fracture risk and bone mass may be dominated by any one or more of these factors, obscuring our ability to detect the link between calcium nutrition and bone health even if that link exists.

Among the nutritional factors, protein intake and dietary fiber are special cases deserving mention. Numerous studies have shown that increases in protein intake will lead to more negative calcium balance (Heaney and Recker, 1982; Lutz, 1984; Johnson *et al.*, 1970; Walker and Linkswiler, 1972; Anand and Linkswiler, 1974; Margen *et al.*, 1974). The effect has been so constant that any study failing to show it may be regarded as suspect. However, high protein intakes are not likely to be very important in the development of low bone mass and skeletal fragility, because variation in calcium intake is almost always parallel with variation in protein intake. The negative effect of high protein intake is offset by the positive effect of the higher calcium intake. This has been supported in two studies, one in which calcium balance was measured in normal subjects on their usual nutrient intake (Heaney and Recker, 1982) and the other in normals who had a conscious increase in their calcium intake in the form of milk (Recker and Heaney, 1985). In the first study, the subjects had more positive calcium balance with higher calcium intakes in spite of the accompanying increase in protein intake. In the second, an average change in calcium intake from 0.697 g/day to 1.471 g/day using a milk supplement resulted in a modest rise in nitrogen intake from 9.941 g/day to 12.941 g/day and an improvement in calcium balance from −0.061 g/day to −0.017 g/day. Nevertheless, the correlation between protein intake and calcium balance was significantly negative ($r = -0.396$, $P < 0.01$) when controlled for calcium intake in a partial correlation. This indicates that increases in calcium intake overwhelm the negative effect of the accompanying increase in protein intake and that variation in protein intake probably does not contribute much to the problem of age-related bone loss in women. It is possible that the relatively high phosphorus content of the milk supplement helped to offset the negative effect of the increased protein intake. However, in studies by Heaney *et al.* (Heaney and Recker, 1982), variation in self-selected phosphorus intake had no independent effect on calcium balance in healthy adult females.

It has been known for some time that dietary fiber has been associated with negative calcium balance (Jowsey, 1977; Slavin and Marlett, 1980; McCance and Widdowson, 1942; Cummings *et al.*, 1979; Kelsay *et al.*, 1979). It is not clear how important this effect is in the population, and it is not clear what mechanism is responsible for this. However, it is not likely that uncharged fibers would complex calcium and therefore decrease its absorption. Accordingly, plant components with high concentrations of carboxylic acid may bind calcium through calcium salt bridge formation. Further, it has been shown that ^{45}Ca binding by fiber extracted from 29 different foods was found to be proportional to the uronic acid content of the fibers, each millimole of uronic acid binding 0.31 mmole of calcium (James *et al.*, 1978). The extent of binding was pH dependent, suggesting that ionization of the carboxyl groups of uronic acids might be responsible. Considerable further work needs to be done in this area.

8. Calcium Intake in the United States

Calcium intake in U.S. females is substantially below the RDA of 800 mg/day. After age 50 the median intake on a given day is less than 500 mg (National Center for Health Sciences, 1971–1974; Carroll *et al.*, 1976–1980), and even more alarming, 25% of U.S. women beyond age 30 consume less than 300 mg on any given day. Further, the trend seems to be toward lower intakes for teenage girls judging from the decline fround between the two HANES surveys done in 1971–1974 and 1976–1980 (National Center for Health Sciences, 1971–1974; Carroll *et al.*, 1976–1980). Given the link between low intakes and bone fragility, these data indicate the presence of a serious calcium nutrition problem.

9. Recommendations

Heaney (1986) has pointed out that one cannot simply dismiss the evidence in favor of a positive effect of calcium intake on bone health even though there are uncertainties in the data. Instead, the data overwhelmingly suggest that there is a link between calcium intake and bone mass in some people but not in others and in some skeletal sites and not in others.

The currently available data support the recommendation of the NIH consensus conference (Consensus Conference, 1984) that calcium intake should be 1000 mg/day in premenopausal women or estrogen-treated postmenopausal women and 1500 mg/day in estrogen-deprived postmenopausal women. There are uncertainties and cautions in this recommendation, and not everyone will require these intake levels. On the other hand, there is minimal risk and expense to the population at large, and the incidence of fractures from osteoporosis is so high that even a modest reduction of say 10% or 20% would be welcome. Recommendations for childhood, adolescence, and young adulthood are made on even more uncertain grounds because of the lack of data. This is unfortunate because the meager data we do have suggest that this may be the most important time to insure adequate calcium intake.

The time seems to be appropriate to recommend a higher calcium intake to the population at large even though the extent of its potential efficacy in reducing fracture risk in the elderly is uncertain and precise estimates of its efficacy may never be known. This is not a very extraordinary recommendation, inasmuch as recent studies of primitive intakes suggest that the diet humans are adapted to contains in excess of 1500 mg/day (Eaton and Konner, 1985).

10. References

Albanese, A. A., Edelson, A. H., Woodhull, J. L., Lorenze, E. J., Jr., Wein, E. H., and Orto, L. A., 1973, Effect of a calcium supplement on serum cholesterol, calcium, phosphorus and bone density of "normal, healthy" elderly females, *Nutr. Rep. Int.* **8:**119–130.

Albanese, A. A., Edelson, A. H., Lorenze, E. J., Jr., Woodhull, M. L., and Wein, E. H., 1975, Problems of bone health in the elderly, *N.Y. State J. Med.* **75:**326–336.

Allen, L. H., 1982, Calcium bioavailability and absorption: A review, *Am. J. Clin. Nutr.* **35:**783–808.

Aloia, J. F., Vaswani, A. N., Yeh, J. K., Ross, P., Ellis, K., and Cohn, S. H., 1983, Determinants of bone mass in postmenopausal women, *Arch. Intern. Med.* **143:**1700–1704.

Anand, C. R., and Linkswiler, H. M., 1974, Effect of protein intake on calcium balance of young men given 500 mg calcium daily, *J. Nutr.* **104:**695.

Anderson, J. J. B., and Tylavsky, F. A., 1984, Diet and osteopenia in elderly Caucasian women, in: *Proceedings of the Copenhagen International Symposium on Osteoporosis* (C. Christiansen, C. D. Arnaud, B. E. C. Nordin, A. M. Parfitt, W. A. Peck, and B. L. Riggs, eds.), Department of Clinical Chemistry, Glostrup Hospital, Copenhagen, pp. 299–304.

Carroll, M. D., Abraham, S., and Dresser, C. M., 1976–1980, *Dietary Intake Source Data, United States,* National Center for Health Statistics, Public Health Service, Hyattsville, MD.

Consensus Conference, 1984, Osteoporosis, *J.A.M.A.* **252:**799–802.

Cummings, H. J., Hill, M. J., Houston, H., Branch, W. S., and Jenkins, D. J. A., 1979, The effect of meat protein and dietary fiber on colonic function and metabolism. I. Changes in bowel habit, bile acid excretion, and calcium absorption, *Am. J. Clin. Nutr.* **32:**2086–2093.

Eaton, S. B., and Konner, M., 1985, Paleolithic nutrition: A consideration of its nature and current implications, *N. Engl. J. Med.* **312:**283–289.

Francis, R. M., Peacock, M., Storer, J. H., Davies, A. E. J., Brown, W. B., and Nordin, B. E. C., 1983, Calcium malabsorption in the elderly: The effect of treatment with oral 25-hydroxyvitamin D_3, *Eur. J. Clin. Invest.* **13:**391–396.

Gallagher, J. C., Riggs, B. L., Eisman, J., Hamstra, A., Arnaud, S. B., and DeLuca, H. F., 1979, Intestinal calcium absorption and serum vitamin D metabolites in normal subjects and osteoporotic patients, *J. Clin. Invest.* **64:**729–736.

Garn, S. M., Solomon, M. A., and Friedl, J., 1981, Calcium intake and bone quality in the elderly, *Ecol. Food Nutr.* **10:**131–133.

Garsdal, O., Christensen, M. S., and Christiansen, C., 1984, Effects of oral calcium, vitamin D_3 and 1-alpha-hydroxy vitamin D_3 on urinary calcium excretion rate and serum PTH in the early menopause, in: *Proceedings of the Copenhagen International Symposium on Osteoporosis* (C. Christiansen, C. D. Arnaud, B. E. C. Nordin, A. M. Parfitt, W. A. Peck, and B. L. Riggs, eds.), Department of Clinical Chemistry, Glostrup Hospital, Copenhagen, pp. 829–833.

Godara, R., Kaur, A. P., and Charanjit, J. B., 1981, Effect of cellulose incorporation in a low fiber diet on fecal excretion and serum levels of calcium, phosphorus, and iron in adolescent girls, *Am. J. Clin. Nutr.* **34:**1083–1086.

Heaney, R. P., 1986, Calcium bone health and osteoporosis, in: Bone and Mineral Research 4 (W. Peck, ed.), Elsevier, Amsterdam, pp. 255–301.

Heaney, R. P., and Recker, R. R., 1982, Effects of nitrogen, phosphorus, and caffeine on calcium balance in women, *J. Lab. Clin. Med.* **99:**46–55.

Heaney, R. P., Recker, R. R., and Saville, P. D., 1978, Menopausal changes in calcium balance performance, *J. Lab. Clin. Med.* **92:**953–963.

Horsman, A., Gallagher, J. C., Simpson, M., and Nordin, B. E. C., 1977, Prospective trial of oestrogen and calcium in postmenopausal women, *Br. Med. J.* **2:**789–792.

Hurxthal, L. M., and Vose, G. P., 1969, The relationship of dietary calcium intake to radiographic bone density in normal and osteoporotic persons, *Calcif. Tissue Res.* **4:**245–256.

James, W. P. T., Branch, W. J., and Southgate, D. A. T., 1978, Calcium binding by dietary fibre, *Lancet* **1:**638–639.

Johnson, N. E., Alcantara, E. N., and Linkswiler, H. M., 1970, Effect of protein intake on urinary and fecal calcium and calcium retention of young adult males, *J. Nutr.* **100:**1425.

Jowsey, J., 1977, Osteoporosis: Dealing with a crippling bone disease of the elderly, *Geriatrics* **32:**41–50.

Kanders, B., Lindsay, R., Dempster, D., Markhard, L., and Valiquette, G., 1984, Determinants of bone mass in young healthy women, in: *Proceedings of the Copenhagen International Symposium on Osteoporosis* (C. Christiansen, C. D. Arnaud, B. E. C. Nordin, A. M. Parfitt, W. A. Peck, and B. L. Riggs, eds.), Department of Clinical Chemistry, Glostrup Hospital, Copenhagen, pp. 337–340.

Kelsay, J. L., Behall, K. M., and Pratgher, E. S., 1979, Effect of fiber from fruits and vegetables on metabolic responses of human subjects. II. Calcium, magnesium, iron, and silicon balances, *Am. J. Clin. Nutr.* **32:**1876–1880.

Lavel-Jeantet, A. M., Paul, G., Bergot, C., Lamarque, J. L., and Ghiania, M. D., 1984, Correlation between vertebral bone density measurement and nutritional status, in: *Proceedings of the Copenhagen International Symposium on Osteoporosis* (C. Christiansen, C. D. Arnaud, B. E. C. Nordin, A. M. Parfitt, W. A. Peck, and B. L. Riggs, eds.), Department of Clinical Chemistry, Glostrup Hospital, Copenhagen, pp. 305–309.

Lawson, D. E. M., Paul, A. A., Black, A. E., Cole, T. J., Mandal, A. R., and Davie, M., 1979, Relative contributions of diet and sunlight to vitamin D state in the elderly, *Br. Med. J.* **6185:**303–305.

Lee, C. J., Lawler, G. S., and Johnson, G. H., 1981, Effects of supplementation of the diets with calcium and calcium-rich foods on bone density of elderly females with osteoporosis, *Am. J. Clin. Nutr.* **34:**819–823.

Lutz, J., 1984, Calcium balance and acid–base status of women as affected by increased protein intake and by sodium bicarbonate ingestion, *Am. J. Clin. Nutr.* **39:**281–288.

Margen, C., Chu, J.-Y., Kaufman, N. A., and Callaway, D. H., 1974, Studies in calcium metabolism. I. The calciuretic effect of dietary protein, *Am. J. Clin. Nutr.* **27:**584.

Matkovic, V., Kostial, K., Simonovic, I., Buzina, R., Brodarec, A., and Nordin, B. E. C., 1979, Bone status and fracture rates in two regions in Yugoslavia, *Am. J. Clin. Nutr.* **32:**540–549.

McCance, R. A., and Widdowson, E. M., 1942, Mineral metabolism of healthy adults on white and brown bread dietaries, *J. Physiol. (Lond.)* **101:**44–85.

Melton, L. J. III, and Riggs, B. L., 1983, Epidemiology of age-related fractures, in: *The Osteoporosis Syndrome* (L. V. Avioli, ed.), Grune & Stratton, New York, pp. 45–72.

National Center for Health Sciences, 1971–1974, *Dietary Intake Source Data. United States* (HEW Publication No. (PHS) 79-1221), National Center for Health Statistics, Hyattsville, MD.

Nilas, L., Christiansen, C., and Rodbro, P., 1984, Calcium supplementation and postmenopausal bone loss, *Br. Med. J.* **289:**1103–1106.

Nilsson, B. E., and Westlin, N. E., 1975, Long-term observations on the loss of bone mineral following Colles' *fracture, Acta Orthop. Scand.* **46:**61–66.

Nordin, B. E. C., 1961, The pathogenesis of osteoporosis, *Lancet* **1:**1011–1014.

Nordin, B. E. C., Wilkinson, R., Marshall, D. H., Gallagher, J. C., Williams, A., and Peacock, M., 1976, Calcium absorption in the elderly, *Calcif. Tissue Res.* **21:**442–451.

Nordin, B. E. C., Horsman, A., Marshall, D. H., 1979a, Calcium requirement and calcium therapy, *Clin. Orthop.* **140:**216–239.

Nordin, B. E. C., Peacock, M., Crilly, R. G., and Marshall, D. H., 1979b, Calcium absorption and plasma $1{,}25(OH)_2D$ levels in postmenopausal osteoporosis, in: *Vitamin D, Basic Research and Its Clinical Application,* Walter de Gruyter, New York, pp. 99–106.

Nordin, B. E. C., Peacock, M., Aaron, J., Crilly, R. G. H., Heyburn, P. J., Horsman, A., and Marshall, D., 1980, Osteoporosis and osteomalacia, *Clin. Endocrinol. Metab.* **1:**177–205.

Pacifici, R., Droke, D., Smith, S., Susman, N., and Avioli, L. V., 1985, Quantitative computer tomographic (QCT) analysis of vertebral bone mass (VBM) in a female population, *Clin. Res.* **33:**615A.

Parfitt, A. M., Gallagher, J. C., Heaney, R. P., Johnston, C. C., Neer, R., and Whedon, G. D., 1982, Vitamin D and bone health in the elderly, *Am. J. Clin. Nutr.* **36:**1014–1031.

Recker, R. R., and Heaney, R. P., 1985, The effect of milk supplements on calcium metabolism, bone metabolism and calcium balance, *Am. J. Clin. Nutr.* **41:**254–263.

Recker, R. R., Saville, P. D., and Heaney, R. P., 1977, Effect of estrogens and calcium carbonate on bone loss in postmenopausal women, *Ann. Intern. Med.* **87:**649–655.

Riggs, B. L., Kelly, P. J., Kinney, V. R., 1967, Calcium deficiency and osteoporosis: Observations in one hundred and sixty-six patients and critical review of the literature, *J. Bone. Joint Surg.* **49A:**915–924.

Riggs, B. L., Wahner, H. W., Dunn, W. L., Mazess, R. B., Offord, K. P., and Melton, L. J. III, 1981, Differential changes in bone mineral density of the appendicular and axial skeleton with aging, *J. Clin. Invest.* **67:**328–335.

Riis, B., Thomsen, K., and Christiansen, C., 1987, Does calcium supplementation prevent postmenopausal bone loss? *N. Engl. J. Med.* **316:**173–177.

Slavin, J. L., and Marlett, J. A., 1980, Influence of refined cellulose on human bowel function and calcium and magnesium balance, *Am. J. Clin. Nutr.* **33:**1932–1939.

Smith, R. W., and Frame, B., 1965, Concurrent axial and appendicular osteoporosis, *N. Engl. J. Med.* **273:**73–78.

Smith, R. W., and Rizek, J., 1966, Epidemiologic studies of osteoporosis in women of Puerto Rico and southeastern Michigan with special reference to age, race, national origin and to other related or associated findings, *Clin. Orthop. Rel. Res.* **45:**31–48.

Sowers, M. F., Wallace, R. B., and Lemke, J. H., 1985, Nutritional and non-nutritional correlates of forearm bone density: A community study, *Am. J. Clin. Nutr.* (in press).

Vintner-Paulsen, N., 1953, Calcium and phosphorus intake in senile osteoporosis, *Geriatrics* **8:**76–79.

Walker, R. M., and Linkswiler, H. M., 1972, Calcium retention in the adult human male as affected by protein intake, *J. Nutr.* **102:**1297.

9

Trace Elements in the Elderly

Metabolism, Requirements, and Recommendations for Intakes

Walter Mertz, Eugene R. Morris, J. Cecil Smith, Jr., Emorn Udomkesmalee, Meira Fields, Orville A. Levander, and Richard A. Anderson

*1. General Aspects**

1.1. Definitions

Trace elements are inorganic micronutrients present in the organism in concentrations of parts per million (μg/g) or parts per billion (ng/g). Such concentrations were not quantifiable by the methods available during the early years of analysis, hence the name trace elements. That expression is now widely accepted, even though modern methods allow adequate quantification even of concentrations as low as fractions of a nanogram per gram.

It has become customary to include among the trace elements those that occur in blood serum or plasma of mammalian species in concentrations of approximately 1 μg/ml or less or, from a nutritional point of view, those with a daily requirement in the healthy adult human of less than 50 mg. That definition comprises elements such as iron, copper, zinc, iodine, chromium, and selenium but excludes the electrolytes and mineral elements sodium, potassium, magnesium, and calcium, which are present in biological materials in much higher concentrations and for which the requirement is greater, in the range of hundreds of milligrams per day.

*This section is by Walter Mertz.

Walter Mertz, Eugene R. Morris, J. Cecil Smith, Jr., Orville A. Levander, and Richard A. Anderson • U.S. Department of Agriculture, ARS, Beltsville Human Nutrition Research Center, Beltsville, Maryland 20705. ***Emorn Udomkesmalee*** • Visiting Scientist from Institute of Nutrition, Mahidol University, Research Center, Ramathibodi Hospital, Bangkok 10400, Thailand. ***Meira Fields*** • Georgetown University, Washington, D.C. 20007.

The trace elements can be discussed in two categories: one for which essential functions have been proven or postulated and another for which such functions have not been established. Essentiality is usually defined on the basis of animal experiments in which a reduction of dietary intake below a certain level must result in a reproducible impairment of a physiological function, reversible or preventable by adequate amounts of the trace element under investigation. Demonstration of essentiality in an animal species does not necessarily indicate essentiality in man, but such demonstration in two or more animal species strengthens the probability that the element under investigation may be essential also for man. Proof of essentiality in man is derived from experiments of nature in which signs of deficiency are associated with low environmental exposure and can be reversed by adequate supplementation. Such evidence is available for the elements fluorine, chromium, iron, copper, zinc, selenium, and iodine (Underwood, 1977). Other elements clearly established as essential in animal experiments, such as manganese and molybdenum, are not known to present nutritional problems in human populations, although low environmental molybdenum levels have been postulated to increase the risk of esophageal cancer.

1.2. Causes of Deficiencies

A deficiency results from an imbalance between the nutritional need of the organism and the amount of biologically utilizable macronutrient in the diet.* Imbalances can arise, therefore, from increased requirements of the organism or from insufficient supply. Inadequate supply can be related to geochemical influences, well known for fluorine, selenium, and iodine: a low concentration of the elements in soil and water is reflected in the daily food and can cause endemic deficiency diseases.

A reduced supply of a biologically available trace element can also result from man's own activities and dietary choices. Many interactions among dietary ingredients determine the biological availability of trace elements. Although few of the known interactions can be quantified as yet, their nutritional impact is no less than the impact of geochemical influences; the biological availability of dietary iron can vary by a factor of at least ten, depending on chemical form and dietary interactions (Monsen *et al.*, 1978).

Man's preferences for partitioned foods (simple sugars, white flour, oils, fats, alcohol) can lead to a significant reduction of essential trace elements in the diet (Schroeder, 1971). Dependence on highly purified parenteral or enteral formulae for medical reasons, especially if over extended periods of time, can induce pronounced deficiencies.

Pathological conditions affecting gastric secretion, especially gastric acidity, can strongly depress the bioavailability of trace elements, as the acidic milieu of the stomach is essential for chemical reactions that keep dietary trace elements in solution. The risk of atrophic gastritis is known to increase with age, and a 31.5% incidence was found in a recent survey of 359 elderly subjects, average age 76 years, in Boston (Krasinski *et al.*, 1986).

*The term diet includes the intake of water. The contribution of airborne elements to the daily intake is negligible in ordinary circumstances.

Table 1. Energy Intake at Different Ages[a] (Average Intake per Individual in a Day)

Age (years)	Males (kcal/day)	Females (kcal/day)
9–11	2000	1865
12–14	2366	1903
15–18	2698	1791
19–22	2569	1621
23–34	2449	1616
35–50	2314	1514
51–64	2148	1522
65–74	1970	1444
75+	1808	1367

[a]From USDA (1980).

Finally, because the intake of trace elements is directly proportional to the total food intake, the substantial decline in food consumption with age reduces the intake of trace elements by approximately one third (Table 1). These latter two influences have substantial importance in elderly populations.

1.3. Present Status of Knowledge

Until recently, most if not all studies of metabolism and requirements of nutrients were performed in young subjects, mainly college students. Although some data relating to nutritional status and nutrient intake of elderly populations have become available, the estimates of requirements or of recommended intakes for the elderly are based on extrapolation from much younger age groups. The uncertainty arising from extrapolations is reflected in the widely different nutritional recommendations for the elderly in different countries. For most nutrients, the Food and Agricultural Organization/World Health Organization neglects the possibility of different needs of the elderly altogether, and their oldest age group for which recommendations are made is that of "adults." Bulgaria, on the other hand, has established a separate category of nutrient requirements for those 90 years and older (Committee 1-5, IUNS, 1983).

Similarly, there is little agreement among countries concerning the ideal nutrient intake of the elderly. Most recommend a reduction of energy intake with advancing age, accompanied by a proportional reduction in the intake of the B vitamins. Some also reduce other nutrients such as vitamin A, β-carotene, calcium, iodine, and iron, and only one country, the Netherlands, recommends an increased nutrient intake (of calcium) for the elderly. Such lack of agreement among nations demonstrates the uncertainties that prevail in attempts to determine requirements and arrive at recommended intakes for the elderly population.

1.4. Health Status and Physiological Function

The two age-related changes that affect nutrient metabolism and requirements most extensively are the decline of lean body mass (Munro, 1985) and, independently or not, the decline in energy requirement and food intake (Table I). Both have important consequences for trace element requirement and status of the elderly.

Trace elements are distributed mainly in the lean body mass, where their concentrations are quite stable during adult age, as shown by several analytical studies of autopsy material (Schroeder *et al.*, 1966, 1970). A diminishing body mass while steady concentrations are maintained indicates a diminishing size of the metabolic pools of these elements. Since it is well established that the obligatory daily loss of trace elements is proportional to the existing pool size, one could conclude that the minimal daily requirements (the amount necessary to replace obligatory losses) would decline somewhat with progressing age. There are two notable exceptions: the concentrations of chromium (Schroeder *et al.*, 1962) and silicon (Carlisle, 1986) appear to decrease in most tissues with age, possibly suggesting inadequate intake; these are discussed separately. In general, however, the concern with trace element imbalances in the tissue of the elderly should be directed more toward accumulation than toward depletion. This has been described in detail for iron.

The decrease of total food intake in the aged (Table I) will result in a proportional reduction of the trace element intake in the absence of substantial qualitative changes in the diet. That reduction could depress the intake of some trace elements, such as zinc, copper, and chromium, to below acceptable levels. It is not known whether an improvement in the quality of the elderly's diet can compensate for the consequences of the reduction in quantity. There may actually be a qualitative deterioration of the diet of many elderly related to dental problems, impairment of taste and smell function, and many other factors.

If there is uncertainty concerning the adequacy of trace element nutritional status of the elderly, there is practically no information on whether and how their nutritional status may affect their various health functions. The decline of many physiological functions with age is well known (Munro, 1985), but there is little agreement which if any of these are determined by nutritional status. Until results of future research allow a more precise conclusion, it is prudent to assume no more than a moderating influence of nutritional status on the rate of decline of physiological functions. Although several studies have suggested that the rate of the age-related changes can be retarded by nutritional intervention, there is as yet no evidence that their direction can be reversed. This is well illustrated by the example of calcium and its role in osteoporosis, discussed in Chapter 8. Another example is that of chromium, which can improve the impaired glucose tolerance of middle-aged, chromium-deficient persons but is relatively ineffective in cases of established diabetes mellitus (Mertz, 1983).

Although it is unlikely that any of the trace elements or its deficiency is the sole causal agent in the etiology of any of the diseases of importance in the aging process, several elements have been identified as interacting with several risk factors (Table II). Their roles, mechanisms of action, and importance relative to other etiological factors are discussed later in this chapter.

1.5. Requirements and Recommended Intakes

Theoretical aspects of requirements and recommended intakes have been discussed elsewhere (Mertz, 1986) and need only be summarized here. There is only one

Table II. Minerals and Trace Elements with a Potential Connection to Chronic Disease

Physiological function	Element	Diseases
Bone formation and maintenance	F, Si, P, Ca, Mn, Cu, Zn	Osteoporosis
Regulation of blood pressure, blood lipids, coagulation, heart function	Na, Mg, K, Ca, Cu, Se, Cd, I	Cardiovascular
Xanthine oxidation	Mo	Gout
Prevention of oxidative damage	Se	Cancer
Nucleic acid metabolism, protein synthesis, cell division	Zn	Impairments of growth, tissue repair, and immune reactions
Regulation of glucose metabolism	Cr	Impairment of glucose tolerance

example of a well-established, quantifiable change of a trace element requirement with aging: the requirement for absorbable iron in women drops sharply with menopause from about 1.8 to 1.0 mg/day. This reduction has great practical significance: whereas an absolute requirement of 1.8 mg is difficult to satisfy by a typical Western diet, that of 1 mg is easily met.

Any additional statements relating to changes of trace element requirements with age would rest on extrapolation from younger age groups or on inferences from age-related physiological changes that may affect requirement. Such inferences are not necessarily conclusive. For example, the decline of efficiency of intestinal absorption for some trace elements that has been demonstrated in aging experimental animals might suggest increased dietary requirements, but it could just as well be the reaction of the aging organism to an overload of an element that has gradually accumulated during the lifetime. In that case, the diminished absorption efficiency would suggest a decreased rather than an elevated requirement.

Any quantification depends strongly on the definition of requirements. It is possible to sort current definitions into three categories. In the first, nutritional requirements are defined as those daily intakes that prevent nutrient-specific clinical deficiencies. The criterion of avoiding deficiencies is a logical one with a good scientific foundation: the induction of a deficiency is the standard method of proving essentiality of any nutrient. On the other hand, the criterion of avoiding gross deficiency does not take into account the consequences of marginal deficiencies that may not be manifested by clinical signs and yet may have some long-term health significance.

The second category of definitions uses the status quo as the main criterion. Meeting the requirement by that definition will result in maintaining the nutritional status and the nutrition-related health status at the existing level. The use of that criterion is well founded logically in all societies with free availability of a varied food supply and a good health status, and it offers many advantages: it avoids many problems of imbalances and interactions that could arise from fortification or supplementation of diets; also, the typical national diet represents the preference of the majority of a population as it has developed over the decades (provided again that an adequate variety of food is available). On the other hand, that approach renounces the expectations for further improving the health status by nutritional means.

The third category uses as its main criterion of requirement the greatest attainable risk reduction for nutrition-related diseases. Many of these become clinically significant in older age; therefore, the third criterion is particularly important for the elderly. The number of nutrients for which requirements can be expressed by this approach is growing, but because the scientific evidence for effects of that kind is "softer" than evidence using clinical signs of deficiency as endpoints, there is controversy as to the scientific acceptability of that requirement concept. A committee of the Food and Nutrition Board, National Research Council/National Academy of Sciences is currently examining these problems. The outcome of these deliberations will be of substantial importance for the elderly.

The concept of risk reduction by nutritional means requires some qualifications and restrictions. First, there is the caution against expecting the cure of diseases when in the best case a nutrient may only retard the rate at which a physiological or biochemical function declines. Many chronic conditions that affect the aged are initiated at a younger age, at which time they may be more amenable to nutritional intervention than later. The most striking example for that statement is the total prevention of even the severest consequences of iodine deficiency by iodine supplementation at an early age together with the recognized irreversibility of severe goiter and cretinism (Herzel and Maberly, 1986). This and other examples lead to the conclusion that nutritional and health status depend on a person's past history at least as much as on present eating habits.

Another important qualification concerns the risk of imbalances that can be created by the use of trace element or mineral supplements. The reduction of food intake with increasing age (Table I) results in an average daily intake of several elements that is markedly below the recommended dietary allowances. The consequences of that deficit for health are not known; that uncertainty may have convinced nearly 50% of the U.S. population of the desirability of nutritional supplements (Stewart *et al.*, 1985). The nature of such supplements* and the frequency of their use by the elderly population are not well defined at present, but it can be surmised that the elderly are subject to the same pressures of advertising that have led in the rest of the population to a changing pattern of interest in individual minerals and trace elements. Periods of great public concern with iron were followed by others in which, successively, zinc, chromium, selenium, and calcium became popular. Each of these periods could create a risk of trace element imbalances. Although that risk is theoretical for chromium and selenium at this time, deleterious effects of supplementation with calcium and zinc have been demonstrated (Dawson-Hughes *et al.*, 1986). Trace element supplements that are balanced, complete, biologically available, and safe are not yet available. Even

*A recent survey in seven western states by questionnaire found that two-thirds of 2451 adults used mineral supplements (Read *et al.*, 1986).

such "ideal" supplements would contain only those trace elements that are accepted as essential and important for man at the time; they are no substitutes for a balanced diet, which furnishes a much wider range of micronutrients than any supplements would. Only if a person's food intake is consistently and grossly inadequate to supply the requirements for energy and other nutrients should trace element supplements be considered, and then in amounts not to exceed the recommended dietary allowances or ranges of safe and adequate intakes.

2. *Individual Elements*

2.1. *Iron**

The bulk of iron in the body is found in the oxygen transport heme proteins, hemoglobin in the red blood cells and myoglobin in muscle. Other heme iron proteins include the cytochromes of the electron transport chain, catalase, which reduces endogenously generated H_2O_2, cytochrome P450, and peroxidases that are involved in detoxifying reactions and hydroxylations (Jacobs and Worwood, 1980). Nonheme iron is present in the active site and as a cofactor for a number of enzymes involved in oxidative metabolism (Bezkorovainy, 1980). Variable amounts of iron may be present as the nonheme iron storage proteins ferritin and hemosiderin.

Body iron homeostasis is mediated by adjusting absorption of dietary iron from the intestinal lumen according to need of the individual (Bothwell *et al.*, 1979). Iron loss, chiefly by sloughed cells from the intestine and skin and hair, is equal in the adult man and nonmenstruating woman, and daily iron needs may be supplied by similar dietary intakes. Because there is no regulated excretion of excess absorbed iron, body iron in excess of metabolic need is stored as ferritin to prevent accumulation of ionic iron (Munro and Linder, 1978). Iron transport in the body is accomplished by transferrin (Morgan, 1974) and to a lesser degree by other nonheme nontransferrin proteins of the blood serum (Bezkorovainy, 1980). The following discussion focuses on consequences of iron deficiency, the incidence of iron deficiency in the elderly, and possible role of iron in the aging process.

2.1.1. *Iron Deficiency*

Frank iron deficiency will produce anemia, i.e., low hemoglobin concentration. Anemia may, however, be caused by other nutritional deficiencies such as several B vitamins, vitamin A, and copper or by pathological conditions not related to nutrition (Reizenstein *et al.*, 1979). Cook and Finch (1979) have proposed the following biochemical indices of iron deficiency: transferrin saturation <16%, free erythrocyte protoporphyrin >100 μg/dl RBC, and absence of iron stores indicated by serum ferritin of <12 ng/dl. The exact values of the biochemical indices are subject to discussion, but a combination of these parameters will aid in establishing a diagnosis of iron deficiency and exclude other reasons for anemia.

*This section is by Eugene R. Morris.

Edgerton *et al.* (1981) found anemic subjects had a low work tolerance compared to nonanemic subjects. Within 24 hr after transfusion they were able to attain a level of work tolerance equivalent to other subjects having equal hemoglobin levels to the posttransfusion level. Presumably this improvement is related to oxygen transport to the tissues, but there may be a nonhemoglobin component of the effects of iron deficiency on work performance (Ohira *et al.*, 1981). Dallman (1974) and Oski (1979) have reviewed some documented nonhematological effects of iron deficiency in tissues of animals. These effects include decreased growth and decreased concentration of iron proteins, notably cytochrome c. Not all these effects have been corroborated in humans.

Whether these changes occur in older animals and humans that were iron replete and subsequently become iron deficient is not clear. Iron supplementation or increased dietary iron intake can alleviate iron deficiency anemia and the tissue effects of iron deficiency with one documented exception. In rats, decreased brain nonheme iron content persists after other parameters have returned to normal values (Dallman *et al.*, 1975). Cognitive functions found to be deficient in the iron-deficient rat were shown to persist in the iron-repleted animal (Weinberg *et al.*, 1979). Webb and Oski (1973) reported lower "Iowa Test" scores for anemic adolescents than for nonanemic peers. Palti *et al.* (1985) found lower "learning achievement" scores for second-grade students who had been anemic in infancy but subsequently were provided with iron supplementation compared to students that had not been anemic in infancy. Both anemic and nonanemic iron-deficient children retained low mental development scores after 6 months of iron treatment (Deinard *et al.*, 1986) despite complete hematological correction. Thus, although Leibel *et al.* wrote in 1979, "there exists no unequivocal demonstration of an adverse effect of iron deficiency on intelligence, learning attention, motivation, or general sense of well-being," Pollitt *et al.* (1985) see support for the hypothesis that iron deficiency adversely affects the learning and problem-solving capacity of school-age children. The question remains, however, do cognitive deficits occur in iron-deficiency-developing during adult years, and do such deficits expressed in childhood persist into adulthood? Tucker *et al.* (1984) reported that higher serum ferritin levels (indicative of higher iron stores) were associated with greater verbal fluency but poorer auditory task performance by college students. Goodwin *et al.* (1983) conclude that "subclinical malnutrition may play a small role in the depression of cognitive function detectable in some elderly individuals," but they did not measure iron status.

The role of iron in immunocompetence of the elderly is an enigma. Microbial survival and infectivity depend on the ability of the microorganism to obtain iron (Weinberg, 1986; Letendre, 1985). Both animals and humans exhibit a hypoferremic response to infectious invasion, which is an important part of disease resistance. In addition, the iron-binding capability of plasma proteins and lactoferrin exerts a bacteriostatic role. For example, lactoferrin, found in mucosal secretions, will retard growth of *Legionella* (Bortner *et al.*, 1986). Ward *et al.* (1986) found human plasma to be bactericidal for *Klebsiella pneumoniae,* but the bactericidal action of plasma or human polymorphs was abolished by the addition of Fe^{3+} or hematin. On the other hand, animal studies have clearly demonstrated depressed immunocompetence in iron-deficient rats (Sherman, 1984). The role of iron status in immunocompetence of humans is not so clear. Chandra *et al.* (1982) provided nutritional therapy to elderly subjects and noted improvement in T-lymphocyte subpopulations and cell-mediated immunity. The therapy was general nutrition and not just iron *per se*. Tests of lymphocyte function were found to be abnormal in iron-deficient children and returned to normal following iron therapy (Macdougall *et al.*, 1975). Although human malnutrition is often more complex than just iron deficiency, iron is considered to serve a singular role in immunocompetence (McMurray, 1982; Beisel, 1982), whereas iron excess may provide an advantage to an invading infectious organism.

2.1.2. *Iron and the Aging Process*

Aspects of the chemistry of the aging process as currently understood are discussed in detail elsewhere in this volume. The relationship of iron to the aging process is thought to reside in the potential formation of oxygen radicals or oxygen-derived free radical species in the presence of ionic iron (Halliwell and Gutteridge, 1986). Mammals possess an efficient system whereby the concentration of ionic iron is held to a minimum. Extracellularly, iron is transported by transferrin, which has a high affinity constant for Fe^{3+}, and haptoglobin and hemopexin in plasma bind and transport free hemoglobin and hemin, respectively, keeping the potential ionic iron to a minimum. Transferrin-bound iron is transferred intracellularly by the membrane transferrin receptor and subsequent endocytosis before the iron is released (Bomford and Munro, 1985). There may be a low concentration of ionic iron during the initial stages of intracellular processing of iron (Young *et al.*, 1985), which could promote oxygen radical formation, but the concentration of ionic iron is kept at a very low level by incorporation into metalloenzymes or the storage protein ferritin (Munro and Linder, 1978).

Changes in certain characteristics of the erythrocyte observed with increase of age may, therefore, simply be membrane phenomena rather than oxidative damage caused by ionic iron. Some erythrocyte changes noted are increase in the sedimentation rate (Sparrow *et al.*, 1981) and increased fragility (Araki and Rifkind, 1980).

Greenberg (1975) studied the pathogenesis of hypophyseal fibrosis and accompanying accumulation of tissue iron in aging. He concluded that fibrous replacement of the gland begins after the fourth decade and that iron is then deposited in the fibrous tissue. Thus, formation of the fibrous tissue is not a consequence of the iron deposition.

2.1.3. *Incidence of Iron Deficiency in the Elderly*

Anemia *per se* is not a satisfactory criterion for establishing the incidence of iron deficiency in the elderly (Lynch *et al.*, 1982). Other indices of iron status must be measured and, in fact, can be used to establish a diagnosis of iron deficiency without determining hemoglobin concentration. Dallman *et al.* (1984) examined data from the second National Health and Nutrition Examination Survey (NHANES II) conducted in the United States. Reference ranges (95% confidence interval) for hemoglobin values were 12.6–17.4 g/dl for men and 11.7–16.1 g/dl for women 65 to 74 years of age. The reference ranges were calculated after excluding individual hemoglobins for any individual exhibiting another biochemical index indicative of iron deficiency. The percentage of hemoglobin values below the 95% range for all races was 4.4% and 3.9% for men and women, respectively. Complete biochemical data were not available for all these individuals, but only about one-half of the postmenopausal anemic women and about 40% of the anemic men had biochemical indices that indicated iron-deficiency anemia. Dallman *et al.* (1984) concluded that inflammatory disease may be responsible for a significant fraction of the anemia seen in the elderly. This leaves about 2% of iron deficiency anemia among elderly men and women. The sampling of NHANES II was designed to be representative of the United States population. The incidence of iron deficiency may differ for selected ethnic or socioeconomic groups.

The importance of measuring several indices of iron status is further illustrated by the findings of Bailey *et al.* (1979). Fourteen percent of a predominately black elderly urban low-income population were found to be anemic. However, serum iron and transferrin saturation were in the normal range, indicating no iron deficiency anemia. The anemia was attributed chiefly to folacin deficiency.

Caution should also be used in interpreting serum ferritin measurements as criteria of iron deficiency. Loria *et al.* (1979) reported that ten of 55 elderly subjects showing an increase in hemoglobin concentration after oral iron therapy had high or normal serum ferritin values. Similarly, Sharma and Roy (1984) found elderly anemic patients with low serum ferritin were iron deficient as assessed by bone marrow examination, whereas six patients with low or absent bone marrow iron stores had serum ferritin within the normal range. Milman *et al.* (1986) studied a group of elderly in Denmark not suffering from diseases associated with inappropriately high serum ferritin. Serum ferritin less than 15 ng/ml (depleted iron stores) was observed in 8% of the men and 10% of the women. Fewer than 3% of either sex exhibited latent iron deficiency (i.e., serum ferritin $<$15 ng/ml and transferrin saturation $<$15%), and none had iron deficiency anemia.

2.1.4. *Iron Nutrition*

Dietary iron intake of the elderly is not extensively documented. In the United States, mean daily intake of men over 55 years of age in NHANES II exceeded 14 mg, and that of women about 10.5 mg (Lynch *et al.*, 1982). The difference between men and women was associated with a difference in caloric intake, both groups consuming a similar nutrient density (mg iron/1000 kcal). Although caloric intakes of men tend to decrease with advancing age (Elahi *et al.*, 1983), the NHANES II data and surveys by Kohrs *et al.* (1978), Garry *et al.* (1982), and Yearick *et al.* (1980) indicate that mean dietary iron intakes of adult men tend to remain high enough to exceed the recommended dietary allowance established by the National Research Council (1980). Women, on the other hand, consume more nearly 10 mg daily, and in one study (Jansen and Harrill, 1977) the mean intake for those over 75 years of age fell to 7.7 mg.

In the absence of gastrointestinal pathology, there is no evidence that the elderly absorb iron less readily than younger persons with the same degree of iron stores (Marx, 1979). Similarly, Turnlund *et al.* (1981, 1982a) found that although iron balance appeared to be negative, absorption of isotopically labeled iron was 0.8 mg daily from a formula diet providing 10 mg of iron daily to healthy men 65 to 75 years of age. From his study, Marx (1979) concluded that the aged may have decreased red cell uptake of iron, which may contribute to anemia in the presence of adequate iron stores. This decreased uptake may be related to the findings of Ibraham *et al.* (1983) that marrow cells from senescent rats showed as much as 40% less *in vitro* erythroid colony growth than did cells from young rat marrow. In this context, Harrison (1975) reported that transplantation of young marrow cells did not improve a defective response to bleeding of old mice.

The food frequency information from NHANES II reveals that older individuals tend to eat less meat and more cereal grain and legume-derived foods than do younger adults (Lynch *et al.*, 1982). Although foods derived from whole cereal grains and legumes are good sources of dietary iron, bioavailability of the iron is low unless the meals contain meat or ascorbic acid (National Research Council, 1980; Lynch, 1984). Bioavailability factors are thought to function in the same manner in the older population as in younger persons, and it appears that an elderly person with low iron stores will respond with increased iron absorption when required. Therefore, the dietary iron requirement of the elderly man and postmenopausal woman is thought to be adequately supplied by a daily intake of 10 mg from a diet of a variety of foods (National Research Council, 1980). If the diet is vegetarian, an intake of 100 mg of ascorbic acid in one or more meals daily will help ensure adequate iron absorption.

2.2. *Zinc**

It is clearly established that zinc is an essential nutrient, necessary for maintaining health throughout life. Several conditions more prevalent in the elderly have been reported to be associated with a compromised zinc status, including decreased taste and smell acuity, suppressed appetite, impaired wound healing, and depressed immunoresponse (Anonymous, 1986a). In addition, the zinc concentration in plasma and other tissues has been reported to be lower in aged individuals compared to younger subjects (Alhava *et al.*, 1977; Schroeder *et al.*, 1967; Lindeman *et al.*, 1971; Pilch and Senti, 1985).

A key factor that could contribute to compromised zinc status in the elderly is the reported drop in caloric consumption and a concomitant reduction of zinc intake (Table III). Indeed, several reports indicate that the daily zinc intake of elderly ranged from 7 to 11 mg for subjects living in the United States (Fosmire *et al.*, 1984), Australia (Flint *et al.*, 1981), Canada (Gibson *et al.*, 1985), Great Britain (Bunker *et al.*, 1982, 1984), and Sweden (Abdulla *et al.*, 1977). Since the present RDA (National Research Council, 1980) for men and women over 51 years of age is 15 mg, the potential of inadequate zinc nutriture in aged individuals would be considerable if the RDA levels are truly required for adequate status.

Although in 1970, Shock (1970) stated that "present evidence indicates that older people do not show significant impairment in the ability to absorb a specific item from the diet," recent data show lower zinc absorption in elderly men compared to younger ones (Turnlund *et al.*, 1986; Bales *et al.*, 1986).

Focusing attention on possible impaired zinc status of the elderly is important

*This section is by J. Cecil Smith, Jr., and Emorn Udomkesmalee.

Table III. Estimated Energy and Zinc Intakes for Adults 55 Years and Older in the NHANES II Survey 1976–1980[a]

Sex	Age (years)	Energy (kcal)	Zinc (mg)
Males	55–64	2071	12.6
Males	65–74	1828	10.6
Females	55–64	1401	8.2
Females	65–74	1295	7.2

[a]Sandstead *et al.* (1982).

because they are the fastest growing portion of the population in the United States and other countries. Projections indicate that the old people of the world will increase by 80% totaling 390 million by A.D. 2000 (Butler and McGuire, 1982). This review emphasizes facets of zinc nutriture relevant to aged individuals, including biological functions, tissue distribution, functional impairments, as well as the challenge of accurate assessment.

2.2.1. Biological Functions

2.2.1a. Enzymes. A biochemical role for zinc was first demonstrated in 1939 when Keilin and Mann (1939) reported zinc to be an integral component of carbonic anhydrase of red blood cells. Since then, numerous other enzymes (estimated to exceed 200) have been shown to require zinc for structural integrity and/or catalysis (Hambidge *et al.*, 1986; Anonymous, 1986b).

The majority of enzymes involved in nucleic acid and protein synthesis are zinc metalloenzymes (Golden, 1982). Therefore, the biochemical and clinical indices of zinc deficiency may appear similar to the conditions of impaired protein synthesis. For instance, suppressed protein synthesis could result in preventing normal growth and development as well as producing dermatitis and impaired wound healing. These conditions, which require increased protein synthesis, have been associated with inadequate zinc nutriture.

2.2.1b. Membrane Integrity. Chvapil (1973) and Bettger and O'Dell (1981) have suggested that another primary function of zinc is to maintain membrane integrity and function and that this role may be as important as the role of zinc in metalloenzymes.

2.2.1c. Bone Formation. The importance of zinc in bone metabolism and physiology has been reviewed (Asling and Hurley, 1963; Calhoun *et al.*, 1974). However, the role of zinc, if any, in maintaining bone strength and integrity, which are considerations of prime concern to the elderly, has yet to be established.

2.2.1d. Immune System. Recent research indicates that zinc is essential for the integrity of general host-defense mechanisms, particularly the cell-mediated or T-cell systems (Fraker *et al.*, 1986). Moreover, in acrodermatitis enteropathica, a congenital zinc deficiency, most patients develop chronic infections (Golden, 1982).

Table IV. Reported Zinc Concentrations in Selected Tissues and Biological Fluids of Adults

Sample	Units	"Frequent" values[a]	"Typical" concentration[b]	"Experimental" values[c]	Literature ranges[d]
Tissue					
Eye: Retina	μg/g				571
Choroid	μg/g		274		562
Prostate	μg/g		120		520
Bone	μg/g		100–250		218
Hair	μg/g	150–250	180	163	100–255
Fingernail	μg/g		151		
Liver	μg/g	40–60	58		141–245
Muscle	μg/g		42		197–226
Kidney	μg/g		37		184–230
Pancreas	μg/g		26		115–135
Heart	μg/g		23		100
Spleen	μg/g		14		
Testis	μg/g		13		
Brain	μg/g		13		
Lung	μg/g		10		67–86
Skin	μg/g				12–80
Biological fluids					
Semen	μg/ml		150	250	
Platelets	μg/g		49		
Leukocyte	μg/10^{10} cells		76–200		
Red blood cell	μg/g	10–13	8–14	11	10–14
Whole blood	μg/ml	6–7	4–8	5.9	
Serum/plasma	μg/ml	0.8–1.1	0.7–1.0	0.89	0.84–1.40
Breast milk	μg/ml	1.5–2.0	0.6–3.0		
Urine	μg/24 hr		300–500	448	400–600
	μg/liter	400–600			
Saliva	ng/ml		50–100	65	

[a]Iyengar (1985). Values based on wet weight.
[b]Hambidge *et al.* (1986). Values based on wet weight.
[c]Baer and King (1984). Values based on wet weight.
[d]Halsted *et al.* (1974). Values based on dry weight.

2.2.2. *Tissue Distribution and Concentration*

Total body zinc for adults has been reported to approximate 2 g (Lutz, 1926), an estimate that has been confirmed by Widdowson *et al.* (1951) and Hambidge *et al.* (1986). Reported tissue concentration of normal adults was estimated to average 30 μg/g with a range of 120 (Hambidge *et al.*, 1986). The greatest zinc concentration in the human body is found in the tissues of the eye (Eckhert, 1983) and prostate (Halsted *et al.*, 1974). In regard to body fluids, semen exceeds others with an average of 250 μg/g (Baer and King, 1984). Table IV indicates the zinc concentrations reported for selected tissues and body fluids of adults.

2.2.2a. Serum/Plasma Zinc Concentrations. Most early studies indicated that serum or plasma zinc concentration was not different for subjects of various age

Table V. Serum Zinc Concentrations for Subjects by Age in the NHANES II Reference Population 1976–1980[a]

	Mean serum zinc (μg/dl)	
Age (years)	Males	Females
3–8	80.6	80.7
9–19	87.8	84.1
20–44	93.0	84.9
45–64	89.1	84.4
65–74	85.6	83.5

[a]Pilch and Senti (1985).

groups, as reviewed by Smith and Hsu (1982, 1984). However, Halsted and Smith (1970) demonstrated that children of 3–13 years had significantly lower plasma zinc concentrations compared to adults of 23–62 years. In addition, a lower plasma zinc was reported in older subjects in a study comparing individuals ranging in age from 20 to 80 years (Lindeman *et al.*, 1971; Lindeman, 1982). More recently, Stiedemann and Harrill (1980) also reported a negative correlation between age and serum zinc of 36 elderly women 67–96 years of age. Analysis of data from 14,770 persons aged 3–74 years in the NHANES II survey (Pilch and Senti, 1985) provides the most definitive reference values concerning serum zinc concentration in different age groups of the U.S. population. Mean serum zinc levels were significantly higher in males than in females in the age range of 9–74 years. In males, the concentration of serum zinc was low during childhood, increased during adolescence, peaked in young adults, and declined in older adults, as indicated in Table V. Although the trend was similar, the difference of serum zinc among various age groups in females was less pronounced.

2.2.2b. Hair Zinc. Hambidge *et al.* (1972) demonstrated a rapid decline in hair zinc for infants 3 months to 4 years; then a gradual increase from 4 to 17 years and a plateau between 17 and 40 years, with the value approximating that at birth. Unfortunately, this report (Hambidge *et al.*, 1972) did not include subjects over 40 years. Klevay (1970) observed a gradual decline of hair zinc in Panamanian subjects during the first decade of life, but no trend with age was noted for adults 20 to 83 years.

2.2.3. *Considerations for Assessment of Zinc Nutriture in the Elderly*

A major limitation for the assessment of zinc nutriture has been and remains the lack of sensitive indices. Several studies assessing zinc status of the elderly (Greger, 1977; Greger and Sciscoe, 1977; Flint *et al.*, 1981; Hutton and Hayes-Davis, 1983) have employed only one parameter such as serum, plasma, or hair zinc concentration. Although serum/plasma zinc concentrations have been most frequently employed, caution should be exercised when interpreting the data, since that parameter alone is insufficient. Likewise, the usefulness of hair zinc for assessing individual status is limited because of lack of reliability.

An initial consideration when evaluating zinc nutriture is to determine the daily zinc intake. Recent studies indicate consumption by elderly living in developed countries to be considerably less than the RDA of 15 mg (Fosmire *et al.*, 1984; Gibson *et al.*, 1985; Bunker *et al.*, 1982; Abdulla *et al.*, 1977; Flint *et al.*, 1981). It is important to note that this recommended intake is identical for adolescents and adults. However, it is probable that the actual requirement is different for the elderly compared to younger age groups. As stated by Munro (1980), the nutrient requirements for older individuals should be separately delineated for different decades, since the energy intake can decrease by 20% between 65 and 85 years. For zinc, it has been suggested that the requirement might be met in the elderly with less than one-half the RDA (Sandstead *et al.*, 1982). However, those estimates were derived using multiple regression analysis combined with the metabolic balance technique. Current thinking indicates that the balance technique is prone to errors in determining actual requirements (Smith, 1987). Nevertheless, numerous studies have failed to show unequivocal evidence of zinc deficiency in elderly populations consuming less zinc than the RDA. In this respect, recent Recommended Nutrient Intakes for Canadians (1983) suggest 9 mg daily for males and 8 mg for females of 50–74 years. The same level was also recommended for those over 74 compared to all subjects of over 13 years on the assumption that they have similar requirements over this age range. Although overt zinc deficiency has not been detected when the elderly are studied, there remains the possibility that less than optimal intake may result in subclinical conditions that are difficult to diagnose. Thus, the elderly should continue to be considered at risk for inadequate zinc nutriture for the following reasons:

1. Decreased food (energy) intake up to 20% over an age span of the 20 years between the ages of 65 and 85 years (McGandy *et al.*, 1966), resulting in decreased intake of many nutrients including zinc (Sandstead *et al.*, 1982).
2. Significantly less absorption of zinc in elderly men compared to younger ones (Turnlund *et al.*, 1986; Bales *et al.*, 1986).
3. Increased susceptibility of the elderly to infection (Duchateau *et al.*, 1981), impaired wound healing and immune responses (Jacob *et al.*, 1985), alteration of taste acuity, ingestion of alcohol and prescribed drugs (Sandstead *et al.*, 1982; Anonymous, 1986a), and reduced dietary quality (McGandy *et al.*, 1986), all of which have been associated with inadequate zinc nutriture.

2.2.4. *Host Defense Mechanisms in the Elderly*

Inadequate nutrition is associated with increased morbidity and mortality, primarily from infectious diseases (Scrimshaw, 1966; Chandra and Newberne, 1977; Suskind, 1977). Specifically, the elderly are a vulnerable population since the aging process itself has been linked with a progressive change in immune competence (Anonymous, 1984). Recently, the essentiality of zinc for the development and maintenance of the immune system has been established (Good *et al.*, 1982; Beisel, 1982; Fraker *et al.*, 1978, 1986; Gershwin *et al.*, 1983). Rao *et al.* (1979) reported an age-dependent effect of zinc on the mitogenic response of human lymphocytes. More direct evidence of zinc in the host defense mechanisms has been demonstrated by studies of humans with documented zinc deficiency, either congenital or acquired (Good *et al.*, 1982; Beisel, 1982; Fraker *et al.*, 1986).

Recently, a few studies have focused specifically on the relationship between zinc and immunologic function in elderly humans. A brief discussion of these follows. Duchateau *et al.* (1981) reported beneficial effects of oral zinc supplementation on the immune response of aged subjects. The investigation involved 30 "healthy" institutionalized subjects whose average age was 80. One-half of the subjects received a zinc supplement (100 mg of elemental zinc) daily for 1 month. Other subjects served as controls without supplementation. The zinc-treatment group showed a pronounced improvement for the delayed skin responses to purified protein derivatives and increased antibody response to tetanus toxin. There was no effect of zinc on the lymphocyte response to three other mitogens. Apparently, no placebo was offered so the study cannot be considered to be double blind.

Wagner *et al.* (1983) evaluated zinc nutriture and delayed dermal hypersensitivity (DDH) in subjects aged 60–97 years. Of the 121 subjects, 22% were anergic (nonresponsive to skin tests). The serum zinc concentration tended to be lower for these anergic subjects compared to the level of those who developed a positive DDH response, namely, 83 versus 92 μg/dl. However, there was no relationship between age and the DDH response. Included in this report was the observation that five anergic females, 64–76 years old, developed a positive DDH after receiving zinc supplementation of 55 mg daily for 4 weeks. The investigators suggested a "positive relationship between zinc nutriture and immunocompetence" in these subjects. One interpretation of the data could be that immunoresponse is a more sensitive indicator of zinc nutriture than serum zinc concentrations. However, before this interpretation can be considered valid, confirmation by double-blind studies involving larger numbers of subjects is necessary.

An earlier report by Stiedemann and Harrill (1980) suggested a relationship between hemagglutination antibody titers and "zinc status" based on dietary intake and serum concentrations in 36 elderly women. However, subjects with lower postimmune titers consumed only slightly less zinc than the group with higher immunoresponse, 6.2 versus 7.8 mg/day, respectively. In addition, serum zinc concentration of all subjects was within the normal range. Thus, the investigators' conclusion that immunocompetence of these elderly women was related to their zinc status should be viewed with reservation.

At present, no definitive conclusion can be drawn regarding a causal relationship between inadequate zinc status and impaired immunologic function. However, this area deserves, and is receiving, increased attention.

2.2.5. *Other Functional Impairments and Skin Abnormalities: Wound Healing*

A primary process in wound healing involves increased protein synthesis necessary for tissue regeneration. Since zinc is essential for protein synthesis, inadequate zinc status could logically limit the rate of healing. The incidence of impaired wound healing increases with advancing age, e.g., decubitus ulcers and post surgical wounds. An earlier study demonstrated a significant increase in the rate of wound healing in postsurgical young men receiving oral zinc supplementation compared to the untreated controls (Pories and Strain, 1966). Later reports provided confirmative evidence for the beneficial effect of zinc supplementation on wound healing (Greaves and Skillen, 1970; Haeger *et al.*, 1972; Van Rij and Pories, 1980). However, other studies have failed to demonstrate that zinc accelerated the healing process (Brewer *et al.*, 1967; Myers and Cherry, 1971; Barcia, 1970). A more recent investigation involved 26 institutionalized subjects, average age of 82 years, selected because of skin lesions "suggestive of chronic zinc deficiency" (Weismann *et al.*, 1978). Seven hypozincemic patients (plasma zinc approximating 60 μg/dl) completed a 4-week zinc supplementation period. No beneficial effect of zinc supplementation on the skin condition of these patients was observed.

The controversies concerning the role of zinc on wound healing could stem from limitations of identifying truly zinc-deficient subjects, inadequate experimental design, as well as a need for longitudinal studies. These difficulties preclude a definitive conclusion regarding a direct beneficial effect of zinc on the healing process.

2.2.6. *Alteration of Taste Acuity*

Impairment of taste acuity has been associated with the aging process (Anonymous, 1986a). Moreover, decreased taste acuity has been noted in mildly zinc-deficient children (Hambidge *et al.*, 1972) and chronic uremic adults with low zinc status undergoing hemodialysis (Mahajan *et al.*, 1980; Atkin-Thor *et al.*, 1978). Greger and Geissler (1978) reported a double-blind study of 49 subjects of average age 75 years. The subjects were divided into two groups, zinc-supplemented and placebo. Daily dietary intake of zinc was estimated to be 7–9 mg during the experiment. The results indicated no significant effect of zinc supplementation on any of the parameters of taste acuity measured. However, there was no indication that the subjects were zinc deficient. Thus, before a conclusion can be drawn regarding the effect of zinc on taste acuity, studies must involve elderly subjects with well-documented zinc deficiency.

2.2.7. *Future Research Needs*

Primary factors deserving additional attention in future investigations include:

1. Expansion and improvement of biochemical/functional indices for evaluating zinc status in the aged population.
2. Better-controlled experimental protocols, i.e., double-blind involving larger numbers of subjects with accurately defined zinc nutriture. These studies should also be of sufficient duration to allow a complete repletion of impaired zinc status.

Specific areas of research focus are recommended as follows:

1. Determine the prevalence of zinc deficiency in the expanding elderly population.
2. Define the actual requirements and optimal intakes for different decades of life.

3. Delineate the effect of long-term medications on zinc nutriture.
4. Increase the effort to explore further the importance of chronic conditions associated with aging processes that may compromise zinc nutriture.
5. Examine possible interactions of hormonal and physiological changes associated with aging and zinc status.

2.3. *Copper**

Copper is an essential trace element for all animal species including man. Environmental deficiencies and toxicities are known to affect cattle and sheep, and either condition can present substantial production problems, depending on the environment. On the other hand, clinically recognizable copper deficiency is not known to occur in adult, healthy men and women; it has been described only in children recovering from protein–energy malnutrition and in subjects maintained on total parenteral nutrition.

When considered in the context of the various aging phenomena, copper is of special interest for three reasons:

1. The copper-dependent enzyme superoxide dismutase plays a key role in the defense against the highly reactive superoxide anion. Free radical damage to the cell structures is the subject of one prominent hypothesis concerning the cause of aging.
2. Experimental copper deficiency in animal species produces a variety of biochemical and physiological changes that are similar to recognized risk factors for cardiovascular diseases in man.
3. Several analytical surveys have demonstrated recently that the copper intake from a typical U.S. diet is considerably less than the estimated range of "safe and adequate intakes." Although this does not indicate a deficiency, there is no assurance that these low intakes are fully adequate, especially when subject to certain adverse interactions with other dietary factors.

These facts together establish copper as an element of substantial interest for study in conjunction with aging process.

2.3.1. *Free Radicals and Aging*

Many theories have been proposed to explain the biological changes associated with the phenomenon of aging; there is considerable evidence that free radicals might play a role (Harman, 1956, 1978; Isenberg, 1964). Free radicals are produced by all cells at random, in enzymatic and nonenzymatic reactions involving molecular oxygen, as a part of normal cellular function. These free radicals are highly reactive because of the presence of unpaired electrons; they can initiate free radical chain reactions, which propagate in biological systems, thereby contributing to the degradation of these systems. Free radicals can attack and damage almost every molecule found in living cells. They can hydroxylate purines and pyrimidines in nucleic acids

*This section is by Meira Fields.

and cause strand scission, resulting in mutation. Free radicals damage cell membranes since membranes contain unsaturated fatty acids, prime targets for lipid peroxidation. Enzymes are inactivated, and cell surface glycoproteins are attacked (Bisby, 1975; Willson, 1978). The damaging effects of free radicals vary considerably, depending on species, age, physiological state, and diet. For example, older populations of human diploid fibroblasts in culture are more sensitive to O_2^- than are the younger ones (Honda and Matsuo, 1980). Other biochemical changes that may be produced by free radical reactions include accumulation of metabolically inactive lipofuscin age pigments (Tappel, 1973), polymerization and cross linking of enzymes and proteins (Tappel, 1973), and oxidative alterations of collagen (LaBella and Paul, 1965) and elastin (LaBella *et al.*, 1966).

2.3.2. Copper and Free Radicals

As a result of the pioneering work of McCord and Fridovich (1969), it has been clearly established that almost all oxygen-utilizing cells contain the enzyme superoxide dismutase (SOD), which brings about a rapid removal of O_2^- at physiological pH values, so preventing it from undergoing other reactions. Three catalytic metals, copper, manganese, and zinc, have been identified as constituents of the SODs. Of these, copper present in the Cu/Zn enzyme is catalytically the most efficient (Fielden and Rotilio, 1984).

Although there is considerable evidence for substantial biochemical changes produced by free radical reactions, there is insufficient information to determine whether they are cause or effect of the aging process. At present there is no evidence in man or animals that copper or SOD retards the aging process or prevents age-related biological changes. Therefore, it little avails the health conscious to eat SOD. The enzyme SOD, which is sold in many health food stores, is useless when taken orally because it will be digested by the gastrointestinal tract. There is no evidence that supplements of various antioxidant compounds prolong the life span of man. Free radical damage has also been suggested to contribute to the age-related etiologies of diseases such as diabetes, cataract, rheumatism, and cancer.

2.3.3. Other Functions of Copper

In addition to its role in superoxide dismutase, copper participates in numerous biochemical processes that are essential for normal structure and function of the organism. Naturally occurring and experimentally produced deficiencies in many animal species have resulted in many pathological disturbances, such as anemia, neutropenia, disturbances of bone growth, defects of myelination of the nervous system, weakening and rupture of heart muscle and aorta, depigmentation of hair or wool, hypercholesterolemia, hyperglycemia, alterations of fatty acid metabolism, and increased susceptibility to infections and oxidative stresses.

The occurrence of these signs as a result of copper deficiency is extremely rare in human subjects; it may be for that reason that the clinical significance of marginally deficient copper intake has not yet been recognized by the medical community.

2.3.4. Copper Requirements

In contrast to conclusions of the older literature that the copper supply by the typical U.S. diet is adequate, more recent studies using sensitive analytical methods have consistently shown intakes below 2 mg/day (the low end of the range of "safe and adequate intakes," National Research Council, 1980). The daily intake of copper of 22 men and women based on direct analysis of the copper content of duplicate samples of food and beverages consumed during a 6-day period averaged 1 mg, and the median daily amount of copper present in ten diets analyzed in several states was 0.78 mg (Holden *et al.*, 1979). Thus, copper nutriture in general in the United States appears to be a matter of concern.

Klevay (1983, 1984) has emphasized that many of the consequences of copper deficiency are recognized as risk factors for cardiovascular diseases, for example, hypercholesterolemia, abnormal glucose tolerance, and electrocardiographic irregularities. It is now well established that the clinical manifestation of copper deficiency in experimental animals is determined by the nature of the dietary carbohydrate (Fields, 1983, 1984). Feeding fructose or sucrose aggravates the deficiency, whereas feeding starch protects, without markedly influencing circulating or tissue concentrations of the element. Although the observations were made in two animal species (rats and pigs) and not yet in human subjects, they may be relevant to the nutritional status of the population of the United States and other industrial societies.

Diets consumed by these populations contain relatively high levels of simple sugars such as fructose and sucrose (Wotecki *et al.*, 1982), which by themselves cause undesirable biochemical changes indicative of increased risk for cardiovascular diseases (Reiser, 1985). The superimposition of these sugars on a low copper status in animals has an effect that is greater than the effect of either sugars or copper status alone. These effects include hypercholesterolemia, hypertriglyceridemia, abnormal glucose tolerance, decreased insulin binding, decreased glucose utilization, anemia, histopathological changes of the myocardium, and sudden death from rupture of the heart (Fields *et al.*, 1983, 1984; Reiser *et al.*, 1983). In all experiments there was no carbohydrate effect when copper intake was adequate.

Although the consumption of copper by the elderly, like that of other nutrients, declines to below the intake of the general population because of decreasing food consumption, there is no evidence for clinically recognizable copper deficiency in the U.S. elderly population. Whether the copper intake is adequate to maintain at optimal levels all of the copper-dependent functions discussed above is unknown. This is true even for such important possibly age-related functions as free radical control and protection of the heart and circulatory system.

Various studies have indicated that elderly subjects receive less than the dietary recommendations for many trace elements because of reduced food intake. In addition, the decreased absorption and/or increased excretion of nutrients in the elderly may aggravate trace element deficiency, particularly in the presence of marginal dietary trace element intake. The bioavailability of copper, which is that proportion of copper that can be absorbed and utilized in a given physiological state, has been relatively neglected. This is, in part, because the field of copper in human research is relatively new. Copper deficiency in the human population is not fully understood because the levels of copper present in many tissues are too low to be measured by flame atomic absorption spectrophotometry and because of the lack of suitable isotopes to use as labels. Labeling is especially important in absorption studies because it permits the separation of a specific feeding from endogenous copper and copper fed at other times.

Various balance studies, using nonradioactive and radioactive stable isotopes, have been conducted in the elderly population at their own homes, institutions, and hospitals. Turnland *et al.* (1982b) studied the absorption of ^{65}Cu in elderly men. The average apparent copper absorption for the metabolic studies in the elderly men was 25.8% ± 3.1 (mean ± SD), which was lower than the 57% reported from an earlier study from the same laboratory using ^{65}Cu in young women. (King *et al.*, 1978). The decrease in copper absorption in the elderly compared to the previous study was suggested to be due to the high levels of egg white protein which was present in that diet. Egg white albumin has also been shown to impair iron absorption (Monsen *et al.*, 1978).

In another study copper, zinc and selenium states of elderly women, as indicated by dietary and biochemical data, appeared adequate (Gibson *et al.*, 1985). These trends were related to the relatively high socioeconomic status of the participants of this study and is consistent with the findings of several national nutrition surveys (Health & Welfare, Canada, 1975) that suggest that nutritional adequacy of the diet is highly related to socioeconomic status. However, both the mean analyzed and the calculated copper intakes (Gibson *et al.*, 1985) were below the U.S. National Research Council (1980) Adequate and Safe range (2–3mg).

Various studies have shown age- and sex-related changes in total plasma copper and ceruloplasmin concentrations. (Massie *et al.*, 1979; Helgeland *et al.*, 1982). Many other studies have been well summarized by Yunice *et al.* (1976). In a recent study the overall body status of copper and zinc of healthy aged individuals living in their own homes and eating self-selected diets was assessed by means of metabolic balance studies (Bunker *et al.*, 1984a). The mean daily dietary copper intake of 20 μmole was 64% of the lower limit of 31.5 μmole set as safe and adequate by the Food and Nutrition Board (1980). The same levels of dietary copper intake have been reported from a study conducted on Swedish pensioners (Abdulla and Svensson, 1979). In addition, the daily intake and retention of copper of these elderly subjects (Bunker *et al.*, 1984a) were lower than for children as measured by a similar technique (Aggett *et al.*, 1983), although the levels of plasma copper were higher in the group of old people than in the group of younger controls (Bunker *et al.*, 1984a). Ceruloplasmin concentrations were not affected by the age differences. This lack of age-related changes in ceruloplasmin levels has been reported before (Yunice *et al.*, 1974). Since the production of ceruloplasmin in the liver is known to be increased by estrogens, its concentration would be expected to fall at menopause. However, the results of Chilvers and Hodgkinson (1985) indicate the opposite. It may be that other factors influence ceruloplasmin synthesis during the aging process.

It is possible that the higher concentration of ceruloplasmin in females compared with males is a consequence of higher rates of lipid peroxidation, since ceruloplasmin has been shown to inhibit lipid autooxidation and to act as an oxygen-derived free radical scavenger (Oberley *et al.*, 1980; Goldstein *et al.*, 1982).

Age-related increases in ceruloplasmin copper concentrations in females can also be related to other aspects of aging. These include certain types of arthritis, which may explain the elevated plasma copper concentrations found in elderly females but not males (Bajpayee, 1975), arteriosclerosis, which is associated with the formation of lipid peroxides as the pathological aging phenomenon (Hirai *et al.*, 1982), and impaired bile excretion (Cohen *et al.*, 1978). A close relationship has been found between lipid peroxides and the aging process (Hirai *et al.*, 1982), and an increase in lipid peroxidation with increasing age has been found in rats as a result of the elevated levels of unsaturated fatty acids (Pinto and Bartley, 1969a). The increases in total lipid concentration at menopause (Wilding, 1974) could explain the reasons for the high concentration of the antioxidant ceruloplasmin and the activity of glutathione peroxidase (Csallany *et al.*, 1981). Plasma glutathione peroxidase activity in rats showed a similar sex difference to that found for ceruloplasmin and was shown to be under hormonal control (Pinto and Bartley, 1969b).

None of the techniques currently used to assess body status of copper is ideal. Measurements of concentrations of copper in biological samples such as plasma, whole body, urine, hair, etc. have all been shown to be inadequate for diagnostic purposes unless the deficiency is gross (Solomons, 1981). Studies with experimental animals have shown that plasma ceruloplasmin activity is nondetectable after feeding a copper-deficient diet (Fields *et al.*, 1986) and therefore is not a suitable parameter to differentiate degrees of severity of copper deficiency. Plasma copper and erythrocyte SOD activity were similar in all copper-deficient rats fed either fructose or starch (Fields *et al.*, 1986). Thus, these parameters alone are not sufficient to differentiate degrees of deficiencies in experimental animals.

In a recent human study, ingestion of a low-copper diet supplying 20% of the calories from fructose as compared to starch did not alter ceruloplasmin activity or serum copper concentrations but did significantly reduce SOD concentration and activity of erythocytes (Reiser *et al.*, 1985). During the study, four of the 22 subjects exhibited heart-related abnormalities (Reiser *et al.*, 1985). In another human study, Klevay *et al.* (1984) have reported that in a healthy young man fed a diet low in copper (0.83 mg/day), as in animals, plasma copper and ceruloplasmin were not as sensitive as erythrocyte SOD in establishing reduced copper status. Although none of the measures of copper status of animals were sufficiently sensitive to demonstrate differences between degrees of severity in copper-deficient animals, those blood indices can be used to differentiate between degrees of copper status under conditions of copper adequacy (Fields *et al.*, 1986).

Alzheimer-type dementia is thought to affect 11% of people over age 65 years (Terry, 1976) and is a common cause and/or contributory cause of death in the United States (Katzman, 1976). Although the etiology of Alzheimer's disease is unknown, there have been associations with aluminum, silicon, and zinc. In a recent study Hershey *et al.* (1985) measured multiple trace elements in brains of 16 Alzheimer patients and 15 non-Alzheimer controls. The lower levels of brain copper in Alzheimer's patients as compared to controls, and the decrease in brain copper with age in that study, may reflect lower proportions of copper-containing proteins or structural compounds.

It is obvious that more data are required in order to establish whether the concentrations of trace metals in tissues and body fluids increase, decrease, or remain unchanged with age. The effects of age-related disorders on the absorption, excretion, bioavailability, and requirements of the essential trace metals, including copper, are largely unexplored. Alterations in the homeostasis of the essential trace elements with age may affect the well-being of the aging individual, which could in turn accelerate the aging process and adversely affect the progression of certain chronic degenerative disorders.

2.4. *Selenium**

More than 30 years ago, Harman (1956) suggested that the aging process may be the result of cumulative deleterious effects of various free radical reactions in the body. That theory still stands today (Harman, 1986; see Section 2.3.1 for details). Consequently, there is continuing interest in the biological role of certain nutrients with antioxidant properties such as selenium in aging and age-associated diseases. The purpose of this section is to summarize our current knowledge concerning selenium as it relates to the nutrition of the elderly.

2.4.1. Selenium Content of Blood and Tissues

The major factor that determines the selenium content of human blood and tissues is the amount consumed in the diet, which in turn reflects the amount of selenium in soils available for uptake by plants in different geographical regions (Levander, 1987). Such geochemical considerations, for example, account for the wide differences in dietary selenium intakes and corresponding blood and hair selenium levels reported from selenium-deficient (Keshan disease) and human selenosis areas of the People's Republic of China (Yang *et al.*, 1983). Although these geographically determined effects are dominant where consumption of locally produced foods is common, other factors such as total parenteral nutrition (Levander and Burk, 1986), special therapeutic diets (Lombeck *et al.*, 1981), certain diseases (Robinson *et al.*, 1979; Miller *et al.*, 1983), and aging also can have an influence on blood and tissue selenium levels.

Investigators from New Zealand, West Germany, and Belgium have shown that selenium levels in whole blood, serum, and plasma, respectively, decline shortly after birth and then gradually approach adult values by adolescence (Thomson and Robinson, 1980; Lombeck *et al.*, 1981; Verlinden *et al.*, 1983). Other cross-sectional reports from a variety of countries indicate little change in the selenium content of blood or blood fractions from about 20 to 60 years of age (Robinson *et al.*, 1979; Miller *et al.*, 1983; Verlinden *et al.*, 1983; McAdam *et al.*, 1984; Thorling *et al.*, 1985). Dickson and Tomlinson (1967) reported a downward trend in the selenium content of blood of Canadians with age, but there were too few individuals in each age group to give definite statistical significance to such a conclusion.

In New Zealand, where dietary selenium is low, the selenium concentration in whole blood declined in subjects more than 60 years old (Robinson *et al.*, 1979), whereas no difference was observed in the whole-blood selenium level between those

*This section is by Orville A. Levander.

over and under 60 years of age in Belgium (Verlinden *et al.*, 1983). Moreover, erythrocyte glutathione peroxidase activity was lower in New Zealand old people than in young adults (Thomson *et al.*, 1977), whereas in Belgians the elderly had higher enzyme activity than the young (Verlinden *et al.*, 1983). These differences in results may be related to variations in the overall selenium status of persons living in different regions of the world.

As in the case of blood, tissue selenium levels are markedly influenced by geochemical factors (Casey *et al.*, 1982), but no systematic study of the effects of aging on tissue selenium concentrations appears to have been done. No clear-cut correlation was seen between age and the selenium content of 44 liver samples obtained at autopsy in Maryland (Levander, 1975), but these specimens were taken from patients who had suffered from a variety of diseases, and no attempt was made to relate disease history to selenium status. Thimaya and Ganapathy (1982) analyzed hair samples from different age groups in the United States and found that the mean selenium content between ages 21 and 60 ranged between 0.59 and 0.62 μg/g, and the mean levels between 61 and 70 and above 70 years of age were 0.55 and 0.62 μg/g, respectively.

2.4.2. *Mode of Action and Metabolism*

The only currently well-characterized biological function of selenium in mammals is as a constituent of glutathione peroxidase, the enzyme responsible for destroying lipid peroxides (Sunde and Hoekstra, 1980). However, several enzymes from microbial systems have been shown to contain selenium (Stadtman, 1981), and evidence is accumulating for the existence of additional selenoenzymes in mammals as well.

Gastrointestinal absorption of dietary selenium is generally considered to be highly efficient; values of 80% or more are commonly reported in the literature (Levander, 1983). Homeostatic regulation does not occur at the gut level but may exist via the kidney (Robinson *et al.*, 1985). One study of dependent North American men 78 to 88 years of age reported mean apparent absorption values of only 49% for dietary selenium, which might suggest some impairment of selenium absorption in the elderly (Stead *et al.*, 1985). Further investigation along these lines is warranted.

2.4.3. *Selenium in Aging and Degenerative Diseases*

Interest in the possible role of selenium in the aging process *per se* is based largely on its antioxidant function via glutathione peroxidase. Csallany *et al.* (1981) reported increased glutathione peroxidase activities in the kidney, heart, and testis of 19-month-old rats and suggested that this might be an adaptive response to increased peroxidative stress that ultimately leads to lower lipofuscin (aging) pigment accumulation in these tissues. Anneren *et al.* (1986) found that the glutathione peroxidase activity in erythrocytes of persons with Alzheimer's disease or senile dementia of Alzheimer's type was higher than that of healthy controls and suggested that this might be a biochemical adaptation to elevated intracellular turnover of superoxide to peroxide in such patients. On the other hand, Meydani *et al.* (1985) concluded that selenium has only a minor role compared with vitamin E in the protection against *ex vivo* and possibly *in vivo* lipid peroxidation in rat cerebrum. Hafeman and Hoekstra (1977) showed that dietary vitamin E was more effective than dietary selenium in decreasing *in vivo* lipid peroxidation in rats as judged by evolution of ethane. Limited clinical benefits have been observed after combined high-dose selenium and vitamin E therapy plus other antioxidants in Finnish patients with neuronal ceroid lipofuscinosis, a disease characterized by the accumulation of lipofuscin pigments in the body (Westermarck and Santavuori, 1984). Megadose selenium and vitamin E treatment has also been reported to result in some improvement of certain mental characteristics of geriatric nursing home residents in Finland (Tolonen *et al.*, 1985).

Recently, attention has turned to the possible role of dietary selenium in the prevention of age-related degenerative human diseases such as cancer or heart disease. Some, but not all, epidemiologic studies have suggested that increased dietary selenium intakes are associated with a decreased incidence of certain forms of cancer (Levander, 1987). However, there are certain discrepancies among these correlations, and the differences are difficult to reconcile. Numerous animal experiments have now shown that, under certain conditions, levels of dietary selenium bordering on the toxic can protect against chemically induced, spontaneous, or transplantable tumors (comprehensively reviewed by Ip, 1985, and Milner, 1985). The biochemical mechanism of this protective effect of selenium is not understood, but apparently glutathione peroxidase is not involved (Ip, 1986; Medina, 1986). On the other hand, a number of other studies indicate that even high levels of selenium intake are not protective against experimental cancer in all animal models (Thompson and Becci, 1979; Beems, 1986; Bergman and Slanina, 1986; Aquino *et al.*, 1985; Le Boeuf *et al.*, 1985; Ankerst and Sjogren, 1982; Birt *et al.*, 1988), and in one case selenium deficiency protected against tumorigenesis (Reddy and Tanaka, 1986). Thus, the possible role of dietary selenium in the etiology and prevention of human cancer is a question still open for further research.

At the present time, the only human disease clearly connected with selenium deficiency is Keshan disease, a cardiomyopathy that affects primarily infants, children, and women of childbearing age in extremely selenium-poor areas of China (Yang *et al.*, 1984). Although selenium deficiency appears to be the basic lesion predisposing to this disease, other factors, such as a virus, may also be involved. The relationship between selenium status and other types of heart disease, such as the cardiovascular disease prevalent in the West, is less certain. A recent review of published prospective epidemiologic studies concluded that no causal relationship could be established between selenium status and the risk of ischemic heart disease (Salonen and Huttunen, 1986). Nevertheless, it was maintained that those studies did not rule out the possibility of an inverse relationship between serum selenium concentrations less than 45 μg/liter and the risk of ischemic heart disease. Animal experiments have indicated that poor selenium nutriture could exacerbate the course of cardiovascular disease by impairing the biosynthesis by the aorta of the platelet antiaggregatory arachidonic acid metabolite prostacyclin (Schoene *et al.*, 1986). No correlation was observed between various parameters of selenium status and traditional cardiovascular risk factors in human studies from England (Ellis *et al.*, 1984) and New Zealand (Robinson *et al.*, 1983). However, selenium supplementation of elderly North American subjects resulted in decreased plasma levels of two platelet proteins associated with *in vivo* aggregability even in the absence of increased red cell or platelet glutathione peroxidase activities

(Stead *et al.*, 1985). Decreased platelet glutathione peroxidase activity was observed in Italian patients with coronary heart disease (Guidi *et al.*, 1986).

2.4.4. Requirements

There has been a great deal of progress in our understanding of human selenium requirements during the past few years (reviewed in Levander, 1986a). Because of the lack of human data, early attempts to estimate human selenium requirements relied heavily on extrapolation from animal experiments (National Research Council, 1980). Since that time, many human studies utilizing a variety of approaches have appeared that allow determination of the human selenium requirement with a fair degree of precision.

One approach used by several investigators is the metabolic balance study, a technique much used in the past to estimate requirements for many trace elements. However, in the case of selenium, international comparisons quickly made it obvious that the amount of selenium needed to achieve balance in a given subject was highly dependent on the subject's historical dietary selenium intake. For example, only 10 μg of selenium per day was sufficient to maintain balance in Chinese men from a Keshan disease area (Luo *et al.*, 1985), whereas 80 μg/day was needed for balance in North American men (Levander and Morris, 1984). This discrepancy was thought to be the result of differences in total body selenium pools because of differences in habitual dietary selenium intakes. Thus, the balance method would not be particularly useful in delineating human selenium requirements.

Another approach used in China was to determine the amount of selenium needed to prevent the appearance of selenium deficiency disease. This was done by comparing dietary selenium intakes in areas with and without Keshan disease. For men, the dietary intakes were 7.7 and 19.1 μg/day in affected and nonaffected areas, respectively (Yang *et al.*, 1987). The latter intake could be considered equivalent to a minimum daily selenium requirement.

The depletion–repletion method was tried both in North America and in China to estimate human selenium requirements. The North American attempt did not succeed because the sizable selenium stores of the subjects prevented their plasma selenium levels from falling to levels commonly found in persons living in low-selenium areas such as New Zealand or Finland even after consuming a diet low in selenium for 7 weeks (Levander *et al.*, 1981). On the other hand, Yang *et al.* (1987) recognized the scientific potential of persons from a Keshan disease area with naturally low selenium stores and supplemented such people with graded doses of selenomethionine. Plasma glutathione peroxidase activity plateaued in those men receiving a total selenium exposure (diet plus supplement) of 40 μg/day or more. Hence, a physiological selenium requirement of 40 μg/day was established for Chinese males of 60 kg body weight.

In order to translate this Chinese value into a figure appropriate for Western societies, certain adjustments would have to be made for differences in body weight. Also, different estimates of requirement would likely be needed for men and women, since men needed more selenium to maintain balance than women (Levander and Morris, 1984), again probably largely because of differences in body weight (and hence body selenium pools). The final step in this process would be to calculate a dietary recommendation by applying the appropriate safety factors to account for individual variation in requirements.

2.4.5. *Dietary Intakes and Nutritional Status of the Elderly*

Mean dietary selenium intakes for healthy adults in the United States range between 80 and 129 μg/day, whereas intakes in Canada appear to be somewhat higher, 113 to 220 μg/day (reviewed in Levander, 1986a). South Dakota, a high-selenium area in the United States, reported some adult intakes in excess of 200 μg/day (Palmer *et al.*, 1983).

Mean dietary selenium intakes among elderly residents of North America are somewhat lower, ranging from 60 to 94 μg/day in the United States and from 78 to 113 μg/day in Canada (Gibson *et al.*, 1983, 1985; Lane *et al.*, 1983; Stead *et al.*, 1985). Dietary selenium intakes in countries with low-selenium soils are less than those in North America, and the intake of the elderly is no exception to this rule. Pensioners in Sweden, for example, consumed only 34 or 28 μg/day for males and females, respectively (Abdulla *et al.*, 1979).

Although certain difficulties arise when attempting to assess selenium status by estimating dietary selenium intake (Levander, 1986b), the selenium status of the North American elderly seems to be satisfactory by this criterion. Certainly, the mean dietary intakes measured in the United States and Canada for old people all fall within the 50- to 200-μg/day range judged safe and adequate by the U.S. National Research Council (1980). Moreover, all these mean intakes exceed the physiological requirement derived by the Chinese even after adjustment for differences in body weight.

Thus, the selenium status of the elderly in North America as judged by dietary selenium intake appears quite satisfactory. This conclusion of course does not take into account diseased persons (Miller *et al.*, 1983), persons with generalized malnutrition (Smith *et al.*, 1986), or patients undergoing total parenteral nutrition (Levander and Burk, 1986). All those situations are specialized cases that require individual attention. On the other hand, even healthy old people living in countries with low-selenium soils would have difficulty in meeting either of the two dietary criteria of selenium status discussed above, as would any members of such populations.

The relative advantages and disadvantages of assessing selenium status by measuring blood, plasma, or hair selenium levels or red cell, plasma, or platelet glutathione peroxidase activities have been discussed elsewhere (Levander, 1985). All of these indices of selenium status have been used to assess selenium status in the North American elderly, and these persons appear to have adequate selenium status by these criteria (Gibson *et al.*, 1983, 1985; Lane *et al.*, 1983; Stead *et al.*, 1985). Furthermore, a supplementation trial conducted in Augusta, Georgia, a low-selenium area of the United States, showed that 200 μg of selenium per day in the form of kelp raised the plasma selenium level of elderly men but had no effect on their erythrocyte or platelet glutathione peroxidase activities (Stead *et al.*, 1985). It was concluded that their usual dietary selenium intake of 60 μg/day was nutritionally adequate for these North American subjects.

As in the case of dietary selenium intakes, blood selenium levels and glutathione peroxidase activities are depressed in persons residing in low-selenium countries, whatever their age group. In some New Zealand elderly, there was an additional decrement in both of these variables because of age (Thomson *et al.*, 1977; Robinson *et al.*, 1979). This suggests that populations whose selenium status is already low because of geochemical factors may be particularly at risk when other unfavorable factors (aging, disease, poor food habits, etc.) are superimposed.

2.4.6. *Conclusions*

Because of its antioxidant function as a constituent of the enzyme glutathione peroxidase, attempts have been made to link selenium with the aging process itself as well as certain age-related chronic degenerative human diseases such as cancer or heart disease. Selenium has been demonstrated to play a role in Keshan disease, but its involvement in other human diseases is less certain. The only dietary standard for selenium currently in existence is the safe and adequate range of 50 to 200 μg/day for adults established by the U.S. National Research Council in 1980.

Nutrition surveys carried out in Canada and the United States indicate that elderly people in these countries with relatively selenium-rich soils have an adequate selenium status as assessed by traditional criteria such as dietary intakes and blood selenium levels and glutathione peroxidase activities. In areas with low-selenium soils (Scandinavia, New Zealand, and certain parts of China), however, old people whose selenium status is already depressed because of geochemical reasons may be particularly at risk with regard to further selenium depletion from other factors.

In China, selenium supplements in the form of pills containing sodium selenite are distributed to children living in low-selenium areas to protect them against Keshan disease (Yang *et al.*, 1984). Based largely on epidemiologic considerations, authorities in Finland have permitted the addition of selenium to fertilizers for use on human food crops in order to fortify the selenium content of the national food supply (Koivistoinen and Huttunen, 1986). In New Zealand, nutritionists have steadfastly denied any deleterious effects of low selenium status on the public health of its population (Robinson and Thomson, 1983), and there are no official programs of selenium supplementation or fortification. In the United States, a recent review concluded that the evidence available at this time does not support recommending diet supplementation with selenium for either life extension or the prevention of cancer (Schneider and Reed, 1985). Each country will have to develop its own national policy concerning the need for, or desirability of, dietary selenium supplementation or fortification.

2.5. *Chromium**

Chromium nutrition is of particular importance to the general population since insufficient dietary chromium is linked to two of the leading causes of poor health in older people, namely, maturity-onset diabetes and cardiovascular disease(s). The nutritional role of chromium in human health and disease has been conclusively demonstrated in three separate studies involving patients on total parenteral nutrition (Jee-

*This section is by Richard A. Anderson.

jeebhoy *et al.*, 1977; Freund *et al.*, 1979; Brown *et al.*, 1986). Specific signs displayed by the patients in the three studies included principally glucose intolerance and impaired insulin function as well as unexpected weight loss, impaired nerve conduction, peripheral neuropathy, negative nitrogen balance, and brain disorders. These symptoms were refractory to exogenous insulin but were alleviated by addition of supplemental chromium to the TPN solutions. In free-living subjects, signs of marginal chromium deficiency, including impaired glucose tolerance, elevated circulating insulin, elevated serum lipids, and reduced levels of HDL-cholesterol, have all been demonstrated to improve following supplemental chromium. Marginal chromium deficiency appears to be widespread, and often 50% or more of the subjects in various studies improve following chromium supplementation (see reviews, Mertz, 1969; Borel and Anderson, 1984).

2.5.1. Intake

The suggested safe and adequate intake for chromium as established by the National Academy of Sciences is 50 to 200 μg per day (National Research Council, 1980). However, dietary chromium intake, even of young subjects eating normal diets, appears to be only half of the minimum suggested intake. In a study involving ten adult males and 22 females, mean daily dietary chromium intake determined for seven consecutive days was 33 ± 3 μg per day (mean ± S.E.) for the males and 25 ± 1 μg for females. Approximately 90% of the daily diets were below the minimum suggested safe and adequate intake, and not one of the subjects had a 7-day average dietary intake meeting the suggested minimum intake (Anderson and Kozlovsky, 1985). In that study conditions were optimized for chromium during the collection, homogenization, and analysis steps. If appropriate steps are not taken, such as elimination of exposure of food samples to stainless steel, erroneously high chromium values will be obtained. For example, if food samples are homogenized in a plastic blender jar but with stainless steel blades, apparent food chromium will depend more on time of blending than on the actual chromium content of the food composite. Leaching of chromium from stainless steel containers used in food preparation is also well documented (Kumpulainen *et al.*, 1979; Offenbacher and Pi-Sunyer, 1983; Anderson and Bryden, 1983). Chromium that leaches from stainless steel during the preparation of foods and beverages may be utilized. For example, Anderson and Bryden (1983) reported that absorption of contaminating chromium in beer samples was similar to that of the chromium found endogenously in beer and other foods.

Recent studies from Finland (Koivistoinen, 1980) and England (Bunker *et al.*, 1984b) reported dietary intakes in the region of 30 μg, similar to those of Anderson and Kozlovsky (1985). Dietary chromium intake is usually in the range of 9 to 15 μg/1000 kcal, so that in excess of 3000–5000 kcal may need to be consumed to obtain the minimum suggested intake. Therefore, as the caloric intake tends to decrease with age, the intake of chromium falls further below the minimum suggested intake.

Changes in food selection as well as preparation also appear to favor decreases in dietary chromium intake. For example, foods that are high in simple sugars are becoming more popular, especially in older individuals (Albanese, 1976), since the taste for sweetness is one of the tastes that is strongest in the elderly. Sweet foods are often eaten at the expense of other more nutritious foods. Sweet foods containing simple sugars are not only low in chromium but also stimulate chromium losses (Kozlovsky *et al.*, 1986). Preparation of foods also may affect chromium intake. For example, foods are often not prepared in stainless steel or iron cookware but rather in Teflon-coated stainless steel, porcelain containers, or microwave cookware, all of which would not contribute exogenous chromium to the foods.

Dietary chromium intake of elderly subjects appears to vary significantly. For example, two groups of elderly subjects in the same city were supplemented with chromium in the form of a high-chromium yeast to determine if elderly subjects were consuming sufficient amounts of dietary chromium. In the first study (Offenbacher and Pi-Sunyer, 1980), elderly subjects (mean age 78) responded to supplemental chromium with improvements in glucose tolerance and serum lipids, thus suggesting that this group of elderly subjects had been consuming suboptimal levels of chromium. Dietary chromium intake was not measured. In a second study performed by the same investigators (Offenbacher *et al.*, 1985), 23 elderly subjects (mean age 73 years) did not respond to supplemental chromium. However, in the second study, nutrition-conscious subjects were selected. These subjects had well-balanced diets containing 100% or more of the suggested intake of eight potentially problem nutrients. Calcium was the only nutrient that did not appear to be consumed at 100% or more of the RDA. Mean chromium intake of this group was 37.1 μg per day. Chromium intake of 85 older free-living Canadian women (59–82 years) was 91 μg (Martinez *et al.*, 1985). However, subjects who showed a positive response to supplemental chromium had a significantly lower median daily chromium intake of 56 μg. Values for chromium intake reported in the Canadian study (Martinez *et al.*, 1985) appear to be too high, based on other values reported for studies that optimized conditions for chromium. Food composites in that study were homogenized using a stainless steel Waring blender coated with Teflon. Teflon coating may not provide complete protection against chromium leaching from the stainless steel.

Absorption of chromium is postulated to decrease with age. This is well documented in rats but not in humans (Doisy *et al.*, 1971). Absorption of orally administered inorganic radioactive chromium by elderly and younger subjects was similar at approximately 0.5%. Chromium absorption by humans appears to be inversely related to dietary chromium intake, thus helping to ensure at least a minimum maintenance level of chromium (Anderson and Kozlovsky, 1985).

Although chromium absorption does not appear to decrease with age, the ability to convert chromium to a usable physiological form may be age dependent. Children responded to inorganic chromium supplementation by an improvement in glucose tolerance within 24 hr (Hopkins *et al.*, 1968; Gurson and Saner, 1971), whereas adult subjects require 1 to 3 months to respond (Glinsmann and Mertz, 1966). This suggests that age may play a role in the ability of the body to convert chromium to a usable form.

2.5.2. Chromium in Aging and Degenerative Diseases

Schroeder *et al.* (1962) reported that the high levels of chromium at birth declined in the first one or two decades of life to adult levels. Kidney and liver appeared to maintain neonatal concentrations until the second decade of life, while lung, aorta, heart, and spleen declined rapidly in the first 45 days following birth. Only in the case of the lung, presumably because of inhalation of chromium in polluted air, did concentrations rise in later life. There have not been any recent comprehensive studies using modern instruments and techniques relating changes in chromium concentrations of human tissues to age.

Values reported in the study of Schroeder *et al.* (1962) are severalfold higher than presently accepted values, and the reader is urged to use caution when forming conclusions based on analytical work involving chromium that does not employ reference materials of verified chromium concentration. Standard reference materials are available from the National Bureau of Standards (Gaithersburg, MD). Other standards of verified chromium concentration with a matrix and chromium concentration similar to those of the samples being analyzed can be obtained from the International Atomic Energy Agency.

Recent studies involving changes in serum and urine concentrations of adult subjects have been completed (Tables VI and VII) using modern instrumentation and techniques to avoid chromium contamination; there does not appear to be any significant difference in serum chromium (Table VI) or urinary chromium excretion for subjects (Table VII) among the decades from 20 to 60-plus years. Although chromium status may be exacerbated with age, there are other factors that tend to mask any aging effects. Similar results are often observed in chromium supplementation studies of subjects of varying ages; for example, subjects even in their 20s and 30s as well as those above 60 years often respond to supplemental chromium (Anderson *et al.*, 1983b), indicating a marginal chromium status.

Hair chromium has been suggested as a possible indicator of chromium status (Hambidge, 1971). Furthermore, hair chromium concentrations can be correlated with age, but usually only for children. For example, the chromium concentration distal from the scalp of an 18-month-old child whose hair had never been cut was 940 ppb, reflecting high levels at birth, but the chromium concentration in the 2-cm region closest to the scalp was only 144 ppb, a value similar to that for older children and

Table VI. Serum Cr Concentration[a] and Aging

Age[b]	Serum Cr (ng/ml) (mean ± S.E.M.) Fasting	90-min post-glucose[c]
20–29 (10)	0.13 ± 0.03	0.14 ± 0.02
30–39 (20)	0.13 ± 0.02	0.12 ± 0.02
40–49 (22)	0.14 ± 0.02	0.12 ± 0.02
50+ (16)	0.12 ± 0.03	0.14 ± 0.03

[a]Serum Cr values for normal free-living subjects. There was no significant difference between serum Cr values for males and females; therefore, sexes were grouped. Subject selection and methods for serum Cr analysis have been reported (Anderson *et al.*, 1985).
[b]Number in parentheses denotes number of subjects.
[c]The "90-min post-glucose" values refer to samples taken 90 min following a glucose challenge (1 g glucose/kg body wt).

Table VII. Daily Urinary Cr Excretion and Aging[a]

Age (years)	Cr excretion (μg/day) (mean ± S.E.M.)
20–29 (7)[b]	0.22 ± 0.06
30–39 (10)	0.23 ± 0.05
40–49 (16)	0.14 ± 0.02
50+ (9)	0.18 ± 0.04

[a]Daily urinary Cr excretion of normal free-living subjects. There was no significant difference in the urinary Cr excretion of male and female subjects; therefore, sexes were grouped. Subject selection and methods for Cr analysis have been reported (Anderson *et al.*, 1983a).
[b]Number in parentheses denotes number of subjects.

adults. Hair chromium content of premature infants may be indicative of gestational age (Hambidge, 1971). Hair chromium content of babies at a gestational age of 32 weeks was six times lower than that of babies at a gestational age of 36 weeks.

It is generally agreed that chromium deficiency may account for certain cases of diabetes and that administration of chromium improves glucose tolerance of hyper- and hypoglycemic subjects, alleviates hypoglycemic symptoms, and improves insulin efficiency and binding (see Mertz, 1969; Borel and Anderson, 1984; Anderson, 1985; Anderson *et al.*, 1987). Insulin-dependent diabetes also affects the chromium content of human tissues. Morgan (1972) reported that hepatic chromium concentration of diabetics was less than that of controls, and the chromium concentration of the pancreas of diabetic subjects was also less than that of controls (Schroeder *et al.*, 1962; Chao *et al.*, 1976). Hair chromium of diabetic children (Hambidge, 1971) and female diabetics (Rosson *et al.*, 1979) was reported to be significantly decreased compared with that of controls. However, reduced concentrations of chromium in the tissues and hair of diabetics are reflected in neither the absorption nor the concentrations of chromium in the urine and serum of diabetics. Indeed, chromium absorption of insulin-dependent diabetics is two to four times greater than that of normal subjects (Doisy *et al.*, 1976), and chromium concentrations of urine and serum of diabetics are significantly greater than those of control subjects (Vanderlinde *et al.*, 1979). Diabetics appear to utilize chromium differently than control subjects; it is postulated that diabetics are unable to convert inorganic chromium to a usable form. Similarly, diabetic mice are unable to utilize inorganic chromium but can utilize chromium in a physiologically active form (Tuman *et al.*, 1978), whereas normal experimental animals as well as humans can utilize both inorganic and preformed biologically active forms of chromium.

Several independent studies have substantiated a role of chromium in decreasing risk factors associated with cardiovascular diseases. Common risk factors of cardiovascular disease include elevated blood lipids, decreased HDL-cholesterol, elevated circulating insulin, impaired glucose tolerance, and diabetes. Chromium has been demonstrated to improve all of these factors in humans (see review Anderson, 1985), therefore lessening the chances of cardiovascular diseases. In experimental animals, supplemental chromium has also been shown to reverse arterial plaque formation (Abraham *et al.*, 1980).

The arterial wall is comprised of insulin-sensitive tissues. Elevated circulating insulin levels lead to proliferation of smooth muscle cells, inhibition of lipolysis, and increased synthesis of cholesterol, phospholipids, and triglycerides (Stout, 1977). Therefore, insufficient dietary chromium, which leads to increased levels of circulating concentrations of insulin and perturbed arterial wall metabolism, increases risk factors associated with cardiovascular diseases. Two independent studies have reported significant differences in the serum chromium of patients with coronary artery diseases (CAD) compared to control subjects (Newman *et al.*, 1978; Simonoff *et al.*, 1984). Serum chromium correlated highly ($P < 0.01$) and inversely with the appearance of coronary artery disease, whereas elevated serum triacylglycerol correlated less significantly, and there was no correlation between other risk factors such as serum cholesterol, blood pressure, or body weight and the incidence of CAD (Newman *et al.*, 1978). Simonoff *et al.* (1984) state that "an upper limit for plasma chromium may be established . . . beyond which CAD may be considered to be extremely unlikely, thus eliminating the need for a certain number of cineangiographic examinations." Although this may be an overestimation of the predictability of serum chromium as an indicator of CAD, it does illustrate the strong inverse correlation of serum chromium and CAD and the subsequent strong beliefs of the researchers. The reader is cautioned, nevertheless, that in both of the previously mentioned studies, serum chromium values are too high based on the presently accepted values, suggesting a need for repetition with more modern methodology.

2.5.3. Conclusions

Chromium is a critical element involved in human health. Degenerative diseases including diabetes and cardiovascular diseases are exacerbated by insufficient intakes of dietary chromium. Dietary chromium intake is approximately half of the suggested intake, and numerous studies involving elderly, middle-aged, and children have reported beneficial effects of supplemental chromium. Beneficial effects include improvements in glucose tolerance for both hyper- and hypoglycemic subjects, alleviation of symptoms of hypoglycemia, improved insulin efficiency, increased insulin receptor number, decreased total cholesterol and triglycerides, and increased HDL-cholesterol. Most subjects respond to inorganic chromium supplementation, but some subjects appear to lose the ability to convert inorganic chromium to a usable form and are therefore dependent on preformed physiologically active chromium complexes. Severity of common degenerative diseases such as maturity-onset diabetes and cardiovascular diseases may be alleviated by proper chromium nutrition.

*2.6. Silicon**

Although a human requirement for silicon can only be inferred from studies in rats and chickens, and no quantitative estimates of a requirement in man can be made, this element is of potential interest in relation to the aging process for three reasons. Silicon is essential for proper bone formation in animals and may play an important, albeit hitherto neglected role in maintaining bone structure throughout the lifetime (Carlisle,

*This section is by Walter Mertz.

1986). Secondly, two investigators have independently theorized that silicon may protect against certain diseases of the vascular system in man (Schwarz *et al.*, 1977; Loeper *et al.*, 1978). Finally, the element has been shown in experimental animals to decline with age in certain organs, such as arterial walls and skin (Loeper *et al.*, 1978).

2.6.1. *Concentration in Biological Materials*

The analytical values reported for silicon in biological tissues are unreliable because of technical difficulties. Data validated by the use of proper reference materials have not yet been published, but concentrations in human tissues have been estimated at between 3 and 60 μg/g wet weight, except for much higher values in lymph nodes. Significantly lower concentration were found in adult rat and rhesus monkey tissues. A recent analytical study estimated the daily silicon intake from a typical British diet at approximately 30 mg; it also identified certain high-silicon foods (barley and oats with 2610 and 4310 μg/g silicon, respectively), whereas fruits, meat, fish, fats, and milk contained considerably less (Bowen and Peggs, 1984). A study in the United States detected a strong dependence of dietary silicon levels on the fiber content: low- and high-fiber diets furnished 21 and 45.8 mg/day respectively (Kelsay *et al.*, 1979).

Silicon is concentrated in organs of high connective tissue content, such as tendons and skin, and strongly bound to glycosaminoglycans, possibly having some cross-linking functions important for the integrity of the tissues.

2.6.2. *Metabolism and Mode of Action*

A silicon requirement was independently established in chickens (Carlisle, 1972) and rats (Schwarz and Milne, 1972b). Feeding purified diets containing 1 μg/g of silicon resulted in growth retardation and disturbances of bone formation in both species. All of the impairments were prevented by including high levels of soluble silicates, 500 μg Si/g of diet. The exact requirement for silicon of the two species studied is not known. Silicon was shown in electron-microprobe studies to accumulate at high concentrations in the line of ossification of new bone together with increasing calcium content. The subsequent demonstration of high concentrations of silicon within the mitochondria of osteoblasts lends further support to the postulate of a strong, possibly regulatory role of silicon in the formation of connective tissue matrix and subsequent calcification.

2.6.3. *Silicon in Aging and Degenerative Diseases*

A group of workers in France (Loeper *et al.*, 1978) have produced data that tend to link silicon to the aging process and to atherosclerosis. The silicon content of the human aorta was found to decrease from a high of 205 ± 44 μg/100 mg of tissue nitrogen in infants to 86 ± 16 in persons aged 40. The same group demonstrated that the arteriosclerotic process itself is associated with a significant decline in the silicon content of the vessels. (Healthy arteries, 180 μg/100 mg nitrogen; moderately pathological vessels, 105; severely sclerotic arteries with lipid and calcium infiltration, 63 μg). High-silicon supplements, 10 mg intravenously and 200 mg/day orally, reduced the incidence and severity of atheromata in cholesterol-fed rabbits.

In contrast to the beneficial effects described here, some compounds of silicon can act as carcinogens. Inhalation of such compounds over extended periods of time can produce fibrosis of the lungs, and in the form of asbestos fibers, malignant tumors in lungs and gastrointestinal tract (Selikoff, 1978). Although asbestosis is a major public health problem, it is not related in any way to the nutritional role of soluble silicon compounds.

Electron-probe studies have demonstrated the presence of high silicon concentrations in the cerebral cortex of patients with Alzheimer's senile dementia. Silicon accumulations are strictly localized and not representative of the overall Si concentration in the whole brain. It is not known whether the silicon foci have etiological significance or whether they are a consequence of prior tissue degeneration (Austin, 1978).

2.6.4. Conclusions

Silicon may play a role in the aging process, but very few data on metabolism and requirement in man are available. Concentrations of the element appear to decline with age and disease in some important tissues, including the heart and aorta of animal species and man. The cardinal sign of deficiency in two animal species is a derangement of bone formation, indicating an essential function of silicon in bone metabolism. The element's effect on calcification in growing bone was most pronounced with low dietary calcium.

No exact dose–response curves for the biological effects of silicon have been established. The requirement of the two animal species studied may lie between 50 and 500 μg/g diet, depending strongly on the chemical form of the silicon compounds present.

The sparsity of dietary information precludes the establishment of a silicon requirement in man or an assessment of the adequacy of dietary intakes.

*2.7. Fluorine**

Fluorine is included in this discussion because of its reported effects on bone health in the elderly, even though its predominant and best-documented effect is that on dental health in the young (World Health Organization, 1970). Fluoride is generally considered to be an essential element on the basis of its proven effects on dental health, although the experimental evidence for essentiality is ambiguous.

2.7.1. Concentrations in Biological Materials

Within a wide range of exposures, the content of fluorine in blood and soft tissues appears to be well regulated, with concentrations ranging from fractions of 1 μg/g to a few micrograms per gram, depending on species (Underwood, 1977). These con-

*This section is by Walter Mertz.

centrations have been found to increase very little with greatly increasing dietary exposures. Excesses are deposited in bones, which can accumulate several hundred micrograms of fluorine per gram; the rest is excreted in the urine (Spencer *et al.*, 1975).

Most foods of vegetable origin present concentrations of fluorine of less than 1 μg/g with the notable exception of tea leaves, which contribute substantial amounts to the fluorine intake of tea drinkers. Seafood, especially small fish eaten with bones, are outstanding sources of dietary fluorine. Very substantial variations of fluorine content occur in water, ranging from nondetectable levels to 15 mg/liter. Many municipal water supplies in the United States maintain a fluorine concentration of 1 mg/liter. The average, typical diet (with only occasional consumption of small fish and tea) would provide less than 1 mg of fluorine per day if the very substantial contribution of water to the daily intake were unavailable. That contribution is not only via drinking water but also by way of what may be an ion-exchange process between cooking water and foods during food preparation. Prepared meals, therefore, reflect strongly the fluorine content of local drinking water, and daily fluorine intakes are consistently higher in fluoridated areas than in those with low fluorine content in the drinking water. In an analysis of daily diets from 12 cities with fluoridated water (0.91 ± 0.23 mg/liter) and four with low fluorine content (0.23 ± 0.18 mg/liter), the total fluorine intake in the former was 2.63 ± 0.57 mg/day compared with 0.91 ± 0.11 mg/day in the latter (Kramer *et al.*, 1974).

2.7.2. *Metabolism and Mode of Action*

Fluorine is a bone-seeking trace element in that intakes in excess of the excretory capacity of the kidneys are deposited in bones and teeth. Concentrations in the soft tissues, including blood, are maintained over a wide range of intakes.

Fluorine exhibits well-defined zones of biological effects. Growth retardation and discoloration of the teeth were reported by one investigator in rats fed diets ranging from 0.04 to 0.46 μg fluorine/g (Schwarz and Milne, 1972a). The reduction of caries incidence in children by fluorine intakes at or above 1.5 mg/day is well documented. This would correspond to a dietary concentration of 3 μg/g or more. The first signs of overexposure, slight mottling of the enamel of the teeth, can be observed with higher intakes in areas where the drinking water contains more than 5 mg/liter, and the clinically serious disease of fluorosis is generally observed in persons consuming much higher amounts, 20 mg or more, over extended periods of time. Resistance against fluorine toxicity, however, appears to depend on the general nutritional status, especially that of calcium (Krishnamachari, 1987).

2.7.3. *Fluorine in Aging and Degenerative Diseases*

The great affinity of this element for bone and teeth where it becomes part of the hydroxyapatite structure raises the question of whether it could play a role in maintaining bone health. Excessive exposure is associated with greatly increased bone density, and high doses of fluorine are used clinically as part of the treatment of osteoporosis. This suggests that a suboptimal fluorine status might predispose to increased bone loss and that adequate fluorine intake might reduce the rate of calcium loss from the skeleton, which can lead to various health hazards in the elderly. Daily supplements of 40 to 60 mg of sodium fluoride corresponding to 18 to 27 mg of fluorine have been used in combination with either calcium and vitamin D or estrogen and calcium treatment in postmenopausal women. The inclusion of fluorine reduced the rate of vertebral fracture occurrence consistently and significantly beyond that obtained by calcium, estrogen, or vitamin D treatment alone (Riggs *et al.*, 1982). In another study (Bernstein *et al.*, 1966), exposure to fluoride concentrations of 4 to 5.8 mg/liter naturally occurring in the drinking water of North Dakota has been associated with a significant reduction in the occurrence of collapsed vertebrae in women aged 55 years and older, as compared with women living in an area with low fluoride concentrations in the drinking water (0.15 to 0.3 mg/liter). This effect was not seen in males. There was also evidence of a reduced incidence of decreased bone density in the residents of the high-fluoride area and of radiologically detectable calcification of the abdominal aorta, which was significant in males (Bernstein *et al.*, 1966). These findings are consistent with the results of a similar, more recent study in Finland (Simonen and Laitinen, 1985).

2.8. *Aluminum**

Aluminum is of potential interest to the elderly for three reasons: (1) intravenous, long-term administration, inadvertently given in the past, has caused two serious chronic diseases, namely, encephalopathy and osteomalacia; (2) aluminum accumulates in certain foci of the brain in patients with Alzheimer's disease; and (3) the element is available in uncontrolled quantities to the public in the form of antacids (Alfrey, 1986).

2.8.1. *Concentration in Biological Materials*

Aluminum is practically ubiquitous in nature; it occurs in the human and animal organism in concentrations of 1 to 50 μg/g of dry weight. The aluminum concentration in the plasma of unexposed persons has been reported as approximately 5 μg/liter. Tissue concentrations are highest in lymph nodes, lungs, and the thyroid and remain constant with increasing age except for lungs and, possibly, for brain, in which there may be a mild increase (Alfrey, 1986). The daily aluminum intake from typical American diets has been reported to range between 5 and 125 mg. Acidic foods or fluids leaching the element from containers or cookware might contribute to the higher intakes. Drinking water can contain extreme levels of 2 to 4 mg/liter. Other potential sources are aluminum compounds used in food processing, such as fillers in cheeses and pickles, baking powder, and aluminum-containing antacid preparations (Greger and Baier, 1983).

2.8.2. *Metabolism and Mode of Action*

Essential functions of aluminum beneficial for health have not been described. Clinically significant toxic effects are known only as a consequence of intravenous

*This section is by Walter Mertz.

application of aluminum, although interactions of ingested aluminum with phosphorus and fluorine have been described and may have long-range adverse health effects (Alfrey, 1986). Urine is the major excretory route for absorbed aluminum; it reflects the very low degree of intestinal absorption.

Aluminum toxicity affecting the brain has been described not too long ago in patients undergoing renal dialysis at clinical centers with high aluminum concentrations in the water. The successes of chelation therapy and the virtual disappearance of the syndrome after the aluminum content of the dialysis water had been controlled provide evidence for an etiological role of the intravenously administered aluminum. It is, however, not clear whether this dialysis encephalopathy bears any resemblance to Alzheimer's disease (senile dementia). Although there is evidence for elevated aluminum levels in the brain in Alzheimer's disease, it is unlikely that aluminum plays a causal role. Its accumulation may be secondary to an underlying, primary pathological process (Alfrey, 1986).

In the past, osteomalacia resulting in reduced mineralization and diminished strength of the bone was often associated with renal dialysis treatment. The condition is believed to be a consequence of high parenteral aluminum exposure. It does not respond to vitamin D therapy but has practically disappeared in renal dialysis patients since routine deionization of the dialysis fluid was begun (Alfrey, 1986).

There remains the important question whether aluminum also exerts its toxicity when it is taken by the oral route, for example, as a constituent of antacids. Aluminum interacts *in vitro* with phosphate to form a poorly soluble precipitate. There is evidence that this reaction also occurs *in vivo* and that aluminum at high intakes interferes with phosphate metabolism and absorption, which is consistent with the frequently observed decrease in urinary phosphorus excretion. Several cases of an osteomalacialike syndrome have been reported in subjects consuming gram quantities of aluminum in antacids over extended periods of time. These cases improved with phosphate repletion. Alfrey (1986) has emphasized that the risk of systemic aluminum toxicity, even from oral application, is greatly increased in persons with impaired renal function.

2.8.3. Aluminum in Aging and Degenerative Diseases

The preceding discussion has presented convincing evidence that parenterally administered aluminum causes a specific type of encephalopathy and osteomalacia. The oral intake of aluminum in antacids, even in relatively small amounts of 1–2 g/day, interferes with phosphorus metabolism and results in a negative calcium balance, especially when the calcium intake is low (Spencer *et al.*, 1982). The combination of aluminum-containing antacids and a low calcium intake is not rare in the elderly. Because impairment of renal function, which increases the risk of systemic aluminum toxicity, is also common in the elderly population, it is prudent for that group to limit the consumption of aluminum-containing antacids. It is not known whether aluminum ingested from normal, dietary sources represents a health risk. A 40-day study did not detect any adverse effects of a high-aluminum diet (125 mg/day) on mineral and trace element balances of human volunteers (Gregor and Baier, 1983).

3. Conclusions*

Although dietary requirements of the elderly for trace elements are not well defined, the available data do allow a tentative classification of the elements discussed above into three groups (Mertz, 1986). The first group comprises elements that are directly involved in age-related diseases and for which the adequacy of intake in the U.S. elderly population should not be taken for granted (calcium, chromium, selenium, and silicon). The second group of elements (zinc, copper, fluorine, and magnesium) is of concern in the elderly because of functions that are at least theoretically important in the protection against age-related diseases and because of uncertainties concerning the adequacy of intake. A third group consists of elements that are not known to pose nutritional problems in the elderly in the United States (manganese, iron, cobalt, molybdenum, and iodine).

The intake of food—and, therefore, of trace elements—declines with increasing age. In addition, impairment of gastric acid secretion may depress bioavailability. It is not known, however, whether these changes result in nutritional inadequacy and health risks.

In view of the uncertainties of the elderly's trace element requirements, it appears prudent to consider both overexposure and inadequate intakes as health risks, as has been demonstrated for iron. These considerations caution against self-supplementation with trace elements; they also emphasize the need for research to determine directly the nutrient requirements of the elderly.

4. References

Abdulla, M., and Svensson, D., 1979, Zinc, *Scand. J. Gastroenterol.* **14**(Suppl. 52):172–175.

Abdulla, M., Jagerstad, M., Norden, A., Qrist, I., and Svensson, S., 1977, Dietary intake of electrolytes and trace elements in the elderly, *Nutr. Metab.* **21**:41–44.

Abdulla, M., Kolar, K., and Svensson, S., 1979, Selenium, *Scand. J. Gastroenterol.* **14**(Suppl. 52):181–184.

Abraham, A. S., Sonnenblick, M., Eini, M., Shemash, O., and Batt, A. P., 1980, The effect of chromium on established atherosclerotic plaques in rabbits, *Am. J. Clin. Nutr.* **33**:2294–2298.

Aggett, P. J., Moore, J., Thorn, J. M., Delves, H. T., Cornfield, M., and Clayton, B. E., 1983, Evaluation of the trace metal supplements for a synthetic low lactose diet, *Arch. Dis. Child.* **58**:433–437.

Albanese, A. A., 1976, Nutrition and health of the elderly, *Nutr. News* **39**:5.

Alfrey, A. C., 1986, Aluminum, in: *Trace Elements in Human and Animal Nutrition, 5th ed.* Volume 2 (W. Mertz, ed.), Academic Press, New York, pp. 399–413.

Alhava, E. M., Olkkonen, H., Puittinen, J., and Nokso-Koivisto, V. M., 1977, Zinc content of human cancellous bone, *Acta Orthop. Scand.* **48**:1–4.

Anderson, R. A., 1985, Chromium requirements and needs in the elderly, in: *Handbook of Nutrition in the Aged,* (R. R. Watson, ed.) CRC Press Inc., Boca Raton, FL, pp. 137–144.

Anderson, R. A., and Bryden, N. A., 1983, Concentration, insulin potentiation and absorption of chromium in beer, *J. Agric. Food Chem.* **31**:308–311.

Anderson, R. A., and Kozlovsky, A. S., 1985, Chromium intake, absorption and excretion of subjects consuming self-selected diets, *Am. J. Clin. Nutr.* **41**:1177–1183.

*This section is by Walter Mertz.

Anderson, R. A., Polansky, M. M., Bryden, N. A., Patterson, K. Y., Veillon, C., and Glinsmann, W., 1983a, Effect of chromium supplementation of urinary Cr excretion of human subjects and correlation of Cr excretion with selected clinical parameters, *J. Nutr.* **113:**276–281.

Anderson, R. A., Polansky, M. M., Bryden, N. A., Roginski, E. E., Mertz, W., and Glinsmann, W., 1983b, Chromium supplementation of human subjects: Effects on glucose, insulin and lipid parameters, *Metabolism* **32:**894–899.

Anderson, R. A., Bryden, N. A., and Polansky, M. M., 1985, Serum chromium of human subjects: Effects of chromium supplementation and glucose, *Am. J. Clin. Nutr.* **41:**571–577.

Anderson, R. A., Polansky, M. M., Bryden, N. A., Bhathena, S. J., and Canary, J. J., 1987, Effects of supplemental chromium on patients with symptoms of reactive hypoglycemia, *Metabolism* **36:**351–355.

Ankerst, J., and Sjogren, H. O., 1982, Effect of selenium on the induction of heart fibroadinomas by adinovirus type 9 and 1,2-dimethylhydrazine-induced bowel carcinogenesis in rats, *Int. J. Cancer* **24:**707–710.

Anneren, G., Gardner, A., and Lundin, T., 1986, Increased glutathione peroxidase activity in erythrocytes in patients with Alzheimers disease/senile dementia of Alzheimer's type, *Acta Neurol. Scand.* **73:**586–589.

Anonymous, 1984, Megadose vitamin supplementation and immunological function in the elderly, *Nutr. Rev.* **42:**46–48.

Anonymous, 1986a, Nutrition and the elderly, *Food Tech.* **40:**81–88.

Anonymous, 1986b, Role of zinc in enzyme regulation and protection of essential thiol groups, *Nutr. Rev.* **44:**309–311.

Aquino, T. M., Porta, E. A., Sablan, H. M., and Dorado, R. D., 1985, Effects of selenium supplementation on hepatocarcinogenesis in rats, *Nutr. Cancer* **7:**25–36.

Araki, K., and Rifkind, J. M., 1980, Age dependent changes in osmotic hemolysis of human erythrocytes, *J. Gerontol.* **35:**499–505.

Asling, C. W., and Hurley, L. S., 1963, The influence of trace elements on the skeleton, *Clin. Orthop.* **27:**213–262.

Atkin-Thor, E., Goddard, B. W., O'Nion, J., Stephen, R. L., and Kolff, W. J., 1978, Hypogeusia and zinc depletion in chronic dialysis patients, *Am. J. Clin. Nutr.* **31:**1948–1951.

Austin, J. H., 1978, Silicon levels in human tissues, in: *Biochemistry of Silicon and Related Problems* (G. Bentz and I. Lindquist, eds.), Plenum Press, New York, pp. 255–265.

Baer, M. T., and King, J. C., 1984, Tissue zinc levels and zinc excretion during experimental zinc depletion in young men, *Am. J. Clin. Nutr.* **39:**556–570.

Bailey, L. B., Wagner, P. A., Christakis, G. J., Araujo, P. E., Appledorf, H., Davis, C. G., Masteryanni, J., and Dinning, J. S., 1979, Folacin and iron status and hematological findings in predominately black elderly persons from urban low-income households, *Am. J. Clin. Nutr.* **32:**2346–2353.

Bajpayee, D. P., 1975, Significance of plasma copper and ceruloplasmin in rheumatoid arthritis, *Ann. Rheum. Dis.* **34:**162–169.

Bales, C. W., Steinman, L. C., Freeland-Graves, J. H., Stone, J. M. and Young, R. K., 1986, The effect of age on plasma zinc uptake and taste acuity, *Am. J. Clin. Nutr.* **44:**664–669.

Barcia, P. J., 1970, Lack of acceleration of healing with zinc sulfate, *Ann. Surg.* **172:**1048–1050.

Beems, R. B., 1986, Dietary selenium and benzo(a)pyrene-induced respiratory tract tumors in hamsters, *Carcinogenesis* **7:**485–489.

Beisel, W. R., 1982, Single nutrients and immunity, *Am. J. Clin. Nutr.* **35:**417–468.

Bergman, K., and Slanina, P., 1986, Effects of dietary selenium compounds on benz(a)pyrene-induced forestomach tumors and whole-blood glutathione peroxidase activities in C_3H mice, *Anticancer Res.* **6:**785–790.

Bernstein, D. S., Sadowski, N., Hegsted, D. M., Guri, C. D., and Stare, F. J., 1966, Prevalence of osteoporosis in high- and low-fluoride areas in North Dakota, *J. A. M. A.* **198:**499–504.

Bettger, W. J., and O'Dell, B. L., 1981, A critical physiological role of zinc in the structure and function of biomembranes, *Life Sci.* **28:**1425–1438.

Bezkorovainy, A., 1980, *Biochemistry of Nonheme Iron*, Plenum Press, New York.

Birt, D. F., Julius, A. D., Runice, C. E., White, L. T., Lawson, T., and Pour, P. M., 1988, Enhancement of N-nitrosobis(2-oxopropyl)amine-induced pancreatic carinogenesis in selenium-fed Syrian golden hamsters under specific dietary conditions, *Nutr. and Cancer* **11:**21–33.

Bisby, R. H., 1975, A pulse radiolysis study of some free radical reactions with erythrocyte membranes, *Biochim. Biophys. Acta* **389:**137–143.

Bomford, A. B., and Munro, H., 1985, Transferrin and its receptor: Their roles in cell function, *Hepatology* **5:**870–875.

Borel, J. S., and Anderson, R. A., 1984, Chromium, in: *Biochemistry of the Essential Ultratrace Elements* (E. Frieden, ed.), Plenum Press, New York, pp. 175–199.

Bortner, C. A., Miller, R. D., and Arnold, R. R., 1986, Bactericidal effect of lactoferrin on *Legionella pneumophilia, Infect. Immun.* **51:**373–377.

Bothwell, T. H., Charlton, R. W., Cook, J. D., and Finch, C. A., 1979, *Iron Metabolism in Man,* Blackwell Scientific Publications, Oxford.

Bowen, H. J. M., and Peggs, A., 1984, Determination of the silicon content of food, *J. Sci. Food Agric.* **35:**1225–1229.

Brewer, R. D., Jr., Mihaldzic, N., and Dietz, A., 1967, The effect of oral zinc sulfate on the healing of decubitus ulcers in spinal cord injured patients, in: *Proceedings 16th Annual Clinical Spinal Cord Injury Conference,* Veterans Administration, Long Beach, CA, pp. 70–72.

Brown, R. O., Forloines-Lynn, S., Cross, R. E., and Heizer, W. D., 1986, Chromium deficiency after long-term total parenteral nutrition, *Dig. Dis. Sci.* **31:**661–664.

Bunker, V. W., Lawson, M. S., Delves, H. T., and Clayton, B. E., 1982, Metabolic balance studies for zinc and nitrogen in healthy elderly subjects, *Hum. Nutr. Clin. Nutr.* **36C:**213–221.

Bunker, V. W., Hinks, L. J., Lawson, M. S., and Clayton, B. E., 1984a, Assessment of zinc and copper status of healthy elderly people using metabolic balance studies and measurement of leucocyte concentrations, *Am. J. Clin. Nutr.* **40:**1096–1102.

Bunker, W., Lawson, M. S., Delves, H. T., and Clayton, B. E., 1984b, The uptake and excretion of chromium by the elderly, *Am. J. Clin. Nutr.* **39:**797–802.

Butler, R. N., and McGuire, E. A. H., 1982, Foreword, symposium on evidence relating selected vitamins and minerals to health and disease in the elderly population, *Am. J. Clin. Nutr.* **36:**977–978.

Calhoun, N. R., Smith, J. C., Jr., and Becker, K. L., 1974, The role of zinc in bone metabolism, *Clin. Orthop.* **103:**212–234.

Carlisle, E. M., 1972, Silicon: An essential element for the chick, *Science* **178:**619–621.

Carlisle, E. M., 1986, Silicon, in: *Trace Elements in Human and Animal Nutrition,* 5th ed., Volume 2 (W. Mertz, ed.), Academic Press, Orlando, pp. 373–390.

Casey, C. E., Guthrie, B. E., Friend, G. M., and Robinson, M. F., 1982, Selenium in human tissues from New Zealand, *Arch. Environ. Health* **37:**133–135.

Chandra, R. K., and Newberne, P. M. (eds.), 1977, *Nutrition, Immunity and Infection,* Plenum Press, New York.

Chandra, R. K., Joshi, P., Au, B., Woodford, G., and Chandra, S., 1982, Nutrition and immunocompetence of the elderly: Effect of short-term nutritional supplementation on cell-mediated immunity and lymphocyte subsets, *Nutr. Res.* **2:**223–232.

Chao, S. S., Kanabrocki, E. L., Moore, C. E., Oester, Y. T., Greco, J., and Von Smolinski, A., 1976, Determination of trace elements in human tissues II. Chromium in the pancreas and in raw and commercial sugar, *Appl. Spectrosc.* **30:**155–159.

Chilvers, D. C., and Hodgkinson, A., 1985, Age and sex-related variations in the distribution of copper and zinc in human plasma, *Trace Elem. Med.* **2:**22–27.

Chvapil, M., 1973, New aspects in the biological role of zinc: A stabilizer of macromolecules and biological membranes, *Life Sci.* **13:**1041–1049.

Cohen, D. I., Illowsky, B., and Linder, M., 1978, Altered copper absorption in tumor-bearing and estrogen-treated rats, *Am. J. Physiol.* **236:**E309–314.

Committee 1-5, International Union of Nutritional Sciences, 1983, Recommended dietary intakes around the world, *Nutr. Abstr. Rev. Clin. Nutr. [A]* **53:**539–1015.

Cook, J. D., and Finch, C. A., 1979, Assessing iron status of a population, *Am. J. Clin. Nutr.* **32:**2115–2119.

Csallany, A. S., Zaspel, B. J., and Ayaz, K. L., 1981, Selenium and aging, in: *Selenium in Biology and Medicine* (J. E. Spallholz, J. L. Martin, and H. E. Ganther, eds.), AVI Press, Westport, CT, pp. 118–131.

Dallman, P. R., 1974, Tissue effects of iron deficiency, in: *Iron in Biochemistry and Medicine* (A. Jacobs and M. Worwood, eds.), Academic Press, New York, pp. 437–475.

Dallman, P. R., Siimes, M. A., and Manies, E. C., 1975, Brain iron: Persistent deficiency following short-term iron deprivation in the young rat, *Br. J. Haematol.* **31**:309–215.

Dallman, P. R., Yip, R., and Johnson, C., 1984, Prevalence and causes of anemia in the United States, 1976 to 1980, *Am. J. Clin. Nutr.* **39**:437–445.

Dawson-Hughes, B., Seligson, F. H., and Hughes, V. A., 1986, Effect of calcium carbonate and hydroxyapatite on zinc and iron retention in postmenopausal women, *Am. J. Clin. Nutr.* **44**:83–88.

Deinard, A. S., List, A., Lindgren, B., Hunt, J. V., and Chang, P.-N., 1986, Cognitive deficits in iron-deficient and iron-deficient anemic children, *J. Pediatr.* **108**:681–689.

Dickson, R. C., and Tomlinson, R. H., 1967, Selenium in blood and human tissues, *Clin. Chim. Acta* **16**:311–321.

Doisy, R. J., Streeten, D. H. P., Souma, M. L., Kalafer, M. E., Rekant, S. L., and Dalakos, T. G., 1971, Metabolism of chromium^{51} in human subjects, in: *Newer Trace Element in Nutrition* (W. Mertz and W. E. Cornatzer, eds.), Marcel Dekker, New York, pp. 155–168.

Doisy, R. J., Streeten, D. H. P., Freiberg, J. M., and Schneider, A. J., 1976, Chromium metabolism in man and biochemical effects, in: *Trace Elements in Human Health and Disease,* Volume II: *Essential and Toxic Elements* (A. S. Prasad and D. Oberleas, eds.), Academic Press, New York, pp. 79–104.

Duchateau, J., Delepesse, G., Vrijens, R., and Collet, H., 1981, Beneficial effects of oral zinc supplementation on the immune response of old people, *Am. J. Med.* **70**:1001–1004.

Eckhert, C. D., 1983, Elemental concentration in ocular tissues of various species, *Exp. Eye Res.* **37**:639–647.

Edgerton, V. R., Ohira, Y., Hettiarachchi, J., Senewiratne, B., Gardner, G. W., and Barnard, R. J., 1981, Elevation of hemoglobin and work tolerance in iron-deficient subjects, *J. Nutr. Sci. Vitaminol.* **27**:77–86.

Elahi, V. K., Elahi, D., Andres, R., Tobin, J. D., Butler, M. G., and Norris, A. H., 1983, A logitudinal study of nutritional intake in men, *J. Gerontol.* **38**:162–180.

Ellis, N., Lloyd, B., Lloyd, R. S., and Clayton, B. E., 1984, Selenium and vitamin E in relation to risk factors for coronary heart disease, *J. Clin. Pathol.* **37**:200–206.

Fielden, E. M., and Rotilio, G., 1984, The structure and mechanisms of Cu/Zn superoxide dismutase, in: *CRC Copper Proteins and Copper Enzymes,* Volume II (R. Lontie, ed.), CRC Press, Boca Raton, FL, pp. 27–63.

Fields, M., Ferretti, R. J., Smith, J. C., and Reiser, S., 1983, Effect of copper deficiency on metabolism and mortality in rats fed sucrose or starch diets, *J. Nutr.* **113**:1335–1345.

Fields, M., Ferretti, R. J., Smith, J. C., and Reiser, S., 1984, The interaction of type of dietary carbohydrates with copper deficiency, *Am. J. Clin. Nutr.* **39**:289–295.

Fields, M., Holbrook, J., Scholfield, D., Rose, A., Smith, J. C., and Reiser, S., 1986, Development of copper deficiency in rats fed fructose or starch: Weekly measurements of copper indices in blood, *Proc. Soc. Exp. Biol. Med.* **181**:120–124.

Flint, D. M., Wahlqvist, M. L., Smith, T. J., and Parish, A. E., 1981, Zinc and protein status in the elderly, *J. Hum. Nutr.* **35**:287–295.

Fosmire, G. J., Manuel, P. A., and Smiciklas-Wright, H., 1984, Dietary intakes and zinc status of an elderly rural population, *J. Nutr. Elderly* **4**:19–30.

Fraker, P. J., DePasquale-Jardieu, P., Zwickl, C. M., and Luecke, R. W., 1978, Regeneration of T-cell helper function in zinc-deficient adult mice, *Proc. Natl. Acad. Sci. U.S.A.* **75**:5660–5664.

Fraker, P. J., Gershwin, M. E., Good, R. A., and Prasad, A., 1986, Interrelationship between zinc and immune function, *Fed. Proc.* **45**:1474–1479.

Freund, H., Atamian, S., and Fischer, J. E., 1979, Chromium deficiency during total parenteral nutrition, *J. A.M.A.* **241**:496–498.

Garry, P. J., Goodwin, J. S., Hunt, W. C., Hooper, E. M., and Leonard, A. G., 1982, Nutritional status in a healthy elderly population: Dietary and supplemental intakes, *Am. J. Clin. Nutr.* **36**:319–331.

Gershwin, M. E., Beach, R., and Hurley, L., 1983, Trace metals, aging, and immunity, *J. Am. Geriatr. Soc.* **31**:374–378.

Gibson, R. S., Anderson, B. M., and Sabry, J. H., 1983, The trace metal status of a group of post-menopausal vegetarians, *J. Am. Diet. Assoc.* **82**:246–250.

Gibson, R. S., Martinez, O. B., and MacDonald, A. C., 1985, The zinc, copper, and selenium status of a selected sample of Canadian elderly women, *J. Gerontol.* **40**:296–302.

Glinsmann, W. H., and Mertz, W., 1966, Effect of trivalent chromium on glucose tolerance, *Metabolism* **15:**510–520.

Golden, M. H. N., 1982, Trace elements in human nutrition, *Hum. Nutr. Clin. Nutr.* **36C:**185–202.

Goldstein, I. M., Kaplan, H. B., Edelson, H. S., and Weissmann, G., 1982, Ceruloplasmin: An acute phase reactant that scavengers oxygen-derived free-radicals, *Ann. N.Y. Acad. Sci.* **389:**368–373.

Good, R. A., Fernandes, G., Garofalo, J. A., Cunningham-Rundles, C., Iwata, T., and West, A., 1982, zinc and immunity, in: *Clinical, Biochemical, and Nutritional Aspects of Trace Elements, Current Topics in Nutrition and Disease,* Volume 6 (A. S. Prasad, ed.), Alan R. Liss, New York, pp. 189–202.

Goodwin, J. S., Goodwin, J. M., and Garry, P. J., 1983, Association between nutritional status and cognitive functioning in a healthy elderly population, *J.A.M.A.* **249:**2917–2921.

Greaves, M. W., and Skillen, A. W., 1970, Effects of long-continued ingestion of zinc sulphate in patients with venous leg ulceration, *Lancet* **2:**889–891.

Greenberg, S. R., 1975, The pathogenesis of hypophyseal fibrosis in aging: Its relationship to tissue iron deposition, *J. Gerontol.* **30:**531–538.

Greger, J. L., 1977, Dietary intake and nutritional status in regard to zinc of institutionalized aged, *J. Gerontol.* **32:**549–553.

Greger, J. L., and Baier, M. J., 1983, Effect of dietary aluminum on mineral metabolism of adult males, *Am. J. Clin. Nutr.* **38:**411–419.

Greger, J. L., and Geissler, A. H., 1978, Effect of zinc supplementation on taste acuity of the aged, *Am. J. Clin. Nutr.* **31:**633–637.

Greger, J. L., and Sciscoe, B. S., 1977, Zinc nutriture of elderly participants in an urban feeding program, *J. Am. Diet. Assoc.* **70:**37–41.

Guidi, G., Schiavon, R., Sheiban, I., and Perona, G., 1986, Platelet glutathione peroxidase activity is impaired in patients with coronary heart disease, *Scand. J. Clin. Lab. Invest.* **46:**549–551.

Gurson, C. T., and Saner, G., 1971, Effect of chromium on glucose utilization in marasmic protein–calorie malnutrition, *Am. J. Clin. Nutr.* **24:**1313–1319.

Haeger, K., Lanner, E., and Magnusson, P. O., 1972, Oral zinc sulphate in the treatment of venous leg ulcers, *J. Vasc. Dis.* **1:**62–69.

Hafeman, D. G., and Hoekstra, W. G., 1977, Lipid peroxidation *in vivo* during vitamin E and selenium deficiency in the rat as monitored by ethane evolution, *J. Nutr.* **107:**666–672.

Halliwell, B., and Gutteridge, J. M. C., 1986, Iron and free radical reactions: Two aspects of antioxidant protection, *Trends Biochem. Sci.* **11:**372–375.

Halsted, J. A., and Smith, J. C., Jr., 1970, Plasma zinc in health and disease, *Lancet* **1:**322–324.

Halsted, J. A., Smith, J. C., Jr., and Irwin, M. I., 1974, A conspectus of research on zinc requirements of man, *J. Nutr.* **104:**345–378.

Hambidge, K. M., 1971, Chromium nutrition in the mother and the growing child, in: *Newer Trace Elements in Nutrition* (W. Mertz and W. E. Cornatzer, eds.), Marcel Dekker, New York, pp. 169–194.

Hambidge, K. M., Hambidge, C., Jacobs, M., and Bauon, J., 1972, Low levels of zinc in hair, anorexia, poor growth and hypogeusia in children, *Pediatr. Res.* **6:**868–874.

Hambidge, K. M., Casey, C. E., and Krebs, N. F., 1986, Zinc, in: *Trace Elements in Human and Animal Nutrition,* 5th ed., Volume 2 (W. Mertz, ed.), Academic Press, New York pp. 1–137.

Harman, D., 1956, Aging: A theory based on free radical and radiation chemistry, *J. Gerontol.* **11:**298–300.

Harman, D., 1978, Free radical theory of aging, nutritional implications, *Age* **1:**145–152.

Harman, D., 1986, Free radical theory of aging: Role of free radicals in the origination and evaluation of life, aging and disease processes, in: *Free Radicals, Aging, and Degenerative Diseases* (J. E. Johnson, D. Harman, R. Walford, and I. Miguel, eds.), Alan R. Liss, Inc., New York, pp. 3–50.

Harrison, D. E., 1975, Defective erythropoietic responses of aged mice not improved by young marrow, *J. Gerontol.* **30:**286–288.

Health & Welfare Canada, 1975, *Report on the Relationship between Income and Nutrition,* Bureau of Nutritional Sciences Health Protection Branch, Ottawa.

Helgeland, K., Haider, T., and Jonsen, J., 1982, Copper and zinc in human serum in Norway: Relationship to geography, sex and age, *Scand. J. Clin. Lab. Invest.* **42:**35–41.

Hershey, C. O., Hershey, L. A., Wongmongkolrit, T., Varnes, A. W., and Breslan, D., 1985, Trace element content of brain in Alzheimer disease and aging, *Trace Elem. in Med.* **2:**40–43.

Hetzel, B. S., and Maberly, G. F., 1986, Iodine, in: *Trace Elements in Human and Animal Nutrition,* 5th ed. (W. Mertz, ed.), Academic Press, New York, pp. 139–208.

Hirai, S., Okamoto, K., and Morimatsu, M., 1982, Lipid peroxides in the aging process, in: *Lipid Peroxides in Biology and Medicine* (K. Yage, ed.), Academic Press, New York, p. 305.

Holden, J. M., Wolf, W. F., and Mertz, W., 1979, Zinc and copper in self-selected diets, *J. Am. Diet. Assoc.* **75:**23–28.

Honda, S., and Matsuo, M., 1980, The sensitivity to hyperbaric oxygen of human diploid fibroblasts during aging *in vitro, Mech. Ageing Dev.* **12:**31–41.

Hopkins, L. L., Jr., Ransome-Kuti, O., and Majaj, A. S., 1968, Improvement of impaired carbohydrate metabolism by chromium (III) in malnourished infants, *Am. J. Clin. Nutr.* **21:**203–211.

Hutton, C. W., and Hayes-Davis, R. B., 1983, Assessment of the zinc nutritional status of selected elderly subjects, *J. Am. Diet. Assoc.* **82:**148–153.

Ibraham, N. G., Lutton, J. D., and Levere, R. D., 1983, Erythroid colony development as a function of age: The role of marrow cellular heme, *J. Gerontol.* **38:**13–18.

Ip, C., 1985, Selenium inhibition of chemical carcinogenesis, *Fed. Proc.* **44:**2573–2578.

Ip, C., 1986, The chemopreventive role of selenium in carcinogenesis, *J. Am. Coll. Toxicol.* **5:**7–20.

Isenberg, I., 1964, Free radicals in tissues, *Physiol. Rev.* **44:**487–517.

Iyengar, G. V., 1985, *Concentrations of 15 Trace Elements in Some Selected Adult Human Tissues and Body Fluids of Clinical Interest from Several Countries: Results from a Pilot Study for the Establishment of Reference Values (February 1985),* Institute of Medicine, Juelich Nuclear Research Center, Juelich, FRG, p. 20.

Jacob, R. A., Russell, R. M., and Sandstead, H. H., 1985, Zinc and copper nutrition in aging, in: *CRC Handbook of Nutrition in the Aged* (R. R. Watson, ed.), CRC Press, Boca Raton, FL, pp. 77–88.

Jacobs, A., and Worwood, M. (eds.), 1980, *Iron in Biochemistry and Medicine II,* Academic Press, New York.

Jansen, C., and Harrill, I., 1977, Intakes and serum levels of protein and iron for 70 elderly women, *Am. J. Clin. Nutr.* **30:**1414–1422.

Jeejeebhoy, K. N., Chu, R. C., Marliss, E. B., Greenberg, G. R., and Bruce-Robertson, A., 1977, Chromium deficiency, glucose intolerance, and neuropathy reversed by chromium supplementation in a patient receiving long-term total parenteral nutrition, *Am. J. Clin. Nutr.* **30:**531–538.

Katzman, R., 1976, The prevalence and malignancy of Alzheimer disease: A major killer, *Arch. Neurol.* **33:**217–220.

Keilin, D., and Mann, T., 1939, Carbonic anhydrase, *Nature* **144:**442–443.

Kelsay, J. L., Behall, K. M., and Prather, E. S., 1979, Effect of fiber from fruits and vegetables on metabolic responses of human subjects, II. Calcium, magnesium, iron, and silicon balances, *J. Sci. Food Agric.* **32:**1876–1880.

King, J. C., Raynolds, W. L., and Margen, S., 1978, Absorption of stable isotopes of iron, copper and zinc during oral contraceptive use, *Am J. Clin. Nutr.* **31:**1198–1203.

Klevay, L. M., 1970, Hair as a biopsy material, I. Assessment of zinc nutriture, *Am. J. Clin. Nutr.* **23:**284–289.

Klevay, L. M., 1983, Copper and ischemic heart disease, *Biol. Trace Elem. Res.* **5:**245–286.

Klevay, L. M., 1984, The role of copper, zinc and other chemical elements in ischemic heart disease, in: *Metabolism of Trace Metals in Man,* Volume 1 (O. W. Rennert and W. Y. Chan, eds.), CRC Press, Boca Raton, FL, pp. 129–157.

Klevay, L. M., Inman, L., Johnson, L. K., Lawler, M., Mahalko, J. R., Milne, D. B., Lukaski, H. C., Boloncuk, W., and Sandstead, H. H., 1984, Increased cholesterol in plasma in a young man during experimental copper depletion, *Metabolism* **33:**1112–1118.

Kohrs, M. B., O'Neal, R., Preston, A., Eklund, D., and Abrahams, O., 1978, Nutritional status of elderly residents in Missouri, *Am. J. Clin. Nutr.* **31:**2186–2197.

Koivistoinen, P. (ed.), 1980, Mineral element composition of Finnish foods: N, K, Ca, Mg, P, S, Fe, Cu, Mn, Zn, Mo, Co, Ni, Cr, F, Se, Si, Rb, Al, B, Br, Hg, As, Cd, Pb and Ash, *Acta Agric. Scand. [Suppl]* **22:**1–171.

Koivistoinen, P., and Huttunen, J. K., 1986, Selenium food and nutrition in Finland, an overview on research and action, *Ann. Clin. Res.* **18:**13–17.

Kozlovsky, A. S., Moser, P. B., Reiser, S., and Anderson, R. A., 1986, Effects of diets high in simple sugars on urinary chromium losses, *Metabolism* **35:**515–518.

Kramer, L., Osis, D., Wiatrowski, E., and Spencer, H., 1974, Dietary fluoride in different areas in the United States, *Am. J. Clin. Nutr.* **27**:590–594.

Krasinski, S. D., Russell, R. M., Samloft, J. M., Jacob, R. A., Dallal, G. E., McGandy, R. B., and Hartz, S. C., 1986, Fundic atrophic gastritis in an elderly population: Effect on hemoglobin and several serum nutritional indicators, *J. Am. Geriatr. Soc. (in press).*

Krishnamachari, K. A. V. R., 1987, Fluorine in: *Trace Elements in Human and Animal Nutrition,* 5th ed. Volume 1 (W. Mertz, ed.), Academic Press, New York, pp. 365–415.

Kumpulainen, J. T., Wolf, W. R., Veillon, C., and Mertz, W., 1979, Determination of chromium in selected United States diets, *J. Agric. Food Chem.* **27**:490–494.

LaBella, F. S., and Paul, G., 1965, Structure of collagen from human tendon as influenced by age and sex, *J. Gerontol.* **20**:54–59.

LaBella, F. S., Vivian, S., and Thornhill, D. P., 1966, Amino acid composition of human aortic elastin as influenced by age, *J. Gerontol.* **21**:550–555.

Lane, H. W., Warren, D. C., Taylor, B. J., and Stool, E., 1983, Blood selenium and glutathione peroxidase levels and dietary selenium of free-living and institutionalized elderly subjects, *Proc. Soc. Exp. Biol. Med.* **173**:87–95.

Le Boeuf, R. A., Laishes, B. A., and Hoekstra, W. G., 1985, Effects of dietary selenium concentration on the development of enzyme-altered liver foci and hepatocellular carcinoma induced by diethylnitrosamine or N-acetylaminofluorene in rats, *Cancer Res.* **45**:5489–5495.

Leibel, R. L., Greenbield, D. B., and Pollitt, E., 1979, Iron deficiency: Behavior and brain biochemistry, in: *Human Nutrition—A Comprehensive Treatise,* Volume 1: *Nutrition, Pre- and Postnatal Development* (M. Winick, ed.), Plenum Press, New York, pp. 383–439.

Letendre, E. D., 1985, The importance of iron in the pathogenesis of infection and neoplasia, *Trends Biochem. Sci.* **10**:166–168.

Levander, O. A., 1975, Selenium and chromium in human nutrition, *J. Am. Diet. Assoc.* **66**:338–344.

Levander, O. A., 1983, Considerations in the design of selenium bioavailability studies, *Fed. Proc.* **42**:1721–1725.

Levander, O. A., 1985, Considerations on the assessment of selenium status, *Fed. Proc.* **44**:2579–2783.

Levander, O. A., 1986a, Selenium, in: *Trace Elements in Human and Animal Nutrition Fifth Edition,* Volume 2 (W. Mertz, ed.), Academic Press, Orlando, FL, pp. 209–279.

Levander, O. A., 1986b, The need for measures of selenium status, *J. Am. Coll. Toxicol.* **5**:37–44.

Levander, O. A., 1987, A global view of human selenium nutrition, *Annu. Rev. Nutr.* **7**:227–250.

Levander, O. A., and Burk, R. F., 1986, Report on the 1986 A.S.P.E.N. research workshop on selenium in clinical nutrition, *J. Parent. Ent. Nutr.* **10**:545–549.

Levander, O. A., and Morris, V. C., 1984, Dietary selenium levels needed to maintain balance in North American adults consuming self-selected diets, *Am. J. Clin. Nutr.* **39**:809–815.

Levander, O. A., Sutherland, B. M., Morris, V. C., and King, J. C., 1981, Selenium balance in young men during selenium depletion and repletion, *Am. J. Clin. Nutr.* **34**:2662–2669.

Lindeman, R. D., 1982, Mineral metabolism in the aging and the aged, *J. Am. Coll. Nutr.* **1**:49–73.

Lindeman, R. D., Clark, M. L., and Colmore, J. P., 1971, Influence of age and sex on plasma and red-cell zinc concentrations, *J. Gerontol.* **26**:358–363.

Loeper, J., Loeper, J., and Fragny, M., 1978, The physiological role of the silicon and its antiatheromatous action, in: *Biochemistry of Silicon and Related Problems* (G. Bendz and I. Lindquist, eds.), Plenum Press, New York, pp. 281–306.

Lombeck, I., Kasperek, K., Feinendegen, L. E., and Bremer, H. J., 1981, Low selenium state in children, in: *Selenium in Biology and Medicine* (J. E. Spallholz, J. L. Martin, and H. E. Ganther, eds.), AVI Press, Westport, CT, pp. 269–282.

Loria, A., Hershko, C., and Konijn, A. M., 1979, Serum ferritin in an elderly population, *J. Gerontol.* **34**:521–524.

Luo, X., Wei, H., Yang, C., Xing, J., Qiao, C., Feng, Y., Liu, J., Lin, Z., Wu, Q., Liu, Y., Stoecker, B. J., Spallholz, J. E., and Yang, S. P., 1985, Selenium intake and metabolic balance of 10 men from a low selenium area of China, *Am. J. Clin. Nutr.* **42**:31–37.

Lutz, R. E., 1926, The normal occurrence of zinc in biologic materials: A review of the literature, and a study of the normal distribution of zinc in the rat, cat, and man, *J. Indust. Hyg.* **8**:177–207.

Lynch, S. R., 1984, Iron, in: *Absorption and Malabsorption of Mineral Nutrients* (N. R. Solomons and I. H. Rosenberg, eds.), Alan R. Liss, New York, pp. 89–124.

Lynch, S. R., Finch, C. A., Monsen, E. R., and Cook, J. D., 1982, Iron status of elderly Americans, *Am. J. Clin. Nutr.* **36:**1032–1045.

Macdougall, L. G., Anderson, R., McNab, G. M., and Katz, J., 1975, The immune response in iron-deficient children: impaired cellular defense mechanisms with altered humoral components, *J. Pediatr.* **86:**833–843.

Mahajan, S. K., Prasad, A. S., Lambujon, J., Abbasi, A. A., Briggs, W. A., and McDonald, F. D., 1980, Improvement of uremic hypogeusia by zinc: A double blind study, *Am. J. Clin. Nutr.* **33:**1517–1521.

Martinez, O. B., MacDonald, A. C., Gibson, R. S., and Bourn, D., 1985, Dietary chromium and effect on chromium supplementation on glucose tolerance of elderly Canadian women, *Nutr. Red.* **5:**609–620.

Marx, J. J. M., 1979, Normal iron absorption and decreased red cell iron uptake in the aged, *Blood* **53:**204–211.

Mason, K. E., 1979, A conspectus of research on copper metabolism and requirements of man, *J. Nutr.* **109:**1979.

Massie, H. R., Colacicco, J. R., and Aiello, V. R., 1979, Changes with age in copper and ceruloplasmin in serum from humans and C57BL/6J mice, *Age* **2:**97–105.

McAdam, P. A., Smith, D. K., Feldman, E. B., and Hames, C., 1984, Effect of age, sex and race on selenium status of healthy residents of Augusta, Georgia, *Biol. Trace Elem. Res.* **6:**3–9.

McCord, J. M., and Fridovich, I., 1969, Superoxide dismutase. An enzymic function for erythrocuprein (hemocuprein), *J. Biol. Chem.* **224:**6049–6053.

McGandy, R. B., Barrows, C. H., Spanias, A., Meredith, A., Stone, J. L., and Norris, A. H., 1966, Nutrient intakes and energy expenditure in men of different ages, *J. Gerontol.* **21:**581–587.

McGandy, R. B., Russell, R. M., Hartz, S. C., Jacob, R. A., Tannenbaum, S., Peters, H., Sahyon, N., and Otradovec, C. L., 1986, Nutritional status survey of healthy noninstitutionalized elderly: Energy and nutrient intakes from three-day diet records and nutrient supplements, *Nutr. Res.* **6:**785–798.

McMurray, D. N., 1982, Iron deficiency and secretory immunity, *Nutr. Res.* **2:**639–640.

Medina, D., 1986, Mechanisms of selenium inhibition of tumorigenesis, *J. Am. Coll. Toxicol.* **5:**21–27.

Mertz, W., 1969, Chromium occurrence and function in biological systems, *Physiol. Rev.* **49:**163–239.

Mertz, W., 1983, Chromium: An ultra-trace element, *Chim. Script.* **21:**71–83.

Mertz, W., 1986, Trace elements and the needs of the elderly, in: *Nutrition and Aging* (M. L. Hutchinson and H. N. Munro, eds.), Academic Press, New York, pp. 71–83.

Meydani, M., Verdon, C. P., and Blumberg, J. B., 1985, Effect of vitamin E, selenium and age on lipid peroxidation events in rat cerebrum, *Nutr. Res.* **5:**1227–1236.

Miller, L., Mills, B. J., Blotcky, A. J., and Lindeman, R. D., 1983, Red blood cell and serum selenium concentrations as influenced by age and selected diseases, *J. Am. Coll. Nutr.* **4:**331–341.

Milman, N., Andersen, H. C., and Pedersen, N. S., 1986, Serum ferritin and iron status in "healthy" elderly individuals, *Scand. J. Clin. Lab. Invest.* **46:**19–26.

Milner, J. A., 1985, Effect of selenium on virally induced and transplantable tumor models, *Fed. Proc.* **44:**2568–2572.

Monsen, E. R., Hallberg, L., Layrisse, M., Hegsted, D. M., Cook, J. D., Mertz, W., and Finch, C. A., 1978, Estimation of available dietary iron, *Am. J. Clin. Nutr.* **31:**134–141.

Morgan, E. H., 1974, Transferrin and transferrin iron, in: *Iron in Biochemistry and Medicine* (A. Jacobs and M. Worwood, eds.), Academic Press, New York, pp. 30–71.

Morgan, J. M., 1972, Hepatic chromium content of diabetic subjects *Metab. Clin. Exp.* **21:**313–316.

Munro, H. N., 1980, Major gaps in nutrient allowances, *J. Am. Diet. Assoc.* **76:**137–141.

Munro, H. N., 1985, Nutrient needs and nutritional status in relation to aging, *Drug Nutr. Interact.* **4:**55–74.

Munro, H. N., and Linder, M. C., 1978, Ferritin: Structure, biosynthesis, and role in iron metabolism, *Physiol. Rev.* **58:**317–396.

Myers, M. B., and Cherry, G., 1971, Pathophysiology and treatment of stasis ulcers of the leg, *Am. Surg.* **37:**167–174.

National Research Council, 1980, *Recommended Dietary Allowances*, 9th ed. National Academy of Sciences, Washington.

Newman, H. A. I., Leighton, R. F., Lanese, R. R., and Freedland, N. A., 1978, Serum chromium and angiographically determined coronary artery disease, *Clin. Chem.* **24:**541–544.

Oberley, L. M., Oberley, T. D., and Buettner, G. R., 1980, Cell differentiation, aging and cancer. The possible roles of superoxide and superoxide dismutases, *Med. Hypoth.* **6**:249–253.

Offenbacher, E. G., and Pi-Sunyer, F. X., 1980, Beneficial effect of chromium-rich yeast on glucose tolerance and blood lipids in elderly subjects, *Diabetes* **29**:919–925.

Offenbacher, E. G., and Pi-Sunyer, F. X., 1983, Temperature and pH effects on the release of chromium from stainless steel into water and fruit juices, *J. Agric. Food Chem.* **31**:89–92.

Offenbacher, E. G., Rinko, C. J., and Pi-Sunyer, F. X., 1985, The effects of inorganic chromium and brewer's yeast on glucose tolerance, plasma lipids and plasma chromium in elderly subjects, *Am. J. Clin. Nutr.* **42**:454–461.

Ohira, Y., Edgerton, V. R., Gardner, G. W., Gunawardena, K. A., Senewiratne, B., and Ikawa, S., 1981, Work capacity after iron treatment as a function of hemoglobin and iron deficiency, *J. Nutr. Sci. Vitaminol.* **27**:87–96.

Oski, F. A., 1979, The nonhematologic manifestations of iron deficiency, *Am. J. Dis. Child.* **133**:315–322.

Palmer, I. S., Olson, O. E., Ketterling, L. M., and Shank, L. E., 1983, Selenium intake and urinary excretion in persons living near a high selenium area, *J. Am. Dietet. Assoc.* **82**:511–515.

Palti, H., Meijer, A., and Adler, B., 1985, Learning achievement and behavior at school of anemic and non-anemic infants, *Early Hum. Dev.* **10**:217–223.

Pilch, S. M., and Senti, F. R., 1985, Analysis of zinc data from the Second National Health and Nutrition Examination Survey (NHANES II), *J. Nutr.* **115**:1393–1397.

Pinto, R. E., and Bartley, W., 1969a, The effect of age and sex on glutathione reductase and glutathione peroxidase activities and on aerobic glutathione oxidation in rat liver homogenates, *Biochem. J.* **112**:109–113.

Pinto, R. E., and Bartley, W., 1969b, The nature of the sex-linked differences in glutathione peroxidase activity and aerobic oxidation of glutathione in male and female rat liver, *Biochem. J.* **115**:449–455.

Pollitt, E., Soemantri, A. G., Yunis, F., and Scrimshaw, N. S., 1985, Cognitive effects of iron-deficiency anaemia, *Lancet* **1**:158.

Pories, W. J., and Strain, W. H., 1966, Zinc and wound healing, in: *Zinc Metabolism* (A. S. Prasad, ed.), Charles C Thomas, Springfield, IL, pp. 378–394.

Rao, K. M., Schwartz, S. A., and Good, R. A., 1979, Age-dependent effect of zinc on the transformation response of human lymphocytes to mitogens, *Cell. Immunol.* **42**:270–278.

Recommended Nutrient Intakes for Canadians, 1983, Department of National Health and Welfare, Canadian Government Printing Centre, Ottawa.

Reddy, B. S., and Tanaka, T., 1986, Interactions of selenium deficiency, vitamin E, polyunsaturated fat, and saturated fat on azoxymethane-induced colon carcinogenesis in male F344 rats, *J. Natl. Cancer Inst.* **76**:1157–1162.

Reiser, S., 1985, Effects of dietary sugars, *Nutr. Health* **3**:203–216.

Reiser, S., Ferretti, R. J., Fields, M., and Smith, J. C., 1983, Role of dietary fructose in the enhancement of mortality and biochemical changes associated with copper deficiency in rats, *Am. J. Clin. Nutr.* **38**:214–222.

Reiser, S., Smith, J. C., Mertz, W., Holbrook, J., Scholfield, D. J., Powell, A. S., Canfield, W. K., and Canary, J. J., 1985, Indices of copper status in humans consuming a typical American diet containing either fructose or starch *Am. J. Clin. Nutr.* **42**:242–251.

Reizenstein, P., Ljunggren, G., Smedby, B., Agenas, I., and Penchansky, M., 1979, Overprescribing iron tablets to elderly people in Sweden, *Br. Med. J.* **2**:962–963.

Riggs, B. L., Seeman, E., Hodgson, S. F., Taves, D. R., and O'Fallon, W. M., 1982, Effect of the fluoride/calcium regimen on the vertebral fracture occurrence in postmenopausal osteoporosis, *N. Engl. J. Med.* **306**:446–450.

Robinson, J. R., Robinson, M. F., Levander, O. A., and Thomson, C. D., 1985, Urinary excretion of selenium by New Zealand and North American human subjects on differing intakes, *Am. J. Clin. Nutr.* **41**:1023–1031.

Robinson, M. F., and Thomson, L. D., 1983, The role of selenium in the diet, *Nutr. Abstr. Rev. Clin. Nutr. [A]* **53**:3–26.

Robinson, M. F., Godfrey, P. J., Thomson, C. D., Rea, H. M., and Van Rij A. M., 1979, Blood selenium and glutathione peroxidase activity in normal subjects and in surgical patients with and without cancer in New Zealand, *Am. J. Clin. Nutr.* **32**:1477–1485.

Robinson, M. F., Campbell, D. R., Sutherland, W. H. F., Herbison, G. P., Paulin, J. M., and Simpson, F. O., 1983, Selenium and risk factors for cardiovascular disease in New Zealand, *N.Z. Med. J.* **96**:755–757.

Rosson, J. W., Foster, K. J., Walton, R. J., Monro, P. P., Taylor, T. G., and Alberti, K. G. M., 1979, Hair chromium concentrations in adult insulin-treated diabetics, *Clin. Chim. Acta* **93**:299–304.

Salonen, J. T., and Huttunen, J. K., 1986, Selenium in cardiovascular diseases, *Ann. Clin. Res.* **18**:30–35.

Sandstead, H. H., Henriksen, L. K., Greger, J. L., Prasad, A. S., and Good, R. A., 1982, Zinc nutriture in the elderly in relation to taste acuity, immune response, and wound healing, *Am. J. Clin. Nutr.* **36**:1046–1059.

Schneider, E. L., and Reed, J. D., 1985, Life extension, *N. Engl. J. Med.* **312**:1159–1168.

Schock, N. W., 1970, Physiologic aspects of aging, *J. Am. Diet. Assoc.* **56**:491–496.

Schoene, N. W., Morris, V. C., and Levander, O. A., 1986, Altered arachidonic acid metabolism in platelets and aortas from selenium-deficient rats, *Nutr. Res.* **6**:75–83.

Schroeder, H. A., 1971, Losses of vitamins and trace minerals resulting from processing and preservation of foods, *Am. J. Clin. Nutr.* **24**:562–573.

Schroeder, H. A., Balassa, J. J., and Tipton, I. H., 1962, Abnormal trace metals in man—chromium, *J. Chron. Dis.* **15**:941–964.

Schroeder, H. A., Nason, A. P., and Tipton, I. H., 1966, Essential trace metals in man: Copper, *J. Chron. Dis.* **19**:1007–1034.

Schroeder, H. A., Nason, A. P., Tipton, I. H., and Balassa, J. J., 1967, Essential trace metals in man: Zinc. Relation to environmental cadmium, *J. Chron. Dis.* **20**:179–210.

Schroeder, H. A., Balassa, J. J., and Tipton, I. H., 1970, Essential trace metals in man: Molybdenum, *J. Chron. Dis.* **23**:481–499.

Schwarz, K., and Milne, D. B., 1972a, Fluorine requirement for growth in the rat, *Bioinorg. Chem.* **1**:331–338.

Schwarz, K., and Milne, D. B., 1972b, Growth-promoting effects of silicon in rats, *Nature* **239**:333–334.

Schwarz, K., Ricci, B. A., Punsar, S., and Karvonen, M. J., 1977, Inverse relation of silicon in drinking water and atherosclerosis in Finland, *Lancet* **1**:538–539.

Scrimshaw, N. S., 1966, Synergistic and antagonistic interaction of nutrition and infections, *Fed. Proc.* **25**:1679–1681.

Selikoff, I. J., 1978, Carcinogenic potential of silica compounds, in: *Biochemistrv of Silicon and Related Problems* (G. Bendz and I. Lindquist, eds.), Plenum Press, New York, pp. 281–306.

Sharma, J. C., and Roy, S. N., 1984, Value of serum ferritin as an index of iron deficiency in elderly anemic patients, *Age Aging* **13**:248–250.

Sherman, A. R., 1984, Iron, infection, and immunity, in: *Nutrition, Disease Resistance, and Immune Function* (R. R. Watson, ed.), Marcel Dekker, New York, pp. 251–266.

Shock, N. W., 1970, Physiologic aspects of aging, *J. Am. Diet. Assoc.* **56**:491–496.

Simonen, O., and Laitinen, O., 1985, Does fluoridation of drinking water prevent bone fragility and osteoporosis? *Lancet* **2**:432–434.

Simonoff, M., Llabador, Y., Hamon, C., Piers, A. M., and Simonoff, G. N., 1984, Low plasma chromium in patients with coronary artery and heart diseases, *Biol. Trace Elem. Res.* **6**:431–439.

Smith, D. K., Teague, R. J., McAdam, P. A., Feldman, D. S., and Feldman, E. B., 1986, Selenium status of malnourished hospitalized patients, *J. Am. Coll. Nutr.* **5**:243–252.

Smith, J. C., 1987, Methods of trace element research, in: *Trace Elements in Human and Animal Nutrition,* 5th ed., Volume 1 (W. Mertz, ed.), Academic Press, New York, pp. 21–56.

Smith, J. C., Jr., and Hsu, J. M., 1982, Trace elements in aging research: Emphasis on zinc, copper, chromium, and selenium, in: *Nutritional Approaches to Aging Research* (G. B. Moment, ed.), CRC Press, Boca Raton, FL, pp. 119–134.

Smith, J. C., Jr., and Hsu, J. M., 1984, Parameters of zinc, copper, chromium, and selenium metabolism in humans of different ages, in: *Nutrition in Gerontology* (J. M. Ordy and D. Harman, eds.), Raven Press, New York, pp. 141–166.

Solomons, N. W., 1981, Nutrition in the nineteen eighties. Constraints on our knowledge, in: *Zinc and Copper in Human Nutrition* (N. Selvey and P. L. White, eds.), Alan R. Liss, New York, pp. 97–127.

Sparrow, D., Rowe, J. W., and Silbert, J. E., 1981, Cross-sectional and longitudinal changes in the erythrocyte sedimentation rate in men, *J. Gerentol.* **36**:180–184.

Spencer, H., Kramer, L., Osis, D., and Wiatrowski, E., 1975, Excretion of retained fluoride in man, *J. Appl. Physiol.* **38:**282–287.

Spencer, H., Kramer, L., Norris, C., and Osis, D., 1982, Effect of small doses of aluminum-containing antacids on calcium and phosphorus metabolism, *Am. J. Clin. Nutr.* **36:**32–40.

Stadtman, T. C., 1981, Bacterial selenoenzymes and seleno-tRNAs, in: *Selenium in Biology and Medicine* (J. E. Spallholz, J. L. Martin, and H. E. Ganther, eds.), AVI Press, Westport, CT, pp. 203–208.

Stead, N. W., Leonard, S., and Carroll, R., 1985, Effect of selenium supplementation on selenium balance in the dependent elderly, *Am. J. Med. Sci.* **290:**228–233.

Stewart, M. L. McDonald, J. T., Levy, A. S., Schucker, R. E., and Henderson, D. P., 1985, Vitamin/mineral supplement use: A telephone survey of adults in the United States, *J. Am. Diet. Assoc.* **85:**1585–1590.

Stiedemann, M., and Harrill, I., 1980, Relation of immunocompetence to selected nutrients in elderly women, *Nutr. Rep. Int.* **21:**931–942.

Stout, R. W., 1977, The relationship of abnormal circulating insulin levels to atherosclerosis, *Atherosclerosis* **27:**1–13.

Sunde, R. A., and Hoekstra, W. G., 1980, Structure, synthesis and function of glutathione peroxidase, *Nutr. Rev.* **38:**265–273.

Suskind, R. M. (ed.), 1977, *Malnutrition and the Immune Response: Kroc Foundation Series,* Volume 7, Raven Press, New York.

Tappel, A. L., 1973, Lipid peroxidation damage to cell components, *Fed. Proc.* **32:**1870–1874.

Terry, R. D., 1976, A brief and selective review, *Arch. Neurol.* **33:**1–5.

Thimaya, S., and Ganapathy, S. N., 1982, Selenium in human hair in relation to age, diet, pathological conditions and serum levels, *Sci. Total Environ.* **24:**41.

Thompson, H. J., and Becci, P. J., 1979, Effect of graded dietary levels of selenium on tracheal carcinomas induced by 1-methylnitrosourea, *Cancer Lett.* **7:**215–219.

Thomson, C. D., and Robinson, M. F., 1980, Selenium in human health and disease with emphasis on those aspects peculiar to New Zealand, *Am. J. Clin. Nutr.* **33:**303–323.

Thomson, C. D., Rea, H. M., Robinson, M. F., and Chapman, O. W., 1977, Low blood selenium concentrations and glutathione peroxidase activities in elderly people, *Proc. Univ. Otago Med. Sch.* **55:**18–19.

Thorling, E. B., Overvad, K., Heerfordt, A., and Foldspang, A., 1985, Serum selenium in Danish blood bank donors, *Biol. Trace Elem. Res.* **8:**65–73.

Tolonen, M., Halme, M., and Sarna, S., 1985, Vitamin E and selenium supplementation in geriatric patients, *Biol. Trace Elem. Res.* **7:**161–168.

Tucker, D. M., Sandstead, H. H., Penland, J. G., Dawson, S. L., and Milne, D. B., 1984, Iron status and brain function: Serum ferritin levels associated with asymmetries of cortical electrophysiology and cognitive performance, *Am. J. Clin. Nutr.* **39:**105–113.

Tuman, R. W., Bilbo, J. T., and Doisy, R. J., 1978, Comparison and effects of natural and synthetic glucose tolerance factor in normal and genetically diabetic mice, *Diabetes* **27:**49–56.

Turnlund, J., Costa, F., and Margen, S., 1981, Zinc, copper, and iron balance in elderly men, *Am. J. Clin. Nutr.* **34:**2641–2647.

Turnlund, J. R., Michel, M. C., Keyes, W. R., King, J. C., and Margen, S., 1982a, Use of enriched stable isotopes to determine zinc and iron absorption in elderly men, *Am. J. Clin. Nutr.* **35:**1033–1040.

Turnlund, J. R., Michel, M. C., Keyes, W. R., Schutz, Y., and Margen, S., 1982b, Copper absorption in elderly men determined by using stable ^{65}Cu, *Am. J. Clin. Nutr.* **36:**587–591.

Turnlund, J. R., Durkin, N., Costa, F., and Margen, S., 1986, Stable isotope studies of zinc absorption and retention in young and elderly men, *J. Nutr.* **116:**1239–1247.

Underwood, E. J., 1977, *Trace Elements in Human and Animal Nutrition,* 4th ed., Academic Press, New York.

U.S. Department of Agriculture, 1980, *Nationwide Food Consumption Survey 1977–1978, Preliminary Report No. 2,* USDA, Washington.

Vanderlinde, R. E., Kayne, F. J., Komar, G., Simmons, M. J., Tsou, J. Y., and Lavine, R. L., 1979, Serum and urine levels of chromium, in: *Chromium in Nutrition and Metabolism* (D. Shapcott and J. Hubert, eds.), Elsevier/North Holland, Amsterdam, pp. 49–57.

Van Rij, A. M., and Pories, W. J., 1980, Zinc in wound healing, in: *Zinc in the Environment,* Volume 2 (J. O. Nriagu, ed.), John Wiley & Sons, New York, pp. 215–236.

Verlinden, M., Van Sprundel, M., Van der Auwera, J. C., and Eylenbosch, W. J., 1983, The selenium status of Belgian population groups. II. Newborns, children, and the aged, *Biol. Trace Elem. Res.* **5**:103–113.

Wagner, P. A., Jernigan, J. A., Bailey, L. B., Nickens, C., and Brazzi, G. A., 1983, Zinc nutriture in cell-mediated immunity in the aged, *Int. J. Vitam. Nutr. Res.* **53**:94–101.

Ward, C. G., Hammond, J. S., and Bullen, J. J., 1986, Effect of iron compounds on antibacterial function of human polymorphs and plasma, *Infect. Immun.* **51**:723–730.

Webb, T. E., and Oski, F. A., 1973, Iron deficiency anemia and scholastic achievement in young adolescents, *J. Pediatr.* **82**:827–830.

Weinberg, E. D., 1986, Iron, infection, and neoplasia, *Clin. Physiol. Biochem.* **4**:50–60.

Weinberg, J., Levine, S., and Dallman, P. R., 1979, Long-term consequences of early iron deficiency in the rat, *Pharmacol. Biochem. Behav.* **11**:631–638.

Weismann, K., Wanscher, B., and Krakauer, R., 1978, Oral zinc therapy in geriatric patients with selected skin manifestions and a low plasma zinc level, *Acta Dermatovener.* **58**:157–161.

Westermarck, T., and Santavuori, P., 1984, Principles of antioxidant therapy in neuronal ceroid lipofuselnosis, *Med. Biol.* **62**:148–151.

Widdowson, E. M., McCance, R. A., and Spray, C. M., 1951, The chemical composition of the human body, *Clin. Sci.* **10**:113–125.

Wilding, P., 1974, Biochemical changes at the menopause, in: *Biochemistry of Women* (A. S. Curry and J. V. Hewitt, eds.), CRC Press, Cleveland, pp. 103–115.

Willson, R. L., 1978, Hydoxyl radicals and biological damage *in vitro:* What relevance *in vivo?* in: *Oxygen Free Radicals and Tissue Damage, CIBA Foundation Symposium (New Series),* No. 65, Excepta Medica, Amsterdam, p. 19.

World Health Organization, 1970, *Fluorides and Human Health,* WHO Monograph Series No. 59, WHO, Geneva, p. 364.

Woteki, C. E., Welsh, S. O., Raper, W., and Marston, R. M., 1982, Recent trends and levels of dietary sugars and other caloric sweetness, in: *Metabolic Effects of Utilizable Carbohydrates* (S. Reiser, ed.), Marcel Dekker, New York, pp. 1–27.

Yang, G. Q., Wang, S., Zhou, R., and Sun, S., 1983, Endemic selenium intoxication of humans in China, *Am. J. Clin. Nutr.* **37**:872–881.

Yang, G., Chen, J., Wen, Z., Ge, K., Zhu, L., Chen, X., and Chen, X., 1984, The role of selenium in Keshan disease, *Adv. Nutr. Res.* **6**:203–231.

Yang, G. Q., Zhu, L., Liu, S., Gu, L., Qian, P., Huang, J., and Lu, M., 1987, Human selenium requirements in China, in: *Selenium in Biology and Medicine, 3rd Symposium* (G. F. Combs, Jr., J. E. Spallholz, O. A. Levander, and J. E. Oldfield, eds.), AVI Press, Westport, CT, pp. 589–607.

Yearick, E. S., Wang, M.-S. L., and Pisies, S. J., 1980, Nutritional status of the elderly: Dietary and biochemical findings, *J. Gerontol.* **35**:663–671.

Young, S. P., Roberts, S., and Bomford, A., 1985, Intracellular processing of transferrin and iron by isolated rat hepatocytes, *Biochem. J.* **232**:819–823.

Yunice, A. A., Lindeman, R. D., Czerwinski, A. W., and Clark, M., 1974, Influence of age and sex on serum copper and ceruloplasmin levels, *J. Gerontol.* **29**:277–281.

Yunice, A. A., Lindeman, R. D., Czerwinski, A. W., and Clark, M., 1976, Effect of age and sex on serum copper and ceruloplasmin levels, in: *The Biomedical Role of Trace Elements in Aging* (J. M. Hsu, R. L. Davis, and R. W. Neithamer, eds.), Eckerd College Gerontology Center, St. Petersberg, FL., pp. 55–71.

10

Vitamin Nutriture and Requirements of the Elderly

Paulo M. Suter and Robert M. Russell

1. Introduction

In 1983, 27 million in the U.S. population (11.7%) were over 65 years of age, and by the year 2050 this number is expected to be nearly double (U.S. Census of Population, 1980). In view of this projection, there is concern for maintaining health and function as late as possible into an individual's life span. In the maintenance of health and prevention of disease, adequacy of nutrition is an important component. At different stages of life, sufficiency of intakes of nutrients is prescribed by the recommended dietary allowances (National Academy of Sciences, 1980), which have been defined as "the levels of intake of essential nutrients considered, in the judgment of the Committee on Dietary Allowances of the Food and Nutrition Board on the basis of available scientific knowledge, to be adequate to meet the known nutritional needs of practically all healthy persons." The basis for this definition is discussed in Chapter 1. In the case of adults, the 1980 RDAs are divided into two age categories, namely, 23–50 years and 51 years upwards. It is, however, unlikely that the nutrient requirements of a 50-year-old adult are the same as those of a person of 23 years, and it is even more improbable that a person of 90 years has the same needs as an individual aged 51 years. Acceptance of these broad categories for RDAs underlines the paucity of data on which to base narrower age bands.

This chapter reviews the published evidence as to the appropriateness of the 1980 RDAs for vitamins for the healthy elderly, defined here as those in the population over 60 years of age, and also assesses the nutritive status of old people in relation to vitamins. The chapter does not deal with the effects of diseases of the elderly on their vitamin status or needs, nor does it speculate on the role of vitamin status on the incidence of chronic diseases associated with aging. Accordingly, the focus of this review is restricted to evaluation of 1980 RDAs from the point of view of preventing

Paulo M. Suter and Robert M. Russell • USDA Human Nutrition Research Center on Aging, Tufts University, Boston, Massachusetts 02111.

vitamin deficiency states from occurring in elderly populations. Interactions of vitamins with other dietary components (e.g., fiber) and therapeutically important drug–vitamin interactions (see also Chapter 14) are summarized.

Although this review uses data from many countries, special attention has been focused on U.S. studies, notably the Health and Nutrition Examination Surveys (HANES I, 1971–1974, and HANES II, 1976–1980), which describe population samples chosen to be representative of the overall U.S. population (HANES I, 1975; HANES II, 1982). A serious limitation of these surveys is that they do not go beyond 74 years. Emphasis has also been placed on the results of the Ten-State Nutrition Survey (TSNS, 1968–1970), which included subjects from five high-income states and five low-income states (TSNS 1972). We have also utilized data from the recent study by Garry *et al.* (1982a) of a group of 300 elderly over 60 years of age who are described as free-living, healthy, well-educated, middle- to upper-class, motivated, health-conscious Caucasians living in Albuquerque, New Mexico. In addition, observations of vitamin intakes by healthy elderly studied in the Boston area are emerging (McGandy *et al.*, 1986) and are referred to where available. Since this review focuses on the appropriateness of the vitamins available from dietary sources, emphasis is placed on data from no-supplement takers, an aspect that is not provided by the HANES and TSNS. Finally, the elderly accumulate an increasing burden of chronic diseases that can result in nutritional deficiencies. As discussed in Chapter 1, groups of elderly screened for debilitating chronic diseases provide the best evidence regarding nutrient needs of the elderly.

There are several criteria for assessing vitamin nutriture. First, dietary intakes of a group of the population can be compared with the RDA for each vitamin. Since the RDAs are intended to cover the needs of populations ranging up to two standard deviations above the mean requirement (see Chapter 1), it follows that intakes moderately below the RDAs are not likely to be associated with deficiency. In surveys of population groups, it is therefore a common practice to express potential inadequacy of the diet in terms of the percentage of people below two-thirds of the RDA for that age and sex. In the case of the HANES data, the percentage of subjects below this critical level is reported separately for sex, income, and race, so that the entries in this review for HANES data are given as a range of percentages according to these subgroups (e.g., in HANES I, depending on sex, race, and income, 18 to 46% of elderly between 65 and 74 years had daily intakes of vitamin B_1 below two-thirds of the RDA for that age). The conclusions to be drawn from nutrient intake data are often restricted by the incomplete analysis of dietary components for many of the vitamins (Hepburn, 1982). Nevertheless, Garry and Hunt (1986) report good correlations between the assessed intakes of some B vitamins by individual elderly in their New Mexico population and their blood levels of these vitamins, e.g., correlation coefficients of 0.59 for plasma ascorbic acid, 0.45 for plasma cobalamin, 0.50 for plasma folate, and 0.49 for erythrocyte folate levels.

Second, a variety of approaches have been used to measure vitamin nutriture biochemically. One can measure the concentrations of the vitamin itself or its metabolites in different body fluids (whole blood, serum, or plasma) and tissues (e.g., red cells, leukocytes, liver). Functional tests, either enzymatic or metabolic, are also frequently available for evaluation of vitamin nutriture. In addition, *in vitro* stimulation assays are available in which a defined amount of the vitamin in coenzyme form is added and the change in enzyme activity is measured. The response is expressed as the percentage increase from baseline or as an activity coefficient. Another example is the tryptophan loading test for assessing vitamin B_6 nutriture. In this test of a metabolic function, urinary output of xanthurenic acid from the administered tryptophan becomes a measure of the adequacy of vitamin B_6 nutriture (Bamji, 1981; Machlin, 1984a; Sauberlich *et al.*, 1984).

2. *The Fat-Soluble Vitamins*

2.1. *Vitamin A*

In addition to its role in maintaining normal vision, vitamin A plays an important part in tissue differentiation and may act as an anticancer agent (Wald, 1968; Diet, Nutrition and Cancer Report, 1982; Willett *et al.*, 1984; Peto *et al.*, 1981; Chytil, 1984). Night blindness, xerophthalmia, and proneness to infection are major symptoms of deficiency. The metabolism of vitamin A and its precursor β-carotene is illustrated in Fig. 1. The carotenoids are vitamin A precursors, and some are converted to retinol with variable efficiency during the absorptive process in the gut mucosa. β-Carotene is the carotenoid with the highest provitamin A activity (Goodman, 1984; Olson, 1984a). Major dietary sources of preformed vitamin A are animal products, whereas carotenoids are mainly found in plants and vegetables (Olson, 1984a). There may be dietary benefits of carotenoids as such in quenching singlet oxygen and in the prevention of DNA damage and cancer initiation; these effects may occur independently of its provitamin A activity. At this time, there is insufficient evidence to factor this information into the RDA calculation for vitamin A. The 1980 RDA for vitamin A is 1000 μg/day retinol equivalents (RE) for adult males and 800 μg/day RE for females [1 RE = 1 μg retinol or 6 μg β-carotene (National Academy of Sciences, 1980)].

The literature shows that, among surveyed elderly groups, there is wide variation in the prevalence of vitamin A intakes below two-thirds of the RDA (Garry *et al.*, 1982a; Bowman and Rosenberg, 1982; Grey *et al.*, 1983; Harrill and Cervone, 1977; Yearick *et al.*, 1980; Stiedemann *et al.*, 1978; Beauchene and Davis, 1979; Kohrs *et al.*, 1978; O'Hanlon and Kohrs, 1978; Steinkamp *et al.*, 1965; Prothro *et al.*, 1976; Dibble *et al.*, 1967; Barr *et al.*, 1983; Vir and Love, 1979). Depending on sex, income, and race, 42% to 65% of the surveyed elderly aged 65–74 years in HANES I had vitamin A intakes below two-thirds of the RDA (Bowman and Rosenberg, 1982). Similar intake data have been reported from the TSNS (1972), which showed a particularly high prevalence (50% intakes $<\frac{1}{2}$RDA) of low vitamin A intakes among Spanish Americans. However, Garry *et al.* (1982a) found only approximately 12% of free-living, wealthy, and healthy Caucasian elderly to have vitamin A intakes below three-fourths of the RDA. In general, elderly men tend to have higher vitamin A intakes than women (Garry *et al.*, 1982a; Bowman and Rosenberg, 1982; Yearick *et al.*, 1980; Stiedemann *et al.*, 1978; Kohrs *et al.*, 1978; Steinkamp *et al.*, 1965; Prothro *et al.*, 1976; MacLeod *et al.*, 1974). However, caution must be exercised in interpreting vitamin A intake data because the vitamin A content of food varies widely, and

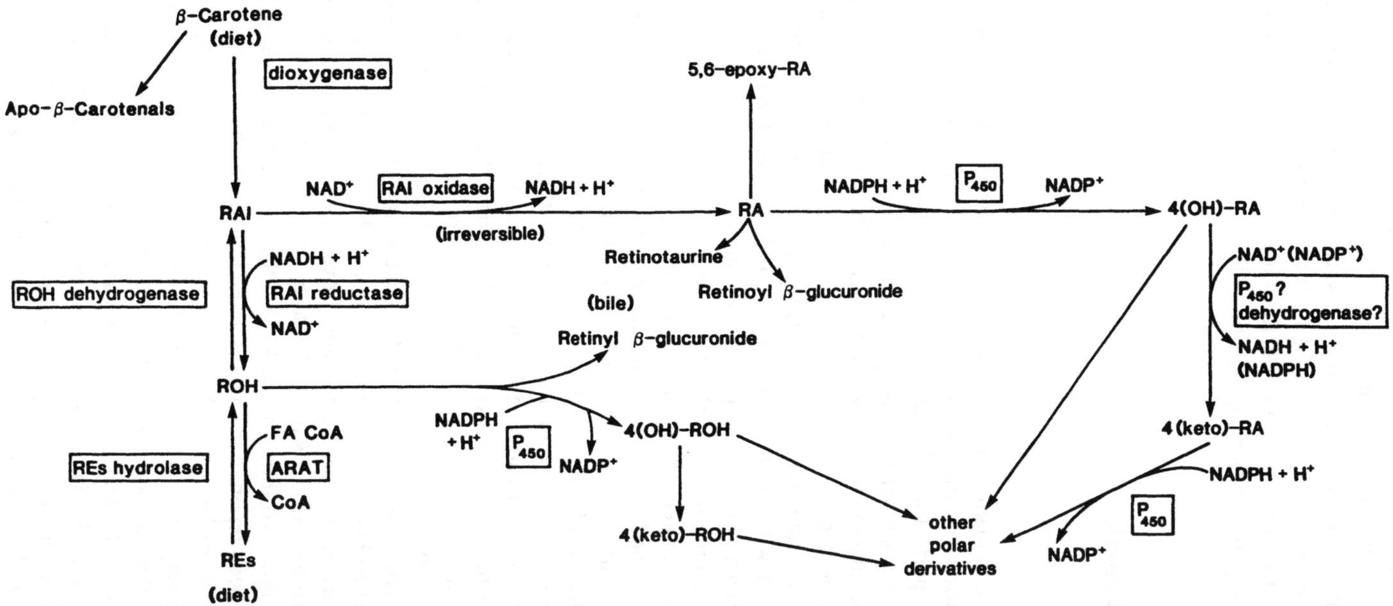

Fig. 1. Absorption and metabolic pathways of vitamin A and carotene. Vitamin A in the rat is absorbed by a non-energy-dependent carrier-mediated system, whereas carotene is absorbed passively. Subsequent metabolism of carotene takes place in the intestinal epithelium and possibly other tissues. Retinyl esters (REs) are taken up from blood and stored in the liver. Retinol (ROH) is secreted by the liver bound to retinol-binding protein (RPB). Transthyretin (TTR) binds holo-RBP, so that retinol finally circulates as a trimolecular complex (retinol-RBP-TTR). Retinyl glucuronides but not retinotaurine appear to have biological activity. The biliary excretion of metabolites is increased in vitamin A overload conditions. RAl, retinaldehyde; RA, retinoic acid; FA, fatty acyl; CoA, coenzyme A; ARAT, acyl-CoA: retinol acyltransferase.

accordingly surveys based on 24-hr recalls are not necessarily representative of long-term eating habits.

From the literature there is no agreement on whether age influences serum or plasma vitamin A or carotene levels (Dibble *et al.*, 1967; Yiengst and Shock, 1949; Kirk and Chieffi, 1948; Leitner *et al.*, 1960; Rafsky *et al.*, 1948; Gillum *et al.*, 1955). Vitamin A is stored in the liver, and fasting serum vitamin A levels are controlled by this store within a narrow range until liver stores are depleted or overwhelmed, when a fall or rise in serum levels, respectively, is seen (Sauberlich *et al.*, 1984; Olson, 1984b). Thus, it is not to be expected that serum levels would closely parallel dietary intake data. In confirmation, only <0.3% of the elderly in HANES I had serum vitamin A levels below 20 μg/dl, whereas 42–65% had vitamin A intakes less than two-thirds of RDA (Bowman and Rosenberg, 1982). Similarly, all of the healthy noninstitutionalized elderly (aged 63–96 years) surveyed by Yearik *et al.* (1980) had normal plasma vitamin A levels, although 22% had vitamin A intakes below two-thirds of the RDA. This goes along with maintenance of liver stores of vitamin A throughout life. One autopsy survey (Hoppner *et al.*, 1968) showed that liver levels of vitamin A are well maintained throughout all age groups regardless of the cause of death. This reflects the general finding of a tendency of liver vitamin A levels to increase in the elderly (Underwood *et al.*, 1970a; Raica *et al.*, 1972).

Yiengst and Shock (1949) could not show an age-related change in vitamin A tolerance curves in humans. However, the relevance of tolerance curves to vitamin A absorption when a mammoth dose of vitamin A is used is uncertain. Contrary to the observations of Fleming *et al.* (1982a), Hollander and Morgan (1979) found increased uptake of vitamin A with age in rats when the intraluminal concentration of vitamin A was kept within the physiological range. Similarly, when physiological doses of vitamin A were fed to humans, a higher peak height on the vitamin A tolerance curves has been reported in old than in young adults (Krasinski *et al.*, 1985a). The increased absorption of vitamin A and the elevated tolerance curves in elderly humans and animals could reflect age-related changes in the unstirred water layer of the intestinal mucosa, resulting in greater penetration by fat-soluble vitamins. Thus, the elderly would be able to maintain stores of vitamin A despite their lower intakes of this vitamin.

Drugs that might interfere with vitamin A status are listed in Table I. Ethanol (Sato and Lieber, 1981; Majumdar *et al.*, 1983) and certain drugs such as phenobarbital can produce a depression of the vitamin A levels in liver tissue, possibly by an acceleration of vitamin A metabolism through induction of microsomal enzymes (Leo *et al.*, 1982, 1984). In animal models it has been shown that vitamin A is important for the metabolism of certain xenobiotics including drugs such as barbiturates. Thus, in animal studies vitamin A deficiency reduced the activities of cytochrome P-450 and hepatic and extrahepatic mixed-function oxidases (Chhabra, 1984; Miranda *et al.*, 1979; Colby *et al.*, 1975). Consequently, vitamin A deficiency could play a role in the development of drug toxicity in the elderly.

In summary, although low vitamin A intakes are common among the elderly, few have plasma levels of retinol below 20 μg/ml, and liver stores are well maintained or even increased throughout life. Thus, from the point of view of preventing deficiency, there is no evidence for significant vitamin A deficiency among senior citizens, and

Table I. Therapeutically Significant Drug–Vitamin Interactions in the Elderly

Drug group	Malabsorption/malutilization	Mechanism
Acid-lowering agents		
Aluminum hydroxide	Malabsorption of vit. A	?Adsorption of vit. A
$NaHCO_3$	Folate malabsorption	Rise in intraluminal pH
Cimetidine	Vitamin B_{12} malabsorption	Inhibition of IF secretion
	Vitamin D	Inhibition of 25-hydroxylase activity in liver
	Folate	Rise in intraluminal pH
Laxatives		
Mineral oil	Vitamin A, K, E, D, and carotene malabsorption	Physical barrier to absorption, decreased micelle formation, solubilization of nutrients, intestinal hurry, loss of structural integrity
Anticonvulsants		
Phenytoin	Folate deficiency	?
Phenobarbital		
Diphenylhydantoin		
Primidone		
Glutethimide	Vitamin B_6	?
	Vitamin D	Enzyme induction
Tranquilizers		
Chlorpromazine	Riboflavin deficiency	Inhibition of hepatic flavokinase, impairment of tissue utilization, increased urinary excretion
Imipramine		
Amitriptyline		
Antidepressants		
Amyltriplyline		
Hydrazine derivatives	Vitamin B_6 deficiency	Vitamin B_6 antagonist
Ipronizaid		
Nialamid		
Isocarboxazid		
Imipramine		
Antihypertensives		
Hydralazine	Vitamin B_6 deficiency	Vitamin B_6 antagonist
Diuretics		
Triamterene	Folate deficiency	Inhibition of dihydrofalate reductase
Ethacrynic acid	Impaired folate metabolism	Impaired cellular uptake
Furosemide		
Antiinflammatory		
Aspirin	Folate deficiency	Displacement of folate from binding proteins, ?increased urinary excretion (clinical significance?)
	Vitamin C	?Increased urinary excretion, decreased uptake in leukocytes and platelets
Miscellaneous		
Potassium chloride (esp. in slow-release preparation)	Vitamin B_{12} malabsorption	Lowers intraluminal pH

indeed it is possible that the vitamin A requirements for the elderly are appreciably lower than those presently recommended.

2.2. *Vitamin D*

Vitamin D is essential for maintaining normal calcium and phosphorus metabolism and bone health. The daily vitamin D requirement is met by ingestion of vitamin D_2 (synthetic ergocalciferol) or D_3 (natural cholecalciferol) and by synthesis of vitamin D_3 in the skin on exposure to sunlight. The 1980 RDA for vitamin D for all adults is 5 μg (200 IU) cholecalciferol per day (National Academy of Sciences, 1980). Unfortified food is, in general, a poor vitamin D source. Deep-sea fish have a high vitamin D content, but meat and eggs are relatively low, and vegetables do not contain the vitamin (Norman and Miller, 1984). In the United States, milk and margarine are fortified with vitamin D_2, whereas in many parts of Europe this is not so. This may be related to the observed higher frequency of osteomalacia in Britain (Campbell *et al.*, 1984). The active form of the vitamin is 1,25-dihydroxyvitamin D [1,25 $(OH)_2D$], which is formed from vitamin D_2 or D_3 by hydroxylation reactions in the liver (25-hydroxylation) and the kidney (1-hydroxylation). The predominant form of vitamin D in plasma is 25-hydroxyvitamin D (25-OH vitamin D), which is bound to a vitamin-D-binding protein (DBP), as are other vitamin D metabolites (Belsey *et al.*, 1974; Daiger *et al.*, 1975). The metabolism of vitamin D and its regulation in relation to calcium and parathyroid hormones has recently been reviewed (Frazier, 1980; Holick and Potts, 1983; Bell, 1985).

It is controversial whether the diet or exposure to the sun is the major source of vitamin D for the elderly (Parfitt *et al.*, 1982; Anwar, 1978; Pittet *et al.*, 1979; Dattani *et al.*, 1984; Conely *et al.*, 1977; Sedrani *et al.*, 1983; Sheltawy *et al.*, 1984; Nayal *et al.*, 1978; Davie and Lawson, 1980; Lawson *et al.*, 1979; Lund and Sorensen, 1979; Omdahl *et al.*, 1982; Beadle, 1977). The daily intake of vitamin D by the elderly is usually below the U.S. RDA (Garry *et al.*, 1982a; MacLeod *et al.*, 1974; Parfitt *et al.*, 1982; Pittet *et al.*, 1979; Newton *et al.*, 1985; Corless *et al.*, 1979; Vir and Love, 1978a; Elsborg *et al.*, 1983; Lonergan *et al.*, 1975). From different studies, 62–74% of the healthy free-living elderly have intakes below two-thirds of the 1980 RDA. Even in a generally well-nourished elderly group in New Mexico, 70% of the males and 74% of the females surveyed by Garry *et al.* (1982a) had intakes below three-fourths of the RDA. Lonergan *et al.* (1975) obtained 1-week dietary histories in free-living elderly in Edinburgh: the daily vitamin D intake for 62- to 74-year-old elderly were about 2.0–3.1 μg cholecalciferol equivalents, and for the 75- to 90-year-old elderly, 1.8–2.4 μg cholecalciferol equivalents, both much less than the recommended 5 μg daily (National Academy of Sciences, 1980). Similar low intakes have been reported by others (Corless *et al.*, 1979; Elsborg *et al.*, 1983; Omdahl *et al.*, 1982). In general, elderly females have been found to have lower vitamin D intakes than males, which is also reflected in their lower serum levels of 25-OHD_3.

Serum 25-OH vitamin D levels, in general, have been shown to decrease with age among nonsupplemented subjects, although levels are maintained within acceptably normal ranges (Baker *et al.*, 1980; Lund and Sorensen, 1979; Parfitt *et al.*, 1982;

Sowers *et al.*, 1986; Dattani *et al.*, 1984; Sedrani *et al.*, 1983; Guggenheim *et al.*, 1979; Tsai *et al.*, 1984; Stamp and Round, 1974; Weisman *et al.*, 1981). Differences in the change with aging may relate to local variations in vitamin D content of foods (including fortification) as well as to exposure to sunlight. From a study of women, Sowers *et al.* (1986) report significant correlations between plasma levels of 25-OHD and individual vitamin D intakes from food ($r = 0.11$), supplement use ($r = 0.21$), and sunlight exposure ($r = 0.26$), but the levels were inversely related to age. Among free-living elderly, 2–40% have been reported to have 25-OH vitamin D levels below 8–10 ng/ml (Lund and Sorensen, 1979; Omdahl *et al.*, 1982; Baker *et al.*, 1980; Weisman *et al.*, 1981), whereas 70–90% of institutionalized and homebound elderly lacking exposure to the sun had 25-OH vitamin D levels below 10 ng/ml (Vir and Love, 1978a; Weisman *et al.*, 1981; Devgun *et al.*, 1981). In a study by Corless *et al.* (1975), chronic care patients aged 60–100 years with low circulating 25 -OH vitamin D had daily vitamin D intakes of less than 2.5 μg vitamin D.

The serum 25-OH vitamin D level reflects vitamin D nutriture, but it is not clear whether diet or exposure to the sun is the major determinant of serum levels in the elderly (Devgun *et al.*, 1981; Toss *et al.*, 1980; Lips *et al.*, 1985; Sowers *et al.*, 1986). The photobiogenesis of vitamin D in the skin is promoted by ultraviolet radiation between the wavelengths 275 and 320 nm (window glass usually absorbs these wavelengths). The synthesis of vitamin D in the skin takes place by photochemical transformation of 7-dehydrocholesterol to provitamin D and thermal isomerization of the provitamin D to vitamin D_3 (cholecalciferol) (Frazier, 1980; Beadle, 1977; Holick and Clark, 1978), hydroxylation in the liver and kidney occurring subsequently. Stamp and Round (1974) reported a seasonal variation of serum 25-OH vitamin D levels in young adults to coincide with the amount of ultraviolet radiation exposure. This seasonal variation also occurs among the elderly (Lawson *et al.*, 1979; Lund and Sorensen, 1979; Omdahl *et al.*, 1982; Stamp and Round, 1974; Lambert-Allardt, 1984). However, it was shown that the seasonal variation of 25-OH vitamin D in the serum is less profound in the elderly as compared to younger subjects (Lund and Sorensen, 1979; Lester *et al.*, 1977). This could reflect less sunlight exposure and/or less efficient synthesis of vitamin D in the skin with aging (Holick and MacLaughlin, 1985; MacLaughlin and Holick, 1985).

There is limited evidence for an age effect on 25-hydroxylation of vitamin D by the liver (Rushton, 1978). More impressive is a marked age-dependent decrease in the capacity to convert 25-OH vitamin D to 1,25-$(OH)_2$ vitamin D in the kidney (Armbrecht *et al.*, 1980a, 1982, 1984; Baksi and Kenny, 1981; Gray and Gambert, 1982). Elderly osteoporotic patients (Slovik *et al.*, 1981; Gallagher *et al.*, 1979), normal healthy elderly (Gallagher *et al.*, 1979; Fujisawa *et al.*, 1984), and aged animals (Armbrecht *et al.*, 1980b) all show lower serum levels of 1,25-$(OH)_2$ vitamin D than younger controls despite normal 25-OH vitamin D levels. The conversion of 25-OH vitamin D to 1,25-$(OH)_2$ vitamin D via 1α-hydroxylase is regulated by parathyroid hormone (PTH) (Mawer *et al.*, 1975; DeLuca, 1972; Garabedian *et al.*, 1972). In humans, serum PTH levels increase with age (Gallagher *et al.*, 1980). Slovik *et al.* (1981) infused PTH into osteoporotic volunteers (aged 50–80 years) and found decreased production of 1,25-$(OH)_2$ vitamin D as compared to normal young adults. A decreased responsiveness of the 1α-hydroxylase to PTH with age has therefore been postulated as the cause of the lower 1,25-$(OH)_2$

vitamin D levels in the elderly. Although plasma binding capacity for 25-OH vitamin D is reduced in the elderly (MacLennan and Hamilton, 1979), this is of little if any physiological consequence, since only a minor proportion of the total binding capacity is used.

There is conflicting evidence for age-related changes in vitamin D absorption (Weisman *et al.*, 1981; Corless *et al.*, 1975; Somerville *et al.*, 1977; Barragry *et al.*, 1978; Krawitt and Chastenay, 1980; Hollander and Tarnawski, 1984; Fleming and Barrows, 1982a; Holt and Dominguez, 1981). Barragry *et al.* (1978) measured [^{3}H]cholecalciferol absorption in geriatric patients (aged 68–94 years) and younger controls. The mean 6-hr plasma [^{3}H]cholecalciferol level expressed as percentage of an oral dose of 15–42 IU vitamin D was 7.6 ± 0.9% of the administered dose in the elderly patients versus 12.2 ± 1.0% in the young subjects. Since vitamin D absorption tests could be influenced by many factors such as body stores of vitamin D or the composition of the administered diet (Barragry *et al.*, 1978; Krawitt and Chastenay, 1980), interpretation of such test results is uncertain. Hollander and Tarnawski (1984) and also Fleming and Barrows (1982a) found no age-related impairment of vitamin D absorption in rats. However, Holt and Domingues (1981), also using a rat model, showed reduced triglyceride and vitamin D absorption with increasing age.

Drugs that interfere with vitamin D metabolism are listed in Table I. A common mechanism of drug interference (e.g., phenobarbital) with vitamin D metabolism is enzyme induction with a consequent increased rate of degradative metabolism of vitamin D (Hahn *et al.*, 1972; Hahn and Avioli, 1984).

In summary, impairment of vitamin D nutriture because of specific age-related changes is common in the elderly population and biochemically reflected in a decrease in 1,25-$(OH)_2$ vitamin D serum levels. These age-related changes include a low vitamin D intake, lack of exposure to the sun, reduced vitamin D synthesis in the skin, impaired hydroxylation of 25-OH vitamin D by the kidney, and alterations in vitamin D metabolism induced by medications. There are, to date, insufficient data to propose an increase in the RDA for vitamin D with aging, and at present no general recommendation for the use of vitamin D supplements in free-living elderly can be given because of potential toxicity from overdoses. However, for institutionalized elderly a combination of low-level vitamin D supplementation of 400 IU/day (10 μg/day), especially during the winter months, and increased sunlight exposure whenever possible may be the best approaches for improving vitamin D status.

2.3. *Vitamin E*

Although vitamin E was identified 50 years ago, its exact function has not yet been fully established. It has been theorized that vitamin E may play an important role as an antioxidizing agent in the aging process (Chen, 1981; Passeri and Proveddini, 1982; Ledvina, 1985). There exists several isomers of vitamin E (α-, β-, γ-, and δ-tocopherols); α-tocopherol is the most active form. Vitamin E is widely distributed in nature, especially good sources being vegetable oils, seeds, grains, and nuts (Machlin, 1984b). The 1980 RDA for vitamin E is 10 mg α-tocopherol equivalents (α-TE) for adult males and 8 mg α-TE for females (National Academy of Sciences, 1980). Vitamin E deficiency in humans is very rare except in subjects with fat malabsorption

(Binder *et al.*, 1965; Farrell, 1980), long-term total parenteral nutrition (Bieri, 1984), or with a selective defect in vitamin E absorption (Harding *et al.*, 1985). Vitamin E is absorbed in the jejunum by a nonsaturable passive diffusion mechanism.

Vitamin E intake data are of uncertain reliability because of the wide variation of the vitamin E content of certain foods and the considerable losses of the vitamin that can take place during food processing and storage. There are few studies on vitamin E intakes by the elderly. Leichter *et al.* (1978) found that the mean vitamin E intake based on 24-hr recalls of free-living elderly Canadians (65–90 years old) was adequate. The study by Garry *et al.* (1982a) of healthy, noninstitutionalized elderly over 60 years of age showed that 46% of the males and 42% of the females had intakes from diet alone of less than three-fourths of the RDA. It may be noted, however, that close to one-third of this upper-middle-class group were taking daily multivitamin supplements containing vitamin E.

There have been several studies on the effect of age on blood tocopherol levels (Leitner *et al.*, 1960; Chieffi and Kirk, 1951; Chen *et al.*, 1977; Lewis *et al.*, 1973; Desai, 1968; Wei-W. and Draper, 1975; Darby *et al.*, 1949; Kelleher and Losowsky, 1978; Vatassery *et al.*, 1971; Barnes and Chen, 1981; Gabriel *et al.*, 1980). Most of the studies have demonstrated an increase of the total serum tocopherol from young adulthood through middle age in healthy people (Leitner *et al.*, 1960; Chieffi and Kirk, 1959; Chen *et al.*, 1977; Lewis *et al.*, 1973; Desai, 1968; Wei-W. and Draper, 1975; Darby *et al.*, 1949; Kelleher and Losowsky, 1978), which can be related to an age-related increase in plasma levels of β-lipoproteins, which carry most of the plasma vitamin E (Kelleher and Losowsky, 1978). However, Vatassery *et al.* (1983) recently was unable to demonstrate a significant correlation between total plasma tocopherol concentration and age (24–91 years) or even between the physiologically more important α-tocopherol and age. Indeed, after age 65, some studies have shown a decline in serum vitamin E levels with advancing age (Wei-W. and Draper, 1975; Barnes and Chen, 1981).

A possible cause for a decline in the plasma tocopherol levels in advanced age might be that vitamin E circulates bound to lipoproteins and, in consequence, vitamin E levels correlated with the total serum lipid levels (Baker *et al.*, 1967). Total serum lipid levels tend to rise until about the age of 60, after which a decline in plasma lipid levels occurs, in part reflecting the increased mortality of hyperlipidemic subject (Horwitt *et al.*, 1972). Similarly, subjects taking antihyperlipidemic drugs have lower serum tocopherol levels (Weiss and Bianchine, 1970; Leonhardt, 1978). Because of this interdependence of vitamin E and blood lipids, it is more appropriate to express the vitamin E serum level relative to the lipid level. In one study involving 48 men aged 24–91 years, Vatassery *et al.* (1983) could demonstrate no decrease in the vitamin E/lipid ratio with age. To date, no large-scale studies have measured the vitamin E/lipid ratio in relation to age. A further reason for declining plasma vitamin E levels with advanced age is illness. For example, Kelleher and Losowsky (1978) reported total serum tocopherol levels below 4.5 μg/ml (below which an increased prevalence of *in vitro* erythrocyte hemolysis occurs) in 38% of acute geriatric hospital admissions over 65 years of age. On the other hand, using the erythrocyte hemolysis test as an indicator of vitamin E deficiency, Tulloch and Sood (1967) could not show an increased prevalence of hemolysis with increasing age in an African population (N =

208, age range 0–71). However, in rats it was demonstrated that the amount of vitamin E needed to prevent erythrocyte hemolysis on exposure to dialuric acid increases threefold from the age of 9–11 weeks to 71–72 weeks of age (Ames, 1972).

The α-tocopherol content of the liver, heart, and adrenal glands of rats increases with age (Weglicki *et al.*, 1969). In the livers of humans killed by accident, Underwood *et al.* (1970b) could not find a change of α-tocopherol content with age (range 2–84 years), which contrasts with the findings of Dju *et al.* (1958), who reported a decrease of total tocopherol in human adipose tissue, skeletal muscle, and liver over the age range 23–93 years. Although the two studies were both done in New York, the contradictory findings might reflect the different assays used (α-tocopherol versus total tocopherol) and the differences in the populations studied. Furthermore, the study of Dju *et al.* (1958) included not only accidental deaths but also patients with cardiovascular disease and chronic alcoholics. A decrease in platelet vitamin E concentration with age has been demonstrated (Vatassery *et al.*, 1983); however, the functional significance of this finding remains uncertain.

There is no evidence for decreased vitamin E absorption with age among healthy elderly. An insignificant difference (72% versus 68%) in mean vitamin E absorption was seen in subjects under 65 versus over 65 years (Kelleher and Losowsky, 1978). A high-polyunsaturated-fatty-acid (PUFA) diet decreases vitamin E absorption in rats, probably by expansion of micellar size (Muralidhara and Hollander, 1977). The clinical significance of this finding remains to be determined, since PUFA-rich foods are, in general, good vitamin E sources. Dietary fiber could reduce vitamin E absorption by removing bile acids, thus inducing fat and vitamin E malabsorption (Doi *et al.*, 1983).

There is evidence based on a bioassay that the vitamin E requirement for the rat increases with age (Berg, 1951; Fuhr *et al.*, 1949; Emerson and Evans, 1939a,b). The bioassay used for the determination of vitamin E requirement in rats is a fertility assay based on the prevalence of fetal resorption in female rats. Fuhr *et al.* (1949), using a fetal resorption assay in pregnant female rats, showed that the vitamin E requirements for maintaining a pregnancy rate of 50% increased tenfold from the maternal age of 3–5 months to the age of 1–2 years. Similar results have been reported by Emerson and Evans (1939b), but Ames (1974) reported an approximately 70-fold increase in the amount of vitamin E necessary to maintain fertility in 59-week-old rats as compared to rats aged 9–11 weeks. Chen (1974) reported that the rate of lipid peroxidation in liver tissue of older rats was significantly higher than in younger rats fed the same vitamin-E-containing diet. The author concluded that the amount of vitamin E needed to protect tissues from peroxidation increases with age and that the requirement may therefore be higher for older subjects. However, Gabriel *et al.* (1980) found no evidence with advancing age (age range 8–64 weeks) for an increased vitamin E requirement to prevent myopathy in the rat. In contrast to the above, Grinna (1976) found it to be more difficult to produce a deficiency state or to deplete the body vitamin E stores in older versus younger rats. Eleven-week-old rats fed a diet low in vitamin E developed deficiency signs after 7 weeks, whereas in rats aged 42 weeks consuming the same diet, the deficiency signs only appeared after 16 weeks. This argues for reduced rat vitamin E requirements with age, possibly because of increased body stores of vitamin E in tissue lipids.

Important drug–vitamin E interactions are listed in Table I. In addition, vitamin E shows antivitamin K activity (Anonymous, 1982a); thus, hypervitaminosis E may cause a prolongation of the prothrombin time with a resulting hemorrhagic syndrome in patients taking warfarin anticoagulants. The exact mechanism of antivitamin K effect of the tocopherols is not known, but it might be mediated by certain tocopherol metabolites such as α-tocopheryl hydroquinones (Rao and Mason, 1975). However, the anticoagulant activity of the tocopherols appears to have little significance in healthy humans (Corrigan, 1982), and even in patients taking warfarin, a vitamin E intake that does not exceed 400 IU per day appears to be safe (Corrigan and Ulfers, 1981). Considering the popularity of high-vitamin-E supplement intakes, however, doses over 400 IU should be discouraged in anticoagulated patients.

In summary, dietary vitamin E intake is below the RDA in up to 60% of the elderly. Although the data are not consistent, there is an increase of total serum tocopherol levels until about the seventh decade of life because of the changing levels of the vitamin E carrier lipoproteins with age. Data on age-related changes in tissue tocopherol levels and requirements in animals are conflicting. The functional significance of lowered platelet vitamin E concentrations with age remains to be determined. There is no compelling evidence at present that tocopherol requirements for aged humans differ from those of young adults, although the effects of increased vitamin E on lipid peroxidation and on platelet function should be clarified for a final verdict.

2.4. *Vitamin K*

Vitamin K is essential for the synthesis of the blood-clotting factors II (prothrombin), VII, IX, and X and thus is essential for maintaining blood coagulation (Suttie and Jackson, 1977). Other vitamin-K-dependent γ-carboxylated proteins have been isolated from different body tissues (e.g., osteocalcin from bone) (Vermeer, 1984). Absorbed vitamin K comes partly from the diet and partly from intestinal bacterial synthesis. The total daily requirement for adult humans from both sources appears to be about 0.03 μg/kg body weight, as determined in a series of experiments by Frick *et al.* (1967) in which blood coagulation in patients with sterile intestinal tracts was studied. There is no RDA for vitamin K, but the range 70–140 mg daily is recommended provisionally as safe (National Academy of Sciences, 1980).

Vitamin K is widely distributed in food, green leafy vegetables providing the best source (Suttie, 1984). Diet-induced vitamin K deficiency is rare but has been occasionally reported in adults (Kark and Lozner, 1939; Colvin and Lloyd, 1977). Kark and Lozner (1939) described prolonged prothrombin times that normalized after oral administration of vitamin K in four patients (aged 49 to 64) with overall poor nutrition but free of liver disease. Vitamin K deficiency is most commonly diagnosed by prolongation of the prothrombin time, which returns to normal after administration of oral or parenteral vitamin K. A recently described test for detecting vitamin K deficiency is the level of circulating abnormal prothrombin, which has a reduced content of γ-carboxyglutamic acid residues (Anonymous, 1982b; Blanchard *et al.*, 1981, 1983). Abnormal prothrombin cannot bind calcium and is therefore inactive in blood coagulation. The radioimmunoassay for abnormal prothrombin is approximately 1000 times more sensitive than the prothrombin time in detecting vitamin K deficiency. Therefore, even mild to moderate vitamin K deficiency may be detectable (Krasinski *et al.*, 1985b).

Information on the vitamin K status of the elderly is practically nonexistent, no population studies having been reported. Overt vitamin K deficiency is probably not common in healthy elderly. However, in a study by Hazell and Baloch (1970), 110 ill patients (aged 56 to 100 years) were examined for vitamin K deficiency using the thrombotest procedure, which depends on all four vitamin-K-dependent clotting factors. Seventy-four percent of these subjects had abnormal thrombotest results; after the oral administration of 20 mg of a vitamin K analogue for 14 days, the test normalized in 62 of the 81 patients with abnormal values.

Evidence for an age-related change in the metabolism of vitamin K stems from the fact that, with increasing age, there is an increased sensitivity to the anticoagulant warfarin in humans and in rats (Hewick *et al.*, 1975; Shepherd *et al.*, 1977; Hayes *et al.*, 1975). At a given warfarin dose, increased inhibition of the synthesis of the vitamin-K-dependent clotting factors is seen with advancing age in humans and in rats. There is, however, no statistically significant difference in warfarin pharmacokinetics (plasma $t_{\frac{1}{2}}$, volume of distribution, plasma warfarin clearance) between different age groups. Decreases in plasma albumin levels with age, with consequent less albumin binding of warfarin and thus higher levels of free drug, could explain increased warfarin sensitivity with age (Hayes *et al.*, 1975). Other possible reasons for the altered sensitivity of the clotting-factor-synthesizing system to warfarin could be a decreased binding affinity to vitamin K with advancing age or depleted vitamin K stores (Shepherd *et al.*, 1977). Alternatively, the elderly might be mildly deficient in vitamin K because of lower vitamin K intakes or altered absorption. It has been shown that it is easier to induce experimental vitamin K deficiency in old rats than in young ones (Doisy, 1961).

Drugs that can interfere with vitamin K are listed in Table I. The vitamin K–vitamin E interaction is discussed in Section 2.3. Dietary requirements for vitamin K need to be determined for all ages, and this can now be done by application of a sensitive test such as the abnormal prothrombin assay at various levels of controlled vitamin K intake. This could also be used for population studies, which are not presently available.

3. *Vitamin C*

Ascorbic acid (vitamin C) is involved in a variety of oxidation reactions and has a necessary role in collagen synthesis. Ascorbic acid is widely distributed in nature, major food sources being citrus fruits, broccoli, kale, and cabbage (Jaffe, 1984). Supplemental ascorbic acid is also widely consumed in large doses. In Western societies, cases of scurvy occur rarely (Connelly *et al.*, 1982). The 1980 RDA for vitamin C is 60 mg per day for both sexes (National Academy of Sciences, 1980). Despite the many food sources of vitamin C, there is a broad range of ascorbic acid intakes by the elderly (Garry *et al.*, 1982a; Harrill and Cervone, 1977; Yearick *et al.*, 1980; Stiedemann *et al.*, 1978; O'Hanlon and Kohrs, 1978; Steinkamp *et al.*, 1965; Dibble *et al.*, 1967; Cheng *et al.*, 1985; Burr *et al.*, 1974b; Bates *et al.*, 1977;

Roderuck *et al.*, 1958; Morgan *et al.*, 1955; Milne *et al.*, 1971; O'Sullivan *et al.*, 1968; Roine *et al.*, 1974; Jacob *et al.*, 1988). In general, dietary intakes of vitamin C decline with increasing age. In HANES I (depending on income and race), 23–42% of the elderly had intakes below 30 mg per day (Bowman and Rosenberg, 1982). Black and white men with incomes below the poverty level had the highest prevalence (42%) of intakes below 30 mg. A similar high prevalence was found among low-income elderly in Ireland (O'Sullivan *et al.*, 1968). In one long-term study (Bates *et al.*, 1977) of 23 elderly individuals studied over 18 months, the mean daily ascorbic acid intake was 36 mg based on daily food records; eight of these (34%) had vitamin C intakes equal to or below 30 mg per day. In contrast, others (Garry *et al.*, 1982a; Gray *et al.*, 1983; Harril and Cervone, 1977; Yearick *et al.*, 1980; Kohrs *et al.*, 1978; Barr *et al.*, 1983) have reported ascorbic acid intakes below 30 mg per day in fewer than 7% of healthy free-living elderly, and in some studies the mean vitamin C intake was above 60 mg/day (Yearick *et al.*, 1980; Kohrs *et al.*, 1978; O'Hanlon and Kohrs, 1978; Morgan *et al.*, 1955). There is no consistent relationship between sex and ascorbic acid concentration in the different body fluids and blood cells.

Several factors such as emotional and environmental stress (National Academy of Sciences, 1980; Baker, 1967), smoking (Pelletier, 1975), certain drugs (e.g., aspirin) (Sahud and Cohen, 1971), as well as age influence the ascorbic acid levels in different human body fluids and tissues. Although the data on aging are conflicting (Roderuck *et al.*, 1958; Morgan *et al.*, 1955; Brook and Grimshaw, 1968; Loh and Wilson, 1971; Kirk and Chieffi, 1953a,b), most studies have demonstrated an inverse correlation between age (the range being early adulthood to old age) and levels of ascorbate in whole blood (Kirk and Chieffi, 1953a), plasma (Burr *et al.*, 1974b; Brook and Grimshaw, 1968; Schorah, 1979; Kataria *et al.*, 1965; Loh, 1972; Schorah *et al.*, 1979), and leukocytes (Loh and Wilson, 1971; Schorah, 1979; Loh, 1972; Schorah *et al.*, 1979; Attwood *et al.*, 1978). A credible reason for the conflicting data is the seasonality of vitamin C intakes, with differences in plasma and leukocyte levels (Bates *et al.*, 1977; Milne *et al.*, 1971; Roine *et al.*, 1974) dependent on the season a study was performed. The mean annual fall of plasma ascorbate levels with age is estimated to be in the range of 0.006 mg/100 ml (Burr *et al.*, 1974b) to 0.008 mg/100 ml (Brook and Grimshaw, 1968). Garry and Hunt (1986) have attributed this to reduced consumption of ascorbic acid as age advances.

Plasma ascorbic acid levels below 0.4 mg/dl are regarded as indicative of deficiency, and levels below 0.2 mg/dl are associated with scurvy. With regard to frequency of low blood and tissue levels, zero to 25% of elderly have been reported to have low (<0.2 mg/dl) serum or plasma ascorbic acid levels (Yearick *et al.*, 1980; Bates *et al.*, 1977; Brin *et al.*, 1965; Baker *et al.*, 1979; Garry *et al.*, 1982c). Morgan *et al.* (1975) reported 58% of acute geriatric hospital admissions to have leukocyte ascorbate levels below 15 $\mu g/10^8$ white blood cells. In hospitalized elderly British women, Andrews *et al.* (1969) also found low levels of leukocyte ascorbic acid, which were only restored to the levels found in young adults by supplementing the diet with 80 mg ascorbic acid daily, implying that total daily intake must have been in excess of 100 mg. In contrast, Garry *et al.* (1982a) found very few of their economically privileged elderly to have low plasma ascorbic acid levels, probably because the majority were taking supplements of ascorbic acid. Garry *et al.* (1982c) concluded that in order to maintain a good plasma level (1.0 mg/dl), elderly women would need 75 mg daily and elderly men would need 150 mg/day. However, long-term ascorbic acid supplementation has failed to improve the clinical status of the elderly (Andrews *et al.*, 1969; Burr *et al.*, 1974a) or has achieved only small increases in plasma protein levels and in body weight (Schorah *et al.*, 1981). Garry and Hunt (1986) have observed that elderly subjects with low plasma ascorbic acid levels have impaired cognitive functioning.

Yavorski *et al.* (1934) found a small decrease in vitamin C tissue levels with age in adrenal glands, brain, pancreas, liver, spleen, kidney, lung, heart, and thymus from subjects aged 0–77 years. However, these tissues had been obtained from hospital autopsies, and it is not known how disease might have influenced the various tissue levels. In contrast, Schaus (1957) found an age-associated decrease in the ascorbate levels only in pituitary tissue and cerebral cortex. In rat tissues, there is a decline in ascorbic acid content with age even though the rat does not depend on external sources of vitamin C (Patniak and Kanungo, 1966). It has been shown by Grimble and Hughes (1968) that older guinea pigs (which, like humans, require vitamin C) have lower catalyzing activity of glutathione dehydroascorbate oxidoreductase (which catalyzes the formation of L-ascorbic acid from dehydroascorbic acid in some body tissues) than do younger controls. The authors conclude that this could be a reason for lower ascorbic acid tissue levels in the elderly.

Regarding ascorbic acid absorption, weak evidence for an alteration in vitamin C absorption and/or metabolism in the elderly comes from the study by Kirk and Chieffi (1953b) in which three of 19 institutionalized subjects (aged 52–84) did not respond to 100 mg of vitamin C supplementation with a rise in plasma ascorbate levels. Recently, Davies *et al.* (1984) have found that oral dosage of ascorbic acid to hospitalized elderly failed to raise plasma ascorbic acid or urinary ascorbic acid output to the extent that occurred in young healthy subjects and concluded that absorption was faulty. These studies should be repeated on healthy, free-living elderly.

Therapeutically significant drug–vitamin interactions are listed in Table I. Ascorbic acid has an important role in drug metabolism and detoxification (Holloway and Peterson, 1984). It has been shown that vitamin-C-deficient guinea pigs have decreased efficiency of oxidative metabolism and thus increased susceptibility to certain drugs such as aminopyrine and ethoxycoumarin (Peterson *et al.*, 1983). There is one vitamin-C–drug interaction that deserves special attention: vitamin C is partly metabolized by sulfate conjugation, although this biotransforming system has only limited capacity. Some drugs (e.g., isoproterenol, salicylates) are also conjugated with sulfate and could reach toxic levels as a result of competitive inhibition (Houston and Levy, 1975) if there is concomitantly a high pharmacological vitamin C intake.

In conclusion, high prevalences of up to 25% low serum and/or plasma ascorbic acid levels among the elderly can be accounted for by poor intake. The data on age-related changes in ascorbic acid plasma, serum, leukocyte, and tissue levels are somewhat conflicting, and there are no reported changes in vitamin C metabolism with age. The best approach to improve ascorbic acid nutriture in the elderly is by encouraging consumption of vitamin-C-rich foods such as fruits. There is at present little evidence for altering ascorbic acid requirement with age.

4. The B Vitamins

The water-soluble vitamins include the B vitamins as well as ascorbic acid. The B complex consists of eight members, namely, thiamin (B_1), riboflavin (B_2), niacin (nicotinic acid, nicotinamide), vitamin B_6, folic acid (folacin), cyanocobalamin (B_{12}), biotin, and pantothenic acid. These chemically different compounds were originally grouped together as the vitamin B complex because they were found in high concentrations in the same foods. It is convenient to continue this classification since their presence in similar dietary sources means that deficiencies often involve more than one member of the group. Several of them occur in cereals such as wheat, where their presence in the outer coats of the grain means that milling depletes the flour of the vitamins. Fortification of flour with thiamin, riboflavin, and niacin since 1940 has provided protection against deficiency of these vitamins expressed in the form of pellagra and other deficiency diseases (see Chapter 1).

Unlike the fat-soluble vitamins, the members of the B complex pass via the portal vein to the liver, where some (riboflavin, niacin, folic acid, vitamin B_{12}, and pantothenic acid) are stored. In the liver also, some of the B-complex vitamins undergo transformation to storage forms (e.g., folic acid polyglutamates), synthesis of metabolites for export to other tissues of the body (e.g., vitamin B_6 metabolites), or recycling via the bile (vitamin B_{12}). The roles of the B vitamins in intermediary metabolism are illustrated in Fig. 2 and discussed by Danford and Munro (1988).

4.1. Thiamin

The metabolically active form of vitamin B_1 (thiamin) takes the form of the coenzyme thiamin pyrophosphate, which plays an important role in decarboxylation reactions such as the decarboxylation of pyruvate. Major features of thiamin absorption and metabolism are illustrated in Fig. 3. Thiamin is widely distributed in food in relatively small concentrations. Vitamin B_1 deficiency occurs mainly in Asian populations for whom polished rice is the staple food. This classical deficiency syndrome of beriberi is rarely seen in Western societies except among chronic alcoholics (Gubler, 1984; Iber *et al.*, 1982; Baum and Iber, 1984). Because of its involvement in energy metabolism, thiamin requirements should decline in the elderly as they reduce their energy consumption. The 1980 RDA advises a minimum of 0.5 mg thiamin per 1000 kcal for adults generally but recommends no less than 1.2 mg thiamin for older men and 1.0 mg for old women even if their energy intakes are below 2000 kcal/day. A concensus report (Iber *et al.*, 1982) has challenged these recommendations as being unnecessarily high for maintaining the thiamin nutriture of the elderly, pointing out that there was no evidence of deficiency when young adults were given 0.3 mg thiamin per 1000 kcal (Sauberlich *et al.*, 1979).

There is a wide variability in vitamin B_1 intakes in elderly populations (Bowman and Rosenberg, 1982; Garry *et al.*, 1982a; Gray *et al.*, 1983; Harrill and Cervone, 1977; Yearick *et al.*, 1980; Stiedemann *et al.*, 1978; Beauchene and Davis, 1979; Kohrs *et al.*, 1978; O'Hanlon and Kohrs, 1978; Steinkamp *et al.*, 1965; Elsborg *et al.*, 1983; Leichter *et al.*, 1978; Iber *et al.*, 1982; Baum and Iber, 1984). From various studies, 0–47% of elderly have thiamin intakes below two-thirds of the RDA (Bowman

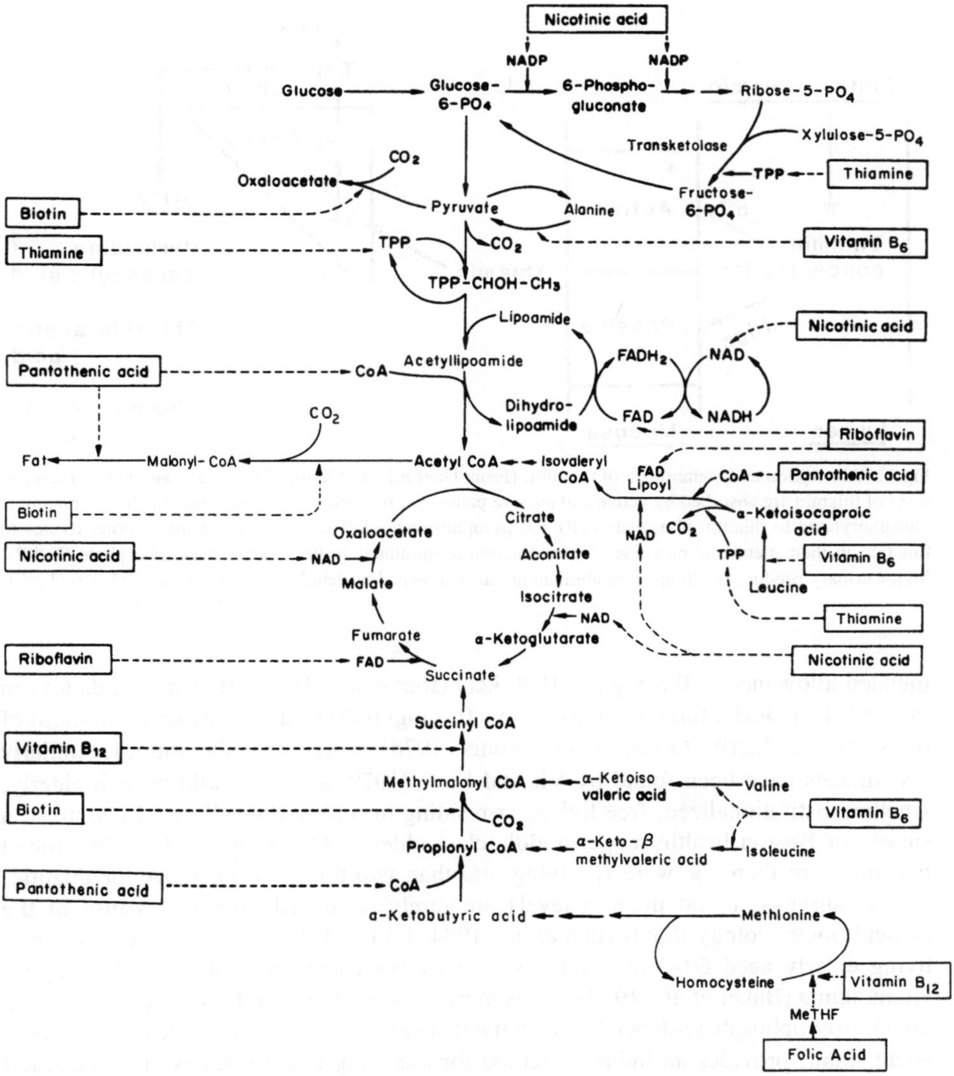

Fig. 2. Coenzyme functions of the B vitamins in some major metabolic pathways. (From Danford and Munro, 1980.)

and Rosenberg, 1982; Gray *et al.*, 1983; Harrill and Cervone, 1977; Yearick *et al.*, 1980; Beauchene and Davis, 1979). In HANES I, 18–46% of elderly aged 65–74 years (depending on race and income) had daily intakes of thiamin below two-thirds of the RDA (Bowman and Rosenberg, 1982). The importance of race and economic status in thiamin intake is clearly reflected in the HANES I data: the highest percentage (46%) of thiamin intake below two-thirds of the RDA was found in black, elderly males with incomes below the poverty level. The thiamin intake per 1000 kcal in HANES I and II, however, was 0.73–0.77 mg and thus above the generally recom-

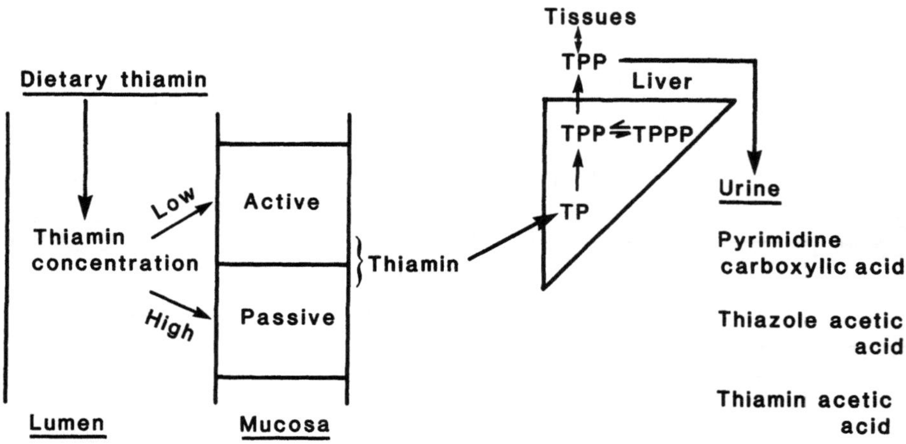

Fig. 3. Absorption and metabolism of thiamin. (From Danford and Munro, 1988.) Low and high concentrations of thiamin are absorbed by active and passive pathways, respectively. On reaching the liver, thiamin is phosphorylated to thiamin phosphate (TP) and pyrophosphate (TPP), the latter passing to other tissues to function in their metabolic processes. Some thiamin accumulates in the liver as the triphosphate (TPPP). Major urinary products of thiamin catabolism are also shown. For details, see Danford and Munro (1988).

mended allowance of 0.5 mg per 1000 kcal (Iber *et al.*, 1982). In contrast, data from the TSNS showed a thiamin intake below 0.4 mg/1000 kcal in more than one-third of the surveyed elderly (O'Hanlon and Kohrs, 1978). Based on 3-day diaries, similarly low intakes have been found by Vir and Love (1979) among Northern Irish elderly, whether institutionalized, free-living, or residing in sheltered dwellings. In contrast, a survey of Boston healthy upper-middle-class elderly (McGandy *et al.*, 1986) found that no more than 5% were receiving less than two-thirds of the RDA for thiamin.

In surveys, blood thiamin levels are rarely measured directly because of the difficult methodology (Sauberlich *et al.*, 1984; Bamji, 1981). However, 11% of free-living elderly aged 60–102 years have been reported to show thiamin blood hypovitaminemia (Baker *et al.*, 1979). Measurement of red blood cell transketolase (TK), a thiamin-pyrophosphate-dependent enzyme that catalyzes reactions in the pentose phosphate shunt, provides an indirect method for assessing thiamin status. The mean red cell TK decreases significantly from birth (5.31 ± 0.98 units) to old age (4.43 ± 1.11 units in 90 to 99-year-old subjects; Markkanen *et al.*, 1969). The clinical and functional consequence of this finding is unclear. With the TK activation coefficient used as an index of thiamin nutriture, 3–15% of healthy, free-living elderly in different surveys had abnormal values (Vir and Love, 1979; Brin *et al.*, 1965; Iber *et al.*, 1982), while 40% of hospitalized elderly had low values (Griffiths *et al.*, 1967).

Another method for assessing thiamin nutriture is the measurement of urinary thiamin excretion. However, no correlation between urinary thiamin excretion and age has been found (Thomson, 1966). Use of urinary thiamin excretion as an index of thiamin status found 0–9% of the elderly in various surveys to have low values (Harrill and Cervone, 1977; Beauchene and Davis, 1979; Leichter *et al.*, 1978; Brin *et al.*, 1965; Fischer *et al.*, 1978), the highest prevalence of low values among HANES-I subjects being found in elderly black men (Lowenstein, 1982). Sick geriatric patients show higher activation coefficients (indicative of deficiency) and a higher prevalence of low urinary thiamin excretion (Vir and Love, 1977c, 1979; Brin *et al.*, 1965; Iber *et al.*, 1982).

There are conflicting data whether age influences thiamin absorption from the gastrointestinal tract (Thomson, 1966; Breen *et al.*, 1985; Draper, 1958; Rafsky and Newman, 1943; Rafsky *et al.*, 1947; Kirk and Chieffi, 1951). Alcohol (an operative factor at all ages) affects thiamin absorption by blocking the egress of thiamin from the mucosal cell and preventing phosphorylation (Leevy, 1982; Hoyumpa *et al.*, 1975; Martin *et al.*, 1985). Also, individuals with a high intake of antithiamin factors (such as caffeic acid and tannic acid, found in coffee and tea, respectively) might be at higher risk for thiamin deficiency (Vimokesant *et al.*, 1982). There are no known age-related changes in thiamin metabolism.

In summary, there is wide variability of thiamin status in the elderly: 0–15% of the elderly show biochemical thiamin deficiency, which is, however, usually related to low dietary intakes. It is concluded that the present RDA for thiamin is adequate for the elderly and that the wide variability in thiamin intakes among the elderly accounts in large part for the variability in biochemical measures of thiamin nutriture among various surveyed elderly groups.

4.2. Riboflavin

The active forms of riboflavin (vitamin B_2) are its coenzymes FMN (flavin mononucleotide) and FAD (flavin adenine dinucleotide), which have an important role in oxidation–reduction reactions. Riboflavin absorption and metabolism are illustrated in Fig. 4. Meat, milk, and milk products are good sources for vitamin B_2, but since

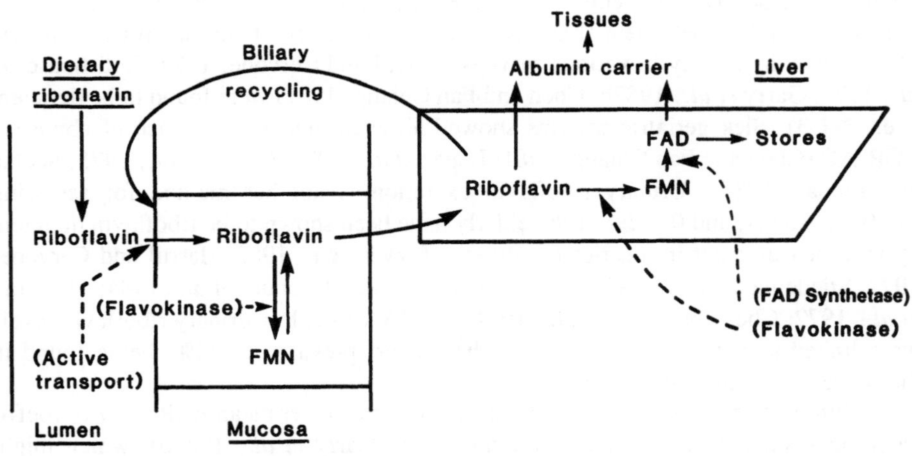

Fig. 4. Absorption and metabolism of riboflavin. (From Danford and Munro, 1988.) Riboflavin is absorbed by active transport and then passes to the liver, where flavokinase transforms part of it to flavin mononucleotide (FMN) and then to flavin adenine dinucleotide (FAD) through the action of FAD synthetase. Both riboflavin and FAD are carried on albumin in the plasma to other tissues. Some hepatic free riboflavin may be recycled via the bile and reabsorption from the intestine. For details, see Danford and Munro (1988).

riboflavin is heat sensitive, large amounts can be destroyed during the cooking process (Foy and Mbaya, 1977). The 1980 RDA for riboflavin is 1.4 mg/day for males and 1.2 mg/day for females over age 50 years (National Academy of Sciences, 1980).

There is a wide spectrum of riboflavin intakes among various elderly populations studied (Bowman and Rosenberg, 1982; Garry *et al.*, 1982b; Gray *et al.*, 1983; Harrill and Cervone, 1977; Yearick *et al.*, 1980; Stiedemann *et al.*, 1978; Kohrs *et al.*, 1978; O'Hanlon and Kohrs, 1978; Vir and Love, 1979), 0–36% being reported to have intakes below two-thirds of the RDA (Bowman and Rosenberg, 1982; Gray *et al.*, 1983; Alexander *et al.*, 1984). In HANES I, depending on race and income, 12–36% of subjects aged 65–74 had riboflavin intakes below two-thirds of the 1974 RDA (Bowman and Rosenberg, 1982), which differed slightly from the 1980 values, being 1.5 mg/day for males and 1.1 mg/day for females. Once again, intake was related to race and income; black elderly males with an income below the poverty level had the highest prevalence (36%) of low intakes. In the TSNS, 19–27% of the elderly grouped by income had intakes below two-thirds of the RDA (Beauchene and Davis, 1979). However, Garry *et al.* (1982a) detected <6% of vitamin B_2 intakes below three-fourths of the RDA among well-educated, healthy elderly aged 60–93. Similarly, all of the healthy residents (aged 70 years or older) in a private women's care facility had mean daily riboflavin intakes of approximately 1.5 times the RDA (Alexander *et al.*, 1984). Rutishauser *et al.* (1979) surveyed the riboflavin status of 23 healthy free-living elderly (aged 72–84 years) over a period of 18 months. The mean daily riboflavin intake over the whole period was 1.0 mg/day for females (range 0.7–1.6 mg/day) and 1.2 mg/day for males (range 0.6–1.7 mg/day), and individual intakes were below the RDA in approximately 75%. Confirming the frequency of low intakes, 18% of the females and 50% of the males had abnormal (i.e., >1.2) glutathione reductase activation coefficients.

Biochemical assessment of deficiency depends on red cell enzyme activation and on urinary riboflavin excretion. With measurement of the erythrocyte glutathione reductase activity coefficient (EGR-AC) used as an index of riboflavin nutriture, 0–28% of healthy elderly in various surveys (Harrill and Cervone, 1977; Rutishauser *et al.*, 1979; Garry *et al.*, 1982b; Chen and Fan Chiang, 1981) were found to be deficient (i.e., >1.3). Sick geriatric patients showed an even higher prevalence of abnormal EGR-AC (Chen and Fan Chiang, 1981; Lopez *et al.*, 1979; Hoorn *et al.*, 1975; Skalka and Prchal, 1981). Urinary riboflavin excretion is another method for assessing riboflavin status, and 0–22% of the elderly have been shown to be riboflavin deficient by this measurement in a series of surveys (Lowenstein, 1982; Harrill and Cervone, 1977; Stiedemann *et al.*, 1978; Fischer *et al.*, 1978; Alexander *et al.*, 1984; Thackray *et al.*, 1972; Chen and Fan Chiang, 1981). In HANES I, low urinary riboflavin levels were linked to poverty and race, with the highest prevalence (20%) being found in black men (Lowenstein, 1982).

With increasing age, there is a tendency towards lower mean EGR activity coefficients independent of sex and riboflavin intake (Garry *et al.*, 1982b), which might indicate lower metabolic vitamin B_2 requirements in the aged, related to their lower energy and protein intakes (Machlin, 1984a). Alternatively, other age-related changes in riboflavin absorption and/or metabolism may occur. However, Said and Hollander (1985) could not show any age difference in vitamin B_2 absorption using everted intestinal sacs prepared from 3- and 26-month-old rats. Weak evidence for changes in riboflavin absorption comes from the study by Vir and Love (1977a), who reported riboflavin deficiency in the elderly despite adequate vitamin B_2 intakes. Regarding tissue levels, Schaus and Kirk (1957) did not find significant age-related changes in the riboflavin concentrations in human cerebral cortex, skeletal muscle, and myocardial muscle.

The riboflavin nutritional status of the elderly is highly variable, the high prevalence of poor riboflavin status in some surveys apparently resulting from poor intake. No proven age-related changes in riboflavin metabolism have been found, and there is presently no evidence to alter vitamin B_2 requirement in the aged. Therapeutically important drug–riboflavin interactions are listed in Table I.

4.3. Niacin

Niacin is the collective term for nicotinic acid and nicotinamide (National Academy of Sciences, 1980). Niacin is a component of the coenzymes nicotinamide adenine dinucleotide (NAD) and nicotinamide adenine dinucleotide phosphate (NADP), which are involved in metabolic reactions of fat, carbohydrate, and amino acid metabolism and tissue respiration. Niacin requirements are expressed as niacin equivalents (NE), since the amino acid tryptophan can be converted to niacin. The 1980 niacin RDA is 16 mg NE per day for males and 13 mg NE per day for females over 50 years of age (National Academy of Sciences, 1980). Meat, nuts, and cereals are good niacin sources; overt niacin deficiency manifests itself as pellagra, rarely seen in the United States today except among alcoholics (Hankes, 1984).

The niacin intakes of the elderly are highly variable (Garry *et al.*, 1982a; Harrill and Cervone, 1977; Yearick *et al.*, 1980; Stiedemann *et al.*, 1978; Beauchene and Davis, 1979; Steinkamp *et al.*, 1965). From 0 to 53% of the surveyed elderly have been reported to have niacin intakes less than two-thirds of the RDA depending on income and race (Bowman and Rosenberg, 1982; Garry *et al.*, 1982a; Gray *et al.*, 1983). In HANES I, the highest prevalence (53%) of low intake values was seen among blacks with incomes below the poverty level, and the lowest prevalence (20%) was seen among white men with incomes above the poverty level. In contrast, all of the healthy, relatively well-off elderly surveyed by Garry *et al.* (1982a) had niacin intakes above the RDA.

Studies on the niacin status of populations are scanty, which in part reflects the lack of good biochemical methods for the evaluation of niacin nutriture (Sauberlich *et al.*, 1984; Bamji, 1981). At present, the only biochemical method of value for assessing niacin status is the urinary excretion of N-methylnicotinamide (NMN) and N-methyl-2-pyridone-5-carboxylamide (2-pyridone). Although measurement of urinary 2-pyridone expressed as the 2-pyridone/NMN ratio is thought to reflect niacin status better, in practice only urinary NMN has been commonly used because of its ease of measurement. By measuring the urinary NMN excretion, biochemical niacin deficiency was detected in 1–50% of heterogeneous elderly populations composed of free-living, institutionalized, and sick individuals (Harrill and Cervone, 1977; Morgan *et al.*, 1975; Bonati *et al.*, 1956). The prevalence of abnormal NMN excretion in urine increases with age and sickness. Rat studies have shown no age-related changes in niacin absorption (Fleming and Barrows, 1982b).

Niacin nutritional status in the elderly thus appears to vary widely, depending on factors such as race and income. Although there is a shortage of data on which to base a conclusion, there is no current evidence that the 1980 RDA for niacin is too low in the case of the elderly. However, more studies are needed before a definitive statement can be made.

4.4. Vitamin B_6

Vitamin B_6 is the collective term for pyridoxine, pyridoxal, and pyridoxamine. Their metabolic interrelationships are illustrated in Fig. 5. Vitamin B_6 is an important cofactor in more than 50 enzymatic reactions such as transamination, deamination, and decarboxylation, most of which are involved in protein metabolism. Vitamin B_6 is widely distributed in food, good sources being meat, poultry, fish, rice, beans, and nuts. Pyridoxine is mainly found in plants, whereas pyridoxal and pyridoxamine occur mainly in animal tissues. Vitamin B_6 is absorbed in the upper jejunum by an active process. Physiologically the active form of vitamin B_6 is pyridoxal phosphate (PLP) (Driskell, 1984; Shideler, 1983). The 1980 RDA for vitamin B_6 is 2.2 mg/day for males and 2.0 mg/day for females, the requirements increasing with a high protein intake with a suggested ratio of 0.02 mg of vitamin B_6 per gram of protein eaten (National Academy of Sciences, 1980). Among the elderly, there is a correlation between protein intake and vitamin B_6 consumption (Munro *et al.*, 1987).

Present data on vitamin B_6 content in food are far from complete. Consequently, intake data are only of limited value for the assessment of vitamin B_6 nutritional status. From a number of surveys, 50–90% of the elderly have low vitamin B_6 intakes as compared to the 1980 RDA (Garry *et al.*, 1982a; MacLeod *et al.*, 1974; Elsborg *et al.*, 1983; Lonergan *et al.*, 1975; Guilland *et al.*, 1984; Vir and Love, 1977b, 1978b; Hampton *et al.*, 1977; Betts and Vivian, 1984; Driskell, 1978; Chrisley and Driskell, 1979). In New Mexico, Garry *et al.* (1982) showed that approximately 85% of healthy free-living middle-income elderly over 60 years had intakes below three-fourths of the 1980 RDA. Guilland *et al.* (1984) reported that approximately half of the residents of a nursing home (all over age 60) had a vitamin B_6 intake of less than 1 mg/day (i.e., less than 50% of the RDA). From various surveys, the vitamin B_6 intake of elderly females is less than that of males (Lonergan *et al.*, 1975; Guilland *et al.*, 1984; Vir and Love, 1978; Betts and Vivian, 1984; Driskell, 1978).

Serum and plasma vitamin B_6 levels are greatly influenced by recent dietary intakes and are thus of uncertain usefulness in assessing vitamin B_6 nutriture. Fasting plasma (Walsh, 1966; Lumeng and Li, 1974; Hamfelt, 1964; Rose *et al.*, 1976) and serum (Anderson *et al.*, 1970) PLP levels have been demonstrated to decrease with age. For example, Rose *et al.* (1976) found a decrease of 0.90 ng/ml per decade in plasma PLP. In consequence, the percentage of low plasma PLP levels increases with age, 3% of a healthy population under 40 years of age showing PLP plasma levels below 5 ng/ml, as compared with 12% in the age group over 80 years. Note that none of the subjects receiving vitamin B_6 supplements had these low values. However, Kheim and Kirk (1967) could not show a significant change in human vascular tissue content of vitamin B_6 over the age range 20–84 years.

An alternative method for assessing vitamin B_6 nutriture is the tryptophan load test. With increasing age there is a diminished capacity to catabolize tryptophan com-

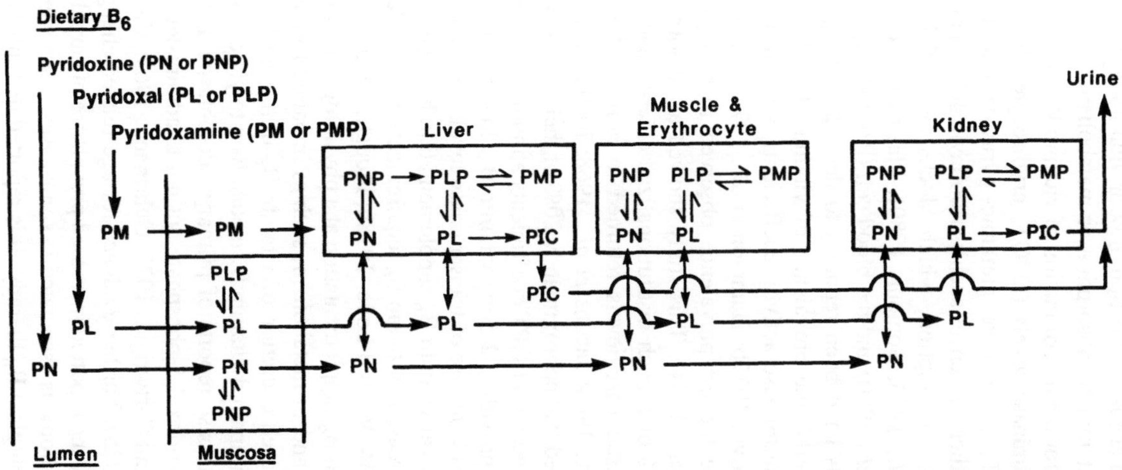

Fig. 5. Absorption and metabolism of vitamin B_6. (From Danford and Munro, 1988.) Following absorption, pyridoxine (PN), pyridoxal (PL), and pyridoxamine (PM) are phosphorylated in the tissues. Most PN is transformed in the liver to PNP, then PLP and PMP. The PLP formed in the liver from dietary PN, PL, and PM provides PL for transport in the blood to some other tissues that do not form it from PN. Pyridoxic acid (PIC) formed in liver and kidney is excreted in the urine as an end-product. For details, see Danford and Munro (1988).

pletely, which is reflected in increased urinary xanthurenic acid excretion after a tryptophan load (Hamfelt, 1964; Ranke *et al.*, 1960). For example, Ranke *et al.* (1960) showed that the mean xanthurenic acid excretion in 24-hr urines after a tryptophan load was approximately 50% higher in 24 elderly people (average age 76 years) than in 20 young adults (average age 25 years). It is not known whether the increase of abnormal tryptophan load tests with age is a reflection of poor vitamin B_6 nutriture or of specific age-related changes in vitamin B_6 absorption or metabolism.

An additional index for the determination of vitamin B_6 status is the measurement of the erythrocyte transaminase levels (EGOT, erythrocyte glutamate–oxaloacetate transaminase, and EGPT, erythrocyte glutamic–pyruvate transaminase), although these are also subject to other influences such as riboflavin deficiency, which depresses serum PLP, and ethanol consumption, which blocks the PLP binding site on the apoenzyme (Leinert *et al.*, 1983; Bonjour, 1980). Plasma concentrations of PLP as well as serum (Ranke *et al.*, 1960) and red blood cell (Rose *et al.*, 1976; Jacobs *et al.*, 1968) transaminase levels have been reported to decline with age. Among various groups of free-living elderly, the prevalence of vitamin B_6 deficiency indicated by abnormal erythrocyte transaminase activity coefficients is about 40% (Chen and Fan Chiang, 1981; Vir and Love, 1977b; Hampton *et al.*, 1977; Driskell, 1984; Chrisley and Driskell, 1979). The highest prevalence observed in a single population was reported by Guilland *et al.* (1984). This study showed an abnormal EGOT activity coefficient (>2.0) in 70% of French institutionalized elderly (aged 60–98 years). In most studies, blood transaminase levels returned to normal after oral vitamin B_6 supplementation (Hamfelt, 1964; Jacobs *et al.*, 1968; Ranke *et al.*, 1960). Vir and Love (1977b) have reported that approximately 20% of their Northern Irish elderly had low transaminase levels and high EGPT coefficients although they were taking a daily multivitamin supplement providing 2.5 mg vitamin B_6. In other studies (Hoorn *et al.*, 1975; Vir and Love, 1978b), failure of transaminase levels and activity coefficients to return to normal on low-level vitamin B_6 supplementation has been reported, supporting the postulate of an increase in vitamin B_6 requirements by the elderly (Hoorn *et al.*, 1975; Guilland *et al.*, 1984; Vir and Love, 1978b; Plough, 1960; Gyorgy, 1971). The lack of response to vitamin B_6 supplementation at a physiological dose might be caused by changes in absorption and/or metabolism, such as impaired formation of pyridoxal phosphate (PLP) or increased excretion of vitamin B_6 in the aged.

Evidence to support impaired vitamin B_6 metabolism to yield pyridoxal phosphate comes from some clinical case reports of primary sideroblastic anemias that are exclusively responsive to pyridoxal-5-phosphate but not to administered pyridoxine as a PLP precursor (Kushner and Cartwright, 1977; Gehrmann, 1965; Mason and Emerson, 1973; Hines and Love, 1975). Further evidence for age-related changes in vitamin B_6 metabolism is provided by the reported increased prevalence of carpal tunnel syndrome (CTS) with age. This syndrome is associated in some cases with vitamin B_6 deficiency and responds to pharmacological B_6 therapy. It is reported that most (85%) of the CTS patients are over 40 years of age and that approximately 30% show biochemical evidence of vitamin B_6 deficiency (Yamaguchi *et al.*, 1965; Folkers *et al.*, 1978; Ellis *et al.*, 1982; Salkeld and Stotz, 1985; Del Tredici *et al.*, 1985). It is not clear whether the age-related increase in prevalence of CTS and of pyridoxine deficiency are coincidental or related.

From animal studies, there is some evidence for age-related changes in vitamin B_6 metabolism (Fonda and Eggers, 1980). When Fonda *et al.* (1980a) injected [^{3}H]pyridoxine into elderly mice, they converted less to PLP and more to pyridoxine and pyridoxic acid. In the brains of senescent (33-month) versus young adult mice (13 months), the same authors showed increased hydrolysis of pyridoxal phosphate (Fonda *et al.*, 1980b). Further, the activity of vitamin B_6-dependent brain aspartate–glutamate oxaloacetate transaminase decreased with increasing age (Fonda *et al.*, 1973). Older animals showed a more rapid vitamin B_6 uptake by the liver (Fonda *et al.*, 1980a). More research is needed for final interpretation of these data.

Drugs commonly used in the elderly that interfere with vitamin B_6 metabolism are listed in Table I. Acetaldehyde from ethanol oxidation accelerates PLP degradation (Driskell, 1984). There is evidence that fiber diminishes the bioavailability of vitamin B_6 (Miller *et al.*, 1979; Leklem *et al.*, 1980). Lindberg *et al.* (1983) showed that the concomitant consumption of 15 g wheat bran with a standard diet decreased the absorption of vitamin B_6 up to 17% in young healthy adults. This finding may be of importance in elderly people with borderline B_6 nutriture who eat high-fiber diets.

In summary, low dietary vitamin B_6 intakes could account for the high prevalence of biochemical B_6 deficiency in the elderly. However, there is evidence to suggest a change in vitamin B_6 metabolism with age in both animals and humans that could result in higher vitamin B_6 requirements. It remains to be shown whether the present vitamin B_6 RDA is adequate for the elderly.

4.5. Folic Acid

Folic acid acts as a donor and acceptor of one-carbon units in biochemical reactions of amino acid and DNA metabolism. Folate absorption and metabolism are illustrated in Fig. 6. Folate is widely distributed in nature, good food sources being vegetables, fruits, and yeast. In nature, folates occur mainly in the reduced form and as polyglutamates, whereas folate in plasma is in the monoglutamate form (5-methyl-H_4-Pte-Glu) (Brody *et al.*, 1984). During the absorptive process in the upper jejunum, folate polyglutamates are hydrolyzed to folate monoglutamates by γ-glutamylpeptidase (conjugase). This process is highly dependent on the intraluminal pH, showing increased activity at a pH of 6.3 (Rosenberg, 1981; Rosenberg *et al.*, 1979; Russell *et al.*, 1979).

The 1980 adult RDA for folate is 400 μg per day for both sexes (National Academy of Sciences, 1980), but surveys show much lower intakes, some of which may reflect incomplete food analysis for folates. Folate intake data for the elderly are scanty, and such reported intakes vary widely (Garry *et al.*, 1982a, 1984; Vir and Love, 1979; MacLeod *et al.*, 1974; Elsborg *et al.*, 1983; Jagerstad and Westesson, 1979; Bates *et al.*, 1980; Rodriguez, 1978). In a healthy, well-cared-for noninstitutionalized population residing in New Mexico, Garry *et al.* (1982a) found that the prevalence of folate intakes below three-fourth of the RDA was 70% in males and 84% in females. In a group of 264 free-living elderly over 65 years, MacLeod *et al.* (1974) reported mean folate intakes to be only 50–65 μg/day, based on 7-day dietary records. Data from the Nutrition Canada Survey (Rosenberg *et al.*, 1982) showed higher mean folate intakes of 130–151 μg/day among elderly over 65 years of age. A Swedish

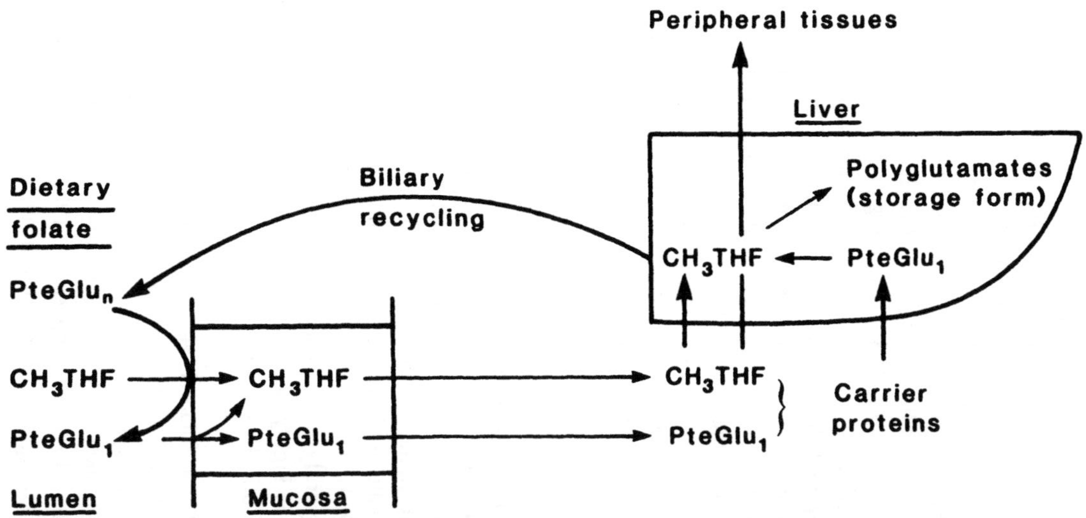

Fig. 6. Absorption and metabolism of folates. (From Danford and Munro, 1988.) Dietary folates lose polyglutamates at the intestinal mucosal cells, where they yield pteroyl monoglutamate ($PteGlu_1$) and methyltetrahydrofolic acid (CH_3THF) for transport to the liver on carrier plasma proteins. The liver avidly takes up $PteGlu_1$ for transformation to CH_3 THF, some of which is stored as polyglutamates, some recycled through the bile, and some passes into the general circulation for uptake by other tissues. For details, see Danford and Munro (1988).

survey (Jagersted and Westesson, 1979) reported a similar picture. Although this all suggests that the elderly have low folate intakes as compared to the RDA, it should be recognized that food tables are relatively incomplete for folate content, so the true consumption may be somewhat higher.

Biochemical methods for assessing folate nutritional status are serum, plasma, and red blood cell folate levels. In the elderly, these are influenced by institutionalization, socioeconomic status, and health status (Lowenstein, 1982; Vir and Love, 1979; Baker *et al.*, 1979; Garry *et al.*, 1984; Runcie, 1979; Bailey *et al.*, 1979; Wagner *et al.*, 1981; Webster and Leeming, 1979; Hurdle and Williams, 1966; Hayes *et al.*, 1985; Magnus *et al.*, 1982; Elwood *et al.*, 1971; Lawrence, 1983). In a review of the published surveys, Rosenberg *et al.* (1982) found 3 to 7% of healthy, free-living elderly to have low plasma/serum folate levels (<3 ng/ml). In HANES I, approximately 6% of the elderly aged 65–74 had serum folate levels below 3 ng/ml (Lowenstein, 1982). Girdwood *et al.* (1967), however, failed to show a significant difference in serum folate levels in a mixed free-living and institutionalized Scottish population of elderly (aged over 65) versus younger controls (aged 20–60). However, higher prevalences (up to 30%) of low values (<3.0 ng/ml) have been reported in heterogeneous free-living and institutionalized elderly populations (Vir and Love, 1979; Webster and Leeming, 1979; Hurdle and Williams, 1966; Magnus *et al.*, 1982; Lawrence, 1983). Evidence that folate intakes below the RDA could be adequate for maintaining normal folate nutriture comes from a Swedish study by Jagerstad and Westesson (1979). In 35 elderly aged 60–67 years, folate intakes were determined and whole-blood folate levels were measured every 2 years during a 6-year period. The initial folate intake of this group was 100–200 μg/day. Despite this low intake as compared to the RDA, normal whole-blood folate levels were found in all but five subjects. In three of the subjects with low blood folate levels, chronic gastritis or pernicious anemia was diagnosed.

Low red blood cell (RBC) folate levels (<140 ng/ml) have been reported in 3–60% of the elderly, depending on socioeconomic and health status (Garry *et al.*, 1984; Bailey *et al.*, 1979; Wagner *et al.*, 1981; Webster and Leeming, 1979; Elwood *et al.*, 1971). Wagner *et al.* (1981) observed low RBC folate values in only 6% of healthy, free-living middle- and upper-class elderly women aged 55–87 years versus 60% of healthy lower-class women of the same age range. In Northern Ireland, Vir and Love (1979) reported low RBC folate levels in 20–60% of free-living elderly aged 65 and over. Liver folate levels measured from hospital autopsy specimens of patients dying from a variety of causes or illnesses decreased from peak levels at age 11 to 30 years of 8.8 ± 2.2 μ/g wet weight to 6.9 ± 2.1 μg/g wet weight at age 80 and over (Hoppner and Lampi, 1980).

Although animal data are conflicting, there is presently no evidence that folic acid absorption is affected by age alone (Runcie, 1979; Ziemlanski *et al.*, 1971; Bhanthumnavin *et al.*, 1974; Elsborg, 1976; Baker *et al.*, 1978; see also Chapter 3). However, folate absorption is impaired in elderly with atrophic gastritis. Atrophic gastritis with resultant hypochlorhydria occurs in 20–50% of the elderly over 60 years. The strong pH dependence of active folate absorption with a pH optimum of 6.3 has been shown by several investigators (Rosenberg, 1981; Russell *et al.*, 1979, 1985). Russell *et al.* (1984) recently showed that subjects with atrophic gastritis malabsorb folate, probably because of the higher intraluminal pH in the proximal GI tract. However, as evidenced by normal erythrocyte folate levels, subjects with atrophic gastritis and hypochlorhydria are not necessarily deficient in folate, possibly because of synthesis of folate by bacteria that have overgrown the nonacidic upper intestinal tract. So far, no consistent age-related changes in folyl conjugase activity have been shown (Kesavan and Noronha, 1983; Bailey *et al.*, 1984). Alcoholics of all age groups are at highest risk of developing folate deficiency (Rosenberg *et al.*, 1982; Russell *et al.*, 1983). Dietary fiber probably does not influence the bioavailability of folic acid (Ristow *et al.*, 1982; Russell *et al.*, 1976; Babu and Srikantia, 1976; Colman *et al.*, 1975). Therapeutically important drug–folate interactions are listed in Table I.

It appears that elderly with folate intakes well below the RDA can maintain normal folate nutriture, which is evidence that the RDA for folate is too high. The few studies that show a high prevalence of biochemical folate deficiency have been among the poor or sick and can be attributed to very low intakes. So far, no consistent age-related changes in folate absorption or metabolism have been described.

4.6. Vitamin B_{12}

Vitamin B_{12} (cobalamin) is required for normal hematopoiesis and for maintaining the integrity of the nervous system. Vitamin B_{12} absorption and metabolism are illustrated in Fig. 7. At the biochemical level, vitamin B_{12} is an important cofactor in the metabolism of folate, the synthesis of methionine, and the conversion of methylmalonyl-CoA to succinyl-CoA, the active coenzymes of vitamin B_{12} being methylcobalamin and 5-deoxyadenosylcobalamin. The major food sources of vitamin B_{12}

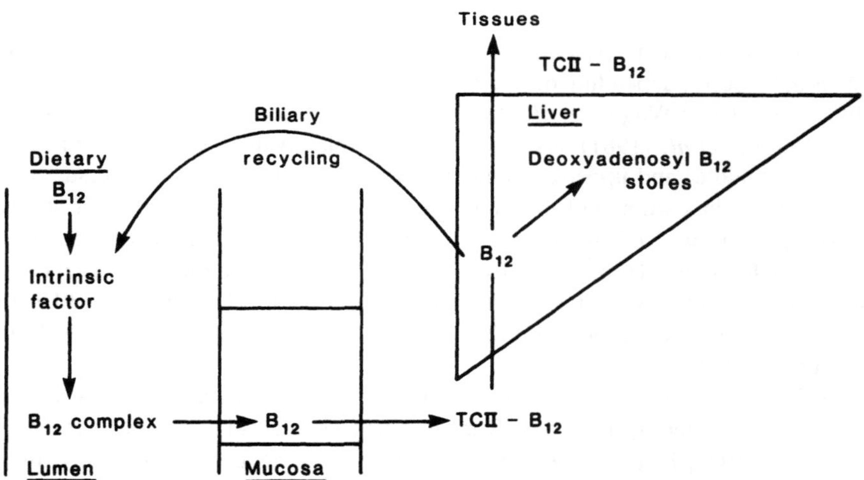

Fig. 7. Absorption and metabolism of vitamin B_{12}. (From Danford and Munro, 1988.) Dietary B_{12} attached to food protein is released by proteolytic digestion and attached to intrinsic factor, which binds the B_{12} to the intestinal mucosa for absorption. In the plasma, B_{12} binds to three transport proteins, notably, transcobalamin II (TC II). In the liver, B_{12} is stored as deoxyadenosyl-B_{12}. For details see Danford and Munro (1988).

are animal products, notably meat, milk, and eggs (Ellenbogen, 1984). The present RDA for vitamin B_{12} is 3.0 μg per day for adults of both sexes (National Academy of Sciences, 1980). Vitamin B_{12} is absorbed by an active process involving binding to intrinsic factor (IF) with subsequent binding of the IF–B_{12} complex to specific receptors in the distal ileum (Ellenbogen, 1984; Seetharam and Alpers, 1985). The most common cause of cobalamin deficiency is cobalamin malabsorption as a result of the lack of IF in pernicious anemia (Zimran and Hershko, 1983). Vitamin B_{12} deficiency from poor dietary intake is uncommon. Although healthy vegetarians might be expected to be at higher risk for deficiency, in practice they rarely show clinical evidence of this (Carmel, 1978; Immerman, 1981).

Vitamin B_{12} intakes of free-living, healthy elderly vary widely (Garry *et al.*, 1982a, 1984; Prothro *et al.*, 1976; Elsborg *et al.*, 1983; Betts and Vivian, 1984). Garry *et al.* (1982a) showed 24% of middle-class male Caucasian elderly and 39% of female Caucasian elderly in New Mexico to have vitamin B_{12} intakes below three-fourths of the RDA. The low risk of clinical and biochemical vitamin B_{12} deficiency associated with a poor dietary intake of vitamin B_{12} is reflected in the data from Prothro *et al.* (1976) in a mainly black healthy, free-living population aged 56 to 85. Although only 8% of the elderly had intakes exceeding two-thirds of the RDA, none had serum vitamin B_{12} levels below 20 pg/ml.

The normal range of fasting serum levels of vitamin B_{12} in humans is 150–900 pg/ml (Sauberlich *et al.*, 1984). Serum and plasma vitamin B_{12} is most commonly measured by microbiological methods or radiodilution assays. Studies done before 1980 using radiodilution assay kits should be interpreted with caution because of the occurrence of "R-binders," which bind vitamin B_{12} analogues, thus producing falsely high vitamin B_{12} values (Ellenbogen, 1984; Anonymous, 1979b). With increasing age of humans and rats, there is a tendency for serum vitamin B_{12} to decline while still within the normal range (Kilpatrick and Withey, 1965; Nyberg *et al.*, 1964; Boger *et al.*, 1955; Gaffney *et al.*, 1957; Chow *et al.*, 1956b; Elsborg *et al.*, 1976; Nielson, 1965; Mollin and Ross, 1952). Mollin and Ross (1952) reported lower serum levels of vitamin B_{12} in the age group 71–93 years versus 15–40 years. Chow *et al.* (1956b) found a decline of serum vitamin B_{12} with age, notably a large drop occurring in subjects after the age of 70 years. Such declines of mean vitamin B_{12} serum levels might result from undetected cases of pernicious anemia and/or vitamin B_{12} malabsorption from atrophic gastritis (*vide infra*). In various surveys, 0% to 23% of free-living elderly were found to have low (150 pg/ml) vitamin B_{12} serum or plasma levels (Garry *et al.*, 1984; Hayes *et al.*, 1985; Magnus *et al.*, 1982; Elwood *et al.*, 1971; Bailey *et al.*, 1980). Nevertheless, several studies have been unable to demonstrate a significant change in serum levels with age (Morgan *et al.*, 1973; Cape and Shinton, 1961; Killander, 1957; Droller and Dossett, 1959; Hitzhusen *et al.*, 1986), and other data on age-related changes of liver vitamin B_{12} content are contradictory (Hsu *et al.*, 1966; McLaren, 1981; Hall, 1982).

Although there is no evidence for altered vitamin B_{12} absorption resulting from advancing age alone (Fleming and Barrows, 1982b; Glass *et al.*, 1956; Chow, 1958; Chernish *et al.*, 1957; Hyams, 1964; Swenseid *et al.*, 1954; Chow *et al.*, 1956a; McEvoy *et al.*, 1982; Doscherholmen *et al.*, 1977), some elderly may have reduced cobalamin absorption because of atrophic gastritis with hypo- or achlorhydria. Atrophic gastritis has been reported in 20–50% of elderly people (Cheli *et al.*, 1980; Kreuning *et al.*, 1978; Hradsky *et al.*, 1966). Using a serological test on an American population, Krasinski *et al.* (1983) found mild to moderate atrophic gastritis in 17% over the age of 60. There are three mechanisms to explain how atrophic gastritis could affect vitamin B_{12} absorption: (1) vitamin B_{12} bound in food cannot be freed because of maldigestion of protein for lack of acid–pepsin digestion (King *et al.*, 1979; Dawson *et al.*, 1984), (2) binding or transformation of vitamin B_{12} to analogues (cobinamides) by bacteria that overgrow in the upper gastrointestinal tract because of the lack of gastric acid (Brandt *et al.*, 1977; Welkos *et al.*, 1981; Gracey, 1979; Giannella *et al.*, 1971; Kistler and Giannella, 1980), and (3) decreased secretion of intrinsic factor (Ardeman and Chanerin, 1966). The exact role of mild to moderate gastric atrophy in the development of vitamin B_{12} deficiency (malabsorption) in the elderly is an area of active investigation.

Therapeutically important vitamin B_{12}–drug interactions are listed in Table I. H-2 blockers (e.g., cimetidine) could influence vitamin B_{12} absorption by lowering gastric acid secretion, and in consequence, subjects on long-term H-2 blocker treatment with concomitant low vitamin B_{12} intakes may be at increased risk for vitamin B_{12} deficiency (Steinberg *et al.*, 1980; Sharpe *et al.*, 1980). The claim that long-term consumption of pharmacological amounts of ascorbic acid simultaneously with marginal vitamin B_{12} intakes can affect vitamin B_{12} nutriture by destroying vitamin B_{12} and/or intrinsic factor has not been confirmed (Watson *et al.*, 1982; Hogenkamp, 1980). Alcoholism (Lindenbaum and Lieber, 1969) and high fiber consumption by increasing fecal excretion (Anonymous, 1979a) could negatively affect vitamin B_{12} status.

In summary, despite the rather high prevalence of low vitamin B_{12} intakes among the elderly, only a minority show low serum plasma levels. The decrease in serum vitamin B_{12} levels with age could be related in part to the increased prevalence of atrophic gastritis with age. No other age-related changes in vitamin B_{12} metabolism have been reported. It remains to be shown whether the vitamin B_{12} requirements in elderly with gastric atrophy are increased and require a larger allowance.

4.7. Biotin

Biotin is an essential cofactor for several carboxylation enzymes such as pyruvate carboxylase, required for conversion of pyruvate to oxaloacetate in the Krebs cycle. Biotin is widely distributed in nature, but the richest food sources are egg yolk, milk, and meat (Bonjour, 1984). Biotin deficiency in humans is very rare but has been reported in long-term total parenteral nutrition (Anonymous, 1981), biotinidase deficiency (Wolf *et al.*, 1985), and individuals consuming diets rich in raw eggs (Sweetman *et al.*, 1981). The estimated safe and adequate dietary biotin intake is in the range of 100–200 μg per day (National Academy of Sciences, 1980). Biotin metabolism has been reviewed recently (Roth, 1981; Dakshinamurti and Bhagavan, 1985).

There are two population studies involving biotin in the elderly. Normal blood levels have been shown in 99% of 473 free-living or institutionalized elderly aged 60–102 (Baker *et al.*, 1979). However, Bonjour (1984) reported significantly lower blood levels in 12 elderly (age not reported) as compared to younger controls. Markkanen and Mustakallio (1963) found a reduction in the urinary excretion of biotin in subjects with achlorhydria because of a possible impairment in release of food-bound biotin in the stomach. The clinical significance of this finding is uncertain.

4.8. *Pantothenic Acid*

Pantothenic acid is the main component of coenzyme A and an important cofactor for acyl group activation reactions. Clearly defined deficiency states of this vitamin have not been described in humans. Pantothenic acid is ubiquitous in nature and therefore widely distributed in food, the richest sources being meat, milk, broccoli, yeast, and bran (Fox, 1984).

Information on pantothenic acid status in different age and population groups is scanty. There is no established RDA for pantothenic acid, but the estimated safe and adequate daily range of intake is set provisionally at 4–7 mg (National Academy of Sciences, 1980). Since the methodology of pantothenic acid analysis in food is poorly developed, intake data are not very reliable in assessing the pantothenic acid nutritional status of an individual or population. However, there is weak evidence that some elderly may have lower pantothenic acid intakes than is currently suggested. Walsh *et al.* (1981) estimated the mean daily pantothenic acid content of a nursing home diet (beverages not included) to be 3.75 mg/day. On the other hand, Srinivasan *et al.* (1981) found an average pantothenic acid intake in elderly institutionalized and non-institutionalized persons to be 5.9 ± 0.3 mg/day, which is more than adequate.

Ishiguro (1961) have demonstrated a decline in blood pantothenic acid levels with increasing age in a rice-eating Japanese population of northern Honshu. More recently, the same investigator has shown only a decline of circulating protein-bound pantothenic acid with age, whereas free pantothenic acid levels remain constant (Ishiguro, 1972). In elderly Americans, no age dependence of blood pantothenic acid level has been shown (Srinivasan *et al.*, 1981). Sugarman and Munro (1980) reported a significantly decreased level of serum pantothenate in old rats as compared to younger rats; however, there was no age-related alteration in tissue uptake of pantothenate. The clinical significance of these changes remains uncertain.

Urinary levels of pantothenic acid have been shown to reflect the dietary intake better than blood levels. Schmidt (1951) showed a lower mean urinary pantothenic acid excretion before and after intramuscular injection of 25 mg pantothenate in elderly subjects (aged 51–82) as compared to younger adults (aged 16–45). In contrast, Srinivasan *et al.* (1981) found no effect of age on mean urinary pantothenic acid excretion in subjects aged 65 to 90 years.

Because of the contradictory data on intake, blood levels, and urinary excretion in relation to age as well as the relatively poor methods for the determination of food pantothenate, no statement can be made at present with regard to the appropriateness of the pantothenic acid requirement for elderly humans.

5. *Conclusion*

The assessment of overall vitamin nutriture in the elderly is complex and difficult. There are difficulties in defining population samples that are representative for various

Table II. Fiber–Vitamin Interactions

Nutrient	Species	Fiber type (amount)	Effect (proposed mechanism)	Reference
Vitamin A	Human	Lignin (12 g in a test meal)	No effect on tolerance curve	Barnard and Heaton (1973)
	Rat	Pectin (3% of diet)	No effect on liver stores	Phillips and Brien (1970)
Vitamin E	Human	Glucomannan (3.9 g with test meal)	Lower vitamin E tolerance curve (bile salt binding to fiber)	Doi *et al.* (1983)
Riboflavin	Human	Single fiber source: coarse or fine bran, cellulose, cabbage with 15 mg riboflavin 5-phosphate (unknown amount fiber)	Increased urinary riboflavin excretion (increased duration of vitamin exposure to absorption sites)	Roe *et al.* (1978)
Vitamin B_6	Human	Wheat bran (15 g for 18 days)	Decreased bioavailability (binding of fiber to vitamin B_6 and/or increased degradation of vitamin B_6)	Lindberg *et al.* (1983)
Folic acid	Human	High-fiber bread with 200 μg pteroylmonoglutamic acid (8.2 g crude fiber)	No influence on absorption	Russell *et al.* (1976)
Vitamin B_{12}	Human	Glucomannan (3.9 g with test meal)	No influence on vitamin B_{12} tolerance curves	Doi *et al.* (1983)
	Rat	Cellulose (10–50%), pectin (5–30%) for 10 weeks	B_{12} malabsorption (binding of fiber to vitamin B_{12})	Cullen and Oace (1978)
Pantothenic acid	Human	Wheat and corn bran (10 g and 20 g, respectively, in basal diet for 6 days)	No influence on blood levels	Trimbo *et al.* (1979)

strata of the elderly population because of unknown variables such as undetected diseases, medications, etc. There are, at present, few controlled metabolic studies in humans related to vitamin metabolism in aging. The criteria used for interpreting the data about vitamin nutriture in the elderly are presently based on normal values derived from young to middle-aged adults, which may not be appropriate. Despite these problems, it appears that the 1980 RDAs are appropriate for the elderly for many vitamins (i.e., vitamin E, thiamin, riboflavin, ascorbic acid, vitamin B_{12}). Impaired nutriture for these vitamins is likely to result from inadequate intakes and not from specific age-related changes in absorption and/or metabolism. There is, however, evidence that the RDAs for vitamin A and folate may be too high in old age, since the elderly maintain a normal biochemical status (e.g., plasma or serum levels) despite intakes well below the RDAs for these vitamins. In contrast, there is evidence that the RDAs for vitamin D and vitamin B_6 may be too low for the elderly. For both vitamins, age-related changes in vitamin metabolism occur that could affect their requirements. For vitamin K, niacin, biotin, and pantothenic acid, there is too little information to judge the adequacy of the present RDAs or the estimated safe and adequate daily dietary intake for the elderly.

An important caveat should be mentioned: there may be specific groups of elderly (e.g., those with atrophic gastritis) whose dietary requirements for particular vitamins may be altered. For example, in elderly people with atrophic gastritis, there may be relative impairment in digestive release of vitamin B_{12} from associated food proteins, thus increasing the dietary requirement for this vitamin. Finally, the interactions of drugs and other dietary components (e.g., fiber) with vitamins play an important role in determining the overall vitamin nutriture in the elderly (Table II). Further research, especially controlled metabolic studies, is needed.

All of these conclusions emphasize that the assessment of the requirements of the elderly for vitamins demands an appreciation of the interactions of the aging process with nutrient needs.

6. References

Alexander, M., Emanuel, G., Golin, T., Pinto, J. T., and Rivlin, R. S., 1984, Relation of riboflavin nutriture in healthy elderly to intake of calcium and vitamin supplements: Evidence against riboflavin supplementation, *Am. J. Clin. Nutr.* **39**:540–546.

Ames, S. R., 1974, Age, parity, and vitamin A supplementation and the vitamin E requirement of female rats, *Am. J. Clin. Nutr.* **27**:1017–1025.

Anderson, B. B., Peart, M. B., and Fulford-Jones, C. E., 1970, The measurement of serum pyridoxal by a microbiological assay using *Lactobacillus casei*, *J. Clin. Pathol.* **23**:232–242.

Andrews, J., Letcher, M., and Brook, M., 1969, Vitamin C supplementation in the elderly: 17-month trial in an old person's home, *Br. Med. J.* **2**:416–418.

Anonymous, 1979a, Dietary fiber and vitamin B-12 balance, *Nutr. Rev.* **37**:116–118.

Anonymous, 1979b, Pitfalls in the diagnosis of vitamin B-12 deficiency by radiodilution assay, *Nutr. Rev.* **37**:313–316.

Anonymous, 1981, Biotin deficiency as a complication of incomplete parenteral nutrition, *Nutr. Rev.* **39**:274–277.

Anonymous, 1982a, Vitamin K, vitamin E and the coumarin drugs, *Nutr. Rev.* **40**:180–182.

Anonymous, 1982b, Abnormal plasma prothrombin in the diagnosis of subclinical vitamin K deficiency, *Nutr. Rev.* **40**:298–300.

Anwar, M., 1978, Nutritional hypovitaminosis-D and the genesis of osteomalacia in the elderly, *J. Am. Geriatr. Soc.* **7**:309–317.

Ardeman, S., and Chanarin, I., 1966, Intrinsic factor secretion in gastric atrophy, *Gut* **7**:99–101.

Armbrecht, H. J., Zenser, T. V., and Davis, B. B., 1980a, Effect of age on the conversion of 25-hydroxyvitamin D_3 to 1,25-dihydroxyvitamin D_3 by kidney of rat, *J. Clin. Invest.* **66**:1118–1123.

Armbrecht, H. J., Zenser, T. V., Gross, C. J., and Davis, B. B., 1980b, Adaptation to dietary calcium and phosphorus restriction changes with age in the rat, *Am. J. Physiol.* **239**:E322–E327.

Armbrecht, H. J., Wongsurawat, N., Zenser, T. V., and Davis, B. B., 1982, Differential effects of parathyroid hormone on the renal 1,25-di-hydroxyvitamin D_3 and 24,25-dihydroxyvitamin D_3 production of young and adult rats, *Endocrinology* **111:**1339–1344.

Armbrecht, H. J., Forte, L. R., and Halloran, B. P., 1984, Effect of age and dietary calcium on renal 25-(OH)D_3 metabolism. serum 1,25-$(OH)_2D_3$, and PTH, *Am. J. Physiol.* **246:**E266–270.

Attwood, E. C., Robey, E., Kramer, J. J., Ovenden, N., Snape, S., Ross, J., and Bradley, F., 1978, A survey of the haematological, nutritional and biochemical state of the rural elderly with particular reference to vitamin C, *Age Aging* **7:**46–56.

Babu, S., and Srikantia, S. G., 1976, Availability of folates from some food, *Am. J. Clin. Nutr.* **29:**376–379.

Bailey, L. B., Wagner, P. A., Christakis, G. J., Araujo, P. E., Appledorf, H., Davis, C. G., Masteryanni, J., and Dinning, J. S., 1979, Folacin and iron status and hematological findings in predominantly black elderly persons from urban low income households, *Am. J. Clin. Nutr.* **32:**2346–2353.

Bailey, L. B., Wagner, P. A., Christakis, G. J., Araujo, P. E., Appledorf, H., Davis, C. G., Dorsey, E., and Dinning, J. S., 1980, Vitamin B-12 status of elderly persons from urban low income households, *J. Am. Geriatr. Soc.* **28:**276–278.

Bailey, L. B., Cerda, J. J., Bloch, B. S., Busby, M. J., Vargas, L., Chandler, C. J., and Halsted, C. H., 1984, Effect of age on poly- and monoglutamyl folacin absorption in human subjects, *J. Nutr.* **114:**1770–1776.

Baker, E. M., 1967, Vitamin C requirements in stress, *Am. J. Clin. Nutr.* **20:**583–590.

Baker, H., Frank, O., Feingold, S., and Leevy, C. M., 1967, Vitamin distribution in human plasma proteins, *Nature* **215:**84–85.

Baker, H., Jaslow, S. P., and Frank, O., 1978, Severe impairment of dietary folate utilization in the elderly, *J. Am. Geriatr. Soc.* **26:**218–221.

Baker, H., Frank, O., Thind, I. S., Jaslow, S. P., and Louria, D. B., 1979, Vitamin profiles in elderly persons living at home or in nursing homes, versus profile in healthy young subjects, *J. Am. Geriatr. Soc.* **27:**444–450.

Baker, M. R., Peacock, M., and Nordin, B. E. C., 1980, The decline in vitamin D status with age, *Age Aging* **9:**249–252.

Baksi, S. N., and Kenny, A. D., 1981, Vitamin D metabolism in aged Japanese quail: Dietary calcium and estrogen effects, *Am. J. Physiol.* **241:**E275–E280.

Bamji, M. S., 1981, Laboratory tests for the assessment of vitamin nutritional status, in: *Vitamins in Human Biology and Medicine* (M. H. Briggs, ed.), CRC Press, Boca Raton, FL, pp. 1–28.

Barnard, D. L., and Heaton, K. W., 1973, Bile acids and vitamin A absorption in man: The effects of two bile acid-binding agents, cholestyramine and lignin, *Gut* **14:**316–318.

Barnes, K. J., and Chen, L. H., 1981, Vitamin E status of the elderly in central Kentucky, *J. Nutr. Elderly* **1:**41–49.

Barr, S. I., Chrysomilides, S. A., Willis, E. J., and Beattie, B. L., 1983, Nutrient intakes of the old elderly: A study of female residents of a long-term care facility, *Nutr. Res.* **3:**417–431.

Barragry, J. M., France, M. W., Corless, D., Gupta, S. P., Switala, S., Boucher, B. K., and Cohen, R. D., 1978, Intestinal cholecalciferol absorption in the elderly and in younger adults, *Clin. Sci. Mol. Med.* **55:**213–220.

Bates, C. J., Rutishauser, I. H. E., Black, A. E., Paul, A. A., Mandal, A. R., and Patnaik, B. K., 1977, Long-term vitamin status and dietary intake of healthy elderly subjects: 2. Vitamin C, *Br. J. Nutr.* **42:**43–56.

Bates, C. J., Fleming, M., Paul, A. A., Black, A. E., and Mandal, A. R., 1980, Folate status and its relation to vitamin C in healthy elderly men and women, *Age Aging* **9:**241–248.

Baum, R. A., and Iber, F. L., 1984, Thiamin—the interaction of aging, alcoholism, and malabsorption in various populations, *World Rev. Nutr. Diet.* **44:**85–116.

Beadle, P. C., 1977, Sunlight, ozone and vitamin D, *Br. J. Dermatol.* **97:**585–591.

Beauchene, R. E., and Davis, T. A., 1979, The nutritional status of the aged in the USA, *Age* **2:**23–28.

Bell, N. H., 1985, Vitamin D-endocrine system, *J. Clin. Invest.* **76:**1–6.

Belsey, R., Clark, M. B., Bernat, M., Glowacki, J., Holick, M. F., DeLuca, H. F., and Potts, J. T., 1974, The physiologic significance of plasma transport of vitamin D and metabolites, *Am. J. Med.* **57:**50–56.

Berg, B. N., 1951, Muscular dystrophy in aging rats, *J. Gerontol.* **11:**134–139.

Betts, N. M., and Vivian, V. M., 1984, The dietary intake of noninstitutionalized elderly, *J. Nutr. Elderly* **3**:3–11.

Bhanthumnavin, K., Wright, J. R., and Halsted, C. H., 1974, Intestinal transport of tritiated folic acid (^{3}H-PGA) in the everted gut sac of different aged rats, *Johns Hopkins Med. J.* **135**:152–160.

Bieri, J. G., 1984, Vitamin E, in: *Present Knowledge in Nutrition,* The Nutrition Foundation, Washington, pp. 226–240.

Binder, H. J., Herting, D. C., Hurst, V., Finch, S. C., and Spiro, H. M., 1965, Tocopherol deficiency in man, *N. Engl. J. Med.* **273**:1289–1297.

Blanchard, R. A., Furie, B. C., Jorgensen, M., Kruger, S. F., and Furie, B., 1981, Acquired vitamin K-dependent carboxylation deficiency in liver disease, *N. Engl. J. Med.* **305**:242–248.

Blanchard, R. A., Furie, B. C., Kruger, S. F., Waneck, G., Jorgensen, M. J., and Furie, B., 1983, Immunoassays of human prothrombin species which correlate with functional coagulant activities, *J. Lab. Clin. Med.* **101**:242–255.

Boger, W. P., Wright, L. D., Strickland, S. C., Gylpe, J. S., and Ciminera, J. L., 1955, Vitamin B-12: Correlation of serum concentration with age, *Proc. Soc. Exp. Biol. Med.* **89**:375–381.

Bonati, B., Nani, S., and Rancati, G. B., 1956, Eliminazione urinaria di vitamine del complesso B nei vecchi, *Acta Vitaminol.* **10**:241–244.

Bonjour, J. P., 1977, Biotin in man's nutrition and therapy—a review, *J. Vitam. Nutr. Res.* **47**:107–118.

Bonjour, J. P., 1980, Vitamins and alcoholism. III. Vitamin B_6, *Int. J. Vitam. Nutr. Res.* **50**:215–230.

Bonjour, J. P., 1984, Biotin, in: *Handbook of vitamins. Nutritional, Biochemical and Clinical Aspects* (L. J. Machlin, ed.), Marcel Dekker, New York, pp. 403–436.

Bowman, B. B., and Rosenberg, I. H., 1982, Assessment of the nutritional status of the elderly, *Am. J. Clin. Nutr.* **35**:1142–1151.

Brandt, L. J., Bernstein, L. H., and Wagle, A., 1977, Production of vitamin B_{12} analogues in patients with small bowel bacterial overgrowth, *Ann. Intern. Med.* **87**:546–551.

Breen, K. J., Buttigieg, R., Iossifidis, S., Lourensz, C., and Wood, B., 1985, Jejunal uptake of thiamin hydrochloride in man: Influence of alcoholism and alcohol, *Am. J. Clin. Nutr.* **42**:121–126.

Brin, M., Dibble, M. V., Peel, A., McMullen, E., Bourquin, A., and Chen, N., 1965, Some preliminary findings on the nutritional status of the aged in Onondaga County, New York, *Am. J. Clin. Nutr.* **7**:240–258.

Brody, T., Shane, B., and Stokstad, E. L. R., 1984, Folic acid, in: *Handbook of Vitamins. Nutritional, Biochemical and Clinical Aspects* (L. J. Machlin, ed.), Marcel Dekker, New York, pp. 459–496.

Brook, M., and Grimshaw, J. J., 1968, Vitamin C concentration of plasma and leukocytes as related to smoking habit, age, and sex of humans, *Am. J. Clin. Nutr.* **21**:1254–1258.

Burr, M. L., Hurley, R. J., and Sweetnam, P. M., 1974a, Vitamin C supplementation of old people with low blood levels, *Gerontol. Clin.* **17**:236–243.

Burr, M. L., Sweetnam, P. M., Hurley, R. J., and Powell, G. H., 1974b, Effects of age and intake on plasma-ascorbic acid levels, *Lancet* **1**:163–164.

Campbell, G. A., Kamin, J. R., Hosking, D. J., and Boyd, R. V., 1984, How common is osteomalacia in the elderly? *Lancet* **1**:386–388.

Cape, R. T. D., and Shinton, N. K., 1961, Serum vitamin B-12 concentration in the elderly, *Gerontol. Clin.* **3**:163–172.

Carmel, R., 1978, Nutritional vitamin B-12 deficiency. Possible contributory role of subtle vitamin B-12 malabsorption, *Ann. Intern. Med.* **88**:647–649.

Cheli, R., Simon, L., Aste, H., Figus, I. A., Nicold, G., Bajtai, A., and Puntoni, R., 1980, Atrophic gastritis and intestinal metaplasia in asymptomatic Hungarian and Italian populations, *Endoscopy* **12**:105–108.

Chen, L. H., 1974, The effect of age and dietary vitamin E on the tissue lipid peroxidation of mice, *Nutr. Rep. Int.* **10**:339–344.

Chen, L. H., 1981, Vitamin E and aging, in: *Handbook of Geriatric Nutrition* (J. M. Hsu, ed.), Noyes, Park Ridge, NJ, pp. 176–187.

Chen, L. H., and Fan Chiang, W. L., 1981, Biochemical evaluation of riboflavin and vitamin B-6 status of institutionalized and noninstitutionalized elderly in central Kentucky, *Int. J. Vitam. Nutr. Res.* **51**:232–238.

Chen, L. H., Hsu, S. J., Huang, P. C., and Chen, J. S., 1977, Vitamin E status of Chinese population in Taiwan, *Am. J. Clin. Nutr.* **30**:728–735.

Cheng, L., Cohen, M., and Bhagavan, H. N., 1985, Vitamin C and the elderly, in: *Handbook of Nutrition in the Aged* (R. R. Watson, ed.) CRC Press, Boca Raton, FL, pp. 157–185.

Chernish, S. M., Helmer, O. M., Fouts, P. J., and Kohlstaedt, K. G., 1957, The effect of intrinsic factor on the absorption of vitamin B-12 in older people, *Am. J. Clin. Nutr.* **5**:651–658.

Chhabra, R. S., 1984, Retinoids and drug-metabolizing enzymes, in: *Drugs and Nutrients. Drug Nutrient Interactions* (D. A. Roe and T. C. Campbell, eds.), Marcel Dekker, New York, pp. 95–117.

Chieffi, M., and Kirk, J. E., 1951, Vitamin studies in middle-aged and old individuals. VI. Tocopherol plasma concentrations, *J. Gerontol.* **6**:17–18.

Chow, B. F., 1958, Vitamin B-12 in relationship to aging, *Gerontologica* **2**:213–221.

Chow, B. F., Gilbert, J. P., Okuda, K., and Rosenblum, C., 1956a, The urinary excretion test for absorption of vitamin B-12. I. Reproducibility of results and agewise variation, *Am. J. Clin. Nutr.* **4**:142–146.

Chow, B. F., Wood, R., Horonick, A., and Okuda, K., 1956b, Agewise variation of vitamin B-12 serum levels, *J. Gerontol.* **11**:142–146.

Chrisley, B. M., and Driskell, J. A., 1979, Vitamin B-6 status of adults in Virginia, *Nutr. Rep. Int.* **19**:553–560.

Chytil, F., 1984, Retinoic acid: Biochemistry, pharmacology, toxicology, and therapeutic use, *Pharmacol. Rev.* **36**(2 Suppl.):93S–100S.

Colby, H. D., Kramer, R. E., Greiner, J. W., Robinson, D. A., Krause, R. F., and Canady, W. J., 1975, Heaptic drug metabolism in retinol-deficient rats, *Biochem. Pharmacol.* **24**:1645–1646.

Colman, N., Green, R., and Metz, J., 1975, Prevention of folate deficiency by food fortification. II. Absorption of folic acid from fortified staple foods, *Am. J. Clin. Nutr.* **28**:459–464.

Colvin, B. T., and Lloyd, M. J., 1977, Severe coagulation defect due to a dietary deficiency of vitamin K, *J. Clin. Pathol.* **30**:1147–1148.

Conely, J., Sumner, D., McKinlay, A., McIntosh, W., and Dunnigan, M. G., 1977, Prevention of vitamin D deficiency in the elderly, *Br. Med. J.* **2**:1668.

Connelly, T. J., Becker, D. O. A., and McDonald J. W., 1982, Bachelor scurvy, *Int. J. Dermatol.* **21**:209–211.

Corless, D., Boucher, B. J., Beer, M., Gupta, S. P., and Cohen, R. D., 1975, Vitamin D status in long-stay geriatric patients, *Lancet* **1**:1404–1406.

Corless, D., Gupta, S. P., Sattar, D. A., Switala, S., and Boucher, B. J., 1979, Vitamin D status of residents of an old people's home and long-stay patients, *Gerontology* **25**:350–355.

Corrigan, J. J., Jr., 1982, The effect of vitamin E on warfarin-induced vitamin K deficiency, *Ann. N.Y. Acad. Sci.* **393**:361–368.

Corrigan, J. J., Jr., and Ulfers, L. L., 1981, Effect of vitamin E on prothrombin levels in warfarin-induced vitamin K deficiency, *Am. J. Clin. Nutr.* **34**:1701–1705.

Cullen, R. W., and Oace, S. M., 1978, Methylmalonic acid and vitamin B-12 excretion of rats consuming diets varying in cellulose and pectin, *J. Nutr.* **108**:640–648.

Daiger, S. P., Schanfield, M. S., and Cavalli-Sforza, L. L., 1975, Group-specific component (gc) proteins bind vitamin D and 25-hydroxyvitamin D, *Proc. Natl. Acad. Sci. U.S.A.* **72**:2076–2080.

Dakshinamurti, K., and Bhagavan, H. (eds.), 1985, Biotin, *Ann. N.Y. Acad. Sci.* **447**:1–441.

Danford, D. E., and Munro, H. N., 1980, The water-soluable vitamins: Vitamin B complex and ascorbic acid, in: *The Pharmacological Basis of Therapeutics*, 6th ed. (L. S. Goodman and A. G. Gilman, eds.), New York, Macmillan, pp. 1560–1582.

Danford, D. E., and Munro, H. N., 1988, Liver in relation to B-vitamins, in: *The Liver: Biology and Pathobiology*, 2nd ed. (I. M. Arias, w. B. Jakoby, H. Popper, D. Schachter, and D. A. Shafritz, eds.), Raven Press, New York, pp. 965–984.

Darby, W. J., Ferguson, M. E., Furman, R. H., Lemley, J. M., Ball, C. T., and Meneely, G. R., 1949, Plasma tocopherols in health and disease, *Ann. N.Y. Acad. Sci.* **52**:328–333.

Dattani, J. T., Exton-Smith, A. N., and Stephen, J. M. L., 1984, Vitamin D status of the elderly in relation to age and exposure to sunlight, *Hum. Nutr. Clin. Nutr.* **38C**:131–137.

Davie, M., and Lawson, D. E. M., 1980, Assessment of plasma 25-hydroxyvitamin D response to ultraviolet irradiation over a controlled area in young and elderly subjects, *Clin. Sci.* **58**:235–242.

Davies, H. E. F., Davies, J. E. W., Hughes, R. E., and Jones, E., 1984, Studies on the absorption of L-xyloascorbic acid (vitamin C) in young and elderly subjects, *Hum. Nutr. Clin. Nutr.* **38C**:463–471.

Dawson, D. W., Sawers, A. H., and Sharma, R. K., 1984, Malabsorption of protein-bound vitamin B-12, *Br. Med. J.* **288**:675–678.

Del Tredici, A. M., Bernstein, A. L., and Chinn, K., 1985, Carpal tunnel syndrome and vitamin B 6 therapy, in: *Vitamin B-6: Its Role in Health and Disease* (J. Leklem and B. Reynolds, eds.) Alan R. Liss, New York, pp. 459–462.

DeLuca, H. F., 1972, Parathyroid hormone as a trophic hormone for 1,25-dihydroxyvitamin D_3, the metabolically active form of vitamin D, *N. Engl. J. Med.* **287**:250–251.

Desai, I. D., 1968, Plasma tocopherol levels in normal adults, *Can. J. Physiol. Pharmacol.* **46**:819–822.

Devgun, M. S., Paterson, C. R., Johnson, B. E., and Cohen, C., 1981, Vitamin D nutrition in relation to season and occupation, *Am. J. Clin. Nutr.* **34**:1501–1504.

Dibble, M. V., Brin, M., Thiele, V. F., Peel, A., Chen, N., and McMullen, E., 1967, Evaluation of the nutritional status of elderly subjects, with a comparison between fall and spring, *J. Am. Geriatr. Soc.* **15**:1031–1061.

Diet, Nutrition, and Cancer Report, 1982, National Academy Press, Washington, pp. 138–144.

Dju, M. Y., Mason, K. E., and Flier, L. J., 1958, Vitamin E (tocopherol) in human tissues from birth to old age, *Am. J. Clin. Nutr.* **6**:50–60.

Doi, K., Matsuura, M., Kawara, A., Tanaka, T., and Baba, S., 1983, Influence of dietary fiber (konjac mannan) on absorption of vitamin B-12 and vitamin E, *Tohoku J. Exp. Med.* **141**:677–681.

Doisy, E. A., Jr., 1961, Nutritional hypoprothrombinemia and metabolism of vitamin K, *Fed. Proc.* **20**:989–994.

Doscherholmen, A., Ripley, D., Chang, S., and Silvis, S. E., 1977, Influence of age and stomach function on serum vitamin B-12 concentration, *Scand. J. Gastroenterol.* **12**:313–319.

Draper, H. H., 1958, Physiological aspects of aging. I. Efficiency of absorption and phosphorylation of radiothiamine, *Proc. Soc. Exp. Biol. Med.* **97**:121–124.

Driskell, J. A., 1984, Vitamin B-6, in: *Handbook of Vitamins. Nutritional, Biochemical and Clinical Aspects* (L. J. Machlin, ed.), Marcel Dekker, New York, pp. 379–401.

Droller, H., and Dossett, J. A., 1959, Vitamin B-12 levels in senile dementia and confusional states, *Gerontol. Clin.* **1**:96–106.

Ellenbogen, L., 1984. Vitamin B-12, in: *Handbook of Vitamins. Nutritional, Biochemical and Clinical Aspects* (L. J. Machlin, ed.), Marcel Dekker, New York, pp. 497–548.

Ellis, J. M., Folkers, K., Levy, M., Shizuknishi, S., Lewandowski, J., Nishi, S., Schubert, H. A., and Ulrich, R., 1982, Response of vitamin B-6 deficiency and the carpal tunnel syndrome to pyridoxine, *Proc. Natl. Acad. Sci. U.S.A.* **79**:7494–7498.

Elsborg, L., 1976, Reversible malabsorption of folic acid in the elderly with nutritional folate deficiency, *Acta Haematol.* **55**:140–147.

Elsborg, L., Lund, V., and Bastrup-Madsen, P., 1976, Serum vitamin B-12 levels in the aged, *Acta Med. Scand.* **200**:309–314.

Elsborg, L., Nielsen, J. A., Bertram, U., Helms, P., Nielsen, K., and Rosenquist, A., 1983, The intake of vitamins and minerals by the elderly at home, *Int. J. Vitam. Nutr. Res.* **53**:321–329.

Elwood, P. C., Shinton, N. K., Wilson, C. I. D., Sweetnam, P., and Frazer, A. C., 1971, Haemoglobin, vitamin B-12 and folate levels in the elderly, *Br. J. Haematol.* **21**:557–563.

Emerson, G. A., and Evans, H. M., 1939a, Restoration of fertility in successively older vitamin E-low female rats, *J. Nutr.* **18**:501–506.

Emerson, G. A., and Evans, H. M., 1939b, Degrees of sterility in female vitamin E-low rats, *Am. J. Physiol.* **126**:484.

Farrell, P. M., 1980, Deficiency states, pharmacological effects and nutrient requirements, in: *Vitamin E, a Comprehensive Treatise* (L. J. Machlin, ed.), Marcel Dekker, New York, pp. 520–620.

Fischer, S., Hendricks, D. G., and Mahoney, A. W., 1978, Nutritional assessment of senior rural Utahns by biochemical and physical measurements, *Am. J. Clin. Nutr.* **31**:667–672.

Fleming, B. B., and Barrows, C. H., Jr., 1982a, The influence of aging on intestinal absorption of vitamins A and D by the rat, *Exp. Gerontol.* **17**:115–120.

Fleming, B. B., and Barrows, C. H., 1982b, The influence of aging on intestinal absorption of vitamin B-12 and niacin in rats, *Exp. Gerontol.* **17**:121–126.

Folkers, K., Ellis, J., Watanabe, T., Saji, S., and Kaji, M., 1978, Biochemical evidence for a deficiency of vitamin B-6 in carpal tunnel syndrome based on a crossover clinical study, *Proc. Natl. Acad. Sci U.S.A.* **75**:3410–3412.

Fonda, M. L., and Eggers, D. K., 1980, Vitamin B-6 metabolism in the blood of young adult and senescent mice, *Exp. Gerontol.* **15**:465–472.

Fonda, M. L., Acree, D. W., and Auerbach, S. B., 1973, The relationship of gamma-aminobutyrate levels and its metabolism to age in brains of mice, *Arch. Biochem. Biophys.* **159**:622–628.

Fonda, M. L., Eggers, D. K., and Metha, R., 1980a, Vitamin B-6 metabolism in the livers of young adult and senescent mice, *Exp. Gerontol.* **15**:457–463.

Fonda, M. L., Eggers, D. K., Auerbach, S., and Fritsch, L., 1980b, Vitamin B-6 metabolism in the brains of young adult and senescent mice, *Exp. Gerontol.* **15**:473–478.

Fox, H. M., 1984, Pantothenic acid, in: *Handbook of Vitamins. Nutrition, Biochemical and Clinical Aspects* (L. J. Machlin, ed.) Marcel Dekker, New York, pp. 437–458.

Foy, H., and Mbaya, V., 1977, Riboflavin, *Prog. Food Nutr. Sci.* **2**:357–394.

Frazier, D. R., 1980, Regulation of the metabolism of vitamin D, *Physiol. Rev.* **60**:551–613.

Frick, P. G., Riedler, G., and Brogli, H., 1967, Dose response and minimal daily requirement for vitamin K in man, *J. Appl. Physiol.* **23**:387–389.

Fuhr, A., Johnson, R. E., Kaunitz, H., and Slanitz, C. A., 1949, Increased tocopherol requirements during the rat's menopause, *Ann. N.Y. Acad. Sci.* **52**:83–87.

Fujisawa, J., Kida, K., and Matsuda, H., 1984, Role of change in vitamin D metabolism with age on calcium and phosphorus metabolism in normal human subjects, *J. Clin. Endocrinol. Metab.* **59**:719–726.

Gabriel, E., Machlin, L. J., Filipski, R., and Nelson, J., 1980, Influence of age on the vitamin E requirement for resolution of necrotizing myopathy, *J. Nutr.* **110**:1372–1379.

Gaffney, G. W., Horonick, A., Okuda, K., Meier, P., Chow, B. F., and Shock, N. W., 1957, Vitamin B-12 serum concentration in 528 apparently healthy human subjects of ages 12–94, *J. Gerontol.* **12**:32–38.

Gallagher, J. C., Riggs, B. L., Eisman, J., Hamstra, A., Arnaud, S. B., and DeLuca, H. F., 1979, Intestinal calcium absorption and serum vitamin D metabolites in normal subjects and osteoporotic patients, *J. Clin. Invest.* **64**:729–736.

Gallagher, J. C., Riggs, B. L., Jerpbak, C. M., and Arnaud, C. D., 1980, The effect of age on serum immunoreactive parathyroid hormone in normal and osteoporotic women, *J. Lab. Clin. Med.* **95**:373–385.

Garabedian, M., Holick, M. F., DeLuca, H. F., and Boyle, I. T., 1972, Control of 25-hydroxycholecalciferol metabolism by parathyroid glands, *Proc. Natl. Acad. Sci. U.S.A.* **69**:1673–1676.

Garry, P. J., and Hunt, W. C., 1986, Biochemical assessment of vitamin status in the elderly: Effect of dietary and supplemental intakes, in: *Nutrition and Aging* (M. L. Hutchinson and H. N. Munro, eds.), Academic Press, Orlando, FL, pp. 117–137.

Garry, P. J., Goodwin, J. S., Hunt, W. C., Hooper, E. M., and Leonard, A. G., 1982a, Nutritional status in a healthy elderly population: Dietary and supplemental intakes, *Am. J. Clin. Nutr.* **36**:319–331.

Garry, P. J., Goodwin, J. S., and Hunt, W. C., 1982b, Nutritional status in a healthy elderly population: Riboflavin, *Am. J. Clin. Nutr.* **36**:902–909.

Garry, P. J., Goodwin, J. S., Hunt, W. C., and Gilbert, B. A., 1982c, Nutritional status in a healthy elderly population: Vitamin C, *Am. J. Clin. Nutr.* **36**:332–339.

Garry, P. J., Goodwin, J. S., and Hunt, W. C., 1984, Folate and vitamin B-12 status in a healthy elderly population, *J. Am. Geriatr. Soc.* **32**:719–726.

Gehrmann, G., 1965, Pyridoxine-responsive anemias, *Br. J. Haematol.* **11**:86–91.

Giannella, R. A., Broitman, S. A., and Zamcheck, N., 1971, Vitamin B-12 uptake by intestinal microorganisms: Mechamisms and relevance to syndromes of intestinal bacterial overgrowth, *J. Clin. Invest.* **50**:1100–1107.

Gillum, H. L., Morgan, A. F., and Sailer, F., 1955, Nutritional status of the aging: V. Vitamin A and carotene, *J. Nutr.* **55**:655–670.

Girdwood, R. H., Thomson, A. D., and Williamson, J., 1967, Folate status in the elderly, *Br. Med. J.* **2**:670–672.

Glass, G. B. J., Goldbloom, A. A., Boyd, L. J., Laughton, R., Rosen, S., and Rich, M., 1956, Intestinal absorption and hepatic uptake of radioactive vitamin B-12 in various age groups and the effect of intrinsic factor preparations, *Am. J. Clin. Nutr.* **4**:124–133.

Goodman, D. S., 1984, Overview of current knowledge of metabolism of vitamin A and carotenoids, *J. Natl. Cancer Inst.* **73**:1375–1379.

Gracey, M., 1979, The contaminated small bowel syndrome: Pathogenesis, diagnosis, and treatment, *Am. J. Clin. Nutr.* **32**:234–243.

Gray, G. E., Paganini-Hill, A., and Ross, R. K., 1983, Dietary intake and nutrient supplement use in a southern California retirement community, *Am. J. Clin. Nutr.* **38**:122–128.

Gray, R. W., and Gambert, S. R., 1982, Effect of age on plasma 1,25-$(OH)_2$ vitamin D in the rat, *Age* **5**:54–56.

Griffiths, L. L., Brocklehurst, J. C., Scott, D. L., Marks, J., and Blackley, J., 1967, Thiamine and ascorbic acid levels in the elderly, *Gerontol. Clin.* **9**:1–10.

Grimble, R. F., and Hughes, R. E., 1968, The glutathione : dehydroascorbate oxidoreductase activity of guinea-pigs from two different age groups, *Life Sci.* **7**:383–386.

Grinna, L. S., 1976, Effect of dietary alpha-tocopherol on liver microsomes and mitochondria of aging rats, *J. Nutr.* **106**:918–929.

Gubler, C. J., 1984, Thiamin, in: *Handbook of vitamins. Nutritional, Biochemical and Clinical Aspects* (L. J. Machlin, ed.), Marcell Dekker, New York, pp. 245–298.

Guggenheim, K., Kravitz, M., Tal, R., and Kaufman, N. A., 1979, Biochemical parameters of vitamin D nutriture in old people in Jerusalem, *Nutr. Metab.* **23**:172–178.

Guilland, J. C., Bereksi-Reguig, B., Lequeu, B., Moreau, D., Klepping, J., and Richard, D., 1984, Evaluation of pyridoxine intake and pyridoxine status among aged institutionalized people, *Int. J. Vitam. Nutr. Res.* **54**:185–193.

Gyorgy, P., 1971, Developments leading to the metabolic role of vitamin B-6, *Am. J. Clin. Nutr.* **24**:1250–1256.

Hahn, T. J., Birge, S. J., Scharp, C. R., and Avioli, L. V., 1972, Phenobarbital-induced alterations in vitamin D metabolism, *J. Clin. Invest.* **51**:741–748.

Hall, C. A., 1982, The luxus vitamins A and B-12: Reply to McLaren, *Am. J. Clin. Nutr.* **35**:772–774.

Hamfelt, A., 1964, Age variation of vitamin B-6 metabolism in man, *Clin. Chim. Acta* **10**:48–54.

Hampton, D. J., Chrisley, B. M., and Driskell, J. A., 1977, Vitamin B-6 status of the elderly in Montgomery County, VA, *Nutr. Rep. Int.* **16**:743–750.

HANES I, 1979, Health and Nutrition Examination Survey. Caloric and selected nutrient values for persons 1–74 years of age, United States, 1971–74, DHEW Publication No. (PHS) 79-1657, National Center for Health Statistics, Hyattsville, MD.

HANES II, 1982, Health and Nutritional Examination Survey No. 2. Dietary intake source data, United States, 1976–80, National Center for Health Statistics, Hyattsville, MD.

Hankes, L. V., 1984, Nicotinic acid and nicotinamide, in: *Handbook of Vitamins. Nutritional, Biochemical and Clinical Aspects* (L. J. Machlin, ed.), Marcel Dekker, New York, pp. 329–378.

Harding, A. E., Matthews, S., Jones, S., Ellis, C. J. K., Booth, I. W., and Muller, D. P. R., 1985, Spinocerebellar degeneration associated with a selective defect of vitamin E absorption, *N. Engl. J. Med.* **313**:32–35.

Harrill, I., and Cervone, N., 1977, Vitamin status of older women, *Am. J. Clin. Nutr.* **30**:431–440.

Hayes, A. N., Willans, D. J., and Skelton, D., 1985, Vitamin B-12 (cobalamin) and folate blood levels in geriatric reference group as measured by two kits, *Clin. Biochem.* **18**:56–61.

Hayes, M. J., Langman, M. J. S., and Short, A. H., 1975, Changes in drug metabolism with increasing age: 1. Warfarin binding and plasma proteins, *Br. J. Clin. Pharmacol.* **2**:69–72.

Hazell, K., and Baloch, K. H., 1970, Vitamin K deficiency in the elderly, *Gerontol. Clin.* **12**:10–17.

Hepburn, F. N., 1982, The USDA national nutrient data bank, *Am. J. Clin. Nutr.* **35**:1297–1301.

Hewick, D. S., Moreland, T. A., Shepherd, A. M. M., and Stevenson, I. H., 1975, The effect of age on the sensitivity to warfarin sodium, *Br. J. Clin. Pharmacol.* **2**:189P–190P.

Hines, J. D., and Love, D., 1975, Abnormal vitamin B-6 metabolism in sideroblastic anemia: Effect of pyridoxal phosphate therapy, *Clin. Res.* **23**:403A.

Hitzhuzen, J. C., Taplin, M. E., Stephenson, W. P., and Ansell, J. E., 1986, Vitamin B-12 levels and age, *Am. J. Clin. Pathol.* **85**:32–36.

Hogenkamp, H. P. C., 1980, The interaction between vitamin B-12 and vitamin C, *Am. J. Clin. Nutr.* **33:**1–3.
Holick, M. F., and Clark, M. B., 1978, The photobiogenesis and metabolism of vitamin D, *Fed. Proc.* **37:**2567–2574.
Holick, M. F., and Potts, J. T., Jr., 1983, Vitamin D, in: *Harrison's Principles of Internal Medicine* (R. G. Petersdorf, R. D. Adams, E. Braunwald, K. J. Isselbacher, J. B. Martin, and J. D. Wilson, eds.), McGraw-Hill, New York, pp. 1944–1949.
Hollander, D., and Morgan, D., 1979, Aging: Its influence on vitamin A intestinal absorption *in vivo* by the rat, *Esp. Gerontol.* **14:**301–305.
Hollander, D., and Tarnawski, H., 1984, Influence of aging on vitamin D absorption and unstirred water layer dimensions in the rat, *J. Lab. Clin. Med.* **103:**462–469.
Holloway, D. E., and Peterson, F. J., 1984, Ascorbic acid in drug metabolism, in: *Drugs and Nutrients: The Interaction Effects* (D. A. Roe and T. C. Campbell, eds.), Marcel Dekker, New York, Basel, pp. 225–295.
Holt, P. R., and Dominguez, A. A., 1981, Intestinal absorption of triglyceride and vitamin D_3 in aged and young rats, *Dig. Dis. Sci.* **26:**1109–1115.
Hoorn, R. K. J., Flikweert, J. P., and Westerink, D., 1975, Vitamin B-1, B-2 and B-6 deficiencies in geriatric patients, measured by coenzyme stimulation of enzyme activities, *Clin. Chim. Acta* **61:**151–162.
Hoppner, K., and Lampi, B., 1980, Folate levels in human liver from autopsies in Canada, *Am. J. Clin. Nutr.* **33:**862–864.
Hoppner, K., Phillips, W. E. J., Murray, T. K., and Campbell, J. S., 1968, Survey of liver vitamin A stores of Canadians, *Can. Med. Assoc. J.* **99:**983–986.
Horwitt, M. K., Harvey, C. C., Dahm, C. J., Jr., and Searey, M. T., 1972, Relationship between tocopherol and serum lipid levels for determination of nutritional adequacy, *Ann. N.Y. Acad. Sci.* **203:**223–236.
Houston, J. B., and Levy, G., 1975, Modification of drug biotransformation by vitamin C in man, *Nature* **255:**78–79.
Hoyumpa, A. M., Jr., Breen, K. J., Schenker, S., and Wilson, F. A., 1975, Thiamine transport across the rat intestine. II. Effects of ethanol, *J. Lab. Clin. Med.* **86:**803–816.
Hradsky, M., Groh, J., Langer, F., and Herout, V., 1966, Chronische gastritis bei jungen und alten personen, histologische und histochemische untersuchung, *Gerontol. Clin.* **8:**164–171.
Hsu, J. M., Kawin, B., Minor, P., and Mitchell, J. A., 1966, Vitamin B-12 concentrations in human tissues, *Nature* **210:**1264–1265.
Hurdle, A. D. F., and Williams, T. C. P., 1966, Folic acid deficiency in elderly patients admitted to hospital, *Br. Med. J.* **2:**202–205.
Hyams, D. E., 1964, The absorption of vitamin B-12 in the elderly, *Gerontol. Clin.* **6:**193–206.
Iber, F. L., Blass, J. P., Brin, M., and Leevy, C. M., 1982, Thiamin in the elderly—relation to alcoholism and to neurological degenerative disease, *Am. J. Clin. Nutr.* **36:**1067–1082.
Immerman, A. M., 1981, Vitamin B-12 status on a vegetarian diet, *World Rev. Nutr. Diet.* **37:**38–54.
Ishiguro, K., 1961, Pantothenic acid and age, *Tohoku J. Exp. Med.* **75:**137–150.
Ishiguro, K., 1972, Aging effect of blood pantothenic acid content in female, *Tohoku J. Exp. Med.* **107:**367–372.
Ishiguro, K., Kobayashi, S., and Kaneta, S., 1961, Pantothenic acid content of human blood, *Tohoku J. Exp. Med.* **74:**65–68.
Jacob, R. A., Otradovec, C. L., Russell, R. M., Munro, H. N., Hartz, S. C., McGandy, R. B., Morrow, F. D., and Sadowski, J. A., 1988, Vitamin C status and nutrient interactions in a health population, *Am. J. Clin. Nutr.* (in press).
Jacobs, A., Cavill, I. A. J., and Hughes, J. N. P., 1968, Erythrocyte transaminase activity. Effect of age, sex, and vitamin B-6 supplementation, *Am. J. Clin. Nutr.* **21:**502–507.
Jaffe, G. M., 1984, Vitamin C, in: *Handbook of Vitamins: Nutritional, Biochemical and Clinical Aspects* (L. J. Machlin, ed.), Marcel Dekker, New York, pp. 199–244.
Jagerstad, M., and Westesson, A. K., 1979, Folate, *Scand. J. Gastroenterol.* **14:**(Suppl 52):196–202.
Kark, R., and Lozner, E. L., 1939, Nutritional deficiency of vitamin K in man, *Lancet* **2:**1162–1164.
Kataria, M. S., Rao, D. B., and Curtis, R. C., 1965, Vitamin C levels in the elderly, *Gerontol. Clin.* **7:**189–190.

Kelleher, J., and Losowsky, M. S., 1978, Vitamin E in the elderly, in: *Tocopherol, Oxygen and Biomembranes* (C. de Duve and O. Hayaishi, eds.), Elsevier/North Holland Biomedical Press, Amsterdam, pp. 311–327.

Kesavan, V., and Noronha, J. M., 1983, Folate malabsorption in aged rats related to low levels of pancreatic folyl conjugase, *Am. J. Clin. Nutr.* **37**:262–267.

Kheim, T., and Kirk, J. E., 1967, Vitamin B-6 content of human arterial and venous tissue, *Am. J. Clin. Nutr.* **20**:702–707.

Killander, A., 1957, The serum vitamin B-12 levels at various ages, *Acta Paediatr.* **46**:585–594.

Kilpatrick, G. S., and Withey, J. L., 1965, The serum vitamin B-12 concentration in the general population, *Scand. J. Haematol.* **2**:220–229.

King, C. E., Leibach, J., and Toskes, P. P., 1979, Clinically significant vitamin B-12 deficiency secondary to malabsorption of protein-bound vitamin B-12, *Dig. Dis. Sci.* **24**:397–402.

Kirk, E., and Chieffi, M., 1948, Vitamin studies in middle-aged and old individuals. I. The vitamin A, total carotene and alpha + beta carotene concentration in plasma, *J. Nutr.* **36**:315–322.

Kirk, J. E., and Chieffi, M., 1951, Effect of oral thiamine administration on thiamine content of the stool, *Proc. Soc. Exp. Biol. Med.* **77**:464–466.

Kirk, J. E., and Chieffi, M., 1953a, Vitamin studies in middle-aged and old individuals. XI. The concentration of total ascorbic acid in whole blood, *J. Gerontol.* **8**:301–304.

Kirk, J. E., and Chieffi, M., 1953b, Vitamin studies in middle-aged and old individuals. XII. Hypovitaminemia C, *J. Gerontol.* **8**:305–311.

Kistler, L. A., and Giannella, R. A., 1980, Relationship of intestinal bacteria to malabsorption, *Prac. Gastroenterol.* **4**:24–44.

Kohrs, M. B., O'Neal, R., Preston, A., Eklund, D., and Abrahams, O., 1978, Nutritional status of elderly residents in Missouri, *Am. J. Clin. Nutr.* **31**:2186–2197.

Krasinski, S., Russell, R. M., Samloff, I. M., Jacob, R. A., Dallal, G. E., McGandy, R. B., and Hartz, S. C., 1983, Prevalence and severity of atrophic gastritis in an elderly population: Effect on serum status of certain nutrients, *Gastroenterology* **84**:1291.

Krasinski, S. D., Russell, R. M., Dallal, G. E., and Dutta, S. K., 1985a, Aging changes vitamin A absorption characteristics, *Gastroenterology* **88**:1715.

Krasinski, S. D., Russell, R. M., Furie, B. C., Kruger, S. F., Jacques, P. F., and Furie, B., 1985b, The prevalence of vitamin K deficiency in chronic gastrointestinal disorders, *Am. J. Clin. Nutr.* **41**:639–643.

Krawitt, E. L., and Chastenay, B. F., 1980, 25-Hydroxy vitamin D absorption test in patients with gastrointestinal disorders, *Calcif. Tissue Int.* **32**:183–187.

Kreuning, J., Bosman, F. T., Kuiper, G., Wal, A. M., and Lindeman, J., 1978, Gastric and duodenal mucosa in healthy individuals, *J. Clin. Pathol.* **31**:69–77.

Kushner, J. P., and Cartwright, G. E., 1977, Sideroblastic anemia, *Adv. Intern. Med.* **22**:229–249.

Lambert-Allardt, C., 1984, The relationship between serum 25-hydroxy-vitamin D levels and other variables related to calcium and phosphorus metabolism in the elderly, *Acta Endocrinol.* **105**:139–144.

Lawrence, V. A., 1983, Demographic analysis of serum folate and folate binding capacity in hospitalized patients, *Acta Haematol.* **69**:289–293.

Lawson, D. E. M., Paul, A. A., Black, A. E., Cole, T. J., Mandal, A. R., and Davie, M., 1979, Relative contributions of diet and sunlight to vitamin D state in the elderly, *Br. Med. J.* **2**:303–305.

Ledvina, M., 1985, Vitamin E in the aged, in: *CRC Handbook of Nutrition in the Aged* (R. R. Watson, ed.), CRC Press, Boca Raton, FL, pp. 89–109.

Leevy, C. M., 1982, Thiamin deficiency and alcoholism, *Ann. N.Y. Acad. Sci.* **378**:316–326.

Leichter, J., Angel, J. F., and Lee, M., 1978, Nutritional status of a select group of free-living elderly people in Vancouver, *Can. Med. Assoc. J.* **118**:40–43.

Leinert, J., Simon, I., and Hotzel, D., 1983, Methoden und deren wertung zur bestimmung des vitamin B-6 versorgungszustandes beim menschen, *Int. J. Vitam. Nutr. Res.* **53**:166–178.

Leitner, Z. A., Moore, T., and Sharman, I. M., 1960, Vitamin A and vitamin E in human blood, *Br. J. Nutr.* **14**:281–287.

Leklem, J. E., Shultz, T. D., and Miller, L. T., 1980, Comparative bioavailability of vitamin B-6 from soybeans and beef, *Fed. Proc.* **39**:558.

Leo, M. A., Lowe, N., and Lieber, C. S., 1982, Decreased hepatic vitamin A after drug administration in men and rats, *Hepatology* **2**:679.

Leo, M. A., Lowe, N., and Lieber, C. S., 1984, Decreased hepatic vitamin A after drug administration in men and in rats, *Am. J. Clin. Nutr.* **40:**1131–1136.

Leonhardt, E. T. G., 1978, Effects of vitamin E on serum cholesterol and triglycerides in hyperlipidemic patients treated with diet and clofibrate, *Am. J. Clin. Nutr.* **31:**100–105.

Lester, E., Skinner, R. K., and Wills, M. R., 1977, Seasonal variation in serum-25-hydroxyvitamin-D in the elderly in Britain, *Lancet* **1:**979–980.

Lewis, J. S., Pian, A. K., Baer, M. T., Acosta, P. B., and Emerson, G. A., 1973, Effect of long-term ingestion of polyunsaturated fat, age, plasma cholesterol, diabetes mellitus, and supplemental tocopherol upon plasma tocopherol, *Am. J. Clin. Nutr.* **26:**136–143.

Lindberg, A. S., Leklem, J. E., and Miller, L. T., 1983, The effect of wheat bran on the bioavailability of vitamin B-6 in young men, *J. Nutr.* **113:**2578–2586.

Lindenbaum, J., and Lieber, C. S., 1969, Alcohol-induced malabsorption of vitamin B-12 in man, *Nature* **224:**806.

Lips, P., Jongen, M. J. M., van Ginkel, F. C., Netelenbos, J. C., and van der Vijgh, W. J. F., 1985, Determinants of vitamin D status in the elderly, in: *Vitamin D. A Chemical, Biochemical and Clinical Update* (A. W. Norman, K. Schaefer, H. G. Grigoleit, and D. V. Herrath, eds.), Walter de Gruyter & Co., Berlin, New York, pp. 1020–1021.

Loh, H. S., 1972, The relationship between dietary ascorbic acid intake and buffy coat and plasma ascorbic acid concentrations at different ages, *Int. J. Vitam. Nutr. Res.* **42:**80–85.

Loh, H. S., and Wilson, C. W. M., 1971, The relationship between leucocyte ascorbic acid and haemoglobin levels at different ages, *Int. J. Vitam. Nutr. Res.* **41:**259–267.

Lonergan, M. E., Milne, J. S., Maule, M. M., and Williamson, J., 1975, A dietary survey of older people in Edinburgh, *Br. J. Nutr.* **34:**517–527.

Lopez, R., Fisher, L. V., and Cooperman, J. M., 1979, Riboflavin deficiency in an aged population, *Fed. Proc.* **38:**451.

Lowenstein, F. W., 1982, Nutritional status of the elderly in the United States of America, 1971–1974, *J. Am. Coll. Nutr.* **1:**165–177.

Lumeng, L., and Li, T. K., 1974, Vitamin B-6 metabolism in chronic alcohol abuse, *J. Clin. Invest.* **53:**693–704.

Lund, B., and Sorensen, O. H., 1979, Measurement of 25-hydroxyvitamin D in serum and its relation to sunshine, age and vitamin D intake in the Danish population, *Scand. J. Clin. Lab. Invest.* **39:**23–30.

Machlin, L. J. (ed), 1984a, *Handbook of Vitamins: Nutritional, Biochemical, and Clinical Aspects,* Marcel Dekker, New York.

Machlin, L. J., 1984b, Vitamin E, in: *Handbook of Vitamins: Nutritional, Biochemical, and Clinical Aspects* (L. J. Machlin, ed.), Marcel Dekker, New York, pp. 99–146.

MacLaughlin, J., and Holick, M. F., 1985, Aging significantly decreases the capacity of human skin to produce vitamin D_3, *J. Clin. Invest.* **76:**1536–1538.

MacLennan, W. J., and Hamilton, J. C., 1979, Plasma binding capacity for 25-hydroxy-vitamin D in the elderly, *J. Clin. Pathol.* **32:**240–243.

MacLeod, C. C., Judge, T. G., and Caird, F. I., 1974, Nutrition of the elderly at home. II. Intakes of vitamins, *Age Aging* **3:**209–220.

Magnus, E. M., Bache-Wiig, J. E., Anderson, T. R., and Melbostad, E., 1982, Folate and vitamin B-12 (cobalamin) blood levels in elderly persons in geriatric homes, *Scand. J. Haematol.* **28:**360–366.

Majumdar, S. K., Shaw, G. K., and Thomson, A. D., 1983, Vitamin A utilization status in chronic alcoholic patients, *Int. J. Vitam. Nutr. Res.* **53:**273–279.

Markkanen, T., and Mustakallio, E., 1963, Absorption and excretion of biotin after feeding minced liver in achlorhydria and after partial gastrectomy, *Scand. J. Clin. Lab. Invest.* **15:**57–61.

Markkanen, T., Heikinheimo, R., and Dahl, M., 1969, Transketolase activity of red blood cells from infancy to old age, *Acta Haematol.* **42:**148–153.

Martin, P. R., Majchrowicz, E., Tamborska, E., Marietta, C., Mukherjee, A. B., and Eckardt, M. J., 1985, Response to ethanol reduced by past thiamine deficiency, *Science* **227:**1365–1368.

Mason, D. Y., and Emerson, P. M., 1973, Primary acquired sideroblastic anemia: Response to treatment with pyridoxal-5-phosphate, *Br. Med. J.* **1:**389–390.

Mawer, E. B., Backhouse, J., Hill, L. F., Lumb, G. A., De Silva, P., Taylor, C. M., and Stanbury, S. W., 1975, Vitamin D metabolism and parathyroid function in man, *Clin. Sci. Mol. Med.* **48:**349–365.

McEvoy, A. W., Fenwick, J. D., Boddy, K., and James, O. F. W., 1982, Vitamin B_{12} absorption from the gut does not decline with age in normal elderly humans, *Age Aging* **11**:180–183.

McGandy, R. B., Russell, R. M., Hartz, S. C., Jacob, R. A., Tannenbaum, S., Peters, H., Sahyoun, N., and Otradovec, C. L., 1986, Nutritional status survey of healthy, non-institutionalized elderly: Nutrient intakes from 3-day diet records and nutrient supplements, *Nutr. Res.* **6**:785–798.

McLaren, D. S., 1981, The luxus vitamins A and B-12, *Am. J. Clin. Nutr.* **34**:1611–1616.

Miller, L. T., Lindberg, A. S., Whanger, P., and Leklem, J. E., 1979, Effect of wheat bran on the bioavailability of vitamin B-6 and the excretion of selenium in men, *Fed. Proc.* **38**:767.

Milne, J. S., Lonergan, M. E., Williamson, J., Moore, F. M. L., McMaster, R., and Percy, N., 1971, Leucocyte ascorbic acid levels and vitamin C intake in older people, *Br. Med. J.* **4**:383–386.

Miranda, C. L., Mukhtar, H., Bend, J. R., and Chhabra, R. S., 1979, Effects of vitamin A deficiency on hepatic and extrahepatic mixed-function oxidase and epoxide-metabolizing enzymes in guinea pig and rabbit, *Biochem. Pharmacol.* **28**:2713–2716.

Mollin, D. L., and Ross, G. I. M., 1952, The vitamin B-12 concentration of serum and urine of normals and of patients with megaloblastic anemias and other diseases, *J. Clin. Pathol.* **5**:129–139.

Morgan, A. F., Gillum, H. L., and Williams, R. I., 1955, Nutritional status of the aging: III. Serum ascorbic acid and intake, *J. Nutr.* **55**:431–448.

Morgan, A. G., Kelleher, J., Walker, B. E., Losowsky, M. S., Droller, H., and Middleton, R. S. W., 1973, A nutritional survey in the elderly: Haematological aspects, *Int. J. Vitam. Nutr. Res.* **43**:461–471.

Morgan, A. G., Kelleher, J., Walker, B. E., Losowsky, M. S., Droller, H., and Middleton, R. S. W., 1975, A nutritional survey in the elderly: Blood and urine vitamin levels, *Int. J. Vitam. Nutr. Res.* **45**:448–462.

Munro, H. N., McGandy, R. B., Hartz, S. C., Russell, R. M., Jacob, R. A., and Otradovec, C. L., 1987, Protein nutriture of a group of free-living elderly, *Am. J. Clin. Nutr.* **46**:586–592.

Muralidhara, K. S., and Hollander, D., 1977, Intestinal absorption of alpha-tocopherol in the unanesthetized rat. The influence of luminal constituents on the absorptive process, *J. Lab. Clin. Med.* **90**:85–91.

National Academy of Sciences, 1980, *Recommended Dietary Allowances*, 9th ed., National Academy Press, Washington.

Nayal, A. S., MacLennan, W. J., Hamilton, J. C., Rose, P., and Kong, M., 1978, 25-Hydroxy-vitamin D, diet and sunlight exposure in patients admitted to a geriatric unit, *Gerontology* **24**:117–122.

Newton, H. M. V., Sheltawy, M., Hay, A. W. M., and Morgan, B., 1985, The relations between vitamin D_2 and D_3 in the diet and plasma $25(OH)D_2$ and $25(OH)D_3$ in elderly women in Great Britain, *Am. J. Clin. Nutr.* **41**:760–764.

Nielson, B., 1965, The blood vitamin B-12 concentration of older patients admitted to a neurological department, *Acta Neurol. Scand.* **41**:513–526.

Nyberg, W., Erikson, A., Forsius, H., and Fellman, J., 1964, Serum vitamin B-12 levels in an isolated island population, *Acta Med. Scand. [Suppl.]* **412**:79–82.

O'Hanlon, P., and Kohrs, M. B., 1978, Dietary studies of older Americans, *Am. J. Clin. Nutr.* **31**:1257–1269.

Olson, J. A., 1984a, Vitamin A, in: *Handbook of Vitamins: Nutritional, Biochemical, and Clinical Aspects* (L. J. Machlin, ed.), Marcel Dekker, New York, pp. 1–44.

Olson, J. A., 1984b, Serum levels of vitamin A and carotenoids as reflectors of nutritional status, *J. Natl. Cancer Inst.* **73**:1439–1444.

Omdahl, J. L., Garry, P. J., Hunsaker, L. A., Hunt, W. C., and Goodwin, J. S., 1982, Nutritional status in a healthy elderly population: Vitamin D, *Am. J. Clin. Nutr.* **36**:1225–1333.

O'Sullivan, D. J., Callaghan, N., Ferriss, J. B., Finucane, J. F., and Hegarty, M., 1986, Ascorbic acid deficiency in the elderly, *Irish J. Med. Sci.* **1**:151–156.

Parfitt, A. M., Gallagher, J. C., Heaney, R. P., Johnston, C. C., Neer, R., and Whedon, G. D., 1982, Vitamin D and bone health in the elderly, *Am. J. Clin. Nutr.* **36**:1014–1031.

Passeri, M., and Proveddini, D., 1982, La vitamina E nella fisiopathologia geriatrica, *Acta Vitam. Enzymol.* **5**:53–63.

Patnaik, B. K., and Kanungo, M. S., 1966, Ascorbic acid and aging in the rat, *Biochem. J.* **100**:59–62.

Pelletier, O., 1975, Vitamin C and cigarette smokers, *Ann. N.Y. Acad. Sci.* **258**:156–168.

Peterson, F. J., Holloway, D. E., Duquette, P. H., and Rivers, J. M., 1983, Dietary ascorbic acid and hepatic mixed function oxidase activity in the guinea pig, *Biochem. Pharmacol.* **32**:91–96.

Peto, R., Doll, R., Buckley, J. D., and Sporn, M. B., 1981, Can dietary beta-carotene materially reduce human cancer rates? *Nature* **290:**201–208.

Phillips, W. E. J., and Brien, R. L., 1970, Effect of pectin, a hypocholesterolemic polysaccharide, on vitamin A utilization in the rat, *J. Nutr.* **100:**289–292.

Pittet, P. G., Davie, M., and Lawson, D. E. M., 1979, Role of nutrition in the development of osteomalacia in the elderly, *Nutr. Metab.* **23:**109–116.

Plough, I. C., 1960, The human requirement for vitamin B-6, *Fed. Proc.* **19:**162.

Prothro, J., Mickles, M., and Tolbert, B., 1976, Nutritional status of a population sample in Macon County, Alabama, *Am. J. Clin. Nutr.* **29:**94–104.

Rafsky, H. A., and Newman, B., 1943, Vitamin B-1 excretion in the aged, *Gastroenterology* **1:**737–742.

Rafsky, H. A., Newman, B., and Jolliffe, N., 1947, The relationship of gastric acidity to thiamine excretion in the aged, *J. Lab. Clin. Med.* **32:**118–123.

Rafsky, H. A., Newman, B., and Jolliffe, N., 1948, A study of the carotene and vitamin A levels in the aged, *Gastroenterology* **8:**612–615.

Raica, N., Jr., Scott, J., Lowry, L., and Sauberlich, H. E., 1972, Vitamin A concentration in human tissues collected from five areas in the United States, *Am. J. Clin. Nutr.* **25:**291–296.

Ranke, E., Tauber, S. A., Horonick, A., Ranke, B., Goodhart, R. S., and Chow, B. F., 1960, Vitamin B-6 deficiency in the aged, *J. Gerontol.* **15:**41–44.

Rao, G. H., and Mason, K. E., 1975, Antisterility and antivitamin K activity of *d*-alpha-tocopheryl hydroquinone in the vitamin E-deficient female rat, *J. Nutr.* **105:**495–498.

Ristow, K. A., Gregory, J. F., and Damron, B. L., 1982, Effects of dietary fiber on the bioavailability of folic acid monoglutamate, *J. Nutr.* **112:**750–758.

Roderuck, C., Burrill, L., Campbell, L. J., Brakke, B. E., Childs, M. T., Leverton, X. R., Chaloupka, M., Jebe, E. H., and Swanson, P. P., 1958, Estimated dietary intake, urinary excretion and blood vitamin C in women of different ages, *J. Nutr.* **66:**15–27.

Rodriguez, M. S., 1978, A conspectus of research on folacin requirements of man, *J. Nutr.* **108:**1983–2103.

Roe, D. A., Wrick, K., McLain, D., and van Soest, P., 1978, Effects of dietary fiber sources on riboflavin absorption, *Fed. Proc.* **37:**756.

Roine, P., Koivula, L., Pekkarinen, M., and Rissanen, A., 1974, Vitamin C intake and plasma level among aged people in Finland, *Int. J. Vitam. Nutr. Res.* **44:**95–106.

Rose, C. S., Gyorgy, P., Butler, M., Andres, R., Norris, A. H., Shock, N. W., Tobin, J., Brin, M., and Spiegel, H., 1976, Age differences in vitamin B-6 status of 617 men, *Am. J. Clin. Nutr.* **29:**847–853.

Rosenberg, I. H., 1981, Intestinal absorption of folate, in: *Physiology of the Gastrointestinal Tract* (L. R. Johnson, ed.), Raven Press, New York, pp. 1221–1230.

Rosenberg, I. H., Selhub, J., and Dhar, G. J., 1979, Absorption and malabsorption of folates, in: *Folic Acid in Neurology, Psychiatry, and Internal Medicine* (M. I. Botez and E. H. Reynolds, eds.), Raven Press, New York, pp. 95–111.

Rosenberg, I. H., Bowman, B. B., Cooper, B. A., Halstead, C. H., and Lindenbaum, J., 1982, Folate nutrition in the elderly, *Am. J. Clin. Nutr.* **36:**1060–1066.

Roth, K. S., 1981, Biotin in clinical medicine—a review, *Am. J. Clin. Nutr.* **34:**1967–1974.

Runcie, J., 1979, Folate deficiency in the elderly, in: *Folic acid in Neurology, Psychiatry, and Internal Medicine* (M. I. Botez and E. H. Reynolds, eds.), Raven Press, New York, pp. 493–499.

Rushton, C., 1978, Vitamin D hydroxylation in youth and old age, *Age Aging* **7:**91–95.

Russell, R. M., Ismail-Beigi, F., and Reinhold, J. G., 1976, Folate content of Iranian breads and the effect of their fiber content on the intestinal absorption of folic acid, *Am. J. Clin. Nutr.* **29:**799–802.

Russell, R. M., Dhar, G. J., Dutta, S. K., and Rosenberg, I. H., 1979, Influence of intraluminal pH on folate absorption: Studies in control subjects and in patients with pancreatic insufficiency, *J. Lab. Clin. Med.* **93:**428–436.

Russell, R. M., Rosenberg, I. H., Wilson, P. D., Iber, F. L., Oaks, E. B., Giovetti, H. C., Otradovec, C. L., Karwoski, P. A., and Press, A. W., 1983, Increased urinary excretion and prolonged turnover time of folic acid during ethanol ingestion, *Am. J. Clin. Nutr.* **38:**64–70.

Russell, R. M., Goldner, B. B., and Krasinski, S. D., 1985, Impariment of folic acid absorption by postpranial antacid in elderly subjects, *Gastroenterology* **88:**1563.

Russell, R. M., Krasinski, S. D., Samloff, I. M., Jacob, R. A., Hartz, S. C., and Brovender, S. R., 1986, Folic acid malabsorption in atrophic gastritis: Compensation by bacterial folate synthesis, *Gastroenterology* **91:**1476–1483.

Rutishauser, I. H. E., Bates, C. J., Paul, A. A., Black, A. E., Mandal, A. R., and Patnaik, B. K., 1979, Long-term status and dietary intake of healthy elderly subjects. 1. Riboflavin, *Br. J. Nutr.* **42**:33–42.

Sahud, M. A., and Cohen, R. J., 1971, Effect of aspirin ingestion on ascorbic acid levels in rheumatoid arthritis, *Lancet* **1**:937–938.

Said, H. M., and Hollander, D., 1985, Does aging effect the intestinal transport of riboflavin? *Life Sci.* **36**:69–73.

Salkeld, R. M. and Stotz, R., 1985, Vitamin B-6 deficiency: An etiological factor of the carpal tunnel syndrome, in: *Vitamin B-6: Its Role in Health and Disease* (J. Leklem and B. Reynolds, eds.), Alan R. Liss, New York, pp. 463–467.

Sato, M., and Lieber, C. S., 1981, Hepatic vitamin A depletion after chronic ethanol consumption in baboons and rats, *J. Nutr.* **111**:2015–2023.

Sauberlich, H. E., Herman, Y. F., Stevens, C. O., and Herman, R. H., 1979, Thiamin requirement of the adult human, *Am. J. Clin. Nutr.* **32**:2237–2248.

Sauberlich, H. E., Skala, H. J., and Dowdy, R. P., 1984, *Laboratory Tests for the Assessment of Nutritional Status,* CRC Press, Boca Raton, FL.

Schaus, R., 1957, The ascorbic acid content of human pituitary, cerebral cortex, heart and skeletal muscle and its relation to age, *Am. J. Clin. Nutr.* **5**:39–42.

Schaus, R., and Kirk, J. E., 1957, The riboflavin concentration of brain, heart, and skeletal muscle in individuals of various ages, *J. Gerontol.* **11**:147–150.

Schmidt, V., 1951, The excretion of pantothenic acid in the urine in young and old individuals, *J. Gerontol.* **6**:132–134.

Schorah, C. J., 1979, An assessment of the prevalence and importance of vitamin C depletion in an urban population, *Int. J. Vitam. Nutr. Res.* **19**:(Suppl):167–177.

Schorah, C. J., Scott, D. L., Newill, A., and Morgan, D. B., 1979, Clinical effects of vitamin C in elderly inpatients with low blood vitamin C levels, *Lancet* **1**:403–405.

Sedrani, S. H., Elidrissy, A. W. T. H., and El Arabi, K. M., 1983, Sunlight and vitamin D status in normal Saudi subjects, *Am. J. Clin. Nutr.* **38**:129–132.

Seetharam, B., and Alpers, D. H., 1985, Cellular uptake of cobalamin, *Nutr. Rev.* **43**:97–102.

Sharpe, P. C., Mills, J. B., Horton, M. A., Hunt, R. H., Vincent, S. H., and Milton-Thomson, G. J., 1980, Histamine H-2 receptors and intrinsic factor secretion, *Scand. J. Gastroenterol.* **15**:377–384.

Sheltawy, M., Newton, H., Hay, A., Morgan, D. B., and Hullin, R. P., 1984, The contribution of dietary vitamin D and sunlight to the plasma 25-hydroxyvitamin D in the elderly, *Hum. Nutr. Clin. Nutr.* **38C**:191–194.

Shepherd, A. M. M., Hewick, D. S., Moreland, T. A., and Stevenson, I. H., 1977, Age as a determinant of sensitivity to warfarin, *Br. J. Clin. Pharmacol.* **4**:315–320.

Shideler, C. E., 1983, Vitamin B-6: An overview, *Am. J. Med. Technol.* **49**:17–22.

Skalka, H. W., and Prchal, J. T., 1981, Cataracts and riboflavin deficiency, *Am. J. Clin. Nutr.* **34**:861–863.

Schorah, C. J., Tormey, W. D., Brooks, G. H., Robertshaw, A., Young, G. A., Talukder, R., and Kelly, J. F., 1981, The effect of vitamin C supplements on body weight, serum proteins, and general health of the elderly, *Am. J. Clin. Nutr.* **34**:871–876.

Slovik, D. M., Adams, J. S., Neer, R. M., Holick, M. F., and Potts, J. T., Jr., 1981, Deficient production of 1,25-dihydroxyvitamin D in elderly osteoporotic patients, *N. Engl. J. Med.* **305**:372–374.

Somerville, P. F., Lien, J. W. K., and Kaye, M., 1977, The calcium and vitamin D status in an elderly female population and their response to administered supplemental vitamin D_3, *J. Gerontol.* **32**:659–663.

Sowers, M. F. P., Wallace, R. B., Hollis, B. W., and Lemke, J. H., 1986, Parameters related to 25-OH-D levels in a population-based study of women, *Am. J. Clin. Nutr.* **43**:621–628.

Srinivasan, V., Christensen, N., Wyse, B. W., and Hansen, R. G., 1981, Pantothenic acid nutritional status in the elderly: Institutionalized and noninstitutionalized, *Am. J. Clin. Nutr.* **34**:1736–1742.

Stamp, T. C. B., and Round, J. M., 1974, Seasonal changes in human plasma levels of 25-hydroxyvitamin D, *Nature* **247**:563–565.

Steinberg, W. M., King, C. E., and Toskes, P. P., 1980, Malabsorption of protein-bound cobalamin but not unbound cobalamin during cimetidine administration, *Dig. Dis. Sci.* **25**:188–191.

Steinkamp, R. C., Cohen, N. L., and Walsh, H. E., 1965, Resurvey of an aging population—fourteen-year follow-up, *J. Am. Diet. Assoc.* **46**:103–110.

Stiedemann, M., Jansen, C., and Harrill, I., 1978, Nutritional status of elderly men and women, *J. Am. Diet. Assoc.* **73:**132–139.

Sugarman, B., and Munro, H. N., 1980, [^{14}C]-Pantothenate accumulation by isolated adipocytes from adult rats of different ages, *J. Nutr.* **110:**2297–2301.

Suttie, J. W., 1984, Vitamin K, in: *Handbook of Vitamins. Nutritional, Biochemical, and Clinical Aspects* (J. L. Machlin, ed.), Marcel Dekker, New York, pp. 147–198.

Suttie, J. W., and Jackson, C. M., 1977, Prothrombin structure, activation, and biosynthesis, *Physiol. Rev.* **57:**1–70.

Sweetman, L., Surh, L., Baker, H., Peterson, R. M., and Nyhan, W. L., 1981, Clinical and metabolic abnormalities in a boy with dietary deficiency of biotin, *Pediatrics* **68:**553–558.

Swendseid, M. E., Gasster, M., and Halsted, J. A., 1954, Absorption of vitamin B-12 in individuals with a functioning gastric mucosa, *Fed. Proc.* **13:**308.

TSNS, 1972, Ten-State Nutrition Survey, 1968–70, Part 5, *Dietary*, Center for Disease Control, Atlanta.

Thackray, G. B., Sharman, I. M., and Hyams, D. E., 1972, Riboflavin status of the elderly, *Proc. Nutr. Soc.* **31:**89A–90A.

Thomson, A. D., 1966, Thiamine absorption in old age, *Gerontol. Clin.* **8:**354–361.

Toss, G., Almqvist, S., Larsson, L., and Zetterqvist, H., 1980, Vitamin D deficiency in welfare institutions for the aged, *Acta Med. Scand.* **208:**87–89.

Trimbo, S., Kathman, J., Kies, C., and Fox, H. M., 1979, Pantothenic acid nutritional status of adolescent humans as affected by dietary fiber and bran, *Fed. Proc.* **38:**556.

Tsai, K. S., Heath, H., Kumar, R., and Riggs, B. L., 1984, Impaired vitamin D metabolism with aging in women, *J. Clin. Invest.* **73:**1668–1672.

Tulloch, J. A., and Sood, N. K., 1967, Vitamin E deficiency in Uganda, *Am. J. Clin. Nutr.* **20:**884–887.

Underwood, B. A., Siegel, H., Weisell, R. C., and Dolinski, M., 1970a, Liver stores of vitamin A in a normal population dying suddenly or rapidly from unnatural causes in New York City, *Am. J. Clin. Nutr.* **23:**1037–1042.

Underwood, B. A., Siegel, H., Dolinski, M., and Weisell, R. C., 1970b, Liver stores of alpha-tocopherol in a normal population dying suddenly and rapidly from unnatural causes in New York City, *Am. J. Clin. Nutr.* **23:**1314–1321.

United States Census of Population, 1980, *Supplementary Reports: Age, Sex, Race and Spanish Origin of the Population by Regions, Divisions and States (PC80-S1-1)*, U.S. Government Printing Office, Washington.

Vatassery, G. T., Alter, M., and Stadlan, E. M., 1971, Serum tocopherol levels and vibratory threshold changes with age, *J. Gerontol.* **26:**481–484.

Vatassery, G. T., Johnson, G. J., and Krezowski, A. M., 1983, Changes in vitamin E concentrations in human plasma and platelets with age, *J. Am. Coll. Nutr.* **4:**369–375.

Vermeer, C., 1984, The vitamin K-dependent carboxylation reaction, *Mol. Cell. Biochem.* **61:**17–35.

Vimokesant, S., Kunjara, S., Rungruangsak, K., Nakornchai, S., and Panijpan, B., 1982, Beriberi caused by antithiamin factors in food and its prevention, *Ann. N.Y. Acad. Sci.* **378:**123–136.

Vir, S. C., and Love, A. H. G., 1977a, Nutritional evaluation of B group vitamins in institutionalised aged, *Int. J. Vitam. Nutr. Res.* **47:**211–218.

Vir, S. C., and Love, A. H. G., 1977b, Vitamin B-6 status of institutionalised and non-institutionalised aged, *Int. J. Vitam. Nutr. Res.* **47:**364–372.

Vir, S. C., and Love, A. H. G., 1977c, Thiamine status of institutionalised and non-institutionalised aged, *Int. J. Vitam. Nutr. Res.* **47:**325–335.

Vir, S. C., and Love, A. H. G., 1978a, Vitamin D status of elderly at home and institutionalised in hospital, *Int. J. Vitam. Nutr. Res.* **48:**123–130.

Vir, S. C., and Love, A. H. G., 1978b, Vitamin B-6 status of the hospitalized aged, *Am. J. Clin. Nutr.* **31:**1383–1391.

Vir, S. C., and Love, A. H. G., 1979, Nutritional status of institutionalised and non-institutionalised aged in Belfast, Northern Ireland, *Am. J. Clin. Nutr.* **32:**1934–1947.

Wagner, P. A., Bailey, L. B., Krista, M. L., Jernigan, J. A., Robinson, J. D., and Cerda, J. J., 1981, Comparison of zinc and folacin status in elderly women from differing socioeconomic backgrounds, *Nutr. Res.* **1:**565–569.

Wald, G., 1968, Molecular basis of visual excitation, *Science* **162:**230–235.

Walsh, J. H., Wyse, B. W., and Hansen, R. G., 1981, Pantothenic acid content of a nursing home diet, *Ann. Nutr. Metab.* **25**:178–181.

Walsh, M. P., 1966, Determination of plasma pyridoxal phosphate with wheat germ glutamic–aspartic apotransaminase, *Am. J. Clin. Pathol.* **36**:282–285.

Watson, W. S., Vallance, B. D., Muir, M. M., and Hume, R., 1982, The effect of megadose ascorbic acid ingestion on the absorption and retention of vitamin B-12 in man, *Scott. Med. J.* **27**:240–243.

Webster, S. G. P., and Leeming, J. T., 1979, Erythrocyte folate levels in young and old, *J. Am. Geriatr. Soc.* **27**:451–454.

Weglicki, W. B., Luna, Z., and Nair, P. P., 1969, Sex and tissue specific differences in concentrations of alpha-tocopherol in mature and senescent rats, *Nature* **221**:185–186.

Weisman, Y., Schen, R. J., Eisenberg, Z., Edelstein, S., and Harell, A., 1981, Inadequate status and impaired metabolism of vitamin D in the elderly, *Israel J. Med. Sci.* **17**:19–21.

Weiss, P., and Bianchine, J. R., 1970, The effect of clofibrate of vitamin E concentrations in the rat, *Atherosclerosis* **11**:203–205.

Wei-Wo, C. K., and Draper, H. H., 1975, Vitamin E status of Alaskan Eskimos, *Am. J. Clin. Nutr.* **28**:808–813.

Welkos, S. L., Toskes, P. P., Baer, H., and Smith, G. W., 1981, Importance of anaerobic bacteria in the cobalamin malabsorption of the experimental rat tlind loop syndrome, *Gastroenterology* **80**:313–320.

Willett, W. C., Polk, B. F., Underwood, B. A., Stampfer, M. J., Pressel, S., Rosner, B., Taylor, J. O., Schneider, K., and Hames, C. G., 1984, Relation of serum vitamins A and E and carotenoids to the risk of cancer, *N. Engl. J. Med.* **310**:430–434.

Wolf, B., Heard, G. S., Jefferson, L. G., Proud, V. K., Nance, w. E., and Weissbecker, K. A., 1985, Clinical findings in four children with biotinidase deficiency detected through a statewide neonatal screening program, *N. Engl. J. Med.* **313**:16–19.

Yamaguchi, D. M., Lipscomb, P. R., and Soule, E. H., 1965, Carpal tunnel syndrome, *Minn. Med.* **48**:22–33.

Yavorsky, M., Almaden, P., and King, C. G., 1934, The vitamin C content of human tissues, *J. Biol. Chem.* **106**:525–529.

Yearick, E. S., Wang, M. S. L., and Pisias, S. J., 1980, Nutritional status of the elderly: Dietary and biochemical findings, *J. Gerontol.* **35**:663–671.

Yiengst, M. J., and Shock, N. W., 1949, Effect of oral administration of vitamin A on plasma levels of vitamin A and carotene in aged males, *J. Gerontol.* **4**:205–211.

Ziemlanski, S., Wartanowicz, M., and Palaszewska, M., 1971, The effect of age and various diets on folic acid absorption in the alimentary tract, *Acta Physiol. Pol.* **22**:241–246.

Zimran, A., and Hershko, C., 1983, The changing pattern of megaloblastic anemia: Megaloblastic anemia in Israel, *Am. J. Clin. Nutr.* **37**:855–861.

11

Role of Fiber in the Diet of the Elderly

David Kritchevsky

1. Introduction

The most common description of dietary fiber uses this term to refer to remnants of plant cells that are not digested by the enzymes of the human alimentary tract (Trowell, 1974). This is a convenient but somewhat misleading description. The term dietary fiber encompasses a variety of substances of different chemical composition and diverse physiological function. In the strictest definition, dietary fiber can be divided into three categories: cellulose, the principal fibrillar component of the plant cell wall; noncellulosic polysaccharides, including pectic substances and hemicelluloses, which form the cell wall matrix; and lignin, an encrusting substance present in the mature plant wall. However, the definition of fiber has been broadened to include plant gums such as guar or tragacanth, agar, and some chemically modified materials such as methylcellulose. All of these substances except lignin are carbohydrate in nature, and all except lignin are degradable (partially or totally) by colonic microflora. The degradation products include hydrogen, methane, carbon dioxide, and short-chain fatty acids—acetic, propionic, and butyric. The actions of fiber as described by Heaton (1983) are:

I.	Food	Solidifier, hardener, water trapper
II.	Mouth	Saliva stimulant, cleaner, work demander
III.	Stomach	Diluter, distender, storage prolonger
IV.	Small intestine	Delayer of absorption, diluter, distender
V.	Large intestine	Diluter, distender, nonbinder, water trapper, bacterial substrate and/or inhibitor
VI.	Stool	Softener, enlarger, strain-preventer.

David Kritchevsky • The Wistar Institute of Anatomy and Biology, Philadelphia, Pennsylvania 19104.

2. *Putative Roles of Fiber in Gastrointestinal Function and Nutrient Availability*

Diets rich in fiber tend to be bulky and require a longer time for ingestion. Haber *et al.* (1977) found that equicaloric amounts of apple, apple sauce, and apple juice were consumed in 17.2, 5.9, and 1.5 min, respectively. McCance *et al.* (1953) found that it took normal subjects 34 min to consume a meal of white bread and 45 min for an equicaloric amount of brown bread. These results suggest that meals high in fiber would be more satiating, and some (Haber *et al.*, 1977; Krotkiewski, 1984) but not all (Bryson *et al.*, 1980) investigators found this to be the case. Gastric emptying is usually delayed by fiber (Holt *et al.*, 1979; Leeds *et al.*, 1981), but, again, this is not a uniform observation (Rydning *et al.*, 1985) and is a function of the type of fiber present in the diet (Kaspar *et al.*, 1985).

Fiber decreases transit time and increases stool weight. This observation has been one of the cornerstones of the "fiber hypothesis" (Burkitt *et al.*, 1972). Walker (1976) compared bowel transit time of South African black and white adults and found the former to exhibit transit times one-half to one-quarter that of the latter and up to threefold greater stool weight. Cummings (1986) reviewed the influence of fiber on fecal output and found the greatest effects to be those of bran or fruit and vegetables and the least effect to be that of pectin (Table I). A specific effect may be hard to recognize, however. In 1936, Williams and Olmsted (1936) fed subjects a variety of fiber-rich substances including cellulose, canned peas, wheat bran, carrots, and cabbage. The observed increases in stool weight could not be correlated with the analytical data (cellulose, lignin, hemicellulose) or with the subjects' perception of the laxative action of the added material.

An increased amount of energy (protein, fat) is lost in the feces of subjects ingesting high-fiber diets (Kelsay *et al.*, 1978, 1981; Cummings *et al.*, 1979a,b), but this is also a function of the type of fiber present in the diet (Slavin and Marlett, 1980; Sandberg *et al.*, 1981, 1983).

Studies on mineral balance are similarly equivocal. The minerals most frequently assayed are calcium, magnesium, iron, and zinc. Recent studies show little effect of fiber-rich foods or of added purified fibers on their availability (Kelsay *et al.*, 1981; Behall *et al.*, 1987).

Table I. Average Increase in Fecal Output per Gram Ingested Fiber[a]

Fiber source	Number of studies	Increase in fecal weight (±S.E.M.) (g/g fiber)
Wheat bran	31	5.7 ± 0.5
Fruits and vegetables	20	4.9 ± 0.9
Oats	3	3.9 ± 1.5
Gums, mucilages	16	3.5 ± 0.7
Corn bran	4	3.4 ± 0.4
Cellulose	6	3.0 ± 0.6
Soy	4	2.8 ± 0.8
Pectin	10	1.3 ± 0.3

[a]After Cummings (1986).

3. Fiber and Aging

The ensuing discussion does not relate to all the nutritional problems of aging, only to those in which dietary fiber may play a pivotal role.

3.1. Relevant Factors Affecting Nutritional Requirements of the Elderly

Lowenstein (1986) has reviewed the factors that may affect nutritional requirements of the elderly. Among the changes in physiology are dental problems. About two-thirds of Americans aged 75 years or older have lost more than half their teeth. The resulting chewing problems affect both quantity and quality of food intake (Heath, 1972). An increasing loss of the senses of taste and smell will reduce stimuli to eating and enjoyment thereof (Meyer and Pudel, 1983). Changes in various processes associated with digestion will result in diminished absorption of necessary nutrients (Bhantamnuvin and Schuster, 1977). Pathological conditions that can affect nutritional requirement include atherosclerosis, cancer, and diabetes. Increased use of various pharmaceutical agents may interfere with absorption of specific nutrients. Psychological factors such as social isolation and depression also influence food intake.

3.2. Role of Dietary Fiber in Chronic Afflictions of the Elderly

Digestive disorders increase with aging (Table II). Many of these problems may be affected by the presence of dietary fiber.

The rate of gastric emptying may (Horowitz *et al.*, 1984) or may not (Moore *et al.*, 1983) be delayed in aging, but in any case the differences are relatively minor. The effect of dietary fiber in slowing gastric emptying has been discussed above. Gastric ulcer is more common among the elderly (Grossman, 1981). Complications such as bleeding and perforation are also more common (Cutler, 1958). Increased dietary fiber has been reported to heal duodenal ulcers (Harju and Larmi, 1985), but there may be other factors operating since diets high (22.6 g/day) or low (8–9 g/day) in fiber

Table II. Prevalence of Chronic Digestive Diseases in the United States[a] (per 1000)

	Age (years)		
Disease	Under 45	45–64	65+
Peptic ulcer	21.4	37.7	30.8
Constipation	12.7	23.6	67.1
Hiatus hernia	8.6	34.3	62.2
Upper G.I.	15.7	29.4	38.5
Gallbladder	1.5	4.4	3.7
Gastritis	8.4	11.4	17.4
Diverticular disease	1.1	13.2	31.0
Gastroenteritis, colitis	5.2	9.7	13.5

[a] After Young and Urban (1986).

promoted the same level of healing (Rydning *et al.*, 1986). However Rydning *et al.* (1982) showed that the recurrence of ulcers in healed subjects was 78% higher on a low-fiber compared to a high-fiber diet.

Constipation is said to be the most common gastrointestinal complaint of the elderly, about half of whom take laxatives despite surveys that suggest that about three-quarters of persons aged 60 years or more have five to seven bowel movements weekly (Connell *et al.*, 1965). There are a number of studies that show that wheat bran, ispaghula, or soy polysaccharide will increase frequency of defecation and stool weight and will obviate the need for laxatives (Clark and Scott, 1976; Smith *et al.*, 1980; Graham *et al.*, 1982; Fischer *et al.*, 1985; Hope and Down, 1986).

Diverticular disease increases with age (Connell, 1975; Parks, 1975). In 1975 Rogers estimated that 15 million people aged 70 or over had colonic diverticula. A similar prevalance has been reported for the United Kingdom (Taylor and Duthie, 1976). Classification of this disease has been attempted by Brodribb (1979) and Mendeloff (1986). Painter *et al.* (1972) showed that diets high in bran could relieve the symptoms of diverticular disease. Eastwood *et al.* (1978) showed that other types of fiber could do so as well. Several reviews have confirmed that diets high in fiber generally relieve diverticular disease (Mitchell and Eastwood, 1976; Brodribb, 1980; Jenkins *et al.*, 1986).

Inflammatory bowel disease is a catch-all phrase that includes ulcerative colitis and Crohn's disease, both of which may occur predominantly in older subjects (Brandt *et al.*, 1982; Shapiro *et al.*, 1981). Use of dietary fiber to treat Crohn's disease has yielded equivocal results (Brandes and Lorenz-Meyer, 1981; Levenstein *et al.*, 1985). Similarly, the use of fiber in treatment of irritable bowel syndrome has yielded positive (Manning *et al.*, 1977) and negative results (Soltoft *et al.*, 1976).

Glen (1981) has reported on the striking increase in gallstone incidence with aging. Thus, gallstones are reported in 10% of people younger than 30, in 25–30% of people aged 50–60; and 55% of persons older than 80. There are reports of treatment of gallstones with high-fiber diets, but concentrations of the chemical triad that makes up the lithogenic index (bile acids, phospholipids, cholesterol) can be affected. Watts *et al.* (1978) and Hansen *et al.* (1983) found diets high in bran or guar gum to reduce bile saturation in normal subjects. Other studies showed that wheat bran (Wechsler *et al.*, 1984) and pectin reduced the lithogenic index, but cellulose and lignin had no effect (Hillman *et al.*, 1986). Pomare *et al.* (1976) and Watts *et al.* (1978) found that diets high in wheat bran (up to 50 g/day) reduced the cholesterol saturation index in subjects with gallstones.

Colon cancer is a significant cause of morbidity and mortality among the elderly. The data on diet, fiber, and colon cancer have been subjected to exhaustive review. In general, international studies support a role for fiber as a protective agent, but case-control studies do not. In a recent review Cummings (1985) stated, "The hypothesis that dietary fiber will prevent large bowel cancer is an intriguing one and worthy of consideration. For a variety of reasons, however, many currently published expidemiological findings, either population or case-control studies, do not support it." In 1982 a select committee of the U.S. National Academy of Sciences concluded: "The committee found no conclusive evidence to indicate that dietary fiber (such as present in fruits, vegetables, grains, and cereals) exerts a protective effect against colorectal cancer in humans'' (Committee on Diet, Nutrition, and Cancer, 1982). Concentration of fecal bile acids is much higher in populations prone to develop colon cancer (Hill *et al.*, 1971; Crowther *et al.*, 1976; Reddy *et al.*, 1978; Jensen *et al.*, 1982). Jensen *et al.* (1982) compared the incidence of colon cancer in urban and rural Danes and Finns and found negative correlations with cereals and total dietary fiber, among other dietary components. Cereals have been correlated with cancer mortality in 38 countries in a study that adjusted for other dietary components (McKeown-Eyssen and Bright-See, 1984). Recent studies (Kuratsune *et al.*, 1986; Walker *et al.*, 1986) have found that populations that exhibit vastly different rates of colon cancer have similar intakes of fiber. Kuratsune compared Japanese, Britons, and Danes, and Walker *et al.*, studied rural and urban blacks, ''coloureds,'' Indians, and whites in South Africa. The question is unsettled, and despite the fact that colon cancer is an important disease entity among the elderly, whatever dietary component this disease entails must be exerting its effect over a lifetime.

Horwitz (1982) has estimated that 16.5% of Americans older than 65 years have diabetes and that this figure may be 26% in those over 85 years of age. Diabetes is one disease in which dietary fiber plays an important therapeutic role. Anderson (1986) summarized results from 23 studies in which a diet supplemented with fiber (wheat bran, guar gum, glucomannan, psyllium, apple fiber, or cellulose) was administered to diabetic subjects. Blood glucose was reduced in 21 of the studies (91.3%). In 23 other studies in which a high-fiber diet (fiber-rich foods) was used, 21 reported reduced blood glucose levels. The insulin requirement in type I (insulin-dependent) diabetic men given a high-carbohydrate, high-fiber diet was reduced by 37.5%, and in type II (non-insulin-dependent) diabetic men it was reduced by 94.7%. Serum or plasma cholesterol and triglyceride levels were usually reduced in men fed the high-fiber diet, the cholesterol change being more consistent.

3.3. *Interaction of Fiber with Important Nutrients*

The dietary levels of calcium (O'Hanlon and Kohrs, 1978; Lowenstein, 1986) and zinc (Sandstead *et al.*, 1982; Greger, 1984) are low in older Americans. Absorption of iron (Freiman and Johnston, 1963) and magnesium (Seelig, 1981) is reduced in the elderly. Lowenstein (1982) reviewed the nutritional status of Americans aged 65–74 using data from NHANES I (National Health and Nutrition Examination Survey), which reviewed data from 3479 in that age group. The data suggested low levels of calcium and iron intake, but evidence of a high incidence of low-iron status could not be adduced from measurements of serum iron or transferrin saturation. In the last decade there have been a number of studies on the effects of dietary fiber on mineral balance in man. Sandstead *et al.* (1978) found no effect of wheat or corn bran on iron, zinc, or copper balance. Cummings *et al.* (1979a,b) found wheat fiber to result in a negative calcium balance but pectin to have no effect. Kies *et al.* (1979) found hemicellulose to exert a negative effect on zinc balance, and Slavin and Marlett (1980) found cellulose to cause negative calcium balance but to have no effect on magnesium balance. In studies using fruits and vegetables or whole-meal bread, Kelsay *et al.* (1981) and Andersson *et al.* (1983) found no effect on calcium, magnesium, iron, or zinc balance. In well-fed adults, fiber seems to have no effect on mineral balance.

Table III. Influence of Dietary Fiber on Nutritional Problems of Aging

Condition	Fiber effect
Gastric emptying	Negative
Ulcers	Positive[a]
Constipation	Positive
Diverticular disease	Positive
Inflammatory bowel disease	Questionable
Gallstones	Positive[a]
Colon cancer	Questionable
Diabetes	Positive
Mineral absorption	Questionable[b]

[a]Probably positive, more data needed.
[b]Probably no effect.

4. Conclusion

Table III presents the balance sheet. Although the effects of fiber are generally beneficial, it should be noted that the results cited were obtained in young adults. In a population such as the elderly, whose food intake may be rather limited, a very high intake of fiber may be deleterious. Consequently, it is best to recommend a daily fiber intake given as a function of caloric intake. A Canadian panel (Expert Advisory Committee, 1985) has suggested that an intake of 15–25 g fiber/1000 kcal might be reasonable.

Perhaps the wisest advice is that given by Dr. Elsie Widdowson (1983): "My recipe for nutrition in extreme old age is well-fitting dentures, portions of ordinary meals, milk to drink with all of them, and anything the individual particularly fancies, whether it be fish, fruit, cake, or chocolate." That and tender loving care.

ACKNOWLEDGMENTS. This work was supported in part by a Research Career Award (HL00734) from the National Institutes of Health and by funds from the Commonwealth of Pennsylvania.

5. References

Anderson, J. W., 1986, Dietary fiber in nutrition management of diabetes, in: *Dietary Fiber: Basic and Clinical Aspects* (G. V. Vahouny and D. Kritchevsky, eds.), Plenum Press, New York, pp. 343–360.

Andersson, H., Nävert, B., Bingham, S. A., Englyst, H. N., and Cummings, J. H., 1983, The effects of breads containing similar amounts of phytate but different amounts of wheat bran on calcium, zinc and iron balance in man, *Br. J. Nutr.* **50:**503–510.

Behall, K. M., Scholfield, D. J., Lee, K., Powell, A. S., and Moser, P. B., 1987, Effect of four refined fibers on apparent mineral balance in adult men, *Am. J. Clin. Nutr.* **46:**307–314.

Bhantumnavin, K., and Schuster, M., 1977, Aging and gastrointestinal function, in: *Handbook of the Biology of Aging* (C. E. Finch and L. Hayflick, eds.), Van Nostrand-Reinhold, New York, pp. 709–723.

Brandes, J. W., and Lorenz-Meyer, H., 1981, Zuckerfreie Diät: Eine neue Perspektive zur Behandlung des Morbus Crohn: Eine randomisierte, kontrollierte Studie, *Z. Gastroenterol.* **19:**1–12.

Brandt, L. J., Boley, S. J., and Mitsudo, S., 1982, Clinical characteristics and natural history of colitis in the elderly, *Am. J. Gastroenterol.* **77**:382–386.

Brodribb, A. J. M., 1979, The treatment of diverticular disease with dietary fibre, in: *Dietary Fibre: Current Developments of Importance to Health* (K. W. Heaton, ed.), Technomic Publishing Company, Westport, CT, pp. 63–73.

Brodribb, A. J. M., 1980, Dietary fiber in diverticular disease of the colon, in: *Medical Aspects of Dietary Fiber* (G. A., Spiller and R. M. Kay, eds.), Plenum Press, New York, pp. 43–66.

Bryson, E., Dore, C., and Garrow, J. S., 1980, Wholemeal bread and satiety, *J. Hum. Nutr.* **34**:113–116.

Burkitt, D. P., Walker, A. R. P., and Painter, N. S., 1972, Effect of dietary fibre on stools and transit times and its role in the causation of disease, *Lancet* **2**:1408–1412.

Clark, A. N. G., and Scott, J. F., 1976, Wheat bran in dyschezia in the aged, *Age Aging* **5**:149–154.

Committee on Diet, Nutrition and Cancer, 1982, *Diet, Nutrition and Cancer,* National Academy Press, Washington.

Connell, A. M., 1975, Applied physiology of the colon: Factors relevant to diverticular disease, *Clin. Gastroenterol.* **4**:23–26.

Connell, A. M., Hilton, C., Lennard-Jones, J. E., and Misiewicz, J. J., 1965, Variation of bowel habits in two population samples, *Br. Med. J.* **2**:1096–1099.

Crowther, J. S., Drasar, B. S., Hill, M. J., Mac Lennan, R., Magnin, D., Peck, S., and Teah-Chan, C. H., 1976, Fecal steroids and bacteria and large bowel cancer in Hong Kong by socioeconomic groups, *Br. J. Cancer* **34**:191–198.

Cummings, J., 1985, Cancer of the large bowel, in: *Dietary Fibre, Fibre-Depleted Foods and Disease* (H. Trowell, D. Burkitt, and K. Heaton, eds.), Academic Press, London, pp. 161–189.

Cummings, J. H., 1986, The effect of dietary fiber on fecal weight and composition, in: *CRC Handbook of Dietary Fiber in Human Nutrition* (G. A. Spiller, ed.), CRC Press, Boca Raton, FL, pp. 211–280.

Cummings, J. H., Southgate, D. A. T., Branch, W. J., Wiggins, H. S., Houston, H., Jenkins, D. J. A., Jivraj, T., and Hill, M. J., 1979a, The digestion of pectin in the human gut and its effect on calcium absorption and large bowel function, *Br. J. Nutr.* **41**:477–485.

Cummings, J. H., Hill, M. J., Jivraj, T., Houston, H., Branch, W. J., and Jenkins, D. J. A., 1979b, The effect of meat protein and dietary fiber on colonic function and metabolism. I. Changes in bowel habit, bile acid excretion, and calcium absorption, *Am. J. Clin. Nutr.* **32**:2086–2093.

Cutler, C. W., Jr., 1958, Clinical patterns of peptic ulcer after sixty, *Surg. Gynecol. Obstet.* **107**:23–30.

Eastwood, M. A., Smith, A. N., Brydon, W. G., and Pritchard, J., 1978, Comparison of bran, ispaghula and lactulose on colon function in diverticular disease, *Gut* **19**:1144–1147.

Expert Advisory Committee, 1985, *Report of the Expert Advisory Committee on Dietary Fibre to the Health Protection Branch,* Health and Welfare, Canada, Ottawa.

Fischer, M., Adkins, W., Hall, L., Scaman, P., Hsi, S., and Marlett, J., 1985, The effects of dietary fibre in a liquid diet on bowel function of mentally retarded individuals, *J. Ment. Defic. Res.* **29**:373–381.

Freiman, R., and Johnston, F. A., 1963, Iron absorption in the healthy aged, *Geriatrics* **18**:716–720.

Glen, F., 1981, Surgical management of acute cholecystis in patients 65 years of age and older, *Ann. Surg.* **193**:56–59.

Graham, D. Y., Moser, S. E., and Estes, M. K., 1982, The effect of bran on bowel function in constipation, *Am. J. Gastroenterol.* **77**:599–603.

Greger, J. L., 1984, Zinc and copper requirements of the elderly, in: *Annual Conference on Trace Substances in Environmental Health 13* (D. Hemphill, ed.), University of Missouri, Columbia, pp. 463–475.

Grossman, M. I., 1981, *Peptic Ulcer: Guide for the Practicing Physician,* Yearbook Publications, Chicago, pp. 10–11.

Haber, G. B., Heaton, K. W., Murphy, D., and Burroughs, L. F., 1977, Depletion and disruption of dietary fibre: Effects on satiety, plasma-glucose and serum insulin, *Lancet* **2**:679–682.

Hansen, W. E., Maurer, H., Vollmer, J., and Bräuning, C., 1983, Guar gum and bile: Effects on Postprandial gallbladder contraction and on serum bile acids in man, *Hepatogastroenterology* **30**:131–133.

Harju, E. J., and Larmi, T. K., 1985, Effect of guar gum added to the diet of patients with duodenal ulcer, *J. Parent. Ent. Nutr.* **9**:496–500.

Heath, M. R., 1972, Dietary selection by elderly persons related to dental state, *Br. Dent. J.* **132**:145–148.

Heaton, K. W., 1983, Dietary fibre in perspective, *Hum. Nutr. Clin. Nutr.* **37C**:151–170.

Hill, M. J., Drasar, B. S., Aries, V. C., Crowther, J. S., Hawksworth, G., and Williams, R. E. D., 1971, Bacteria and the aetiology of cancer of the large bowel, *Lancet* **1**:95–100.

Hillman, L. C., Peters, S. G., Fisher, C. A., and Pomare, E. W., 1986, Effects of the fibre components pectin, cellulose, and lignin on bile salt metabolism and biliary lipid composition in man, *Gut* **27**:29–36.

Holt, S., Heading, R. C., Carter, D. C., Prescott, L. F., and Tothill, P., 1979, Effect of gel fibre on gastric emptying and absorption of glucose and paracetamol, *Lancet* **1**:636–639.

Hope, A. K., and Down, E. C., 1986, Dietary fibre and fluid in the control of constipation in a nursing home population, *Med. J. Aust.* **144**:306–307.

Horowitz, M., Maddern, G. J., Chatterton, B. E., Collins, P. J., Harding, P. E., and Shearman, D. J. C., 1984, Changes in gastric emptying rates with age, *Clin. Sci.* **67**:213–218.

Horwitz, D. L., 1982, Diabetes and aging, *Am. J. Clin, Nutr.* **36**:803–808.

Jenkins, D. J. A., Wolever, T. M. S., Jenkins, A. L., Thompson, L. U., Rao, A. V., and Francis, T., 1986, The glycemic index: Blood glucose response to foods, in: *Dietary Fiber: Basic and Clinical Aspects* (G. V. Vahouny and D. Kritchevsky, eds.), Plenum Press, New York, pp. 167–179.

Jensen, O. M., MacLennan, R., and Wahrendorf, J., 1982, Diet, bowel function, fecal characteristics and large bowel cancer in Denmark and Finland, *Nutr. Cancer* **4**:5–19.

Kaspar, H., Eilles, C., Reiners, C., and Schrezenmeir, J., 1985, The influence of dietary fiber on gastric transit time, *Hepatogastroenterology* **32**:69–71.

Kelsay, J. L., Behall, K. M., and Prather, E. S., 1978, Effect of fiber from fruits and vegetables on metabolic response of human subjects. I. Bowel transit time, number of defecations, fecal weight, urinary excretions of energy and nitrogen and apparent digestibilities of energy, nitrogen and fat, *Am. J. Clin. Nutr.* **31**:1149–1153.

Kelsay, J. L., Clark, W. M., Herbst, B. J., and Prather, E. S., 1981, Nutrient utilization by human subjects consuming fruits and vegetables as sources of fiber, *J. Agric. Food Chem.* **29**:461–465.

Kies, C., Fox, H. M., and Beshgetoor, D., 1979, Effect of various levels of dietary hemicellulose on zinc nutritional status of men, *Cereal Chem.* **56**:133–136.

Krotkiewski, M., 1984, Effect of guar gum on body-weight, hunger ratings and metabolism in obese subjects, *Br. J. Nutr.* **52**:97–105.

Kuratsune, M., Honda, T., Englyst, H. N., and Cummings, J. H., 1986, Dietary fiber in the Japanese diet as investigated in connection with colon cancer risk, *Jpn. J. Cancer Res.* **77**:736–738.

Leeds, A. R., Ralphs, D. N. L., Ebred, F., Metz, G., and Dilwari, D. B., 1981, Pectin and the dumping syndrome: Reduction of symptoms and plasma volume change, *Lancet* **1**:1075–1078.

Levenstein, S., Prantera, C., Luzi, C., and D'Ubaldi, A., 1985, Low residue or normal diet in Crohn's disease: A prospective controlled study in Italian patients, *Gut* **26**:989–993.

Lowenstein, F. W., 1982, Nutritional status of the elderly in the United States of America 1971–1974, *J. Am. Coll. Nutr.* **1**:165–177.

Lowenstein, F. W., 1986, Nutritional requirements of the elderly, in: *Nutrition, Aging and Health* (E. A. Young, ed.), Alan R. Liss, New York, pp. 61–89.

Manning, A. P., Heaton, K. W., Harvey, R. F., and Uglow, P., 1977, Wheat fibre and irritable bowel syndrome: A controlled trial, *Lancet* **2**:417–418.

McCance, R. A., Prior, K. M., and Widdowson, E. M., 1953, A radiological study on the rate of passage of brown and white bread through the digestive tract of man, *Br. J. Nutr.* **7**:98–104.

McKeown-Eyssen, G. E., and Bright-See, E., 1984, Dietary factors in colon cancer: International relationships, *Nutr. Cancer* **6**:160–170.

Mendeloff, A. I., 1986, Thoughts on the epidemiology of diverticular disease, *Clin. Gastroenterol.* **15**:855–877.

Meyer, J. E., and Pudel, V., 1983, Das Essverhalten im Alter und seine Konsequenzen fur die Ernahrung, *Z. Gerontol.* **16**:241–247.

Mitchell, W. D., and Eastwood, M. A., 1976, Dietarv fiber and colon function, in: *Fiber in Human Nutrition* (G. A., Spiller and R. J. Amen, eds.), Plenum Press, New York, pp. 185–206.

Moore, J. G., Tweedy, C., Christian, P. E., and Datz, F. L., 1983, Effect of age on gastric emptying of liquid–solid meals in man, *Dig. Dis. Sci.* **28**:340–344.

O'Hanlon, P., and Kohrs, M. B., 1978, Dietary studies of older Americans, *Am. J. Clin. Nutr.* **31**:1257–1269.

Painter, N. S., Almeida, A. Z., and Colebourne, K. W., 1972, Unprocessed bran in treatment of diverticular disease of the colon, *Br. Med. J.* **2:**137–140.

Parks, T. G., 1975, Natural history of diverticular disease of the colon, *Clin. Gastroenterol.* **4:**53–69.

Pomare, E. W., Heaton, K. W., Low-Beer, T. S., and Espiner, H. J., 1976, The effect of wheat bran upon bile salt metabolism and upon the lipid composition of bile in gallstone patients, *Am. J. Dig. Dis.* **21:**521–536.

Reddy, B. S., Hedges, A. R., Laakso, K., and Wynder, E. L., 1978, Metabolic epidemiology of large bowel cancer: Fecal bulk and constituents of high-risk North American and low-risk Finnish populations, *Cancer* **43:**2832–2838.

Rogers, A. I., 1975, *Colonic Diverticular Disease,* Hoechst-Roussel Pharmaceuticals, Somerville, NY, pp. 1–20.

Rydning, A., Berstad, A., Aadland, E., and Odegaard, B., 1982, Prophylactic effect of dietary fibre in duodenal ulcer disease, *Lancet* **2:**736–739.

Rydning, A., Berstad, A., Berstad, I., and Hertzenberg, L., 1985, The effect of guar gum and fiber-enriched wheat bran on gastric emptying of a semisolid meal in healthy subjects, *Scand. J. Gastroenterol.* **20:**330–334.

Rydning, A., Weberg, R., Lange, O., and Berstad, A., 1986, Healing of benign gastric ulcer with low-dose antacids and fiber diet, *Gastroenterology* **91:**56–61.

Sandberg, A. S., Andersson, H., Hallgren, B., Hasselblad, K., and Isaksson, B., 1981, Experimental model for *in vivo* determination of dietary fibre and its effect on the absorption of nutrients in the small intestine, *Br. J. Nutr.* **45:**283–294.

Sandberg, A. S., Ahderinne, R., Andersson, H., Halgren, B., and Hulten, L., 1983, The effect of citrus pectin on the absorption of nutrients in the small intestine, *Hum. Nutr. Clin. Nutr.* **37C:**171–183.

Sandstead, H. H., Munoz, J. M., Jacob, R. A., Klevay, L. M., Reck, S. J., Logan, G. M., Jr., Dintzis, F. R., Inglett, G. E., and Shuey, W, C., 1978, Influence of dietary fiber on trace element balance, *Am. J. Clin. Nutr.* **31:**S180–S184.

Sandstead, H. H., Henricksen, L. K., Greger, J. L., Prasad, A. S., and Good, R. A., 1982, Zinc nutriture in the elderly in relation to taste acuity, immune response and wound healing, *Am. J. Clin. Nutr.* **36:**1046–1059.

Seelig, M. S., 1981, Magnesium requirements in human nutrition, *Magnesium Bull.* **1:**26–47.

Shapiro, P. A., Peppercorn, M. A., Antionoli, D. A., Joffe, N., and Goldman, H., 1981, Crohn's disease in the elderly, *Am. J. Gastroenterol.* **76:**132–137.

Slavin, J. L., and Marlett, J. A., 1980, Influence of refined cellulose on human bowel function and calcium and magnesium balance, *Am. J. Clin. Nutr.* **33:**1932–1939.

Smith, R. G., Rowe, M. J., Smith, A. N., Eastwood, M. A., Drummond, E., and Brydon, W. G., 1980, A study of bulking agents in elderly patients, *Age Aging* **9:**267–271.

Soltoft, J., Gudmand-Hoyer, E., Krag, B., Kristensen, E., and Wulff, H. R., 1976, A double-blind trial of the effect of wheat bran on symptoms of irritable bowel syndrome, *Lancet* **1:**270–272.

Taylor, I., and Duthie, H. L., 1976, Bran tablets and diverticular disease, *Br. Med. J.* **1:**988–990.

Trowell, H. C., 1974, Definitions of fibre, *Lancet* **1:**503.

Walker, A. R. P., 1976, Gastrointestinal diseases and fiber intake with special reference to South African populations, in: *Fiber in Human Nutrition* (G. A. Spiller and R. J. Amen, eds.), Plenum Press, New York, pp. 241–261.

Walker, A. R. P., Walker, B. F., and Walker, A. J., 1986, Faecal pH, dietary fibre intake, and proneness to colon cancer in four South African populations, *Br. J. Cancer* **53:**489–495.

Watts, J. M., Jablonski, P., and Toouli, J., 1978, The effect of added bran to the diet in the saturation of bile in people without gallstones, *Am. J. Surg.* **135:**321–324.

Wechsler, J. G., Swobodnik, W., Wenzel, H., Heuchemer, T., Nebelung, W. Hutt, V., and Ditschuneit, H., 1984, Ballaststoffe vom Typ Weizenkleie senken Lithogenität der Galle, *Deutsch. Med. Wochenschr.* **109:**1284–1288.

Widdowson, E. M., 1983, Age, sex and nutrition, *Nutr. Bull.* **8:**117–121.

Williams, R. D., and Olmsted, W. H., 1936, The effect of cellulose, hemicellulose and lignin on the weight of the stool: A contribution to the study of laxation in man, *J. Nutr.* **11:**433–449.

Young, E. A., and Urban, E., 1986, Aging, the aged and the gastrointestinal tract, in: *Aging and Health* (E. A. Young, ed.), Alan R. Liss, New York, pp. 91–131.

III

Other Aspects of the Nutrient Status of the Elderly

12

Factors Affecting Nutritional Status of the Elderly

Mary Bess Kohrs, Dorice M. Czajka-Narins, and James W. Nordstrom

1. Introduction

A complete assessment of nutritional status includes determination of dietary intake, anthropometric measurements, biochemical measurements, and clinical assessment. The state of the art in assessing nutrition status through each of these parameters has been reviewed recently by Kohrs and Czajka-Narins (1986). In interpreting data on the elderly, the advantages and limitations of the methods for dietary intake and anthropometric measurement need to be taken into consideration as well as the limitations of the current biochemical methods.

A major factor influencing nutritional status is decreased consumption of foods with adequate concentrations of nutrients. Many factors play a role in determining dietary intake (Fig. 1). Socioeconomic, psychological, ethnic, physiological, and pathological factors all influence dietary intake, interacting in a complex and intertwining manner. For example, financial stress can lead to depression, which in turn adversely affects dietary intake. In turn, inadequate intake can lead to protein–calorie malnutrition, which in itself can cause anorexia, depression, and apathy, ultimately setting up a vicious cycle.

Likewise, a disease process may affect nutritional status by affecting food intake and/or by affecting absorption or metabolism of a specific nutrient. Finally, nutrient intake may be an intervening variable that will affect the management of disease. For example, good nutritional status produced by maintaining the child with cancer with parenteral nutrition is associated with greater tolerance to treatment (Coates *et al.*, 1986). An example more relevant to the elderly is the influence of improved nutritional status with increased caloric intake on morbidity and mortality from decubitus ulcers (Breslow *et al.*, 1987).

Mary Bess Kohrs • Department of Community Health Sciences, University of Illinois–Chicago, Chicago, Illinois 60612. ***Dorice M. Czajka-Narins*** • Department of Physiology and Biophysics, University of Health Sciences/Chicago Medical School, North Chicago, Illinois 60064. ***James W. Nordstrom*** • Human Nutrition Research Program, Lincoln University, Jefferson City, Missouri 65101.

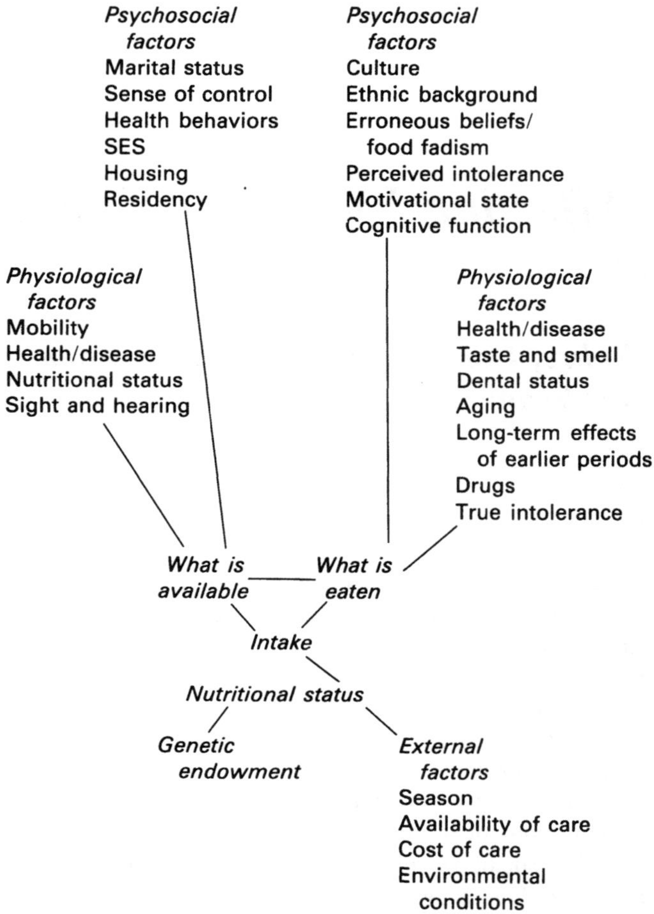

Fig. 1. Major factors in determining food intakes of the elderly. Although most lines should point in both directions and there should be many lines between factors indicating interactions, these have not been included in the interest of simplifying the diagram and emphasizing the major relationships.

A major problem with much research on the elderly is the failure to recognize the heterogeneity among older, nondiseased individuals for many physiological and cognitive characteristics. Emphasis on "normal" focuses attention on typical or usual. However, for any measure that shows average decline with age, one can find elderly individuals who have minimal or no loss as well as those with substantial loss as compared to the average of their younger-aged counterparts. Rowe and Kahn (1987) categorize those elderly individuals as having aged successfully with regard to that particular variable. They designate as "usual aging" typical nonpathological age-linked losses. Further, they suggest that the effects of aging itself have been overemphasized and the role of diet, exercise, and other factors underestimated. Perhaps along with the usual descriptive statistics, investigators should report the percentage of elderly having values within the normal range for the contrast (younger) group.

Another difficulty that arises from failure to recognize heterogeneity in the elderly is the frequent failure to use appropriate statistics to determine the true role of age. Many investigators analyze their data by dealing with all elderly subjects as one group although the age range may be as much as 30 to 40 years. Failure to use multivariate statistical techniques to determine the true effect of age complicates interpretation of the data. For example, the mean weight of elderly women aged 65 to 99 years was 65.3 kg. However, when grouped by 5-year age intervals, the mean weight decreased from 69.6 kg for those aged 65–69 years to 59.5 kg for those 80–84 years of age (Czajka-Narins *et al.*, 1988). By linear regression analysis, age was a significant factor in the weight of these women.

Finally, many investigators fail to give mean or median ages not only for the population of elderly subjects but also for the contrast group. Giving means and standard deviations of groups, such as "elderly adults, mean age 82.8 years, S.D. 5.8; young adults, mean age 24.4 years, S.D. 3.47" (Bartoshuk *et al.*, 1986) provides the readers with a much better idea of the distribution of age than the ranges of 74–93 and 20–30 years, respectively. On the other hand, a figure that plots percentage of overweight females 65–74 years of age by poverty status and shows an incidence of 45% for those below the poverty line and 30% for those above the poverty line (Joint Nutrition Monitoring Evaluation Committee, 1986) may not give enough information. Mean ages are not given for the groups, so we do not know how much, if anything, age contributes to the difference either directly or as part of an interaction, possibly through differential mortality in the two groups.

In this chapter, the effects of the major determinants on nutritional status are examined whenever possible by looking at each aspect of nutritional status—dietary intake, anthropometry, biochemical measurements, and clinical findings. In general, many of the factors that affect nutritional status are estimated or measured in only a few studies.

2. *Sociological Factors*

2.1. *Socioeconomic Status*

Traditionally, socioeconomic status (SES) has included three main variables: education, income, and occupation. Together these influence a whole range of nutrition-related behaviors, including but not limited to food preferences, mobility, and food preparation facilities. For example, SES has long been known to be related to obesity, with those in lower SES categories having a higher prevalence of obesity (Kohrs *et al.*, 1979). Little, however, is known about the relationship of SES to obesity among the elderly. Calasanti and Hendricks (1986) have termed the SES factor "access to opportunity." In drawing conclusions about the effect of SES on nutritional status and food intake of the elderly, one must remember that the elderly are a heterogeneous group coming from a diversity of backgrounds and with a lifetime of environmental and social experiences. Relatively little is known about the influence of SES on biochemical measurements of nutritional status.

2.1.1. Income

Income is considered to be a major determinant of dietary intake and nutritional status. Frequently, information on income is not available because of the sensitivity of respondants to providing actual numbers. Therefore, in many studies income is estimated from geographical location or census data. When participants in a congregate meal program for the elderly were asked what problems they encountered regarding foods and total diet, 36% of the 170 responded "expenses" (Van Zandt and Fox, 1986). Participation in the group meals program was said to help control food costs and allow the participants to stay within their food budget. Table I shows the relationship of income and dietary intake of calories and iron among white, elderly subjects in three major nutrition surveys. Income appears to have an influence on caloric intake, which is the major contributor to the lower intake of dietary iron to the point that the mean intake of iron by low-income elderly women in all three surveys is below the recommended dietary allowance (RDA) (Food and Nutrition Board, 1980). Although the mean intake of iron for men is above the RDA, approximately 45% of the low-income men in NHANES-II had iron intakes below 5.9 mg/day (Carroll *et al.*, 1983).

Multivariate analysis of the NHANES-I data for the 65- to 74-year age group showed that a low poverty index ratio was significantly related to a low hemoglobin.

Table I. Mean Dietary Intake of White Elderly Subjects According to Income[a]

Survey group[b]	Energy (kcal)	Iron	
		mg daily	mg/1000 kcal
Males			
NHANES II, 1976–1980			
All incomes	1829	14.1	7.9
Low income	1602	11.4	7.3
NHANES I, 1971–1974[c]			
PIR > 1	1850	12.5	6.8
PIR < 1	1706	11.3	6.6
TSNS, 1968–1970			
High income	2181	15.0	6.9
Low income	1937	12.2	6.3
Females			
NHANES II, 1976–1980			
All income	1295	10.2	8.2
Low income	1223	9.6	8.2
NHANES I, 1971–1974[c]			
PIR > 1	1342	9.6	7.1
PIR < 1	1212	8.1	6.7
TSNS, 1968–1970			
High income	1513	10.5	6.9
Low income	1442	9.5	6.6

[a]Adapted from Kohrs *et al.* (1984) and Carroll *et al.* (1983).
[b]NHANES, National Health and Nutrition Examination Survey; TSNS, Ten-State Nutrition Survey; NHANES 65–74 years; TSNS, 59 years upwards.
[c]PIR, Poverty Index Ratio.

Age within this grouping was not a significant factor, but those who had trouble eating were also more likely to have low hemoglobins than those without these difficulties. Data on elderly in Missouri (O'Hanlon *et al.*, 1983; Kohrs *et al.*, 1978) and Massachusetts (McGandy *et al.*, 1986) have also shown significant decreases in nutrient intake with low income status. Data were not analyzed to determine the interaction of age and income.

A recent study of low-income blacks aged 60–94 years in Washington, D.C. revealed that 33% of the women and 48% of the men had hemoglobin values less than 12 and 14 g/dl, respectively (Macarthy *et al.*, 1986). The direct effect of age was not evaluated statistically. Based on serum ferritin concentrations below 20 ng/ml, 21% of the men and 23% of the women had iron deficiency. Statistically significant correlations were obtained between average daily intake of iron and serum ferritin and hemoglobin concentrations. The prevalence of anemia in this population was 23%, higher than that reported for urban blacks in Florida, 14% (Bailey *et al.*, 1979). Almost 80% of the participants in the Washington survey had annual incomes of $4000 or less. Only one subject had an income greater than $9000. Poverty in later life plagues blacks, especially females. Approximately one-third of the black and one-quarter of the Hispanic elderly have incomes below the poverty level (Calasanti and Hendricks, 1986).

2.1.2. *Education/Occupation*

Education is related to nutritional status. Multivariate analysis of data for the 65- to 74-year-old subjects in NHANES-I showed that less education of the subject and the head of the household was associated with a low hemoglobin concentration (Singer *et al.*, 1982). In this context, years of education was the only variable related to low transferrin saturation. In an assessment of the dietary intake of Missourians participating in the Title VII federally funded Nutrition Program for Older Americans, education was related to consumption of calories, iron, thiamin, and niacin as estimated by dietary histories independent of income (O'Hanlon *et al.*, 1983). One-day food records (comparing cross-sectionally those who ate a meal at the program site to those who did not participate) demonstrated that participation in the program erased the difference in total daily dietary intake for calories and protein related to education (Kohrs *et al.*, 1979). In Massachusetts, mean intake of calcium and several nutrients was lower for elderly individuals with less education (McGandy *et al.*, 1986). In the Washington study of low-income, elderly blacks discussed earlier, 71% of those studied had completed only elementary school (Macarthy *et al.*, 1986).

There are no data that independently relate nutritional status to occupation.

2.2. Housing

Table II lists the various types of housing in which the elderly may reside. Although there may be some interchangeability between two adjacent types, the most restrictive are generally at the top of the list, the least at the bottom. A whole host of factors influence the housing that elderly persons maintain, including income, health, marital status, and general family and social structure. In addition, the relationship of housing to nutritional status may be secondary to mobility, available transportation,

Table II. Impact of Types of Housing and Support Services on Nutrient Intake of the Elderly[a]

Institutional
Hospital/nursing facilities
General hospital
Chronic care facility
Skilled nursing facility
Intermediate care facility
Housing
Group home
Foster home
Boarding house
Congregate care home
Retirement village
Community
Rehabilitation hospital
Day care
Congregate meals
Home bound
Visiting nurse
Homemaker
Home health aids
Meals-on-wheels
Independent living
Congregate meals
Senior citizen center

[a]The general trend is from highly restrictive at the top to situations with very little or no restriction at the bottom. There may be some interchangeability between adjacent listings.

accessibility of local grocery stores, and even fear of susceptibility to crime as the neighborhood changes character.

O'Hanlon *et al.* (1983) showed that those elderly who lived alone in federally funded housing had a lower intake of calories, iron, thiamin, and riboflavin than those who lived with others in privately owned housing. Comparing intake of elderly women in three nursing homes and private homes, Harrill *et al.* (1976) also found intake of calories, calcium, and thiamin to be below that recommended. The caloric intake of women in nursing homes varied among the three homes from about 75% to 100% of the RDA. Women in private homes had a caloric intake comparable to the lowest nursing home. Baker *et al.* (1979) found circulating levels of thiamin, vitamin C, and vitamin B_{12} to be lower in noninstitutionalized elderly compared to both institutionalized elderly and a younger population.

In England, Morgan *et al.* (1986) studied 450 elderly women in six groups spanning a wide range of physical dependency from active with good mobility to a group in which the majority were immobile. Mean ages of the groups ranged from 73 years for the active women to 84 years for those institutionalized for chronic physical or mental disability. Anthropometric and biochemical measures of nutritional status were obtained for all six groups, and dietary intake for four groups. Data were compared to a pooled sample of three groups of younger persons; mean ages of the three groups were 40, 36, and 35 years. Mean triceps skinfold measurements of the active elderly were significantly higher than those for both a younger population and all of the other elderly groups. Plasma vitamin C and prealbumin were significantly higher in the active elderly and for those who attended a day center than for groups of patients who were currently hospitalized or who had recently been hospitalized. Relationships were found between energy, protein, and vitamin C intakes and body weight, plasma protein concentrations, and vitamin C concentrations, respectively. All the above data suggest that low nutrient intakes contribute to poor anthropometric and biochemical measures of nutritional status.

2.3. Residency

Akin *et al.* (1986) conducted an extensive analysis of the data from the 1977–1979 Nationwide Food Consumption Survey of individuals 65 to 74 years old. The results showed that, using cluster analysis of the food patterns, individuals could be categorized into light eaters, heavy eaters, or consumers of large amounts of alcoholic beverages, salty snack products, animal fat products, legumes, or sweets and desserts. Residency was a key factor characterizing the various eating patterns. Light eaters, especially older women, appeared to consume inadequate intakes of energy, calcium, magnesium, and vitamin B_6. Being southern significantly increased one's likelihood of being in a light-eater cluster in three of the six age–sex categories. Nonsoutherners or urbanites were more likely to consume large amounts of alcohol. Heavy dessert eaters were more likely to be rural residents in four age–sex cohorts.

2.4. Marital Status/Children

Traditionally, marital status has been thought to influence dietary intake and nutritional status. Schaefer and Keith (1982) found that single elderly women had a better quality of diet than married elderly. With increasing age, however, the quality of the diet of single women was less good. This was not true for married couples. Analysis of NHANES-I data showed that dietary patterns of older men living with a spouse were better than those living alone or with a person other than a spouse (Davis *et al.*, 1985). Diets of older women were not associated with living arrangements as strongly as those of the men. Other studies (Kohrs *et al.*, 1978; O'Hanlon *et al.*, 1983) did not show an effect of marital status on dietary intake as measured by 1-day food records or dietary histories. However, analysis of the anthropometric data for this large study did show that obesity, as measured by relative weight (average weight for height for age and sex divided by weight for height of 18- to 24-year-olds: Roberts, 1966), was correlated to marital status and education (Table III).

When examining living arrangements, researchers frequently lump all single individuals, ignoring or oblivious to the fact that some may choose to live alone while others are forced to live alone. Never-married elderly are not necessarily socially isolated, but many experience some loneliness and do suffer from the effects of loss in late life (Rubinstein, 1987). There may be no difference among the various types of

Table III. The Influence of Age, Education, and Nutritional Status on Relative Weight of Elderly[a]

Category	Mean relative weight (%)[b]
Age (years)	
59–70	115.3
70–75	115.0
>75	108.2
Education (years)	
<9	111.8
9–12	117.8
>12	107.8
Marital status	
Married	114.8
Single	110.2

[a]M. B. Kohrs and J. Nordstrom (unpublished data, 1987).
[b]Average weight for height for age and sex divided by the weight for height of 18- to 24-year-olds (Roberts, 1966).

singles with regard to nutrition; however, this has yet to be determined. Elderly "isolates" generally partake of meals that involve less preparation (Edwards, 1983), but this has not been shown to affect nutritional status.

The presence or absence of children may also make a difference in nutritional status. Reviewing evidence from several studies, Litwak and Longino (1987) suggest that older people lacking strong informal support groups, such as children, tend to die at an earlier age or enter institutions at earlier stages of health decline. Analyzing migration trends of older persons, they classify postretirement moves into three categories, the second of which is to be near a primary caretaker. The average age at this move is obviously older than that at the first move, which is in the immediate postretirement period.

2.5. Erroneous Beliefs and Food Faddism

Several studies suggest that a large proportion of the elderly consume vitamin and mineral supplements to the extent that in one study the cost of the supplements was reported to be as much as 20% of a monthly income of $300 (Read and Graney, 1982). Both of the surveys in Missouri demonstrated that close to one-third of the subjects consumed one or more vitamin and mineral supplements (Kohrs *et al.*, 1978, 1980). In the evaluation of the Title VII Nutrition Program for Older Americans, significantly more of those who were nonparticipants at the time of the first survey consumed vitamin and mineral supplements and yet had poorer nutritional status than those who were regular participants (Kohrs *et al.*, 1980). The average age and mobility were similiar in both groups. Of approximately 600 elderly surveyed in seven Western states, 60% used supplements (Sheehan *et al.*, 1987). More users of supplements had

Table IV. Mean Days Indoors and in Bed because of Illness Related to Frequency of Vitamin C Use[a]

	Respondents' use of vitamin C pills		
Category	Never	Occasionally	Daily
Number of subjects	1526	874	634
Mean days indoors[b]	7.9	9.4	12.8
Mean days in bed[b]	3.9	5.2	6.9

[a]From Shapiro *et al.* (1983).
[b]$P < 0.001$ (Kruskal-Wallis test) for each category.

some college education and higher income than nonusers and tended to use health food stores, books, and chiropractors as sources of information. More users believed that the quality of food has declined in the last 10 years. In an earlier study (Yung *et al.*, 1984), education and average income were also associated with greater use of health foods. The more committed users bought more sugar-free and salt-free items in health food stores, but the item cited most frequently was vitamins.

Use of supplements may arise from a perceived need rather than a real need. Some people who do not feel well for whatever reason may believe that vitamins will help and can't hurt. Shapiro *et al.* (1983) found that the patterns of vitamin C intake were related to physical health status. More of those in poor physical health, as measured by days indoors and days in bed, had higher intakes of vitamin C supplements than those who were healthier (Table IV). However, intake of vitamin C was influenced by many factors other than state of health. Respondents who did not eat breakfast or who smoked cigarettes had lower vitamin C intakes.

The elderly have several misconceptions regarding nutrition. For example, health food products were thought to give "more pep and energy," make one healthier, and prevent and treat arthritis (Grotkowski and Sims, 1978). Half the respondents in another study (Rountree and Tinklin, 1975) said that gelatin was one of the best sources of protein, and 88% believed that natural vitamins were better than synthetic vitamins. On the other hand, 80% knew meat was a good source of protein. Seventy-five percent could identify good sources of ascorbic acid, but only 25% knew its function.

2.6. Season

Since the elderly have mobility problems as well as problems in finding transportation, a reasonable assumption is that those who live in the North, particularly in rural areas, may have a problem in winter consuming adequate amounts of fruits and vegetables and potentially other perishable items that must be purchased frequently. Dibble *et al.* (1967) looked at the effects of season on nutritional status using biochemical measurements. The primary findings were that plasma carotene and urinary excretion of riboflavin were higher during fall than spring, suggesting a greater consumption of fruits and vegetables with carotene and of foods containing riboflavin such as milk products during the summer. The findings of Kim and Caldwell (1986) are consistent with these findings—more persons had inadequate dietary intakes during the winter of energy, vitamin A, and calcium. However, they did not report biochemical measurements, the most objective indicators of nutritional status.

Surprisingly, even when mobility is not a problem, as in institutionalized patients, some seasonal effects have been identified in England (Davies *et al.*, 1986). In one type of nursing home, serum 25-hydroxyvitamin D_3 increased between spring and autumn. In two other types of facilities there was no change. The intake of vitamin D was suboptimal at all three types of institutions. The incidence of deficiency, defined as <12.5 nmole of serum 25-hydroxyvitamin D_3, varied with season and type of institution (from 11.7% in one in the autumn to 47% in another in the spring). Analyzing samples obtained on admission to a hospital, Bouillon *et al.* (1987) found seasonal variations in total and free 1,25-dihydroxycholecalciferol concentrations. There were no seasonal variations in serum calcium or phosphorus; however, values were significantly lower for the elderly subjects (mean age 78 years) than for a younger group (mean age 39 years). The effect of permanent mild deficiency on bone homeostasis was not addressed in this study.

3. Psychological Factors

Depending on viewpoint, ethnicity and culture can be included in either the social or psychological section. There is a lack of conceptual clarity regarding ethnicity. It has been variously conceptualized as culture, inequality, and traditional ways of thinking and behaving (Rosenthal, 1986). Nonetheless, cultural and ethnic backgrounds, independent of SES, certainly have an influence on nutritional status.

3.1. Ethnic/Cultural Factors

Comparison of the percentages of blacks and whites with low values for hemoglobin and dietary intake of iron during the NHANES-I survey in Tables V and VI shows that a much larger proportion of black subjects have lower hemoglobin values. Twice as many of the males had low serum iron values. Among the low-income black males in the Ten-State Nutrition Survey, 54.6% had low intakes of iron compared to 45% of the white men. Table VII shows the percentage of black and white subjects participating in the NHANES-II survey with low hematological parameters. The results are similar with a similar magnitude of difference for the proportions of blacks and whites with low hemoglobins. One and one-half times as many black females had low values for transferrin saturation, which is a more specific indicator of iron deficiency anemia. Twice as many black females also had low values for mean corpuscular volume, another indicator of iron deficiency anemia.

Although the NHANES-I and -II do include elderly who are black, there are very little data on the nutritional status of this population in urban areas, particularly low-income areas. One study, conducted in Florida (Bailey *et al.*, 1979), showed that as many as 54% of this group had low red blood cell folate levels, currently the best indicator available to evaluate folate status. A large proportion of the same group also had low dietary zinc intakes and serum zinc concentrations (Wagner *et al.*, 1980).

Table V. Hematological Parameters and Dietary Iron Intake for Elderly White Subjects over 59 Years in Four Surveys[a]

	Number	Mean Hb (g/dl)	Mean iron intake (mg/day)	Percentage of low values		
				Hb[b]	Serum iron[c]	Dietary iron[d]
Missouri, 1975						
Males	97	15.1	12.7	18	8	26
Females	223	14.0	11.1	9	4	55
NHANES I, 1971–1974						
Males	1293	15.4	11.3	15	6	52
Females	1426	14.1	8.1	5	5	74
Missouri, 1973						
Males	53	14.6	15.0	21	33	—
Females	66	13.7	10.5	11	15	—
TSNS, 1968–1970						
Males	281	14.5	12.2	23	29	45
Females	347	13.3	9.5	10	15	70

[a]From Kohrs *et al.* (1984).
[b]Males, <14.0 g/dl; females, <12.0 g/dl.
[c]Males, <60 μg/dl; females, <40 μg/dl.
[d]Males and females, <10 mg/day.

Macarthy *et al.* (1986) found that 41% of their low-income elderly subjects living in Washington, D.C. consumed less than the recommended dietary allowance for iron. More subjects had low hemoglobin concentrations than were deficient in iron (defined as low serum iron), suggesting that there were other underlying deficiencies contributing to the low hemoglobin.

Even more limited is the availability of information on other minorities: Hispanic,

Table VI. Percentage of Elderly Black Subjects over 59 Years with Low Hematological Values or Intakes of Dietary Iron[a]

Survey groups	Dietary iron[b]	Hb[c]	Serum iron[d]
NHANES I, 1971–1974			
Males	56.2	41	11
Females	77.3	20	5
TSNS, 1968–1970			
High income			
Males	53.3	8	—
Females	76.0	24	—
Low income			
Males	54.6	65	—
Females	75.6	26	—

[a]From Kohrs, *et al.* (1984).
[b]Males, <14.0 g/dl; females, <12.0 g/dl.
[c]Males and females, <10 mg/day.
[d]Males, <60 μg/dl; females, <40 μg/dl.

Table VII. Percentage of Subjects 65–74 Years Old with Abnormal Hematological Values According to Sex and Race in NHANES II (1976–1980)[a]

	Percentage of low values					
Survey groups	Hct[b]	Hb[c]	MCV[d]	MCH[e]	Serum iron[f]	Transferrin saturation[g]
White males	62.3	20.7	11.1	28.7	8.3	5.7
White females	16.5	4.0	2.3	36.3	1.5	8.3
Black males	52.4	53.4	11.4	55.7	15.6	9.2
Black females	32.0	21.7	5.0	64.4	0.6	11.0

[a]From Kohrs and Czajka-Narins (1986) based on data from Fulwood *et al.* (1982).
[b]Males, 42%; females, 38%.
[c]Males, less than 14 g/dl; females, less than 12 g/dl.
[d]Mean corpuscular volume; both sexes, less than 80 μm^3.
[e]Mean corpuscular hemoglobin; both sexes, less than 30 pg.
[f]Males, less than 60 μg/dl; females, less than 40 μg/dl.
[g]Males, less than 20%; females, less than 15%.

Oriental, and Native American. The lack of information on Hispanics has led to the special Hispanic Health and Nutrition Survey, from which information should be available shortly. Kim *et al.* (1984) reported that a large proportion of the Korean elderly consumed inadequate amounts of calcium. The Ten-State Nutrition Survey, 1968–1970, did include Hispanic and black elderly. Table VIII shows the percentages of low values for hemoglobin, serum iron, and vitamins A and C in those groups compared to whites (Shank, 1974). Nevertheless, evaluation of dietary intakes of Hispanic and Caucasian elderly in Houston did not confirm an inadequate intake of vitamins A and C based on two consecutive 24-hr recalls (Hart and Little, 1986). However, neither the demographic data on the subjects nor the characteristics of the

Table VIII. Percentage of Low-Income Elderly White, Black, and Spanish-American Subjects over 59 Years with Abnormal Values for Serum Albumin and Vitamins A and C in the Ten-State Nutrition Survey[a]

	Percentage of low values		
	Serum albumin[b]	Serum vitamin A[c]	Serum vitamin C[d]
White males	6.2	0.0	12.8
White females	11.1	0.0	1.8
Black males	21.4	0.0	8.6
Black females	14.6	0.0	10.0
Spanish-American males	17.9	13.0	13.6
Spanish-American females	17.6	0.0	0.0

[a]From Shank (1974).
[b]Serum albumin <3.5 g/dl.
[c]Serum vitamin A <20 g/dl.
[d]Serum vitamin C <0.2 mg/dl.

Table IX. Intake of Vitamin A, Vitamin/Mineral Supplements, and Food Categorized as High Sugar or Empty Caloric by Persons over 75 Years Old Either Not Participating (0) in the Nutrition Program for Older Americans in Missouri or Participating Once a Week (1) or More Frequently (2–5 times)[a]

Intake	Participation in program[b]		
	0	1	2–5
Daily vitamin A intake			
IU	9,560[c] ± 929	9,240[c] ± 694	11,934[c] ± 749
Percentage RDA	215[c] ± 8	187[d] ± 6	265[c] ± 6
Servings/day	0.58[c] ± 0.08	0.41[d] ± 0.06	0.73[c] ± 0.06
Nonfood supplement[b]	0.000[c] ± 0.002	0.000[c] ± 0.002	0.010[d] ± 0.003
High-sugar foods[b]	5.20[c] ± 0.40	3.83[d] ± 0.30	3.80[d] ± 0.33
Empty-calorie foods[b]	4.42[c] ± 0.37	2.65[d] ± 0.27	2.80[d] ± 0.30

[a]From Czajka-Narins *et al.* (1987). Data are means ± S.E.M.
[b]Number of times consumed per week.
[c,d]Different letters in a row indicate statistically significant differences ($P < 0.05$).

neighborhoods where the congregate meal sites were located were reported. Betts and Crase (1986) compared the dietary intake based on 3 day food records from 20 urban American Indians to that of elderly white persons from the same geographic area and of the same age range, although mean ages were not given for either group. Although many in both groups had insufficient energy and inadequate intakes of vitamin A and calcium, the elderly Indians consumed a higher total intake of energy, protein, fat, and niacin than the white elderly. Unfortunately, anthropometric data were not given.

The Nutrition Program for Older Americans, now Title IIIc of the Older Americans Act, was funded to meet the social needs of the elderly person because it was recognized that persons socially isolated and/or living alone were less likely to have incentive and/or were unable to prepare food for themselves. Thus, the meals were provided in a congregrate setting and were mandated to provide other supportive services such as assistance with shopping and transportation, nutrition education, health and welfare counseling, and consumer education. Kohrs *et al.* (1978, 1979, 1980) demonstrated that participation in the program resulted in an improvement in nutritional status through improved dietary intake, which was reflected in biochemical assessment for this group. The program not only helped all persons over 59 years old but also was beneficial to those over 75 years old, a group often neglected in studies of the nutritional status of the elderly. Table IX shows the association of participation in the program with estimated mean intake of vitamin A, percentage RDA, and food groups from persons over 75 in this study (Czajka-Narins *et al.*, 1987).

3.2. Cognitive Functioning

In an attempt to see if there was an association between cognitive function and nutritional status, Goodwin *et al.* (1983) evaluated the nutritional status of 304 individuals by determining dietary intake and concentrations of nutrients in the blood and comparing the scores on the Wechsler Memory Test and on the Halstead–Reitan

Categories Tests (a measure of abstract thinking and problem-solving ability—a sensitive indicator of minimal changes in mental status) of those with highest and lowest dietary and blood nutrient values. Verbal memory was correlated with blood levels of vitamin C and riboflavin. Persons with lower blood concentrations of vitamin C, riboflavin, folate, and vitamin B_{12} did significantly worse on the Halstead–Reitan Categories Test. The authors were unable to conclude from their data whether poor performance on cognitive function tests was caused by the suboptimal nutritional status or vice versa. However, poor cognition may still contribute to poor nutritional status.

Although the subjects in the above study were assessed to have poor cognitive function, one confounding variable in dementia is an apparent loss in cognitive function in the elderly as a result of depression. Certainly, one of the major criteria of depression is excessive weight loss or gain. Thus, depression is recognized as leading to apathy, anorexia, and weight loss, potentially culminating in poor nutritional status. Malnutrition is also known to lead to anorexia, depression, and apathy. Thus, a vicious cycle is set up in an elderly person starting out with depression caused by some losses associated with aging, such as loss of physical health, friends, and spouse as well as changes in occupational status.

3.3. Sense of Control and Health-Related Behaviors

Changes in options for control over circumstances and/or environment may profoundly affect emotional and physical health by a number of possible mechanisms, such as stress resistance, physiological responses, and behavior relevant to health. In older individuals this relationship between health and a sense of control may grow stronger. Rodin (1986) reviewed the evidence for this relationship, which may be important to ultimate nutritional status. When control of their activity is restricted, there are detrimental effects on the health of many older people. The preferred amount of control is highly variable, and for some too much control may cause increased stress and worry. People high in perceived control may be healthier because they are more likely to take actions that enhance health. These actions include obtaining health information from various sources, interacting actively with health care providers, and adhering better to health regimens. A reduced sense of control and poor health are associated with low social status.

Despite a number of limitations inherent in studies based on telephone interviews, Bausell (1986) obtained some interesting data regarding health behaviors (Table X). Compared to a younger population 18–64 years of age, those 65 and older were more likely to avoid salt, fat, and sugar and to consume foods rich in fiber and calcium. However, the older group was less likely to exercise regularly and perceived themselves as having less control over their future health. These data are encouraging, but there is still room for substantial improvement of behaviors.

3.4. Hypochondriasis and Perceived Intolerance

Hypochondriacal reactions, i.e., anxious preoccupations with bodily functions, increase significantly with age (Busse, 1976). These are more likely to occur in women between 60 and 70 years of age. Busse (1976) suggested that this increased concern with bodily function results from interactions among the recognition of changes that

Table X. Percentage of Elderly versus Nonelderly Complying with Health-Improving Behaviors[a]

Behavior[b]	65 and over (%)	Under 65 (%)
Have dental checkups	54	77
Avoid salt	65	50
Avoid fat	74	52
Consume fiber	69	58
Avoid cholesterol	58	40
Avoid sugar	60	50
Consume calcium	58	49
Maintain recommended weight	25	23
Exercise regularly	23	36

[a]Adapted from Bausell (1986).
[b]All comparisons are statistically significant ($P < 0.001$) except weight maintained.

accompany age, an increase in social stress and personal losses, and a decline in social opportunities.

Digestive problems resulting from food ingestion have been reported since the days of Hippocrates. Food intolerance, real or imagined, is a discomfort of the gastrointestinal tract resulting from the ingestion of food or a dietary component. Regardless of whether the intolerance is real or perceived, the end result is a decreased intake of a particular food. In a study of acceptance of foods by elderly women living either in private homes or in nursing homes, Harrill *et al.* (1976) found that 13 (22%) of the subjects avoided certain foods because of effects on the digestive system. In an investigation of symptoms of milk intolerance in 87 healthy elderly persons, Rovick and Scrimshaw (1979) found that some intolerances may be psychosomatic in nature. Zimmerman and Krondl (1986) examined perceived intolerances of 66 elderly participants of the Meals on Wheels program to 17 cooked and 14 raw vegetables. Forty percent of the subjects reported that they suffered from one or more food intolerances; 18% had vegetable intolerances. Digestive problems were the second most common food-related problem for 170 participants in a congregrate meal program (Van Zandt and Fox, 1986). Almost one-quarter (24%) indicated that they had digestive problems. Unfortunately, none of these studies examined the actual effect of intolerance on nutritional status, nor did they relate the frequency of intolerance to age.

3.5. Food Preferences

Food preference is a very complex matter that includes not only smell and taste but also temperature, consistency, texture, and appearance (Holt *et al.*, 1987). Krondl *et al.* (1982) reported that in addition to flavor perception, health belief was a strong motive for food selection. For 13 of the 14 marker foods, for example, 2% fat milk, whole-wheat bread, frozen fish fillets, beef liver, winter squash, margarine, and tea, there was a significant association between health belief and use. Price, convenience, and prestige were far less important. Perceived ease of chewing was related to the acceptability of foods among elderly persons with the most severe dentition losses in the Veteran's Administration Longitudinal Study of Oral Health (Wayler *et al.*, 1982, 1984). Familiarity and habit may also play roles in preferences for certain foods.

4. Physiological Factors

Physiologically, aging has been characterized as a decrease in function. Although this may be generally true, the rate at which functions change, as we are learning more and more, is variable.

4.1. Health

Noninstitutionalized elderly can be roughly classified as "well" or "frail," each category encompassing a broad range of wellness or frailty. "Frail" elderly are difficult to access, so research data on this subset are extremely limited. Defining "frail" is another problem; usually no definition is given. In one study, "frail" elderly attending an adult day-care center ranged in weight from 97 to 215 pounds and in age from 60 to 90 years (Ludman and Newman, 1986). Only 27.8% of the total population (75) reported their health as good or excellent; 39.5% rated their health as fair, and 32.9% as poor. Data were not analyzed relative to age. Elderly persons who ate a variety of foods had a better health rating (Krondl, 1979). Preliminary data from the National Health Interview Survey (Kovar, 1986) revealed that only one-third of the noninstitutionalized elderly surveyed perceived their health status as fair or poor, one-third as good, and the final third as very good or excellent. With increasing age the percentage who perceive their health as fair or poor increased from 32% in those 65–74 years of age to 38.4% of those 85 and over. The sample size of elderly in the survey was almost 6000, thus providing good estimates of the U.S. elderly population, estimated to be over 26 million.

4.2. Motor Performance and Mobility

Data from many studies support the "aging curve" for many physical functions including reaction time, balance, flexibility, and grip strength. Performance was generally perceived to improve with age to mid-20s, level off for a period, and decline at a gradual or marked rate. Individuals who maintain an active life style may not experience these typical declines. Physically active elderly perform more like younger individuals than like their inactive age peers (Rikli and Busch, 1986). Motor performance tends to be more highly related to lifelong physical activity level than to age, reinforcing the adage "'Tis better to wear out than rust out." Having better movement and reaction times and keeping active may enable some elderly to be more mobile as well as to feel better. Exton-Smith (1980) concluded from several studies that disability has a greater influence on nutrient intake than age alone.

Ability to perform home management activities changes with age. The percentage of individuals who have difficulty preparing meals increases from 3.5% for those aged 65–69 years to 26.1% for those 85 years and older (Dawson *et al.*, 1987). For shopping the percentages are 1.9 and 37, respectively. The proportion of individuals who have four to six home activities that are difficult also increases dramatically among the oldest of the elderly, those 85 years and upwards.

4.3. Senses

4.3.1. Taste and Smell

Krondl *et al.* (1982) demonstrated that taste (flavor) perception was the strongest motive in determining food use by the elderly. Other studies have shown that the modality of flavor is influenced by odor, cognitive function (the ability to learn and improve a score), and taste sensation. Among elderly subjects, odor and cognitive characteristics are important determinants of recognition of taste (Murphy, 1985).

The importance of odors on intake has long been recognized. In one study, only 32% of 256 "normal" elderly subjects (mean age 70.8 years) were found to have olfactory ability comparable to that of young adults (Newman *et al.*, 1960). In a further 25%, olfaction was slightly diminished, and for the remaining, olfaction was greatly diminished. Schiffman and Covey (1984) found that elderly subjects required as a detection threshold concentrations of food flavors such as cherry and lemon that were at least 11 times as great as those for younger subjects. Decreased sensitivity to food odors results in less appreciation of foods. All her subjects were nonsmokers; mean age was 81.4 years.

Bartoshuk *et al.* (1986) found that both elderly (mean age 82.8 years) and young (mean age 24.4 years) rated moderate and strong tastes similarly, although the perception of intensity of some of the most concentrated standards was slightly less in the elderly. The elderly had a higher taste threshold for mild stimuli, suggesting to the investigators the presence of mild dysgeusia. Weiffenbach *et al.* (1986) found significant age-related changes in the basic taste qualities using ANOVA and regression analysis on data from a population that ranged in age from 23 to 88 years.

Although the declines in the sensitivity of older persons to sweet and salty tastes have been assumed, very little has been done to document the effect of change in taste with age on actual food consumption. Mattes-Kulig and Henkin (1985) did document lower energy consumption and intakes of persons with dysgeusia due to influenza. However, they were unable to show any effect of hypogeusia on nutrient intake. The severity of the dysgeusia was also related to anthropometric indicators of malnutrition. Table XI shows the major taste studies of the elderly and also includes comments on interrelating factors (Booth *et al.*, 1982; Kohrs, 1985).

There are several problems with interpretation of studies of taste. According to Mattes (1986), there are three principal measures of taste—threshold sensitivity, suprathreshold sensitivity (the ability to discriminate between two concentrations of a tastant in above-threshold concentrations), and preferences (appeal of tastes or foods). Threshold sensitivity includes detection thresholds and recognition thresholds. Measures of taste preference may relate to dietary practices better than sensitivity responses (Mattes and Mela, 1986). To taste, one must have receptors that are accessible, "healthy" receptors, and adequate neural transport and processing of the signal. To keep the oral mucosa healthy requires adequate amounts of niacin, riboflavin, thiamin, pyridoxine, pantothenic acid, folic acid, vitamin B_{12}, vitamin A, vitamin C, iron, zinc, and intrinsic factor for B_{12} absorption. Modest deficits of several of these nutrients

Table XI. Summary of Studies on Changes in Sensitivity to the Basic Tastes with Advancing Age[a]

Investigators	Number of subjects	Basic tastes[b] Salt	Sweet	Bitter	Sour	Comment
Richter and Campbell (1940)	174	*	D	*	*	Thresholds three times higher than young subjects
Hinchcliffe (1958)	200	D	D	*	*	No sex differences
Cooper *et al.* (1959)	100	D	D	D	D	Sharpest decline after age 50; sour decline after age 60 No sex or smoking differences
Balogh and Lelkes (1961)	150	D	D	I	N	Marked increase in bitter for smokers
Kalmus and Trotter (1962)	110	*	*	D	*	Tested phenylthiocarbamide sensitivity in same subjects after 10–15 years
Glanville *et al.* (1964)	676	*	*	D	D	Greatest decline in males
Kaplan *et al.* (1965)	395	*	*	D	*	All smokers; found no age or sex differences in nonsmokers
Hermel *et al.* (1970)	118	N	D	D	D	No statistical analysis
Grzegorczyk *et al.* (1979)	76	D	*	*	*	Elevated salivary sodium concentration
Weiffenbach *et al.* (1982)	81	D	N	D	N	Sex effect for sour
Moore *et al.* (1982)	71	D	*	*	*	Highly variable thresholds for elderly
Bales *et al.* (1986)	62	D	D	*	*	Taste acuity not related to hair or dietary zinc

[a]Adapted from Booth *et al.* (1982).
[b]D, decrease; I, increase; N, no difference; *, not tested.

may alter taste. Finally, in assessing preferences of young compared to older individuals, there are differences in lifetime availability of foods and traditional cooking methods that need to be addressed.

4.3.2. *Vision and Hearing*

Frequency of hearing impairments increases from 23% in those 65–74 years of age to 48% in those 85 years and older (Havlik, 1986). For vision impairments these values are 9.5% and 26.8%, respectively. Hearing impairment by itself was a less important factor in the ability of the individual to get out than when combined with a vision impairment (Havlik, 1986). Cataracts are a frequent cause of disability in older persons, increasing in prevalence with age (Kahn *et al.*, 1977). Cataracts are responsible for more than one-third of severe visual impairments and more than one-quarter of milder ones. To examine the impact of cataract surgery on measures of patient function, 246 elderly patients (mean age 72 years at time of surgery) were reexamined 4 months and 1 year after surgery (Applegate *et al.*, 1987). Patients' self-rating of their activities, such as driving a car, improved. Improvement in objective changes of function, such as mental function, were more remarkable. The patients who had the greatest improvements in the various study categories were those who had the greatest improvement in visual impairment. Those patients in whom the activities-of-daily-living scale declined had no improvement in percentage of visual impairment. Unfortunately, no measures of nutritional status were included in this study.

4.4. Dental Status

Dental status has been assumed to affect nutrient intake, but there is relatively little information in this area. Geissler and Bates (1984) critically evaluated the literature published through mid-1983. Loss of a single molar can lead to a 25–33% decrease in efficiency of mastication (Yurkstas, 1954). Intake of residents of a veterans' home was evaluated before and after they were fitted with dentures (Anderson, 1971). Frequency of eating protein foods, vitamin-C-rich foods, or cooked dark green and yellow vegetables was unchanged. The number of servings of crisp raw vegetables consumed was increased, and servings of bread and cereals decreased, after the men were fitted with dentures. Osterberg and Steen (1982) correlated three different classifications for dental status with low dietary intakes of nutrients as measured by the classical method of Burke (1947). A significantly large number of persons among those with poor dental status consumed inadequate amounts of nutrients—25% and 40% of the men and women in class C compared to 0 and 20%, respectively, in those with good dental status. McGandy *et al.* (1986) found that among elderly males, wearing dentures was associated with lower dietary quality. Mean bone density and serum ascorbic acid were lower in elderly denture wearers compared to those having their own teeth (Lee *et al.*, 1981). Those having their own teeth may have been younger; mean ages were not given.

In another study, women with dentures had higher hemoglobin concentrations than women with no natural teeth and no dentures (Bates *et al.*, 1971). The women with dentures were slightly younger than those of the other groups, complicating interpretation. Serum folic acid and B_{12} values were similar for all groups. Many elderly with either poor natural teeth or ill-fitting dentures learn to compensate for problems of chewing. Others learn to avoid pain by removing ill-fitting dentures while eating. Inadequate chewing may result in gastric irritation (Geissler and Bates, 1984).

4.5. Chronic Disease

The drugs used to treat disease as well as the disease process itself may affect the nutritional status of elderly persons directly, usually by reducing the dietary intake of nutrients, and indirectly through the disease processes, which may affect absorption

Table XII. Percentage of Elderly Persons Treated for Disease Who Have Significant Associations of Disease with Unacceptable Blood Values among Subjects over 59 Years with Selected Diseases and Controls without These Diseases[a]

	Percentage with unacceptable values							
	Hematocrit		Hemoglobin		Serum iron		Serum vitamin A	
Disease	With	Without	With	Without	With	Without	With	Without
Anemia	23.5[c]	9.9	23.5[c]	8.5	6.0	5.3	16.7	13.2
Hay fever			20.6[b]	9.6	15.2[c]	4.4		
Allergy							24.5[c]	11.4
Hernia					15.5[b]	5.4		
Liver							50.0[c]	12.9
Hypertension							18.8[b]	10.3
Stroke					29.3[c]	8.7		

[a]M. B. Kohrs and J. Norstrom (unpublished data).
[b]$P < 0.005$ for comparison between those with and without disease.
[c]$P < 0.001$ for comparison between those with and without disease.

and/or utilization (see Chapter 13). Anemia, for example, can be caused by inadequate dietary intake of a variety of nutrients including iron, folic acid, and vitamin B_{12} (Kohrs *et al.*, 1984). However, blood loss and disease can also lead to anemia. The anemias of chronic infection, kidney disease, and thyroid disease have long been recognized by the medical community. Often, nutrient intakes are insufficient for a combination of reasons, as happens in persons with chronic renal failure who are being treated by dialysis. Their appetite is depressed, they have taste changes, and they require special diets that are not palatable. The combined effect is a low dietary intake, compounding the effects of the disease on the anemia (Norris *et al.*, 1985). Nordstrom *et al.* (1982) found that 16% of the elderly women and 3% of the elderly men in their survey in Missouri consumed less than 67% of the RDA for dietary iron. According to Dallman *et al.* (1984), only 4% of those aged 65–74 in the NHANES-II survey had anemia, half (2%) resulting from iron deficiency. Thus, it is likely that the anemia found in elderly persons is a result of multiple etiologies, including nutritional deficits.

Table XII shows the association between a reported history of medical problems and low values for biochemical measures of nutritional status of persons participating in the 1975 Missouri Nutrition Survey of the federally funded Nutrition Program for Older Americans (M. B. Kohrs and J. Nordstrom, 1987, unpublished data). As shown in Table XII, there was a significantly larger percentage of persons with low serum iron among those who were treated for anemia, hay fever, hernia, and stroke than among those not treated for these diseases. A larger percentage of persons treated for allergies, liver disease, and high blood pressure had low serum vitamin A compared to those who were not. An example of the impact of chronic disease on adequacy of protein and energy intakes is described in Chapter 8.

4.5.1. *Metabolic Diseases*

Andres studied changes in body composition with aging and reported that moderate overweight is not associated with a higher mortality in the elderly (Andres, 1980).

Kohrs and Tobben (1982) found similar results for the elderly subjects participating in the evaluation of the Nutrition Program for Older Adults in Missouri in 1975. Although obesity as measured by body mass index was significantly associated ($P < 0.0001$) with heart disease (identified as a positive response to a question regarding intake of prescription drugs) among men 59 to 69 years old, this association did not hold up among those over 69 years old. As expected, gallbladder disease was associated significantly with body mass index among subjects of the younger age category (59–69 years old), but a significant association was also found for gallbladder and obesity among the older subjects. Surprising findings in this study were the lack of any relationships between obesity and diabetes for any of the elderly age groups and between obesity and heart disease among subjects older than 69 years. The absence of association between diabetes and obesity was puzzling in light of the strong evidence that shows such an association between obesity and other diseases among middle-aged individuals. Several factors were considered to influence the finding for diabetes. First, there may have been different standards among physicians diagnosing diabetes among the elderly. Second, weight control is important as a part of the treatment of non-insulin-dependent diabetes. Third, a report from the Framingham study also showed that obesity ceased to be related to heart disease among persons over 75 (Castelli *et al.*, 1981). Finally, a significant factor for those over 75 years may be that individuals who were obese and at risk had already died, leaving those who were better adapted to overweight.

The underlying metabolic changes in other diseases can affect nutrient utilization. Thus, uremia can also alter glucose and lipid metabolism (Barch *et al.*, 1987). The carbohydrate intolerance of this syndrome results from tissue resistance to insulin and decreased cellular uptake and utilization of energy-yielding metabolites. Individuals with uremia may also develop hypertriglyceridemia.

4.5.2. *Diseases That Affect Function*

Neuromuscular diseases such as cerebrovascular accidents, myasthenia gravis, and multiple sclerosis may lead to inadequate mastication and difficulty in swallowing and thus make the actual process of eating more difficult. Weak and unsteady hands can make it difficult for elderly persons to cut food or prepare it for eating. Many elderly may get tired and give up before they consume enough calories and nutrients. Severe arthritis can reduce the mobility of the elderly, making it more difficult for them to shop. Arthritis can also make it impossible for some elderly to open cans and containers as well as to cut food.

4.5.3. *Interrelated Deficiencies*

The preceding discussion emphasizes the multifactorial nature of the relationship between nutrient deficiency and other factors affecting the elderly. Thus, anemia is a symptom for which there may be one cause or for which several causes may coexist. Iron deficiency was found to coexist with pernicious anemia in 25 (20.7%) of 121 patients for whom data obtained at the time of diagnosis could be evaluated (Carmel *et al.*, 1987). Iron deficiency developed over the next 14 months in another 27 patients (22.3%) in this study. For 17 of the patients, a cause was found for the iron deficiency, but for the majority the cause was not identified.

4.6. Drugs

Therapeutic drugs are extensively used by the elderly. The rate of metabolism of drugs may be different in the elderly and directly or indirectly reduce food intake. For example, the plasma half-life of diazepam (Valium®) increases substantially from 55 hr in persons 50 years of age to as long as 90 hr in those 80 years of age (Klotz *et al.*, 1975). Antacids containing aluminum hydroxide combine with phosphates in the intestine, which results in phosphorus depletion and mobilization of the mineral from bone. Abuse of these antacids can therefore result in metabolic bone disease. Abuse of mineral oil as a laxative can decrease absorption of the fat-soluble vitamins and calcium. With the heavy use of medications by the elderly, drug–nutrient interactions are an important issue. For a comprehensive discussion of the effects of drugs on nutritional status and nutrient utilization, see Chapter 14 in this volume.

5. Aging in Relation to Nutritional Status

Average caloric intake decreases about 600 kcal/day from age 30 to age 80 in one cross-sectional study of men of high socioeconomic status (McGandy *et al.*, 1966). In a group of elderly women living alone, the decline in overall energy intake accelerated from age 70 to age 80 by 19% (Exton-Smith, 1980). However in a study of healthy, free-living elderly aged 60 to 90 years, energy and protein intakes on a body-weight basis were not associated with age (McGandy *et al.*, 1986; Munro *et al.*, 1987). An important determinant in this reported decline may be the concurrent increase in immobilizing diseases and disabilities during this decade and consequent reduced physical activity. Exton-Smith (1980) found that elderly women who maintained their health status had similar intakes approximately 7 years after the original study.

According to preliminary data from the 1984 National Health Interview Survey (Kovar, 1986), the percentage of the population having no limitation of activity decreases with age from 62% for those 65–74 years old to 40% among those aged 85 years. At the same time, the percentage of the total population who spent 28–365 days in bed increased from 9.9% in the younger group to 13.9% in the older group. Those who were confined to bed increased from 1.6% in the 75- to 84-year-olds to 3.4% in the group who were 85 years and older. These data should be evaluated in light of the estimate that approximately 25% of people over age 85 years are in nursing homes and that the health of people in nursing homes is generally poor. The percentage of those "unable to perform usual activity" rose from 8.6% in the 75- to 84-year-olds to 22.0% in those 85 years and older. Most of the studies of the elderly do not separate out data on those 85 years of age and older or analyze trends in relation to age. It should, however, be noted that in industrial societies, reduced energy intake begins in middle age, and the low levels of old age are part of this continuum (McGandy *et al.*, 1966).

Longitudinal data on the elderly are rare. The 10-year follow-up of subjects surveyed in NHANES-I, 1971–1975, has taken place, and an initial report has been published (Madans *et al.*, 1986). The data obtained in the follow-up should provide significant information. Lee (1987) presented 4-year follow-up data on 26 elderly females. Statistically significant decreases occurred in both hemoglobin and hematocrit without any change in estimated intake of iron. Mean serum cholesterol also remained unchanged. Tsui *et al.* (1987) compared the dietary intake of 131 subjects in 1985 to intake data on the same subjects obtained ten years earlier. The general trends were decreased fat and protein intake and increased carbohydrate intake. One of the earliest longitudinal studies to assess nutritional status of the elderly in San Mateo, California was summarized by Exton-Smith (1980). In that study, total intake decreased with no significant difference in the proportion of calories from carbohydrate, protein, and fat. Individuals who initially had a low intake of protein tended to keep the same pattern.

Immune response appears to decline with age, but how much of this decline is related to the aging processes or results from mild deficiency of one or more nutrients is debatable (see Chapter 4). Supplementing institutionalized, healthy, elderly women (mean age 78 years) with 400 mg of ascorbic acid daily resulted in increased concentrations of IgG and complement component C3 after 4 and 12 months of supplementation and of IgM after 12 months (Ziemlanski *et al.*, 1986). A positive correlation was also found between serum ascorbic acid concentration and serum concentrations of IgG and C3. This study is difficult to interpret for several reasons. Data on serum ascorbic acid concentrations are not given, nor has a role for ascorbic acid in immunity been defined. In this context, Schlenker *et al.* (1973) noted a positive relationship between length of life of the women in their study and intake of ascorbic-acid-rich diets.

6. *Effects of Long-Term Nutrition on Aging*

Although animal studies testify to the effects of long-term dietary restriction on prolonging survival of animals (see Chapter 2), long-term relationships are difficult to establish, but some work has begun. We frequently state that the health and nutritional status of the elderly is a sum of all their previous life experiences, but there are little data on the relationships of health in middle age, health as a young adult, health as an adolescent, and health as an infant to the incidence of disease in the elderly. The relationship of infant health to subsequent death from ischemic heart disease was explored indirectly by Barker and Osmond (1986) by examining the correlation between the frequency of neonatal and infant mortality in various groups in England and Wales and the subsequent death rate from heart disease 40 to 55 years later. There was a consistently high correlation between infant mortality rates, particularly neonatal deaths, regardless of geographic region, in all age groups and in both sexes, with death from ischemic heart disease. The highest infant mortality rates and also the deaths from heart disease were among those of lowest socioeconomic status. The authors postulate that nutritional practices during pregnancy played a predominant role in subsequent susceptibility to heart disease. Nonhuman primates would be an ideal model to study such a hypothesis.

Recently, the relationship of nutritional status of participants in the congregrate meal program measured in 1975 to mortality over a subsequent 10-year period was investigated (Kohrs *et al.*, 1980; Tsui *et al.*, 1986). Those who died from coronary heart disease had significantly lower serum magnesium and serum iron than those who died from other causes (Tsui *et al.*, 1986). Hypomagnesemia has been suggested as a factor in cardiac arrhythmias and sudden death (Altura *et al.*, 1981). The significance of the Missouri study is that the subjects were normal and free from heart disease at the time of nutritional assessment. Exton-Smith (1977) reports a study in Britain in which low intakes of vitamin C by men and low plasma pyridoxine levels were associated subsequently with early death.

Schlenker *et al.* (1973) found that women who were accustomed to consuming large amounts of thiamin had a lower incidence of death from cardiovascular diseases. As mentioned earlier, women who had diets that contained abundant ascorbic acid also lived longer. Low plasma and leukocyte concentrations of ascorbic acid in healthy elderly or those with chronic diseases are largely caused by a low intake and not by changes in absorption or metabolism (Newton *et al.*, 1985).

Ostfeld (1976) noted that low values for hemoglobin were associated with a high incidence of stroke in older pensioners living in the Chicago area. Although iron-deficiency anemia is not recognized as a major nutritional problem among the elderly, it may be more prevalent among certain subgroups. In the analysis of the Missouri data by Tsui *et al.* (1986), iron intake was not related to coronary heart disease. However, over one-half of the subjects consumed less than the RDA for iron as measured by 1-day food records (Nordstrom *et al.*, 1982). In a study of subjects 60 to 94 years of age maintaining recommended body weight, exercise and not smoking were related to increased longevity (Palmore, 1970). More recently carotene intake from green and yellow vegetables has been linked to decreased risk of cancer deaths among an elderly population (Colditz *et al.*, 1985).

7. Conclusion

Nutrition research on the aged and aging should have as a goal maintenance of full function for as long as possible. To achieve this goal, understanding the relative role of the socioeconomic and other factors discussed here and how they change over time is important for all those currently working with or planning for the elderly and their nutrition. Identification of what is usual aging will aid in the development of strategies to help more people age successfully.

Although many of the factors discussed here potentially have a negative impact on nutritional status, remember that the population of elderly is very heterogeneous and is changing in composition and characteristics. At one end of this age spectrum, the number and percentage of the population who are 85 years of age and older are increasing. These individuals are much more likely to be fragile, are more prone to disease, and are more likely to have psychosocial problems and less support from family structure. On the other hand, the new cohort of young old are better educated and reach this period in better health than previous cohorts (Jones, 1986). Therefore, successive age cohorts will score differently at the same chronological age. A study of health indicators revealed a substantial and consistent improvement of relative health of the elderly between 1961 and 1981, suggesting that factors increasing life expectancy also tend to improve health and reduce disability (Palmore, 1986). With increasing age, more of the elderly are using various community services. The percentage of individuals using senior center meals and home-delivered meals increases from 7.6% and 1.2%, respectively, for those 65–74 years of age to 9.3% and 3.2%, respectively, for those 75 years of age and older (Stone, 1986). These and other programs for the elderly may have contributed to the improved health.

8. References

Akin, J. S., Guilkey, D. K., Popkin, B. M., and Fanelli, M. T., 1986, Cluster analysis of food consumption patterns of older Americans, *J. Am. Diet. Assoc.* **86**:616–624.

Altura, B. M., Altura, B. T., Carells, A., and Turlapaty, P. D., 1981, Hypomagnesemia and vasoconstriction: Possible relationship to etiology of sudden death, ischemic heart disease and hypertensive vascular diseases, *Artery* **9**:212–231.

Anderson, E. L., 1971, Eating patterns before and after dentures, *J. Am. Diet. Assoc.* **58**:421–426.

Andres, R., 1980, Effect of obesity on total mortality, *Int. J. Obesity* **4**:381–386.

Applegate, W. B., Miller, S. T., Elam, J. T., Freeman, J. M., Wood, T. O., and Gettlefinger, T. G., 1987, Impact of cataract surgery with lens implantation on vision and physical function in elderly patients, *J.A.M.A.* **257**:1064–1066.

Bailey, L., Wagner, P. A., Christakis, G. J., Araujo, P. E., Appledorf, H., Davis, C. G., Masteryanni, J., and Dinning, J. S., 1979, Folacin and iron and hematological findings in predominantly black elderly persons from urban low-income households, *Am. J. Clin. Nutr.* **32**:2346–2356.

Baker, H., Frank, O., Thind, I. S., Jaslow, S., and Louria, D. B., 1979, Vitamin profiles in elderly persons living at home or in nursing homes, versus profile in healthy young subjects, *J. Am. Geriatr. Soc.* **27**:444–450.

Bales, C. W., Steinman, L. C., Freeland-Graves, J. H., Stone, J. M., and Young, R. K., 1986, The effect of age on plasma zinc uptake and taste acuity, *Am. J. Clin. Nutr.* **44**:664–669.

Balough, K., and Lelkes, K., 1961, The tongue in old age, *Gerontol. Clin.* **3**(Suppl.):38–54.

Barch, D. H., Fox, C. C., and Mobarhan, S. A., 1987, Effects of chronic disease on nutrition, *Nutr. Int.* **3**:79–86.

Barker, D. J. P., and Osmond, C., 1986, Infant mortality, childhood nutrition, and ischaemic heart disease in England and Wales, *Lancet* **1**:1077–1081.

Bartoshuk, L. M., Rifkin, B., Marks, L. E., and Bars, P., 1986, Taste and aging, *J. Gerontol.* **41**:51–57.

Bates, J. F., Elwood, P. C., and Foster, W., 1971, Studies relating mastication and nutrition in the elderly, *Gerontol. Clin.* **13**:227–239.

Bausell, R. B., 1986, Health-seeking behavior among the elderly, *Gerontologist* **26**:556–559.

Betts, N. M., and Crase, C., 1986, Nutrient intake of urban elderly American Indians, *J. Nutr. Elderly* **5**:11–18.

Booth, P., Kohrs, M. B., and Kamath, S., 1982, Taste acuity and aging: A review, *Nutr. Res.* **2**:95–109.

Bouillon, R. A., Auwerx, J. H., Lissens, W. D., and Pelemans, W. K., 1987, Vitamin D status in the elderly: Seasonal substrate deficiency causes 1,25-dihydroxycholecalciferol deficiency, *Am. J. Clin. Nutr.* **45**:755–763.

Breslow, R., Hallfrisch, J., Moser, P. B., Maney, D., Muller, D., and Goldberg, A., 1987, Nursing home patients, *Fed. Proc.* **46**:4042.

Burke, B. S., 1947, The dietary history as a tool in research, *J. Am. Diet. Assoc.* **23**:1041–1046.

Busse, E. W., 1976, Hypochondriasis in the elderly: A reaction to social stress, *J. Am. Geriatr. Soc.* **24**:145–149.

Calasanti, T. M., and Hendricks, J., 1986, A sociological perspective on nutrition research among the elderly: Toward conceptual development, *Gerontologist* **26**:232–239.

Carmel, R., Weiner, J. M., and Johnson, C. S., 1987, Iron deficiency occurs frequently in patients with pernicious anemia, *J.A.M.A.* **257**:1081–1083.

Carroll, M. D., Abraham, S., and Dresser, C. M., 1983, *Dietary Intake Source Data. United States, 1976–80,* Vital and Health Statistics, Series 11–231, DHHS Pub. No. (PHS) 83-1681, Washington.

Castelli, W. P., Dawber, T. R., Gordon, R., and Kannel, W. B., 1981, Lipoproteins, cardiovascular disease and death: The Framingham study, *Arch. Intern. Med.* **141**:1128–1131.

Coates, T. D., Rickard, K. A., Grosfels, J. L., and Westman, R. M., 1986, Nutritional support of children with neoplastic disease, *Surg. Clin. North Am.* **66**:1197–1212.

Colditz, G. A., Branch, L. G., Lipnick, R. J., Willett, W. C., Rosener, B., Posner, B. M., and Hennekens, C. H., 1985, Increased green and yellow vegetable intake and lowered cancer deaths in an elderly population, *Am. J. Clin. Nutr.* **41:**32–36.

Cooper, R. M., Bilash, I., and Zubek, J. P., 1959, The effect of age on taste sensitivity, *J. Gerontol.* **14:**56–58.

Czajka-Narins, D. M., Kohrs, M. B., Tsui, J., and Nordstrom, J., 1987, Nutritional and biochemical effects of nutrition programs in the elderly, *Clin. Geriatr. Med.* **3:**275–287.

Czajka-Narins, D. M., Tsui, J., Kohrs, M. B., and Nordstrom, J. A., 1988, Anthropometric assessment of an elderly population, (in press).

Dallman, P. R., Yip, R., and Johnson, C., 1984, Prevalence and causes of anemia in the United States, 1976–1980, *Am. J. Clin. Nutr.* **39:**437–445.

Davies, M., Mawer, E. B., Hann, J. T., and Taylor, J. L., 1986, Seasonal changes in the biochemical indices of vitamin D deficiency in the elderly: A comparison of people in residential homes, long-stay wards and attending a day hospital, *Age Ageing* **15:**77–83.

Davis, M. A., Randall, E., Forthofer, R. N., Lee, E. S., and Margen, S., 1985, Living arrangements and dietary patterns of older adults in the United States, *J. Gerontol.* **40:**434–442.

Dawson, D., Hendershot, G., and Fulton, J., 1987, *Aging in the Eighties: Functional Limitations of Individuals 65 and Over. NCHS Advance Data from Vital and Health Statistics No. 133,* DHHS Pub. No. (PHS) 87-1250, Public Health Service, Hyattsville, MD.

Dibble, M. V., Brin, M., Thiele, V. F., Peal, A., Chen, N., and McMullen, E., 1967, Evaluation of the nutritional status of elderly with a comparison between fall and spring, *J. Am. Geriatr. Soc.* **15:**1031–1061.

Edwards, S. J., 1983, Nutrition and lifestyle, in: *Nutrition in the Middle and Later Years* (E. B. Feldman, ed.), John Wright-PSG, Boston, pp. 1–32.

Exton-Smith, A. N., 1977, Vitamin status of the elderly, in: *Nutrition of the Aged* (K. A. Farmer, ed.), University of Calgary, Calgary, Alberta, pp. 1–20.

Exton-Smith, A. N., 1980, Nutrition status: Diagnosis and prevention of malnutrition, in: *Metabolic and Nutritional Disorders in the Elderly* (A. N. Exton-Smith, and F. I. Caird, eds.), John Wright and Sons, Bristol, pp. 66–76.

Food and Nutrition Board, 1980, *Recommended Dietary Allowances,* 9th ed., National Research Council, Washington.

Fulwood, R., Johnson, C. L., Bryner, J. D., Cunter, E. W., and McGrath, C. R., 1982, *Hematological and Nutrition Biochemistry Reference Data for Persons 6 Months–74 Years of Age: 1976–1980,* DHHS Publ. No. (PHS) 83-1682, Washington.

Geissler, C. A., and Bates, J. F., 1984, The nutritional effects of tooth loss, *Am. J. Clin. Nutr.* **39:**478–489.

Glandville, E. V., Kaplan, A. R., and Rischer, R., 1964, Age, sex, and taste sensitivity, *J. Gerontol.* **19:**474–478.

Goodwin, J. S., Goodwin, J. M., and Garry, P. J., 1983, Association between nutritional status and cognitive functioning in a healthy elderly population, *J.A.M.A.* **249:**2917–2921.

Grotkowski, M. L., and Sims, L. S., 1978, Nutritional knowledge, attitudes, and dietary practices of the elderly, *J. Am. Diet. Assoc.* **72:**499–511.

Grzegorczyk, P. B., Jones, S. W., and Mistretta, C. M., 1979, Age-related differences in salt taste acuity, *J. Gerontol.* **34:**834–840.

Harrill, I., Erbes, E., and Schwartz, C. S., 1976, Observations on food acceptance by elderly women, *Gerontologist* **16:**349–355.

Hart, W. D., and Little, S., 1986, Comparison of diets of elderly Hispanics and Caucasians in the urban southewest, *J. Nutr. Elderly* **5:**21–29.

Havlik, R. J., 1986, Aging in the eighties: Impaired senses for sound and light in persons age 65 years and over, in: *NCHS Advance Data from Vital and Health Statistics,* No. 125, DHHS Pub. No. (PHS) 86-1250, Public Health Service, Hyattsville, MD.

Hermel, J., Schonwetter, S., and Samueloff, S., 1970, Taste sensation and age in man, *J. Oral Med.* **25:**39–42.

Hinchcliffe, R., 1958, Clinical quantitative gustometry, *Acta Otolaryngol.* **49:**453–466.

Holt, V., Kohrs, M. B., and Nordstrom, J. W., 1987, Food preferences of older adults, *J. Nutr. Elderly* **6:**47–55.

Joint Nutrition Monitoring Evaluation Committee, 1986, *Nutrition Monitoring in the United States: A Progress Report,* USHHS and USDA, DHHS Publ. No. (PHS) 86-1255, Hyattsville, MD.

Jones, E., 1986, The elderly: A new generation, *Ageing Soc.* **6**:313–331.

Kahn, H. A., Liebowitz, H. M., and Ganley, J. P., 1977, The Framingham Eye Study: Outline and major prevalence findings, *Am. J. Epidemiol.* **106**:17–32.

Kalmus, H., and Trotter, W. R., 1962, Direct assessment of the effect of age on P.T.C. sensitivity, *Ann. Hum. Genet.* **25**:145–149.

Kaplan, A. R., Glanville, E. V., and Discher, R., 1965, Cumulative effect of age and smoking on taste sensitivity in males and females, *J. Gerontol.* **20**:334–337.

Kim, S. K., and Caldwell, N. R., 1986, Dietary status of elderly persons living in an urban community during winter and summer seasons, *J. Nutr. Elderly* **5**:5–21.

Kim, K., Kohrs, M. B., Twork, R., and Grier, M. R., 1984, Dietary calcium intakes of elderly Korean-Americans, *J. Am. Diet. Assoc.* **84**:164–175.

Klotz, U., Avant, G. R., Hoyumpa, A., Schenker, S., and Wilkinson, G. R., 1975, The effects of age and liver disease on the disposition and elimination of diazepam in adult man, *J. Clin. Invest.* **55**:347–359.

Kohrs, M. B., 1985, What is normal aging? Part XIII: Age related changes in taste acuity, *Geriatr. Med. Today* **4**:88–93.

Kohrs, M. B., and Czajka-Narins, D. M., 1986, Assessing the nutritinal status of the elderly, in: *Nutrition, Aging and Health* (E. A. Young, ed.), Alan R. Liss, New York, pp. 25–69.

Kohrs, M. B., and Tobben, C. K., 1982, Association of obesity with disease among the elderly, *Nutr. Rep. Int.* **25**:533–541.

Kohrs, M. B., Preston, A., O'Neal, R., Eklund, D., and Abrahams, O., 1978, Nutritional status of elderly residents in Missouri, *Am. J. Clin. Nutr.* **31**:2186–2197.

Kohrs, M. B., Wang, L. L., Eklund, D., Paulsen, B., and O'Neal, R., 1979, The association of obesity with socioeconomic factors in Missouri, *Am. J. Clin. Nutr.* **32**:2120–2128.

Kohrs, M. B., Nordstrom, J., Plowman, E. L., O'Hanlon, P., Moore, C., Davis, C., Abrahams, O., and Eklund, D., 1980, Association of participation in a nutritional program for the elderly with nutritional status, *Am. J. Clin. Nutr.* **33**:2643–2656.

Kohrs, M. B., Kapica-Cyborski, C., and Czajka-Narins, D. M., 1984, Iron and chromium nutriture in the elderly, in: *Trace Substances in Environmental Health—XVIII* (D. D. Hemphill, ed.), University of Missouri, Columbia, pp. 476–486.

Kovar, M. G., 1986, *Aging in the Eighties: Age 65 Years and Over and Living Alone, Contacts with Family, Friends and Neighbors, NCHS Advance Data from Vital and Health Statistics,* No. 116, DHHS Pub No (PHS) 86-1250, Public Health Service, Hyattsville, MD.

Krondl, M., 1979, Perceived food intolerance, *J. Can. Diet. Assoc.* **40**:264–269.

Krondl, M., Lau, D., Yurkiw, M. A., and Coleman, P. H., 1982, Food use and perceived food meanings of the elderly, *J. Am. Diet. Assoc.* **80**:523–528.

Lee, C. J., 1987, Nutritional status of elderly females: 4-year follow-up study, *Fed. Proc.* **46**:900.

Lee, C. J., Johnson, G. H., and Lawler, G. S., 1981, Some clinical indices of nutrition and health status among elderly Kentucky residents volunteering to be surveyed: Comparison by sociological factors, life-styles and health characteristics, *Nutr. Res.* **1**:47–62.

Litwak, E., and Longino, C. F., 1987, Migration patterns among the elderly: A developmental perspective, *Gerontologist* **27**:266–272.

Ludman, E. K., and Newman, J. M., 1986, Frail elderly: Assessment of nutrition needs, *Gerontologist* **26**:199–202.

Macarthy, P. I., Johnson, A. A., and Walters, C. S., 1986, Iron nutritional status of selected elderly black persons in Washington, D.C., *J. Nutr. Elderly* **6**:3–11.

Madans, J. H., Kleinman, J. C., Cox, C. S., Barbano, H. E., Feldman, J. J., Finucane, F. F., and Cornoni-Huntley, J., 1986, 10 years after NHANES-I: Report of initial followup, 1982–84, *Public Health Rep.* **101**:465–473.

Mattes, R. D., 1986, Effects of health disorders and poor nutritional status on gustatory function, *J. Sens. Stud.* **1**:275–290.

Mattes, R. D., and Mela, D. J., 1986, Relationships between and among selected measures of sweet taste preference and dietary intake, *Chem. Sens.* **11**:523–539.

Mattes-Kulig, D. A., and Henkin, R. I., 1985, Energy and nutrient consumption of patients with dysgeusia, *J. Am. Diet. Assoc.* **85**:822–826.

McGandy, R. B., Barrows, C. H., Spanias, A., Meredith, A., Stone, J. L., and Norris, A. H., 1966, Nutrient intakes and energy expenditure in men of different ages, *J. Gerontol.* **21**:581–587.

McGandy, R. B., Russell, R. M., Hartz, S. C., Jacob, R. A., Tannenbaum, S., Peters, H., Sahyoun, N., and Otradovec, M. A., 1986, Nutritional status survey of healthy noninstitutionalized elderly: Energy and nutrient intakes from three day records and nutrient supplements. *Nutr. Res.* **6**:785–798.

Moore, L. M., Nielsen, C. R., and Mistretta, C. M., 1982, Sucrose taste thresholds: Age related differences, *J. Gerontol.* **37**:64–69.

Morgan, D. B., Newton, H. M. V., Schorah, C. J., Jewitt, M. A., Hancock, M. R., and Hullin, R. P., 1986, Abnormal indices of nutrition in the elderly: A study of different clinical groups, *Age Aging* **15**:65–76.

Munro, H. N., McGandy, R. B., Hartz, S. C., Russell, R. M., Jacob, R. A., and Otradovec, C. L., 1987, Protein nutriture of a group of free-living elderly, *Am. J. Clin. Nutr.* **46**:586–592.

Murphy, C., 1985, Cognitive and chemosensory influences on age-related changes in the ability to identify blended foods, *J. Gerontol.* **40**:47–52.

Newman, E. G., Dovenmuehle, R. H., and Busse, E. W., 1960, Alterations in neurologic status with age, *J. Am. Geriatr. Soc.* **8**:915–917.

Newton, H. M. V., Schorah, C. J., Habibzadeh, N., Morgan, D. B., and Hullin, R. P., 1985, The cause and correction of low blood vitamin C concentrations in the elderly, *Am. J. Clin. Nutr.* **42**:656–659.

Nordstrom, J. W., Abrahams, O. G., and Kohrs, M. B., 1982, Anemia among noninstitutionalized white elderly, *Nutr. Rep. Int.* **25**:97–105.

Norris, S. H., Kohrs, M. B., and Kurtzman, N. A., 1985, Protein–calorie malnutrition in chronic hemodialysis patients, *Kidney Int.* **27**:168.

O'Hanlon, P., Kohrs, M. B., Hilderbrand, E., and Nordstrom, J., 1983, Socioeconomic factors and dietary intake of elderly Missourians, *J. Am. Diet. Assoc.* **82**:646–653.

Osterberg, T., and Steen, B., 1982, Relationship between dental status and dietary intake in 70-year-old males and females in Goteborg, Sweden: A population study, *J. Oral Rehab.* **9**:509–521.

Ostfeld, A. M., 1976, Nutritional aspects of stroke, particularly in the elderly, in: *Nutrition, Longevity and Aging* (M. Rockstein and M. L. Sussman, eds.), Academic Press, New York, pp. 27–52.

Palmore, E., 1970, Health practices and illness among the aged, *Gerontologist* **10**:313–316.

Palmore, E. B., 1986, Trends in the health of the aged, *Gerontologist* **26**:298–302.

Read, M. H., and Graney, A. S., 1982, Food supplement usage by the elderly, *J. Am. Diet. Assoc.* **80**:150–153.

Richter, C. P., and Campbell, K. H., 1940, Sucrose taste thresholds of rats and humans, *Am. J. Physiol.* **128**:291–297.

Rikli, R., and Busch, S., 1986, Motor performance of women as a function of age and physical activity level, *J. Gerontol.* **41**:645–649.

Roberts, J., 1966, *Weight by Height and Age of Adults: 1960–1962. Vital and Health Statistics,* National Center for Health Statistics, Public Health Service, Publ. no. 1000, Series 11, No. 14, Washington.

Rodin, J., 1986, Aging and health: Effects of the sense of control, *Science* **233**:1271–1276.

Rosenthal, C. J., 1986, Family supports in later life: Does ethnicity make a difference? *Gerontologist* **26**:19–24.

Rountree, J. L., and Tinklin, G. L., 1975, Food beliefs and practices of selected senior citizens, *Gerontologist* **15**:537–540.

Rovick, M. H., and Scrimshaw, N. S., 1979, Comparative tolerance of elderly from differing ethnic backgrounds to lactose-containing and lactose-free dairy drinks: A double blind study, *J. Gerontol.* **34**:191–196.

Rowe, J. W., and Kahn, R. L., 1987, Human aging: Usual and successful, *Science* **237**:141–149.

Rubinstein, R. L., 1987, Never married elderly as a social type: Re-evaluating some images, *Gerontologist* **27**:108–113.

Schaefer, R. B., and Keith, P. M., 1982, Dietary quality of married and single elderly, *J. Am. Diet. Assoc.* **81**:30.

Schiffman, S. S., and Covey, E., 1984. Changes in taste and smell with age: Nutritional aspects, in: *Nutrition in Gerontology* (D. Harman and R. Alfin-Slater, eds.), Raven Press, New York, pp. 43–64.

Schlenker, E. D., Feurig, J. S., Stone, L. H., Ohlson, M. A., and Mickelsen, O., 1973, Nutrition and health of older people, *Am. J. Clin. Nutr.* **73:**1111–1119.

Shank, R. E., 1974, Nutrition and aging, in: *Epidemiology of Aging* (A. M. Ostfeld and D. C. Gibson, eds.), DHEW Publ. No. (NIH) 75-711, NIH, USDHEW, Bethesda, MD, pp. 215–222.

Shapiro, L. R., Samuels, S., Breslow, L., and Camacho, T., 1983, Patterns of vitamin C intake from food and supplements: Survey of an adult population in Alameda County, California, *Am. J. Public Health* **73:**773–778.

Sheehan, E. T., Read, M., and DeLette, A. C., 1987, Vitamin and food supplement practices of the elderly in seven western states, *Fed. Proc.* **46:**3405.

Singer, J. D., Granahan, P., Goodrich, N. N., Meyers, L. D., and Johnson, C. L., 1982, *Diet and Iron Status, a Study of Relationships: United States, 1971–74, Vital and Health Statistics Series 11,* No. 229, DHHS Pub. No. (PHS) 83-1679, Washington.

Stone, R., 1986, *Aging in the Eighties: Age 65 Years and Over—Use of Community Services. Advance Data from Vital and Health Statistics,* No. 124, DHHS Pub. No. (PHS) 86-1250, Public Health Service, Hyattsville, MD.

Tsui, J. C., Nordstrom, J. W., and Kohrs, M. B., 1986, Relationship of copper and magnesium nutriture to mortality in the elderly, in: *Trace Substances in Environmental Health—XX* (D. D. Hemphill, ed.), University of Missouri, Columbia, pp. 36–43.

Tsui, J. C., Nordstrom, J. W., Holt, V., and Kohrs, M. B., 1987, Changes in nutrient intakes and food consumption patterns in older adults between 1975 and 1985, *Fed. Proc.* **46:**900.

Van Zandt, S., and Fox, H., 1986, Nutritional impact of congregate meals programs, *J. Nutr. Elderly* **5:**31–43.

Wagner, P. A., Krista, M. L., Bailey, L. B., and Christakis, G. J., 1980, Zinc status of elderly black Americans from urban, low-income households, *Am. J. Clin. Nutr.* **33:**1771–1777.

Wayler, A. H., Kapur, K. K., Feldman, R. S., and Chauncey, H. H., 1982, Effects of age and dentition status on measures of food acceptability, *J. Gerontol.* **37:**294–299.

Wayler, A. H., Muench, M. E., Kapur, K. K., and Chauncey, H. H., 1984, Masticatory performance and food acceptability in persons with removable partial dentures, full dentures and intact natural dentition, *J. Gerontol.* **39:**284–289.

Weiffenbach, J. M., Baum, B. J., and Burghauser, R., 1982, Taste thresholds: Quality specific variation with human aging, *J. Gerontol.* **37:**372–377.

Weiffenbach, J. M., Cowan, B. J., and Baum, B. J., 1986, Taste intensity perception in ageing, *J. Gerontol.* **41:**460–468.

Yung, L., Contento, I., and Gussow, J. D., 1984, Use of health foods by the elderly, *J. Nutr. Educ.* **16:**127–131.

Yurkstas, A. A., 1954, The effect of missing teeth on masticatory performance and efficiency, *J. Prosthet. Dent.* **4:**120–126.

Ziemlanski, S., Wartanowicz, M., Klos, A., Raczka, A., and Klos, M., 1986, The effects of ascorbic acid and alpha-tocopherol supplementation on serum proteins and immunoglobulin concentrations in the elderly, *Nutr. Int.* **2:**245–249.

Zimmerman, S. A., and Krondl, M. M., 1986, Perceived intolerance of vegetables among the elderly, *J. Am. Diet. Assoc.* **86:**1047–1051.

13

Anthropometric Approaches to the Nutritional Assessment of the Elderly

William Cameron Chumlea, Alex F. Roche, and Maria L. Steinbaugh

1. The Importance of Anthropometry in a Nutritional Assessment

The nutritional assessment of an elderly person needs to include data from medical and dietary histories, laboratory measurements, immune-testing results, and anthropometry in order to evaluate present nutritional status or changes in nutritional status as completely as is practical. Anthropometry can also be used to evaluate trends in nutritional status and to help to monitor the effects of nutritional intervention. This chapter discusses the importance of anthropometry in the assessment of nutritional status in the elderly.

Anthropometry provides noninvasive indirect information about the amounts of adipose and muscle tissues in the body. The extreme conditions of these body stores, e.g., obesity or emaciation, and rapid changes in these stores are a concern to those responsible for the health care of the elderly (Kemm and Allcock, 1984; Fanelli, 1987). The prevalence of obesity increases among the elderly with the loss of mobility (Patrick *et al.*, 1982) and places an increased burden on the locomotive and cardiovascular systems in addition to its effects on pulmonary function (Borkan *et al.*, 1986). Emaciation increases the risk of morbidity and mortality, partly because it is frequently associated with depressed immune function (Mitchell and Lipschitz, 1982c; Fanelli, 1987).

2. Relationships among Body Measurements and Age

Despite the need for the establishment of appropriate anthropometric reference data to evaluate nutritional assessments of the elderly, there have been only a few

William Cameron Chumlea and Alex F. Roche • Division of Human Biology, Department of Pediatrics, Wright State University School of Medicine, Dayton, Ohio 45435. ***Maria L. Steinbaugh*** • Nutrition Education, Ross Laboratories, Columbus, Ohio 43216.

studies of nutritional status in the elderly using anthropometric data or more direct measures of body composition (Young *et al.*, 1963; Durnin and Womersley, 1974; Steen *et al.*, 1977, 1979; Chumlea *et al.*, 1984b; Bastow, 1982; Fanelli, 1987). Also, there is limited knowledge of the relationships among body circumferences, subcutaneous adipose tissue thicknesses, and total body fat in the elderly. It appears that the relationships among measures of subcutaneous adipose tissue thickness (triceps and subscapular skinfolds) and total or percentage body fat are stronger and more meaningful in young adults than in the elderly (Chumlea *et al.*, 1984b). Correlations of triceps, subscapular, or suprailiac skinfolds with total or percentage body fat in older adults are less than corresponding values reported for younger adults (Wessel *et al.*, 1963; Stoudt *et al.*, 1965; Ward *et al.*, 1975; Noppa *et al.*, 1979; Roche *et al.*, 1981), but correlations of waist or abdominal circumference with total body fat are larger than corresponding values in younger adults (Ward *et al.*, 1975; Chumlea *et al.*, 1984b). These differences in the associations among body composition variables between young and elderly adults result in part from the fact that measures of body size and fatness are affected by the normal physiological effects of aging such as a reduction in stature (Rossman, 1977), changes in the amount and distribution of subcutaneous adipose tissue (Norris *et al.*, 1963; Wessel *et al.*, 1963; Young *et al.*, 1963; Novak, 1972; Durnin and Womersley, 1974; Forbes, 1976; Borkan and Norris, 1977; Fisher *et al.*, 1978), and alterations in tissue elasticity (Grahame, 1970) and compressibility (Himes *et al.*, 1979). Moreover, the selection of a sample of "healthy" elderly persons who have aged "successfully" for base-line data is hampered by the increased prevalence of degenerative diseases that influence the variability in body measurements (Exton-Smith, 1982; Rowe and Kahn, 1987). Consequently, many study samples of the elderly are biased.

If accepted traditional measures of body size do not provide adequate estimates of nutritional status or of the effects of nutritional intervention in older adults, then other measurements should be considered. For example, an increase in abdominal circumference with age may be a reflection of a shortening of the trunk because of osteoporosis or other spinal deformities in elderly women (Arnold *et al.*, 1966; Laitiner, 1978). It can be hypothesized that the abdomen would increase in girth as the length of the trunk decreases. In support of this hypothesis, the abdominal circumference of elderly women is negatively and significantly correlated with sitting height (Chumlea *et al.*, 1984b). Also, a significant negative correlation between age and calf circumference in elderly men and not women may result from general loss of muscle in response to the reported greater reduction in physical activity among men than women as they age (Fentem *et al.*, 1976; MacLenman *et al.*, 1980; Patrick *et al.*, 1982).

3. *Problems with Anthropometry in the Elderly*

The taking of all body measurements in the elderly should be considered carefully. This is because methods of collecting body measurements in nutritional assessments of many elderly persons have not been entirely satisfactory. Common anthropometric techniques are effective in nutritional assessments of many of those elderly persons who are ambulatory, but these same measurements become increasingly difficult to collect in older elderly persons and those who are disabled. Among the elderly, observer errors for body measurements increase, and more so for circumferences and skinfolds of the trunk (Chumlea *et al.*, 1984a). This may be caused in part by the redistribution of adipose tissue so that there are increasing amounts on the trunk at older ages (Borkan and Hults, 1983). Also, in picking up a skinfold in the elderly, the separation of subcutaneous adipose tissue from the underlying fascia and muscle is not clearly discernible. Greater compressibility and/or poor tissue separation for skinfolds in the elderly can significantly affect reliability (Bowman and Rosenberg, 1982).

In a nutritional assessment, a single observer repeating each measurement is effective, but two observers measuring independently is a preferable practice (Cameron, 1978). Regardless of whether one or two observers are employed, it is important to specify a set limit on the range of intra- or interobserver differences and to repeat measurements if these limits are exceeded (Chumlea *et al.*, 1984a). In one study of the elderly, interobserver differences exceeded preset limits for the first pair of body measurements in 27% of the elderly compared to only 19% for younger adults, and the mean absolute interobserver errors for almost all the anthropometric variables were consistently greater than those for the younger participants. Remeasuring those individuals in each group for whom the interobserver errors exceeded preset limits reduced the prevalence of large interobserver errors to about 8% in each group (Chumlea *et al.*, 1984a). In using anthropometry to assess the nutritional status of elderly persons, close attention needs to be given to techniques that minimize measurement errors.

For the very old who are chairbound or are bedfast because of arthritis, accidents, disease, or surgery, or for those who are unable to stand with the positioning recommended for standard anthropometry, the collection of accurate and reliable anthropometric data can be difficult. Some measurements, e.g., stature, are clearly inapplicable (Vir and Love, 1980; Bastow, 1982). In many situations, the nutritional assessment of an elderly person can be improved by the use of recumbent measurements because errors associated with mobility are reduced. Methods of recumbent anthropometry collected from nonambulatory or ambulatory elderly persons are as reliable as those for standing anthropometry. If corresponding recumbent and standing measures are taken at the exact same body sites and with the same basic methodology, there are no systematic differences between paired values (Chumlea *et al.*, 1985c).

Identifying nonambulatory elderly persons who are unusual in their amounts of adipose tissue or muscle or are experiencing changes in weight is as important for their health as is the corresponding identification of ambulatory elderly persons (Laubach *et al.*, 1981; Mitchell and Lipschitz, 1982a; Chumlea *et al.*, 1985c, 1987). In order to measure nonambulatory elderly persons, however, accepted anthropometric techniques have to be adapted to unusual body positions (Cameron, 1978). Many nonambulatory persons are confined to wheelchairs during the day, and it may appear easier to measure such individuals while they remain seated. Except for midarm circumference, however, measurements are more reliably collected if the elderly person is removed from the wheelchair and placed in a recumbent position (Chumlea *et al.*, 1985b). It is difficult to position an elderly individual properly who is sitting in a wheelchair or to change the position of or remove parts of the wheelchair to take a measurement. All these difficulties contribute to poor measurement reliability. The advantages to measuring elderly persons in a recumbent position, as compared to measuring them seated in their wheelchairs, could be expected to produce even greater error differences in a clinical setting than in a research setting. Recumbent anthropometry can provide reliable nutritional assessments of elderly persons regardless of their levels of mobility (Chumlea *et al.*, 1985b).

4. Recommended Measurements

4.1. Stature

The measurement of stature requires a measuring device that includes a flat, vertical surface and some form of right-angled headboard. The movable measuring rod attached to many upright platform scales does not yield accurate measurements. The elderly person should be able to stand upright without assistance and wear minimum clothing so that posture can be seen clearly. The elderly person being measured needs to stand up straight, with bare heels close together, legs straight, arms at the sides, and shoulders relaxed. In many elderly persons, large amounts of adipose tissue on the buttocks allow only the heels and buttocks to touch the measuring wall. It is more important that the elderly person stand erect than that all body parts make contact with the wall.

The elderly person looks straight ahead so that the line of vision is perpendicular to the body, and the headboard is lowered onto the crown of the head (Fig. 1). The person being measured should take a deep breath, and stature at maximum inspiration is recorded. The measurer's eyes should be level with the headboard to avoid errors caused by parallax, and this may require the measurer to stand on a stool. Stature is recorded immediately to the nearest 0.1 cm, and two measurements taken in immediate succession should agree within 1.0 cm.

In some elderly persons, the spinal column may be so curved that the headboard cannot be positioned on the crown of the head. When stature cannot be measured, knee height, a recumbent measurement, can be used to estimate stature.

4.2. Weight

Weight is the most commonly recorded body measurement. Body weight is a critical measurement in assessing nutritional status (Butterworth and Blackburn, 1975; Heber, 1986). Weight is a gross measure of the mass of body tissues and fluids, and serial measures of weight can record changes in these body constituents. Increases in body weight may indicate developing obesity or edema, whereas decreases in body weight can signify the presence, severity, or progress of disease or a nutritional disorder. Despite the nutritional importance of measures of body weight, it has been reported that body weight was not recorded in about 22% of cases of adults receiving nutritional support because the patients were nonambulatory or too ill or equipment was not available or was unreliable (Guenter *et al.*, 1982).

Ambulatory elderly persons can be weighed on an upright balance beam scale (Fig. 2), but spring-type bathroom scales should not be used because they are not accurate enough for clinical purposes. If an elderly person can only sit, a movable

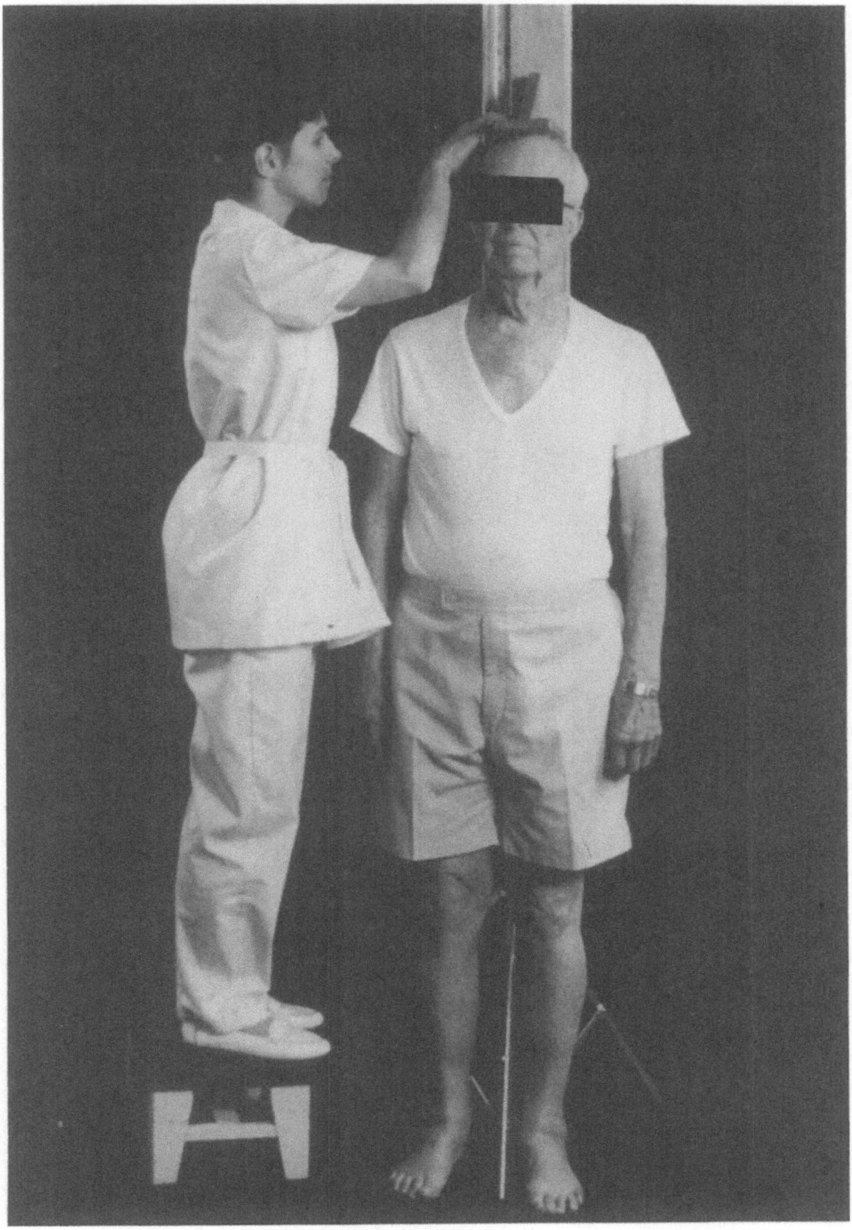

Fig. 1. Measurement of stature. (Printed with permission of Ross Laboratories, Columbus, Ohio.)

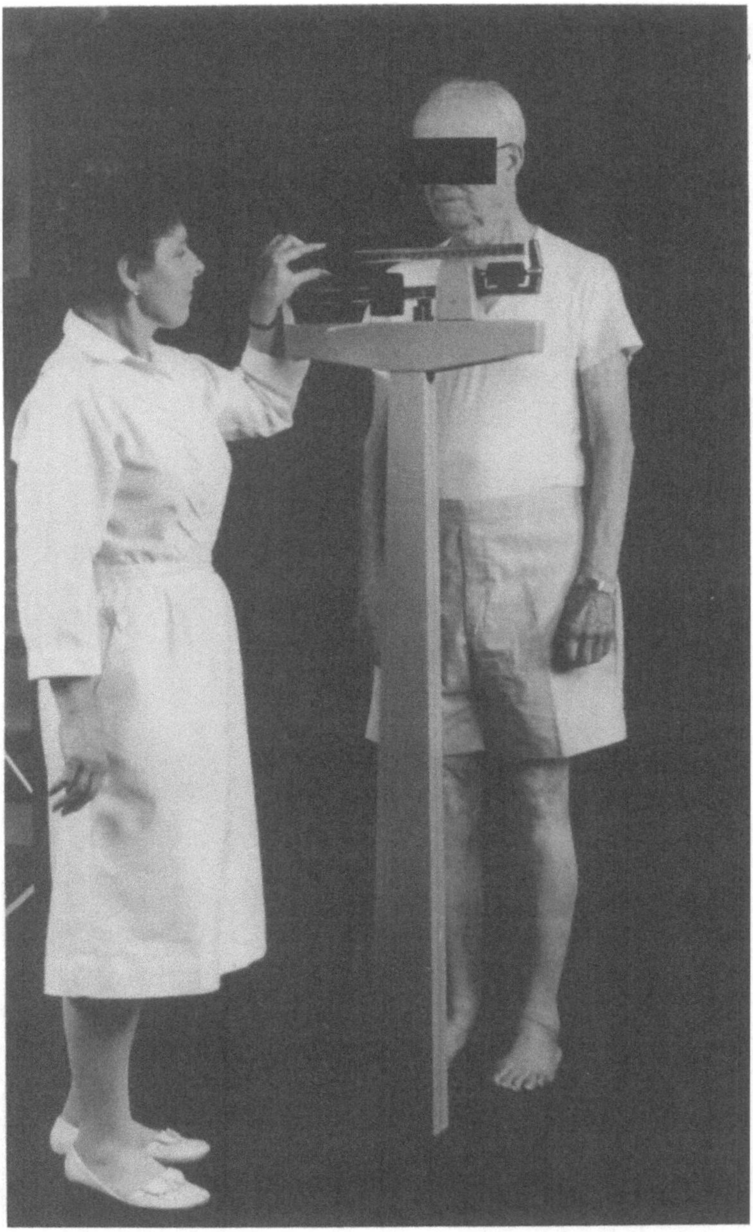

Fig. 2. Measurement of weight with a beam balance scale. (Printed with permission of Ross Laboratories, Columbus, Ohio.)

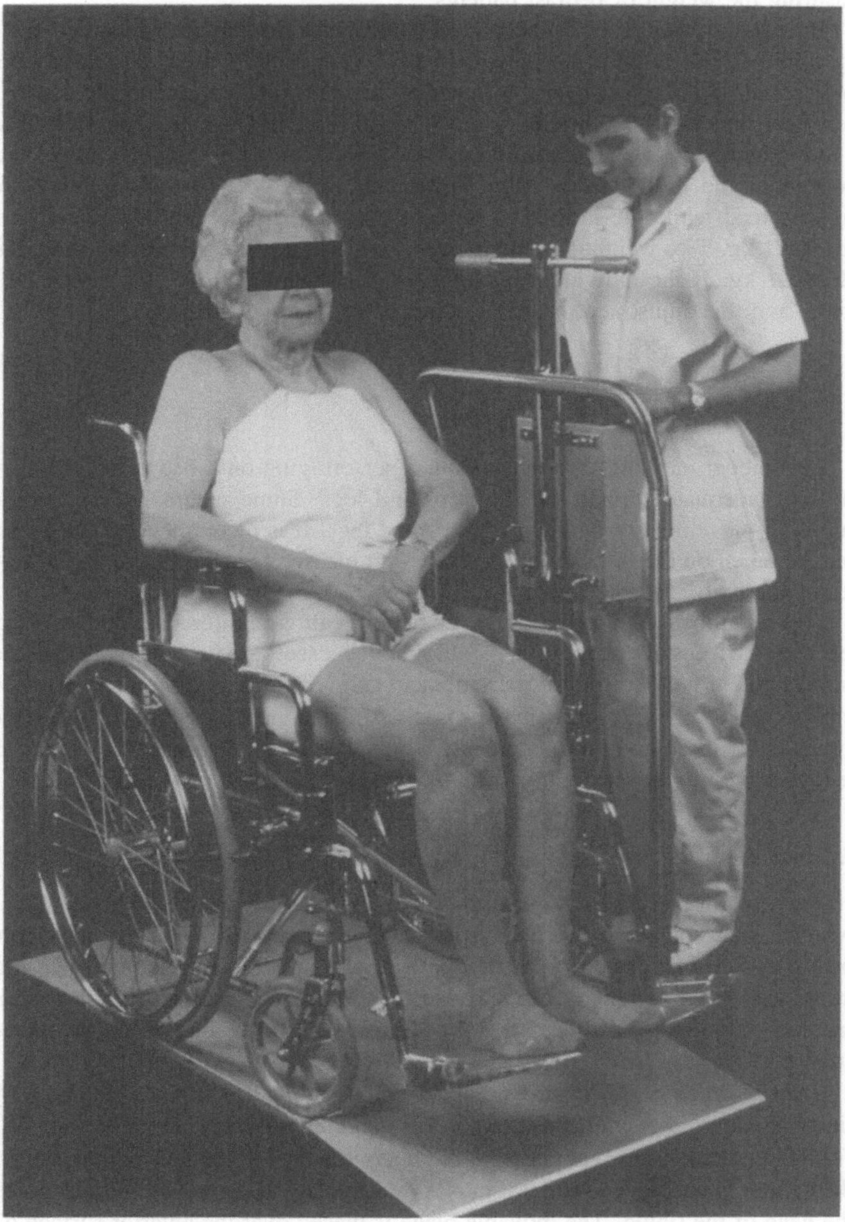

Fig. 3. Measurement of weight with a wheelchair scale. (Printed with permission of Ross Laboratories, Columbus, Ohio.)

wheelchair balance beam scale can be used (Fig. 3), and bed scales are available for measuring the weight of bedfast patients.

Preferably, weight should be recorded nude after the subject has voided and with only minimal underclothing or gown. If a platform scale is used, the elderly person should stand with the feet over the center of the platform. If a chair scale is used, the elderly person should sit upright in the center of the chair. When a bed scale is used, the individual is positioned comfortably in the weighing sling, and the sling is raised slowly until the individual is fully suspended. Regardless of the equipment used, weight is read while the individual remains still and is recorded immediately to the nearest 0.1 kg. Two weight measurements taken in immediate succession should agree within 0.1 kg. If the individual is clothed in undergarments, 0.1 kg should be subtracted, and this adjustment noted next to the recorded weight.

5. *Recumbent Measurements*

Recumbent measures are taken from a person lying on a bed or an examination table with adequate support for the arms and legs. Some recumbent measurements require the movement or bending of arms and legs. It is recommended that measurements be taken on the left side of the body, but measurers should have access to both sides of the body.

Five recumbent measurements, knee height, calf circumference, midarm circumference, and triceps and subscapular skinfold thicknesses, are presented. This sequence minimizes the time required for measurement and reduces any discomfort or inconvenience to the elderly person being measured. A detailed description of the standard techniques for these body measurements is found in the *Anthropometric Standardization Reference Manual* from the Airlie Conference (Lohman *et al.*, 1988).

5.1. *Knee Height*

Knee height is used to estimate the stature of an elderly person who cannot stand or who has such spinal curvature that a measurement of stature would be misleading or impossible. Knee height does not change with age in adults and is highly correlated with stature. Knee height is needed also to compute an estimate of body weight. Equations to estimate stature and body weight from knee height are presented in Section 6.

Knee height is best measured with a specific sliding broad-blade caliper.* Lying supine, the elderly person bends the left knee and left ankle each to a 90° angle (Fig. 4). The fixed blade of the caliper is placed under the heel of the left foot, and the shaft of the caliper is positioned so that it passes over the lateral malleolus and just posterior to the head of the fibula. The movable blade is placed over the anterior surface of the left thigh above the condyles of the femur, about 4.0 cm proximal to the patella. The

*Caliper available from Medical Express, 5150 S.W. Griffith Dr., Beaverton, OR 97005, 800-633-3676.

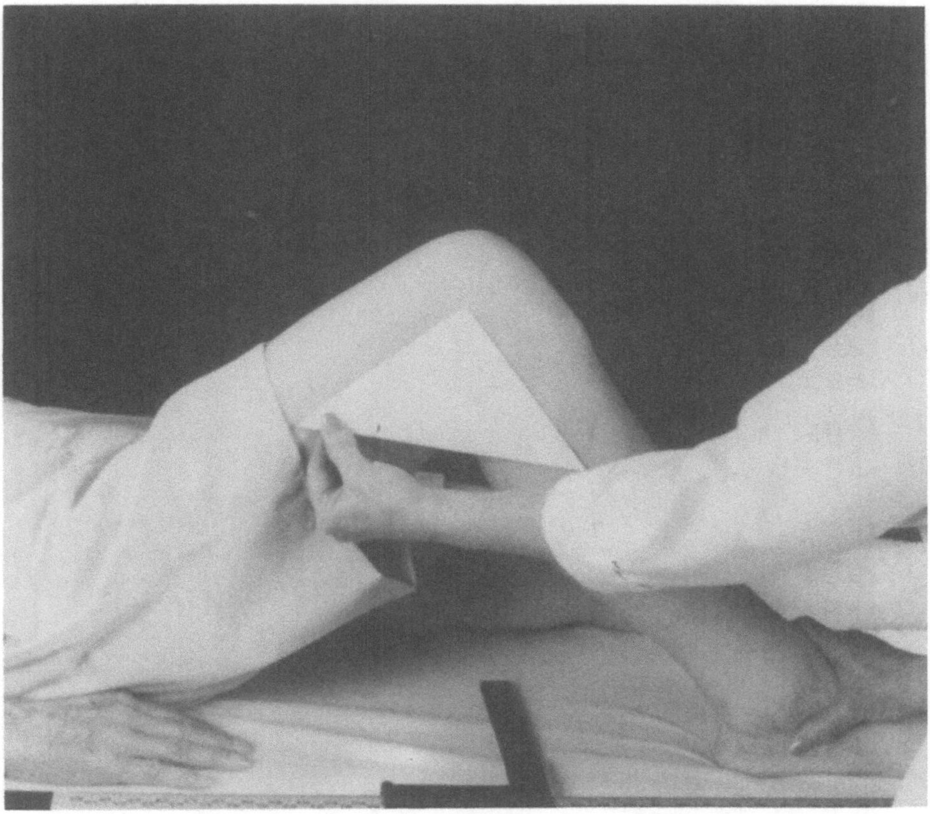

Fig. 4. Position of the left knee at a 90° angle for the measurement of knee height. (Printed with permission of Ross Laboratories, Columbus, Ohio.)

shaft of the caliper is held parallel to the shaft of the tibia, and pressure is applied to compress the tissues (Fig. 5). Measurements are recorded to the nearest 0.1 cm, and two measurements taken in immediate succession should agree within 0.5 cm.

5.2. *Calf Circumference*

Calf circumference is measured with the body in the same position as when measuring knee height. This measurement is taken with an inelastic, flexible measuring tape. With the left knee at a 90° angle, the tape is placed around the calf, and the loop of tape is moved up and down the calf to locate the largest circumference (Fig. 6). The tape is pulled snug around the calf but should not be so tight as to compress the tissues. This measurement is recorded to the nearest 0.1 cm, and successive measurements should agree within 0.5 cm.

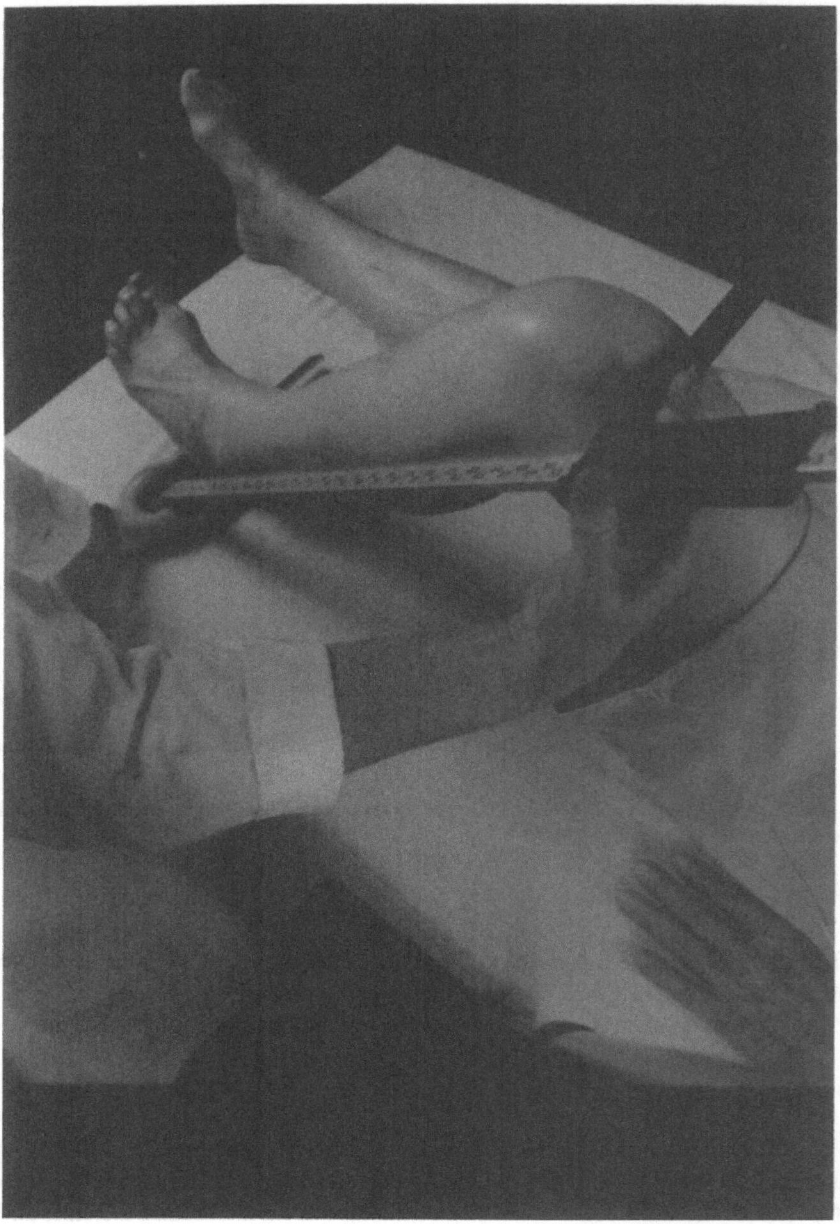

Fig. 5. Position of the Mediform sliding caliper for the measurement of knee height. (Printed with permission of Ross Laboratories, Columbus, Ohio.)

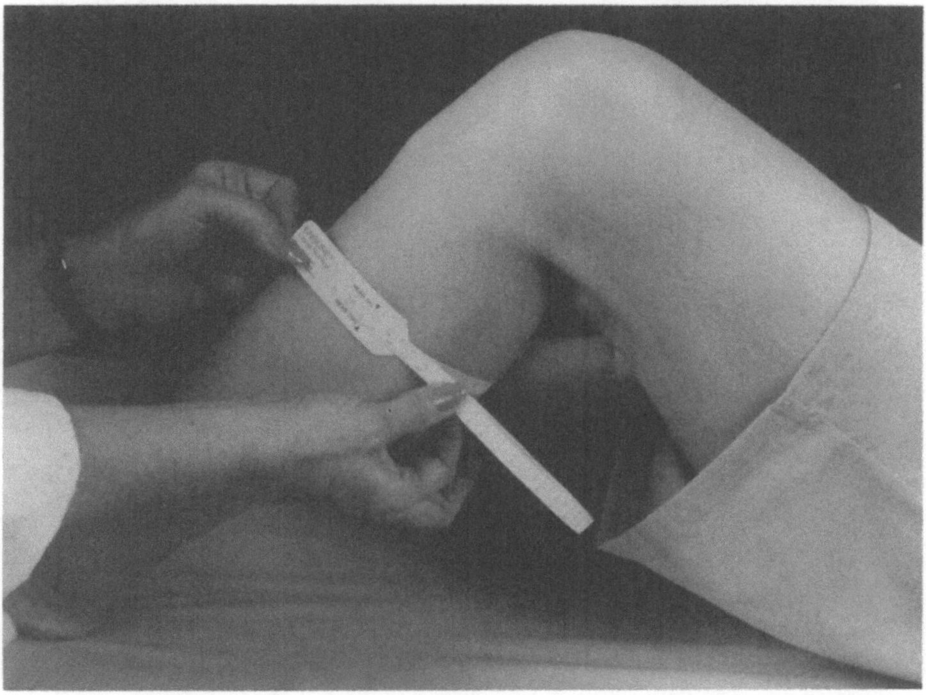

Fig. 6. Measurement of calf circumference. (Printed with permission of Ross Laboratories, Columbus, Ohio.)

5.3. Midarm Circumference

The circumference of the upper arm is measured at its midpoint. The midpoint is located after the left arm is bent to a 90° angle at the elbow and the forearm is placed palm down across the trunk. The upper arm should be approximately parallel to the trunk. Using an insertion tape,* the measurer identifies and marks the midpoint of the arm, halfway between the tip of the acromial process and the tip of the olecranon process (Fig. 7). The skin should be marked at this point before the arm is repositioned for the circumference measurement.

The left arm is then extended alongside the body with the palm facing upward. The arm should be raised slightly off the surface of the bed or examination table by placing a sandbag or towel under the elbow (Fig. 8). The person's hand is placed through the loop of an inelastic, flexible tapemeasure. The tape is placed at the marked midpoint and pulled just snug around the arm, but not so tight that the tissues are compressed (Fig. 9). This measurement is recorded to the nearest 0.1 cm, and successive measurements should agree within 0.5 cm.

*Insertion tapes available from Ross Laboratories, 625 Cleveland Avenue. Columbus, OH 43215, 614-227-3333.

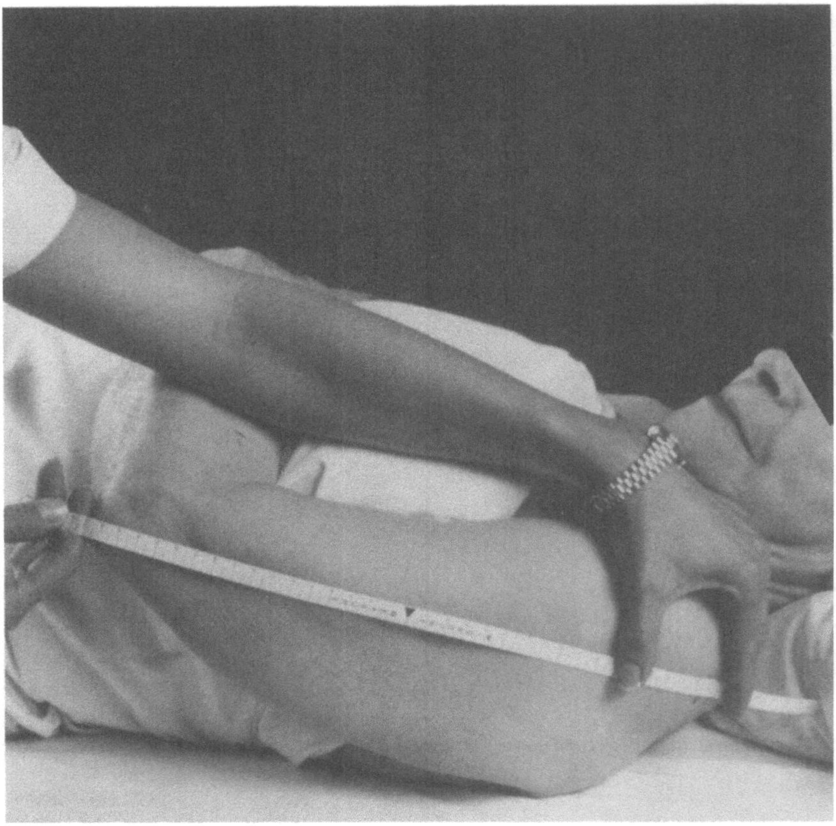

Fig. 7. Locating the midpoint of the upper arm with an insertion tape. (Printed with permission of Ross Laboratories, Columbus, Ohio.)

5.4. Triceps Skinfold Thickness

This measurement is taken while the elderly person lies on the right side, with the right arm extending from the front of the body. The trunk should be in a straight line, and the legs bent and tucked up slightly. The left arm rests along the trunk, palm down (Fig. 10). An imaginary line through the acromion processes should be perpendicular to the bed. There are a variety of skinfold calipers available for measuring subcutaneous adipose tissue thickness. A listing of these can be found in the *Anthropometric Standardization Manual* (Lohman *et al.*, 1988).

The triceps skinfold thickness measurement is taken on the back of the left arm over the triceps muscle, at the level marked as the midpoint for the circumference measurement. Values of repeated triceps skinfold thickness measurements can vary markedly if they are made at different sites.

The measurer gently grasps a double fold of skin and subcutaneous adipose tissue between the fingers and thumb at least 1.0 cm from the marked level. The fold of skin must be on the back of the arm, in the midline, and parallel to the long axis of the upper

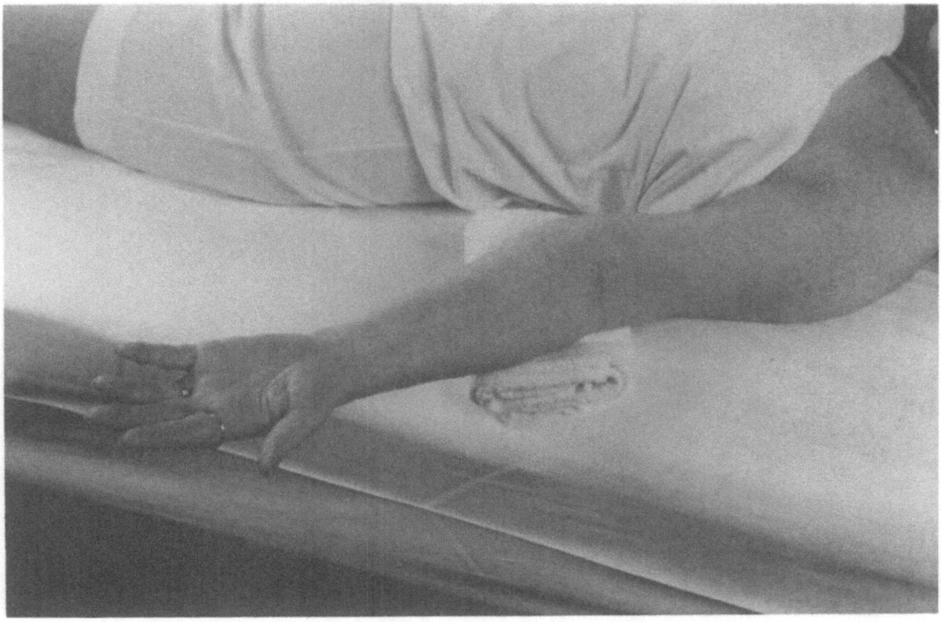

Fig. 8. The position of the arm for measuring midarm circumference. Note pad under elbow to support arm. (Printed with permission of Ross Laboratories, Columbus, Ohio.)

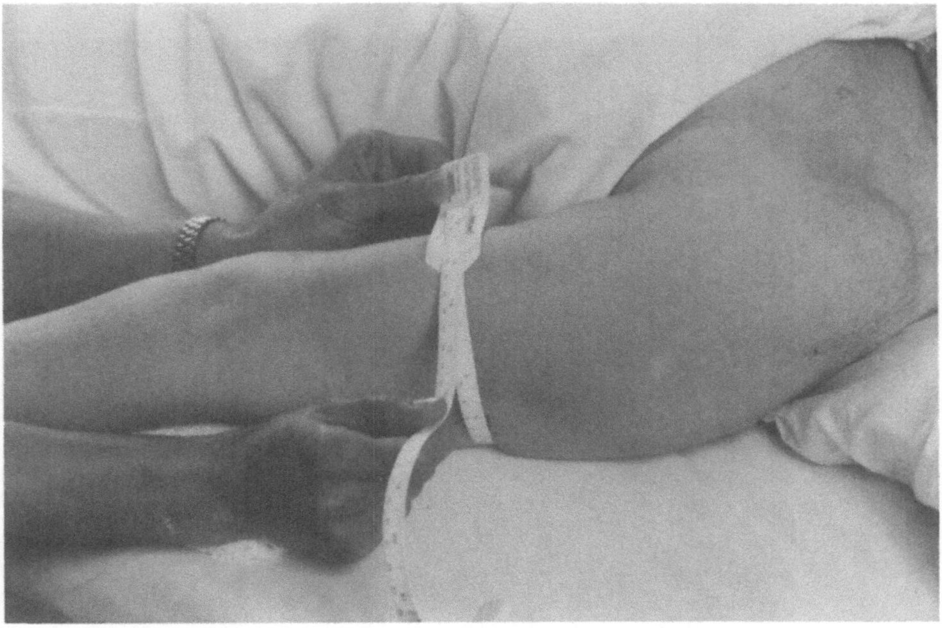

Fig. 9. Measurement of midarm circumference. (Printed with permission of Ross Laboratories, Columbus, Ohio.)

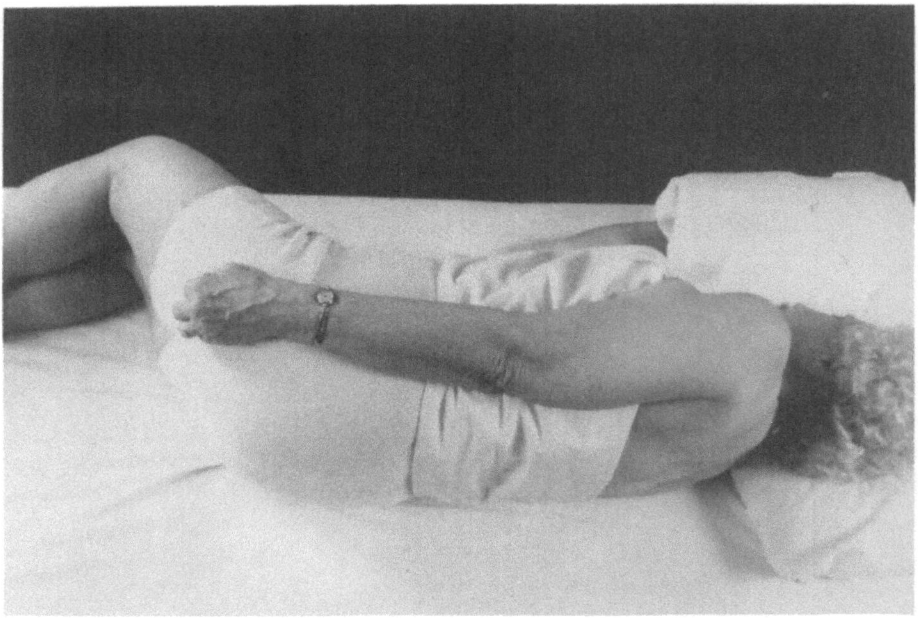

Fig. 10. Position of the body for triceps and subscapular skinfold measurements. (Printed with permission of Ross Laboratories, Columbus, Ohio.)

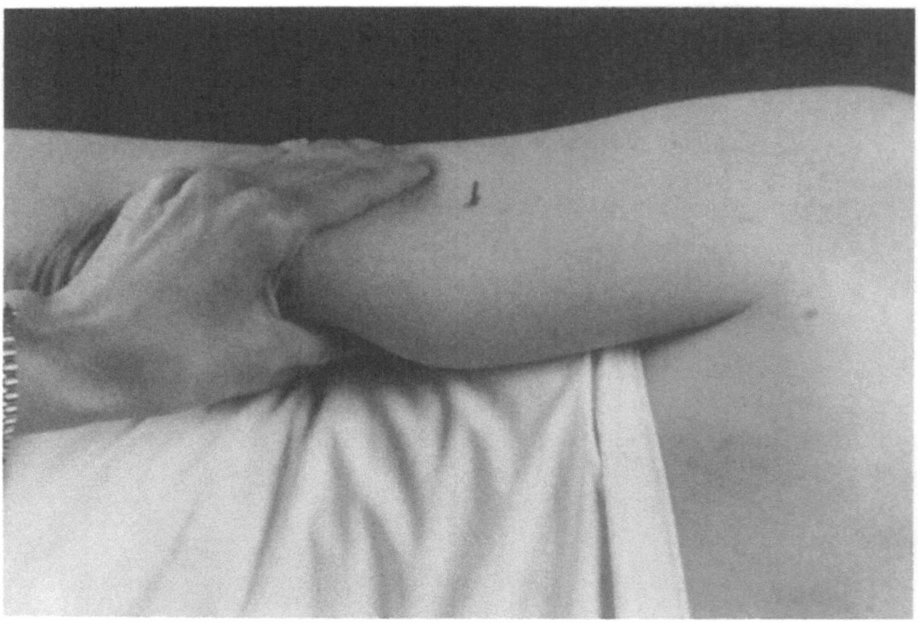

Fig. 11. Grasping the triceps skinfold. (Printed with permission of Ross Laboratories, Columbus, Ohio.)

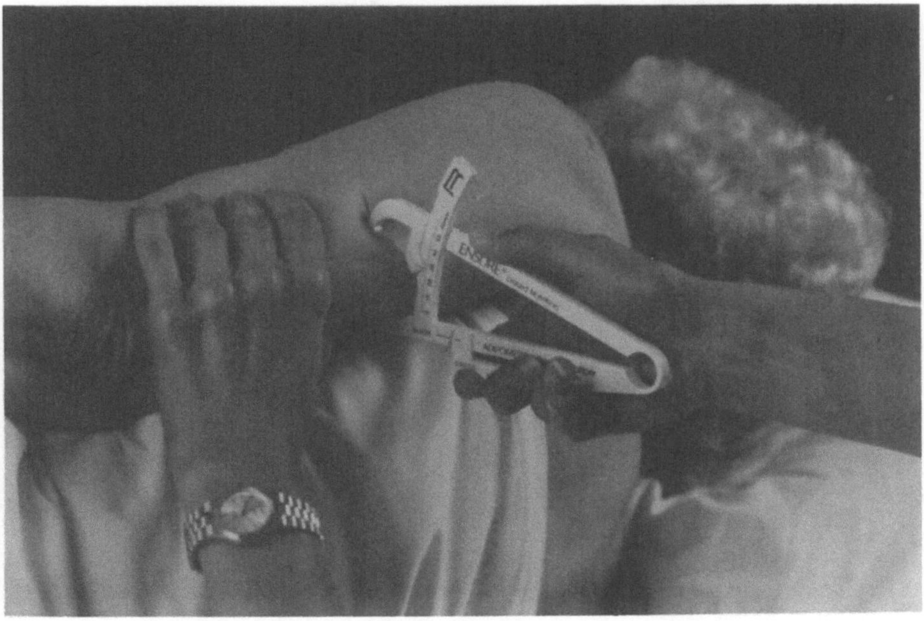

Fig. 12. Measuring the triceps skinfold. (Printed with permission of Ross Laboratories, Columbus, Ohio.)

arm (Fig. 11). The skinfold is grasped to separate the subcutaneous adipose tissue from the underlying muscle. The skinfold is held while the jaws of the caliper are placed perpendicular to the length of the skinfold at the level of the marked midpoint (Fig. 12). In order to avoid errors from parallax, the measurer should bend down to read the caliper.

After about 3 sec, the measurement is read and recorded to the nearest 0.2 mm with a Holtain caliper, and successive measurements should agree within 4 mm. In some elderly persons, the skinfold caliper may take longer to stabilize, particularly if the tissue is edematous.

5.5. Subscapular Skinfold Thickness

This measurement is taken with the elderly person in the same body position as for the measurement of triceps skinfold thickness. Subscapular skinfold thickness is measured just posterior to the inferior angle of the left scapula. The measurer gently grasps a double fold of skin and subcutaneous adipose tissue between the fingers and thumb, on a line from the inferior angle of the left scapula to the left elbow (Fig. 13). Grasping the skinfold separates subcutaneous adipose tissue from the underlying muscle. The skinfold is held while the caliper is positioned perpendicular to the length of the skinfold. The jaws of the caliper are applied medial to the fingers, at a point lateral to and just inferior to the inferior angle of the scapula (Fig. 14). After about 3 sec, the measurement is read and recorded to the nearest 0.2 mm with a Holtain caliper, and successive measurements should agree within 4 mm.

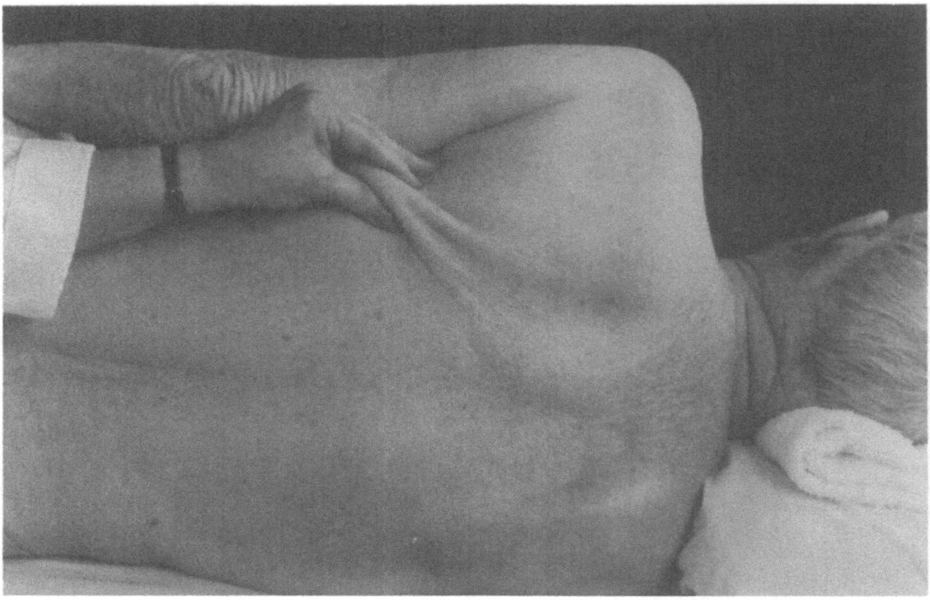

Fig. 13. Grasping the subscapular skinfold. (Printed with permission of Ross Laboratories, Columbus, Ohio.)

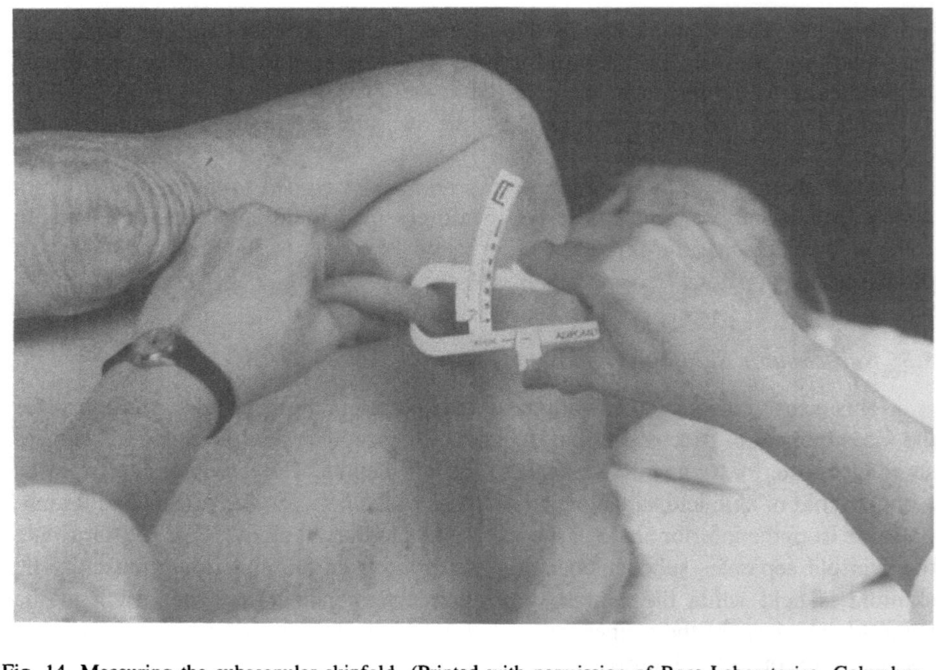

Fig. 14. Measuring the subscapular skinfold. (Printed with permission of Ross Laboratories, Columbus, Ohio.)

6. Derived Measurements and Indices of Nutritional Status

Once stature and weight and/or the recumbent measurements have been taken, these data can be used to derive additional quantitative indexes that can be used in the assessment of nutritional status of the elderly. Estimates of stature and body weight can be computed if they have not been measured. An index of obesity can be derived by dividing weight by stature squared (W/S^2), and midarm muscle area can be calculated also. These computed measurements are derived easily and accurately using a calculator and the appropriate formulas, or all measurements except body weight can be estimated from appropriate nomograms.

6.1. Stature from Knee Height

Knee height is used to estimate the stature of an elderly person who is bedfast or chairbound or who has such spinal curvature that an accurate stature measurement cannot be obtained. The estimated stature value can then be used in indexes such as W/S^2 or in estimates of basal energy expenditure (Harris and Benedict, 1919; Benedict, 1928; Boothby *et al.*, 1936; Dubois, 1936; Blackburn *et al.*, 1977; Long *et al.*, 1979).

The computation of an estimate of stature requires the person's knee height, age, and sex. There is one formula for men and another for women. The knee height measurement is recorded in centimeters, and age is rounded to the nearest whole year; the computed value of stature is (in centimeters):

$$\text{Stature for men} = [2.02 \times \text{knee height}] - [0.04 \times \text{age}] + 64.19$$

$$\text{Stature for women} = [1.83 \times \text{knee height}] - [0.24 \times \text{age}] + 84.88$$

Like knee height, arm span is highly correlated with stature, changes little with age, and has been proposed as a substitute for a measure of stature (Brown and Wigzell, 1963; Dequeker *et al.*, 1969). This is not recommended because arm span is too difficult to measure reliably in nonambulatory elderly persons or those with significant chest or spinal deformities (Mitchell and Lipschitz, 1982b). Total arm length has also been recommended as a substitute for stature in indices of nutritional status because it can be measured in the nonambulatory elderly, does not change with age, and is highly correlated with stature ($r = 0.68$; Mitchell and Lipschitz, 1982b). Knee height is preferred to total arm length because it is a component of stature, and it is more highly correlated with stature than total arm length or other arm-length measurements (Zoreb *et al.*, 1963). Also, the interobserver reliability for knee height is better than that for arm-length measurements (Chumlea *et al.*, 1985a).

The 90% error bounds for the estimated stature of an individual who has a knee height equal to the mean is ± 6.36 cm for men and ± 5.82 cm for women. For individuals with knee heights at plus or minus two standard deviations from the mean, the errors for the estimated statures are the same for men and women. These estimation equations were not developed from a nationally representative sample of elderly persons in the United States, so caution is needed when they are applied to other groups of elderly persons (Chumlea *et al.*, 1985a).

6.2. Weight from Anthropometry

Weight can be estimated for an elderly person from anthropometric data when it cannot be measured directly because of infirmity or fractures requiring traction or casting. Like estimates of stature, estimates of weight can also be used in indexes such as W/S^2 or estimates of energy expenditure using the Harris–Benedict (1919) equation. The estimate of weight requires measurement of calf circumference (*calf C*), knee height (*knee H*), midarm circumference (*MAC*), and subscapular skinfold thickness (*subsc SF*). Most of these measures are in common clinical use and are known to be important in assessing anthropometric nutritional status in the elderly (Blackburn *et al.*, 1977; Chumlea *et al.*, 1985a,c, 1986; Lohman *et al.*, 1988). There are separate equations for men and women.

$$\text{Body weight for men} = (0.98 \times \textit{calf C}) + (1.16 \times \textit{knee H}) + (1.72 \times \textit{MAC}) + (0.37 \times \textit{subsc SF}) - 81.69$$

$$\text{Body weight for women} = (1.27 \times \textit{calf C}) + (0.87 \times \textit{knee H}) + (0.98 \times \textit{MAC}) + (0.4 \times \textit{subsc SF}) - 62.35$$

This method of predicting the body weight of an elderly person with known error makes use of body measurements that are indices of the actual constituents of body composition. Therefore, they are useful apart from their application to the estimation of weight. All these measurements can be collected regardless of an elderly person's level of mobility. Substantial changes in these body measurements should correspond to changes in weight. The equations to estimate weight have a 95% probability of predicting the weight of an elderly man or woman to within plus or minus 8.96 kg or 7.60 kg, respectively (Chumlea *et al.*, 1988).

Besides the equations presented here, there are other equations for predicting the weight of elderly persons that use only two or three body measurements. Although this allows the selection of an equation based on the measurements that can be collected for an individual, the errors of prediction are larger with the use of fewer than four predictor variables or if insufficient attention is given to measurement technique (Chumlea *et al.*, 1988).

6.3. Weight Divided by Stature Squared

Weight divided by stature squared (W/S^2) is an index of obesity and is the best simple indicator of total body fat. It is also an excellent indicator of the amount of body fat expressed as a percentage of body weight (percentage body fat; Roche *et al.*, 1981). A young person with a high W/S^2 value has a greater chance of having more body fat than a person with a relatively low W/S^2 value. Some do not consider W/S^2 useful in many elderly persons because stature decreases in the elderly with age (Dequeker *et al.*, 1969), so interrelations based on present stature are problematic. Depending on the degree of spinal curvature, stature may be a measure of questionable value in some elderly individuals or impossible to measure in others. Since stature can be reliably estimated from knee height and age (Chumlea *et al.*, 1985a), W/S^2 can be used as an index of the degree of obesity in almost all elderly persons. The complete interpretation of W/S^2 in the elderly is uncertain as yet, because the statistical associations between W/S^2 and body fatness from densitometry have not been determined in large representative samples of the elderly.

The W/S^2 index is calculated by first multiplying the elderly person's stature (in meters) by itself and then dividing this number into the person's weight (in kilograms). The amount is then multiplied by 10,000 (10^4) to move the decimal point.

6.4. Midarm Muscle Area

Midarm muscle area (*MAMA*) is an index of the amount of muscle or lean tissue in the body. Lean tissue is metabolically active and useful in determining drug dosages and basal metabolic rates. The computation of midarm muscle area is based on measurements of midarm circumference and triceps skinfold thickness. Because midarm circumference is measured in centimeters and triceps skinfold thickness in millimeters, the latter is converted to centimeters by dividing by 10 in the following formula to compute midarm muscle area:

$$\text{Midarm muscle area (cm}^2) = [\text{midarm circumference (cm)} - \pi \times (\text{triceps skinfold thickness (mm)}/10)^2]/4\pi$$

The use of this formula with recumbent measurements is appropriate because there is no systematic difference between corresponding standing and recumbent measurements (Chumlea *et al.*, 1985b). It has been shown, however, that MAMA calculated from the present formula is an overestimate when compared to actual values from computerized tomographic cross sections at the midpoint of the upper arm in adults (Heymsfield *et al.*, 1979, 1982). Because of these findings, Heymsfield and associates recommend the use of corrected formulas for estimates of *MAMA* and "available *MAMA*," adjusting for the cross-sectional area of bone, but these have not been proven valid in the elderly (Heymsfield, *et al.*, 1982).

7. Interpreting Anthropometric Data in a Nutritional Assessment

The anthropometric data and the indices W/S^2 and *MAMA* can help to identify those nonambulatory elderly persons who may be at nutritional risk for obesity or have inadequate protein reserves. A complete anthropometric nutritional assessment record for an elderly person consists of a combination of tabulated and plotted measurements. After measurements are taken, they should be recorded on an appropriate chart, along with any information relevant to measurement problems or the techniques used (Chumlea *et al.*, 1987; Fig. 15). This simplifies the comparison of current data with previous data. Plotting the data immediately facilitates communication with the elderly individual or caretaker about nutritional status, possible intervention, and follow-up. If any value appears unusual in view of earlier findings, the elderly person should be remeasured to verify the current data. An actual change in an anthropometric finding

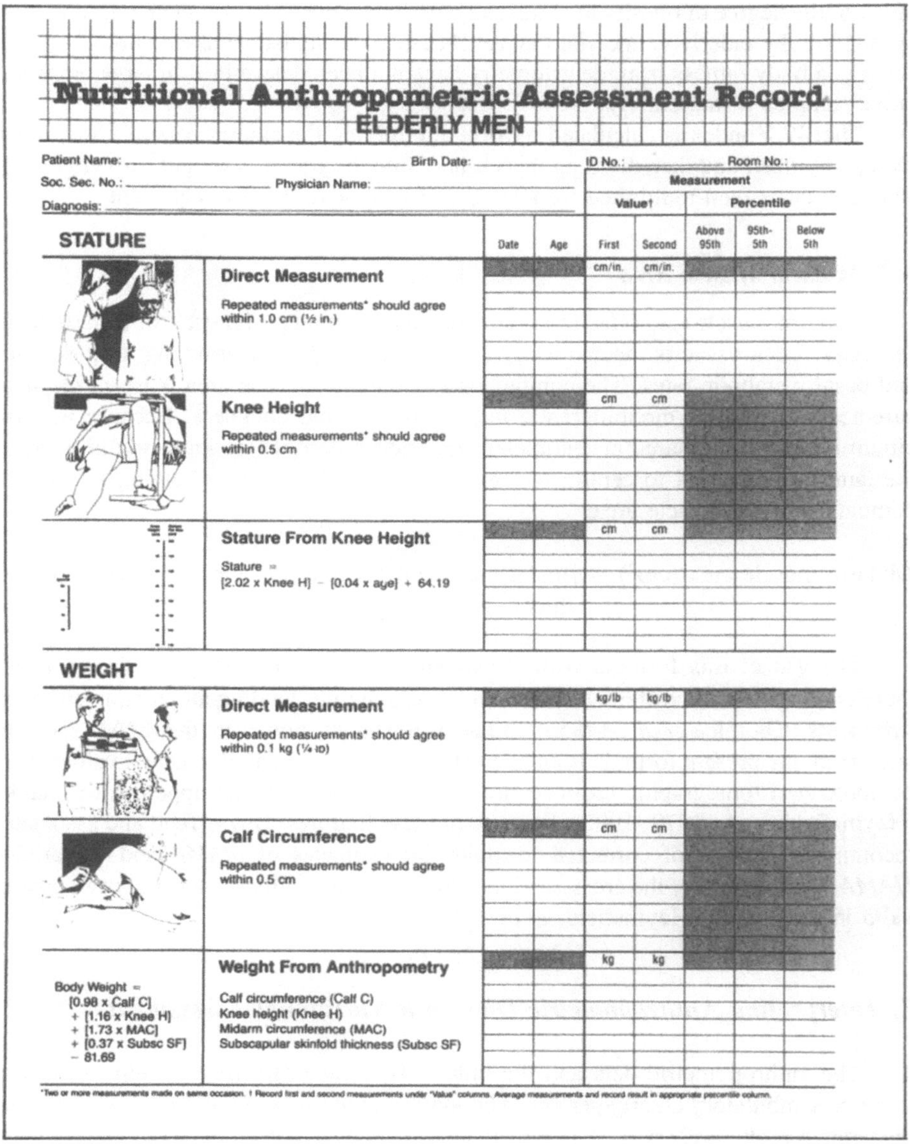

Nutritional Anthropometric Assessment Record
ELDERLY MEN

Patient Name: Birth Date: ID No.: Room No.:
Soc. Sec. No.: Physician Name:
Diagnosis:

Date | Age | Measurement: Value† (First, Second) | Percentile (Above 95th, 95th–5th, Below 5th)

STATURE

Direct Measurement
Repeated measurements* should agree within 1.0 cm (½ in.)
cm/in. cm/in.

Knee Height
Repeated measurements* should agree within 0.5 cm
cm cm

Stature From Knee Height
Stature = [2.02 x Knee H] − [0.04 x age] + 64.19
cm cm

WEIGHT

Direct Measurement
Repeated measurements* should agree within 0.1 kg (¼ lb)
kg/lb kg/lb

Calf Circumference
Repeated measurements* should agree within 0.5 cm
cm cm

Weight From Anthropometry
Body Weight = [0.98 x Calf C] + [1.16 x Knee H] + [1.73 x MAC] + [0.37 x Subsc SF] − 81.69
Calf circumference (Calf C)
Knee height (Knee H)
Midarm circumference (MAC)
Subscapular skinfold thickness (Subsc SF)
kg kg

*Two or more measurements made on same occasion. † Record first and second measurements under "Value" columns. Average measurements and record result in appropriate percentile column.

Fig. 15. Recording record for anthropometric data on an elderly man. (Printed with permission of Ross Laboratories, Columbus, Ohio.)

can signal a potential shift in nutritional status. Such a change would have been missed if earlier measurements had not been available for comparison.

The anthropometric nutritional assessment data for an elderly person are more informative, however, if they are plotted on reference charts for elderly individuals. An example of these charts for men is presented in Fig. 16. Anthropometric nutritional

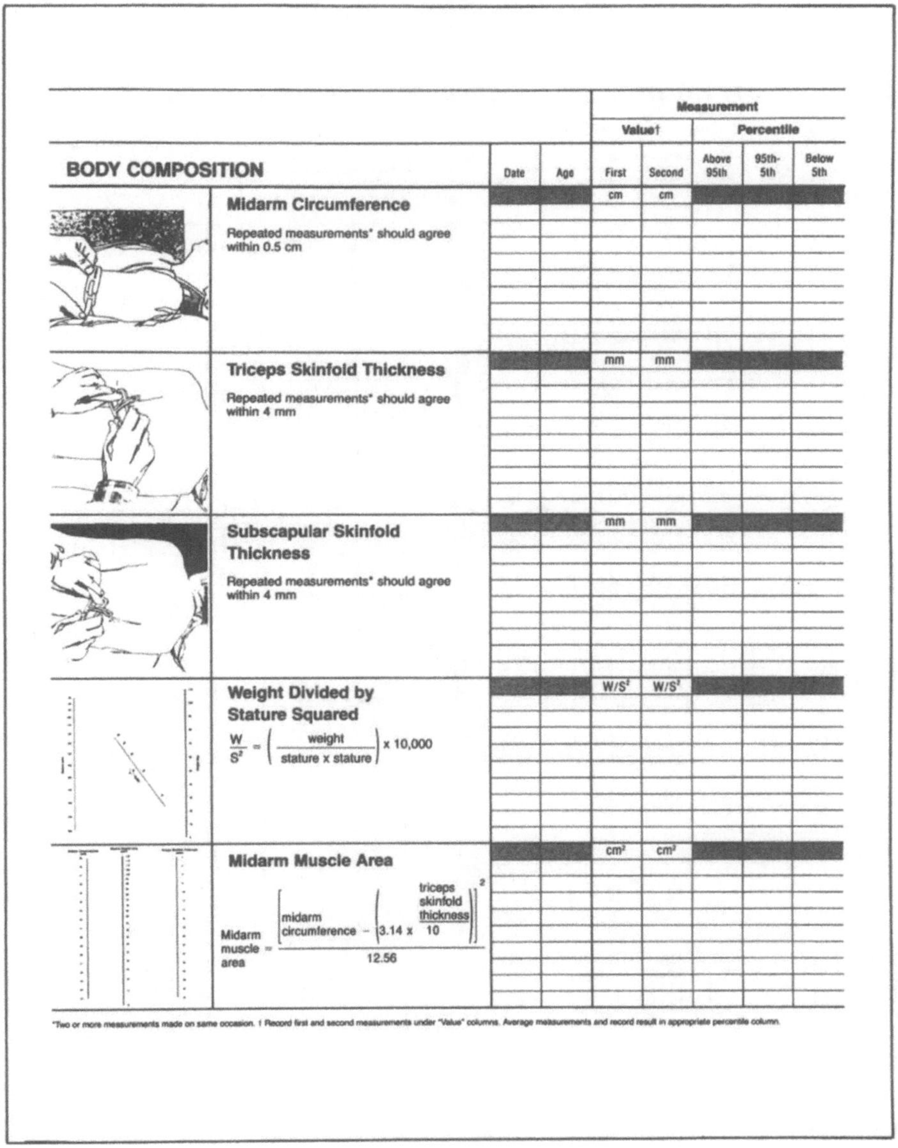

BODY COMPOSITION		Date	Age	Measurement: Value† First	Second	Percentile: Above 95th	95th-5th	Below 5th
	Midarm Circumference Repeated measurements* should agree within 0.5 cm			cm	cm			
	Triceps Skinfold Thickness Repeated measurements* should agree within 4 mm			mm	mm			
	Subscapular Skinfold Thickness Repeated measurements* should agree within 4 mm			mm	mm			
	Weight Divided by Stature Squared $\frac{W}{S^2} = \left(\frac{\text{weight}}{\text{stature} \times \text{stature}}\right) \times 10{,}000$			W/S²	W/S²			
	Midarm Muscle Area $\text{Midarm muscle area} = \frac{\left[\text{midarm circumference} - \left(3.14 \times \frac{\text{triceps skinfold thickness}}{10}\right)\right]^2}{12.56}$			cm²	cm²			

*Two or more measurements made on same occasion. † Record first and second measurements under "Value" columns. Average measurements and record result in appropriate percentile column.

Fig. 15. *(continued)*

assessment charts are used to plot an individual's nutritional anthropometric values at any year between ages 65 and 90 years. Plotting serial nutritional anthropometric values can reveal an abnormal change that warrants further evaluation (Chumlea *et al.*, 1987). Unusual values and/or patterns of change in nutritional anthropometry are useful in identifying, as early as possible, those elderly persons who need diagnostic tests and nutritional intervention. Serial assessment can also help monitor the effective-

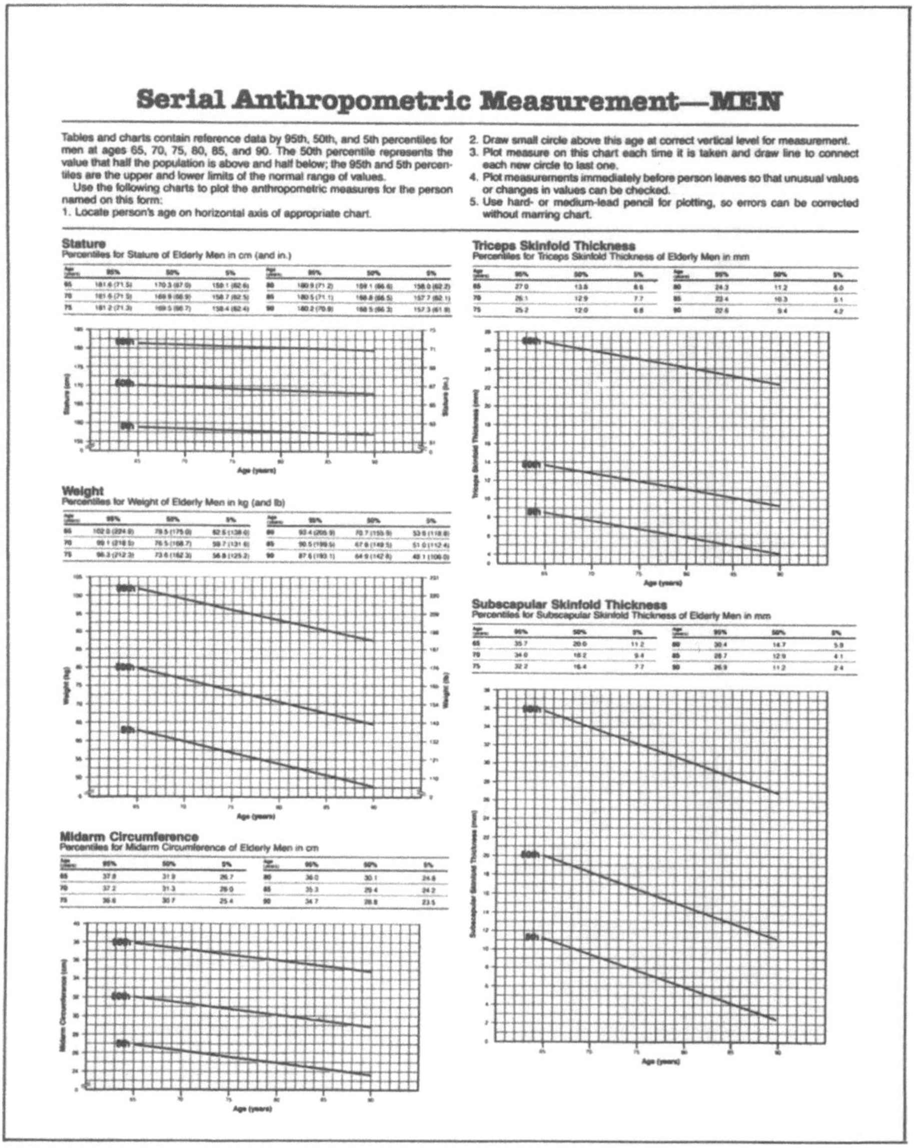

Serial Anthropometric Measurement—MEN

Tables and charts contain reference data by 95th, 50th, and 5th percentiles for men at ages 65, 70, 75, 80, 85, and 90. The 50th percentile represents the value that half the population is above and half below; the 95th and 5th percentiles are the upper and lower limits of the normal range of values.

Use the following charts to plot the anthropometric measures for the person named on this form:

1. Locate person's age on horizontal axis of appropriate chart.
2. Draw small circle above this age at correct vertical level for measurement.
3. Plot measure on this chart each time it is taken and draw line to connect each new circle to last one.
4. Plot measurements immediately before person leaves so that unusual values or changes in values can be checked.
5. Use hard- or medium-lead pencil for plotting, so errors can be corrected without marring chart.

Stature
Percentiles for Stature of Elderly Men in cm (and in.)

Age (years)	95%	50%	5%
65	181.6 (71.5)	170.3 (67.0)	159.1 (62.6)
70	181.6 (71.5)	169.9 (66.9)	158.7 (62.5)
75	181.2 (71.3)	169.5 (66.7)	158.4 (62.4)
80	180.9 (71.2)	169.1 (66.6)	158.0 (62.2)
85	180.5 (71.1)	168.8 (66.5)	157.7 (62.1)
90	180.2 (70.9)	168.5 (66.3)	157.3 (61.9)

Weight
Percentiles for Weight of Elderly Men in kg (and lb)

Age (years)	95%	50%	5%
65	102.0 (224.9)	79.5 (175.0)	62.5 (138.0)
70	99.1 (218.5)	76.5 (168.7)	59.7 (131.6)
75	96.3 (212.3)	73.6 (162.3)	56.8 (125.2)
80	93.4 (205.9)	70.7 (155.9)	53.9 (118.8)
85	90.5 (199.5)	67.8 (149.5)	51.0 (112.4)
90	87.6 (193.1)	64.9 (142.8)	48.1 (106.0)

Midarm Circumference
Percentiles for Midarm Circumference of Elderly Men in cm

Age (years)	95%	50%	5%
65	37.8	31.9	26.7
70	37.2	31.3	26.0
75	36.6	30.7	25.4
80	36.0	30.1	24.8
85	35.3	29.4	24.2
90	34.7	28.8	23.5

Triceps Skinfold Thickness
Percentiles for Triceps Skinfold Thickness of Elderly Men in mm

Age (years)	95%	50%	5%
65	27.0	13.5	6.6
70	26.1	12.9	7.7
75	25.2	12.0	6.8
80	24.3	11.2	6.0
85	23.4	10.3	5.1
90	22.6	9.4	4.2

Subscapular Skinfold Thickness
Percentiles for Subscapular Skinfold Thickness of Elderly Men in mm

Age (years)	95%	50%	5%
65	35.7	20.0	11.2
70	34.0	18.2	9.4
75	32.2	16.4	7.7
80	30.4	14.7	5.9
85	28.7	12.9	4.1
90	26.9	11.2	2.4

Fig. 16. Charts for plotting anthropometric data for an elderly man. (Printed with permission of Ross Laboratories, Columbus, Ohio.)

ness of nutritional intervention. Similar national reference data for a representative sample of persons aged 75 years and older are lacking, and the only reference data for recumbent anthropometry are those reported here (Chumlea *et al.*, 1985c, 1987). These data were collected from 269 elderly white men and women who were free-living voluntary ambulatory residents at four establishments for the elderly in southwest Ohio. Each participant walked to one testing area, but health questionnaires and physical examinations were not conducted.

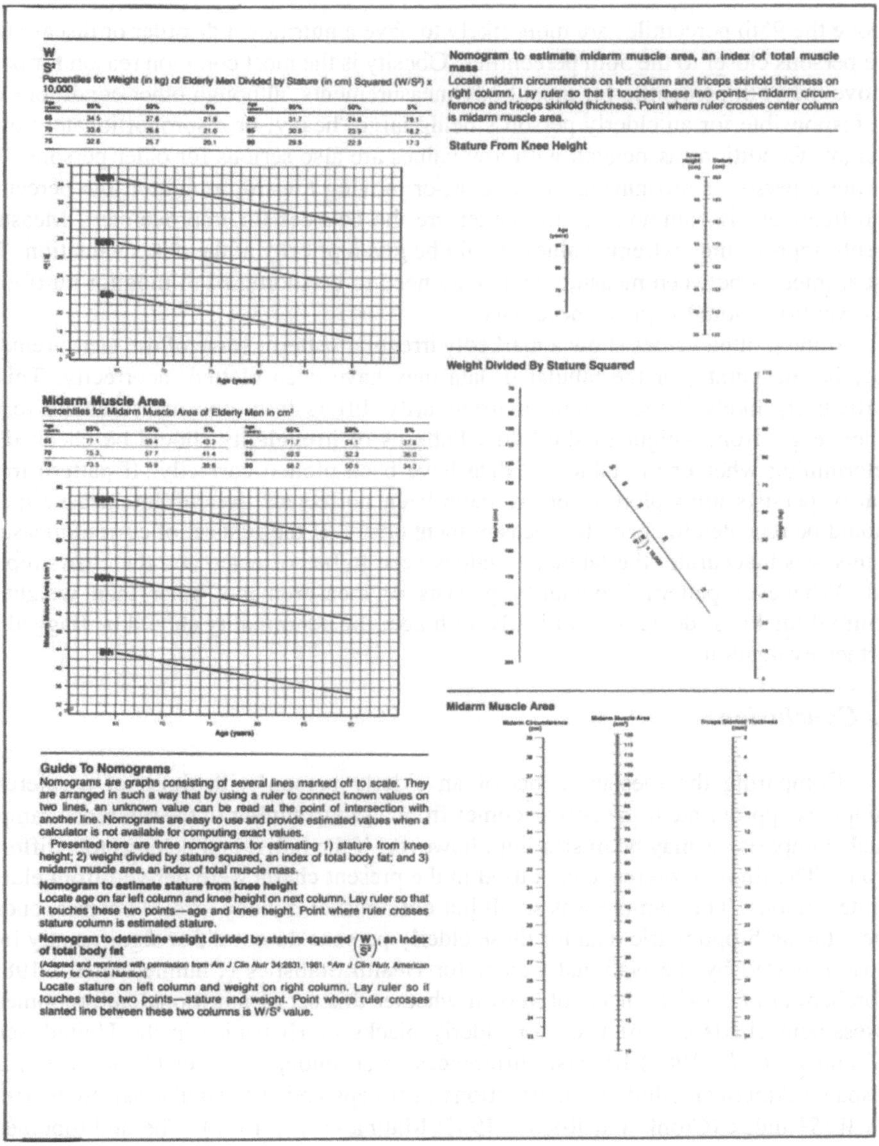

Fig. 16. (*continued*)

8. The Significance of Extremes of Body Size in the Elderly

Body measurements are distributed in an adult population in a continuous manner, with a gradation of individuals from the shortest to the tallest and from the leanest to the fattest. One needs to be concerned about a person near one of the extremes because of the complex interaction of an elderly individual's nutrient intake, body composition, activity level, and state of health. Accurate records of nutritional anthropometric data are important because persons near the extremes, those below the fifth percentile or above the 95th percentile, are more likely to have a nutritional disorder or disease than are persons closer to the 50th percentiles. Obesity is the most common reason for being above the 95th percentile for most body measurements, although other conditions can be responsible for an elderly person's being large, heavy, or disproportionately overweight. Conditions associated with low values are also serious for older persons. The earlier a person is recognized as being at, or moving toward, a high or low percentile and treatment is commenced, the better are the chances for improvement. Measurements approaching extreme values should be given priority at the next evaluation. The usual interval between measurements may need to be shortened to monitor nutritional intervention should it prove necessary.

If the plotted values show a markedly irregular pattern, some of the measurements may be inaccurate, or the tabulated data may have been plotted incorrectly. This is particularly likely if the pattern of irregularity differs from one measurement to another, e.g., from weight to skinfolds. Patterns of irregularity should be checked by determining whether the tabulated data have been plotted correctly. If pattern irregularity persists after plotting errors have been corrected, the current measurements should be repeated to check for measurement errors. If the first set of current measurements was inaccurate, the tabulated values need to be corrected and the charts replotted. Whenever pattern irregularity persists or measurements other than weight or skinfold thickness decrease erratically with age, the abnormality should be flagged for further evaluation.

9. Conclusion

Comparing the measurements of an elderly person with those of a reference sample is appropriate if the person comes from a group similar to the reference sample. Such comparisons may be misleading, however, if the individual belongs to a different group. The limited reference data used in the present charts were derived from elderly white persons. This sample was small but not unusual in body size. At corresponding ages, the anthropometric data for these elderly persons do not differ significantly from those reported by the National Center for Health Statistics (Chumlea *et al.*, 1985c; Abraham *et al.*, 1978). It is not known whether this set of nutritional anthropometric assessment charts can be used for elderly blacks or Hispanics in the United States (Chumlea *et al.*, 1987) because differences exist among younger black, white, and Hispanic American adults in distributions of triceps and subscapular skinfolds and in the W/S^2 index (Cronk and Roche, 1982; Malina *et al.*, 1983). The anthropometric techniques, indices, and limited reference data presented here, when combined with the other components of a nutritional assessment, can provide a very good picture of the nutritional status or change in nutritional status for an elderly person regardless of his or her level of mobility. Although these reference data are not completely applicable to black and Hispanic elderly persons, they can be used effectively to monitor changes in the nutritional status of elderly persons regardless of race.

10. References

Abraham, S., Johnson, C. L., and Najjar, M. F., 1978, *Weight and Height of Adults 18–74 Years of Age, Vital and Health Statistics Series 11* No. 211, DHEW Publication No. (PHS) 79-165, Rockville, MD.

Arnold, J. S., Bartley, M. H., Tont, S. A., and Jenkins, D. P., 1966, Skeletal changes in aging and disease, *Clin. Orthop.* **49:**17–37.

Bastow, M. D., 1982, Anthropometrics revisited, *Proc. Nutr. Soc.* **41:**381–388.

Benedict, F. G., 1928, Basal metabolism data on normal men and women (series II) with some considerations of the use of prediction standards, *Am. J. Physiol.* **85:**607–613.

Blackburn, G. L., Bistrian, B. R., Maini, B. S., Schlamm, H. T., and Smith, M. F., 1977, Nutritional and metabolic assessment of the hospitalized patient, *J. Parent. Ent. Nutr.* **1:**11–22.

Boothby, W. M., Berkson, S. R., and Dunn, H. L., 1936, Studies of the energy metabolism of normal individuals: A standard for basal metabolism with nomogram for clinical application, *Am. J. Physiol.* **116:**468–473.

Borkan, G. A., and Hults, D. E., 1983, Change in body fat content and distribution during aging, *Am. J. Phys. Anthrop.* **60:**175.

Borkan, G. A., and Norris, A. H., 1977, Fat distributions and the changing body dimensions of the adult male, *Hum. Biol.* **49:**495–514.

Borkan, G. A., Sparrow, D., Wisniewski, C., and Vokonos, P. S., 1986, Body weight and coronary disease risk: Patterns of risk factor change associated with long-term weight change, *Am. J. Epidemiol.* **124:**410–419.

Bowman, B. B., and Rosenberg, I. H., 1982, Assessment of the nutritional status of the elderly, *Am. J. Clin. Nutr.* **35:**1142–1151.

Brown, O. T., and Wigzell, F. W., 1963, The significance of span as a clinical measurement. Conference on Medical and Surgical Aspects of Aging, in: *Current Achievements in Geriatrics,* Cassell, London, pp. 246–251.

Butterworth, C. E., and Blackburn, G. L., 1975, Hospital malnutrition, *Nutr. Today* **10:**8–18.

Cameron, N., 1978, The methods of auxological anthropometry, in: *Human Growth,* Volume 2, *Postnatal Growth* (F. Falkner and J. M. Tanner eds.), Plenum Press, New York, pp. 35–90.

Chumlea, W. C., Roche, A. F., and Rogers, E., 1984a, Replicability for anthropometry in the elderly, *Hum. Biol.* **56:**329–337.

Chumlea, W. C., Roche, A. F., and Webb, P., 1984b, Body size, subcutaneous fatness and total body fat in older adults, *Int. J. Obesity* **8:**313–317.

Chumlea, W. C., Roche, A. F., and Steinbaugh, M. L., 1985a, Estimating stature from knee height for persons 60 to 90 years of age, *J. Am. Geriatr. Soc.* **33:**116–120.

Chumlea, W. C., Roche, A. F., Steinbaugh, M. L., and Mukherjee, D., 1985b, Errors of measurement for methods of recumbent nutritional anthropometry in the elderly, *J. Nutr. Elderly* **5:**3–11.

Chumlea, W. C., Steinbaugh, M. L., Roche, A. F., Mukherjee, D., and Gopalaswamy, N., 1985c, Nutritional anthropometric assessment in elderly persons 65 to 90 years of age, *J. Nutr. Elderly* **4:**39–51.

Chumlea, W. C., Roche, A. F., and Mukherjee, D., 1986, Some anthropometric indices of body composition for elderly adults, *J. Gerontol.* **41:**36–39.

Chumlea, W. C., Roche, A. F., and Mukherjee, D., 1987, *Nutritional Assessment in the Elderly Through Anthropometry,* Ross Laboratories, Columbus, OH.

Chumlea, W. C., Guo, S., and Roche, A. F., 1988, Prediction of body weight for the nonambulatory elderly, *J. Am. Diet. Assoc.* **88:**564–568.

Cronk, C. E., and Roche, A. F., 1982, Race- and sex-specific reference data for triceps and subscapular skinfolds and weight/stature.^{2}, *Am. J. Clin. Nutr.* **35:**347–354.

Dequeker, J. V., Baeyers, J. B., and Claessens, J., 1969, The significance of stature as a clinical measurement of aging, *J. Am. Geriatr. Soc.* **17:**169–179.

Dubois, E. F., 1936, *Basal Metabolism in Health and Disease,* 3rd ed., Lea & Febiger, Philadelphia.

Durnin, J. V. G. A., and Womersley, J., 1974, Body fat assessed from total body density and its estimation from skinfold thickness: Measurements on 481 men and women aged from 16 to 72 years, *Br. J. Nutr.* **32:**77–97.

Exton-Smith, A. N., 1982, Epidemiological studies in the elderly: Methodological considerations, *Am. J. Clin. Nutr.* **35:**1273–1279.

Fanelli, M. T., 1987, The ABC's of nutritional assessment in older adults, *J. Nutr. Elderly* **6:**33–40.

Fentem, P. H., Jones, P. R. M., MacDonald, I. C., and Scriven, P. M., 1976, Changes in the body composition of elderly men following retirement from the steel industry, *J. Physiol. (Lond.)* **258:**29P–30P.

Fisher, S., Hendricks, D. G., and Mahoney, A. W., 1978, Nutritional assessments of senior rural Utahns by biochemical and physical measurements, *Am. J. Clin. Nutr.* **31:**667–672.

Forbes, G. B., 1976, The adult decline in lean body mass, *Hum. Biol.* **48:**161–173.

Grahame, R., 1970, A method for measuring human skin elasticity *in vivo* with observations on the effects of age, sex and pregnancy, *Clin. Sci.* **39:**223–238.

Guenter, P. A., Moore, K., Crosby, L. O., Buzby, G. P., and Mullen, J. L., 1982, Body Weight measurement of patients receiving nutritional support, *J. Parent. Ent. Nutr.* **6:**441–443.

Harris, J. A., and Benedict, F. G., 1919, *A Biometric Study of Basal Metabolism in Man,* Carnegie Institute of Washington, Washington.

Heber, D., 1986, Assessing nutritional status of the elderly, *Diagnosis* **8:**41–62.

Heymsfield, S. B., Olalson, R. P., Kutner, M. H., and Nixon, D. W., 1979, A radiographic method of quantifying protein–caloric malnutrition, *Am. J. Clin. Nutr.* **32:**693–702.

Heymsfield, S. B., McManus, C., Smith, J., Stevens, V., and Nixon, D. W., 1982, Anthropometric measurement of muscle mass: Revised equations for calculating bone-free arm muscle area, *Am. J. Clin. Nutr.* **36:**680–690.

Himes, J. H., Roche, A. F., and Siervogel, R. M., 1979, Compressibility of skinfolds and the measurement of subcutaneous fatness, *Am. J. Clin. Nutr.* **32:**1734–1740.

Kemm, J. R., and Allcock, J., 1984, The distribution of supposed indicators of nutritional status in elderly patients, *Age Aging* **13:**21–28.

Laitiner, O., 1978, Osteoporosis, nature, treatment and possible future trends, *Public Health Rev.* **7:**169–195.

Laubach, L. L., Glaser, R. M., and Suryaprasad, A. G., 1981, Anthropometry of aged male wheelchair-dependent patients, *Ann. Hum. Biol.* **8:**25–29.

Lohman, T., Martorell, R., and Roche, A. F. (eds.), 1988, *Anthropometric Standardization Reference Manual* Human Kinetics, Champaign, IL.

Long, C. L., Schaffel, N., and Gieger, J. W., 1979, Metabolic response to injury and illness: Estimation of energy and protein needs from indirect calorimetry and nitrogen balance, *J. Parent. Eng. Nutr.* **3:**452–456.

MacLenman, W. J., Hall, M. R. P., Timothy, J. I., and Robinson, M., 1980, Is weakness in old age due to muscle wasting? *Age Aging* **9:**188–192.

Malina, R. M., Little, B. B., Stern, M. P., Gaskill, S. P., and Hazuda, H. P., 1983, Ethnic and social class differences in selected anthropometric characteristics of Mexican American and Anglo adults: The San Antonio heart study, *Hum. Biol.* **55:**867–883.

Mitchell, C. O., and Lipschitz, D. A., 1982a, The effects of age and sex on the routinely used measurements to assess the nutritional status of hospitalized patients, *Am. J. Clin. Nutr.* **36:**340–349.

Mitchell, C. O., and Lipschitz, D. A., 1982b, Arm length measurement as an alternative to height in nutritional assessments of the elderly, *J. Parent. Ent. Nutr.* **6:**226–229.

Mitchell, C. O., and Lipschitz, D. A., 1982c, Detection of protein caloric malnutrition in the elderly, *Am. J. Clin. Nutr.* **35:**398–406.

Noppa, H., Anderson, M., Bengtsson, C., Bruce, A., and Isaksson, B., 1979, Body composition in middle-aged women with special reference in the correlation between body fat mass and anthropometric data, *Am. J. Clin. Nutr.* **32:**1388–1395.

Norris, A. H., Lundy, T., and Shock, N. W., 1963, Trends in selected indices of body composition in men between the ages 30 and 90 years, *Ann. N.Y. Acad. Sci.* **110:**623–639.

Novak, L. P., 1972, Aging, total body potassium, fat-free mass and cell mass in males and females between ages 18 and 85 years, *J. Gerontol.* **27:**438–443.

Patrick, J. M., Baasey, E. J., and Fentem, P. H., 1982, Changes in body fat and muscle in manual workers and at the retirement, *Eur. J. Appl. Physiol.* **49:**187–196.

Roche, A. F., Siervogel, R. M., Chumlea, W. C., and Webb, P., 1981, Grading body fatness from limited anthropometric data, *Am. J. Clin. Nutr.* **34:**2831–2838.

Rossman, I., 1977, Anatomic and body composition changes with aging, in: *Handbook of the Biology of Aging* (C. E. Finch and L. Hayflick, eds.), Van Nostrand, New York, pp. 189–221.

Rowe, J. W., and Kahn, R. L., 1987, Human aging: Usual and successful, *Science* **237:**143–149.

Steen, B., Bruce, A., Isaksson, B., Levin, T., and Ivanborg, A., 1977, Body composition in 70-year-old males and females in Gothenburg, Sweden—a population study, *Acta Med. Scand.* [*Suppl.*] **611:**87–112.

Steen, G. B., Isaksson, B., and Svanberg, A., 1979, Body composition at 70 and 75 years of age. A longitudinal population study, *J. Clin. Exp. Gerontol.* **1:**185–200.

Stoudt, H. W., Damon, A., McFarland, R. A., and Roberts, J., 1965, *Weight, Height and Selected Body Dimensions of Adults, Vital and Health Statistics Series 11,* DHEW Publication No. (PHS) 1000, Rockville, MD.

Vir, S. C., and Love, A. H. G., 1980, Anthropometric measurements in the elderly, *Gerontology* **26:**1–8.

Ward, G. M., Krzywicki, H. J., Rahman, D. P., Quaas, R. L., Nelson, R. A., and Consolazio, C. F., 1975, Relationship of anthropometric measurements to body fat as determined by densitometry, potassium-40, and body water, *Am. J. Clin. Nutr.* **28:**162–169.

Wessel, J. A., Ufer, A., Van Huss, W. D., and Cederquist, D., 1963, Age trends of various components of body composition and functional characteristics in women 29–69 years, *Ann. N.Y. Acad. Sci.* **110:**608–622.

Young, C. M., Blondin, J., Tensuan, R., and Fryer, J. H., 1963, Body composition studies of "older" women thirty to seventy years of age, *Ann. N.Y. Acad. Sci.* **110:**589–607.

Zoreb, P. A., Prime, F. J., and Harrison, A., 1963, Estimation of height from tibial length, *Lancet* **1:**195–196.

14

Drug–Nutrient Interactions in the Elderly

Daphne A. Roe

1. Classification of Drug–Nutrient Interactions and Their Effects

Drug–nutrient interactions include physicochemical, physiological, and pathophysiological events that are inherent to drug usage (Roe, 1985a). These events, which are summarized in Table I, may affect the disposition of drugs and nutrients.

1.1. Physicochemical Interactions

Physicochemical interactions that occur in the gastrointestinal tract between food components and drugs may alter rates of drug transit, drug dissolution, absorption, or metabolism as well as the digestion, absorption, and metabolism of nutrients. The dissolution of a drug may be promoted by dietary fat, by alcohol, or by intentional food additives that are surface-active agents. Dissolution of griseofulvin, a fat-soluble drug, is promoted by fats such as corn oil or other dietary fats. Antihistamine capsules are dissolved faster when there is concurrent ingestion of alcohol. The rate and extent of absorption of phenacetin are enhanced by polysorbate 80, which is used as an emulsifier in ice cream and frozen custard (Becker *et al.*, 1974; Benarde, 1971; Kabasakalian *et al.*, 1970; Prescott *et al.*, 1970). Drug absorption may be reduced when the drug forms an insoluble precipitate with a food component, when a chelate is formed, or when the drug is adsorbed onto dietary fiber. For example, aluminum hydroxide forms an insoluble phosphate precipitate when taken with phospate-containing food. Tetracycline forms chelates with divalent and trivalent cations in food, including calcium and iron. Lithium carbonate may be adsorbed onto dietary fiber (Eastwood and Mitchell, 1976; Insogna *et al.*, 1980; Lotz *et al.*, 1968; Neuvonen *et al.*, 1971; Roe, 1984a). Furthermore, drugs will not be absorbed when components of the drug formulation interact with enteral formula constituents to form an insoluble gel (Cutie *et al.*, 1983). Indeed, many physicochemical reactions between drugs and nutrients reduce the

Daphne A. Roe • Division of Nutritional Sciences, Cornell University, Ithaca, New York 14853.

Table I. Classification of Drug–Nutrient Interactions

Event	Interaction	Site	Outcome
Physicochemical	1. With food; with beverage	Stomach	Drug dissolution quicker or slower
	2. With nutrient or non-nutrient component of food	Intestine	Drug absorption quicker, slower, enhanced, reduced; nutrient absorption quicker, slower, enhanced, reduced
Physiological	1. With gastric emptying	Stomach	Changed rate of drug–nutrient absorption
	2. With intestinal motility	Intestine	Changed rate/extent of drug–nutrient absorption
	3. With digestion	Stomach, intestine	Enhanced digestion, maldigestion
	4. With absorption	Intestine	Malabsorption
	5. With splanchnic blood flow	Portal vein	Drug or nutrient metabolism quicker or slower
	6. With hepatic enzymes	Liver	Drug or nutrient metabolism enhanced or reduced
	7. With plasma proteins	Blood	Drug or nutrient binding and distribution altered
	8. With renal secretory mechanisms	Kidney	Drug clearance promoted or retarded
Pathophysiological	1. Enterocyte	Intestine	Maldigestion
	2. Hepatocyte	Liver	Malutilization of nutrients and drug toxicity
	3. Erythrocyte precursors	Bone marrow	Nutritional anemia
	4. Nephron	Kidney	Mineral loss

amount of drug that is absorbed to an extent that insufficient drug is absorbed to produce the desired clinical effect. Examples of physicochemical interactions that seriously reduce drug absorption are shown in Table II.

1.2. Physiological Interactions

Physiological interactions between drugs and nutrients encompass events in which either a nutrient or a drug, through specific physiological or pharmacological effects,

Table II. Physicochemical Interactions That Reduce Drug Absorption

Interaction	Example
Chelation	Tetracycline absorption reduced by dietary calcium
Hydrolysis	Penicillin absorption reduced by drug instability in "full" stomach because of long drug exposure to gastric acidity
Precipitation	Phenytoin absorption reduced by enteral formula constituents

Table III. Physiological Interactions between Drugs and Nutrients[a]

Interaction	Example
Related to drug absorption	Promotion of propranolol uptake by dietary protein, which enhances splanchnic blood flow
Related to drug metabolism	Increased rate of theophylline metabolism induced by dietary protein

[a]Viswanathan and Welling (1984).

affects disposition of another. For example, drug uptake can be reduced when the absorption mechanism for that drug is competitive with that of a nutrient. Drug metabolism in the gastrointestinal tract may be promoted by nutrients present in the intestine, which can either influence the microflora present and therefore affect the metabolism of drugs by bacteria or actually induce drug-metabolizing enzymes in the intestinal mucosa (Anderson *et al.*, 1982; Hathcock, 1985). Conversely, the absorption of a nutrient will be impaired if a drug suppresses gastric digestion of the food source of that nutrient. Examples of important physiological interactions between drugs and nutrients are shown in Table III.

1.3. Pathophysiological Effects

Pathophysiological effects of drugs can markedly affect the disposition of nutrients. Acute and chronic toxic effects of drugs on the intestine, liver, or kidney can cause nutrient depletion. Drug-induced malabsorption, impaired utilization of nutrients, or excessive nutrient losses via the renal tract are among the major adverse outcomes of these effects (Fichman *et al.*, 1971; Hahn and Halsted, 1979b). Examples of drug-induced tissue damage or organ pathology that causes malnutrition are shown in Table IV.

Table IV. Drug-Induced Organ Pathology Causing Nutritional Deficiencies

Site of pathology	Example
Intestine (enterocyte)	Chronic folate deficiency induced by methotrexate (Trier, 1962)
Liver (hepatocyte)	Vitamin K deficiency induced by alcohol (Mezey, 1978)
Kidney	Magnesium depletion induced by gentamicin (Barr *et al.*, 1975)

Table V. Drug–Nutrient Interactions and Their Adverse Effects in the Elderly

Interaction	Adverse effect
Incompatibility of phenothiazine liquid formulation with enteral formula	Reduced drug absorption and effect (Cutie *et al.*, 1983)
Glucocorticoid-induced hyperglycemia	Loss of diabetes control (Thomas, 1984)
Furosemide-induced hypokalemia	Digoxin toxicity (Lamy, 1986a)

2. Drug–Nutrient Interactions in the Elderly

2.1. Etiology and Outcomes of Drug–Nutrient Interactions in the Elderly

A high prevalence of drug–nutrient interactions with unwanted outcomes has been documented in the elderly (Roe, 1984b). Characteristics of the elderly that explain the high prevalence of drug–nutrient interactions include effects of aging, the prevalence of chronic disease in older people, their drug-taking habits, and their diets. However, other factors that may provide an explanation of drug–nutrient interactions in the elderly include inappropriate drug prescription, drug misuse, or lack of communication between the drug prescriber and the meal provider so that drug times and meal times conflict. Common problems secondary to drug–nutrient interactions include lack of response to rational drug therapy, loss of disease control, unwanted change in body weight, acute toxic reactions, and drug-induced nutritional deficiencies. Specific problems occurring as a result of drug–nutrient interactions in the elderly and the drugs responsible for these adverse effects are shown in Table V.

2.2. Effects of Aging on Drug Disposition

Aging *per se* produces changes in pharmacokinetics, i.e., drug absorption, disposition, and elimination, and in pharmacodynamics, i.e., the biological and pharmacological effects of drugs. For drug absorption to occur in the gastrointestinal (GI) tract, it must be presented to the absorptive surface of the mucosa in an appropriate form, the local chemical milieu must be right, and the mechanism for absorption must be intact. Although changes in the GI tract occur with aging, including reduction in gastric acidity and reduction in splanchnic blood flow, these changes do not appear to affect the absorption of most drugs. Most drugs are absorbed by a process of passive absorption, which is unaffected by aging.

A few drugs are absorbed by a process of active transport, and their absorption may be reduced by age-related declines in the efficiency of these mechanisms. However, most of the drugs in this category are, in fact, nutrients, such as calcium, or chemical analogues of nutrients (Robertson, 1984).

Drugs are transported in the plasma as free drug or as drug bound to plasma proteins. Most of the drug binding is to plasma albumin. Plasma albumin levels decline as a phenomenon of aging (Greenblatt, 1979). However, although lower plasma albumin levels result in a decline in the number of drug-binding sites, the mild decline in plasma albumin levels that occurs with normal aging does not appear to have a significant effect on drug binding. On the other hand, changes in body composition including those in the percentage of body water, in lean body mass, and in body fat can affect drug disposition. The apparent volume of distribution of a drug is conventionally expressed as the volume of fluid into which the drug appears to be distributed with a concentration that is equivalent to that of plasma. There is an age-related decline in the apparent volume of distribution of drugs such as ethanol and acetaminophen and an increased volume of distribution of highly lipid-soluble drugs such as lidocaine and diazepam. In the case of diazepam, the mean volume of distribution is twice as great in an 80-year-old individual as it is in a 20-year-old (Robertson, 1984). Increased diazepam toxicity in the elderly may be explained by excessive accumulation of the drug and its metabolites in body fat. Conversely, age-related decreases in lean body mass could result in higher and potentially toxic concentrations of digoxin, which is bound to skeletal and cardiac muscle (Roberts and Caird, 1976).

Rates of hepatic drug metabolism may be slowed by aging. However, effects of aging on drug metabolism vary between individuals and between drugs (Cusack and Denham, 1984).

The rate of renal excretion of drugs declines with aging, and this decline parallels the age-related decline in renal function (Rowe *et al.*, 1976). For drugs such as digoxin, which are primarily excreted by glomerular filtration, the decline in efficiency of renal excretion follows the decline in creatinine clearance (Cusack *et al.*, 1979). Tubular secretory function also declines with aging, and this is associated with slowed excretion of drugs such as penicillin and cephalosporin antibiotics, which are primarily excreted by this mechanism (Leikola and Vartia, 1957).

Implications of these changes in drug disposition that occur with aging include an increased risk of drug-induced mineral depletion as a result of the prolongation of nephrotoxic effects. Tissue responsiveness to drugs is also affected by aging. However, aging effects may result in increased or decreased drug effects. Confusion and disorientation are greater with sedatives and hypnotics (MacLennan *et al.*, 1984). These pharmacodynamic changes with aging imply a need to adjust drug dosages relative to body weight to reduce drug toxicity. Certain pharmacodynamic effects of aging have more direct nutritional implications. For example, there is a greater inhibition of vitamin-K-dependent clotting factors following warfarin administration, which can result in hemorrhage unless the drug dose is appropriately lowered. Linkages between age-related effects in drug disposition and drug–nutrient interactions are shown in Table VI.

Table VI. Relationships between Age-Related Changes in Drug Disposition and Drug–Nutrient Interactions

Age-related change	Risk of drug–nutrient interaction
Slowed renal excretion of drugs	Increased risk of cephalosporin-induced vitamin K deficiency (Sattler *et al.*, 1986)
Increase drug in body fat	Increased risk of diazepam toxicity (Klotz *et al.*, 1975)

Table VII. Multiple Health Problems as Risk Factors for Drug–Nutrient Interactions

Concurrent health problems	Risk of drug–nutrient interaction
Hypertension and diabetes	Hyperglycemia caused by thiazides (Brown and Brown, 1967)
Arthritis, heart disease, and renal disease	Hyperkalemia caused by analgesic (indomethacin) and amiloride (Lamy, 1986b)

2.3. *Effects of Geriatric Disease on the Incidence of Drug–Nutrient Interactions*

Although it is well documented that the elderly take more drugs than people in other age groups (Hyams, 1984a; Roe, 1983; World Health Organization, 1981), drug-prescribing practices of physicians for the elderly relative to specific geriatric diseases have received limited coverage in recent literature on drug usage (Christopher *et al.*, 1978). However, drug–nutrient interactions occurring in elderly patients are closely linked to the primary and secondary health problems present. The obvious implication is that the risk of drug–nutrient interactions with cardiac drugs only exists for the cardiac patient, and so on. However, for the elderly the multiplicity of health problems creates additional risk. For example, it has recently been shown that in a frail elderly population, prescriptions for thiazide diuretics were as common for those with diabetes as for those without this disease (D. A. Roe, E. Frongillo, and B. Rauschenback, unpublished data). Thiazide diuretics can cause hyperglycemia in diabetics, and therefore use is unwarranted. However, thiazide prescription, though inappropriate, is explained by the coexistence of hypertension and diabetes. Thus, the risk of drug–nutrient interactions with adverse outcomes is enhanced in the elderly because they may be receiving drugs for the management of several diseases. In controlling one disease with a drug (e.g., hypertension with a thiazide), a risk of drug–nutrient interaction is created relative to another disease, diabetes (Moser, 1984; Murphy *et al.*, 1982). Examples of multiple diagnoses as risk factors for drug–nutrient interactions are shown in Table VII.

2.4. *Effects of Diet and Nutrient Supplements on the Risk of Drug–Nutrient Interactions in the Elderly*

In many elderly the risk of drug–nutrient interactions is related to the wrong spacing of drug times relative to meal times (e.g., administration of tetracycline within 2 hr after a meal containing milk) (Petrick and Kleinman, 1975). Other diet-related factors that increase the risk of drug–nutrient interactions in the elderly include special diet prescription, use of liquid formula supplements, intake of vitamin and mineral supplements, intake of dietary fiber supplements, and nasogastric formula feeding. Examples of drug–nutrient interactions that result from diet-related factors are shown in Table VIII.

When and what food is consumed can strongly influence drug efficacy and safety. Generalizations about the need for nutritional support or restriction can impose unwarranted or even life-threatening health risks on frail elderly. The decision to give high-protein formula supplements to elderly emphysematous patients on theophylline can

Table VIII. Drug–Nutrient Interactions Related to Special Diets and Diet Supplements

Interaction	Special diet	Adverse outcome
Theophylline–protein	High protein	Bronchodilator effect lost, greater wheezing (Kappas *et al.*, 1976)
Griseofulvin–fat	Low fat	Persistent fungus infection (Crounse, 1961)
Digoxin–formula	Continuous enteral infusion	Congestive heart failure (Cutie *et al.*, 1979)
Riboflavin–glucose polymer	Caloric supplement	Enhanced vitamin absorption (Roe, 1984a)
Phenytoin–folate	Vitamin supplement	Loss of seizure control (Mattson *et al.*, 1973)

lead to wheezing and respiratory distress because the protein in the formula increases the rate of metabolism of theophylline and therefore decreases the period of symptom control (Feldman *et al.*, 1980). Severe or even moderate sodium restriction in an elderly person on lithium carbonate can cause lithium toxicity through retention of the lithium salt (Hyams, 1984b). The risk of these events is related to changes in diet prescription or nutrient supplement prescription after drug orders have been made. To be more explicit, it can be stated that new diet orders for elderly patients on drugs need to be made with the understanding that the change in food or nutrient with the new diet can alter the drug dose required.

3. Drug–Nutrient Interactions and Chronic Disease Status

3.1. Drug–Nutrient Interactions in Elderly Cardiac Patients

3.1.1. Mineral Depletion

Mineral depletion is the most common type of drug-induced disorder in elderly cardiac patients, not only because of diuretic use but also because of other risk factors. Indeed, sodium, potassium, and magnesium depletion are usually multifactorial, with risk factors including use of several drugs having this effect, intake of diets or formula feeds that fail to supply mineral requirements, presence of catabolic disease that increases mineral losses (particularly calcium losses), renal impairments, and alcohol abuse, which causes excessive renal loss of both potassium and magnesium (Lindeman, 1986).

Although many physicians and nurses are of the opinion that all elderly cardiac patients with recurrent congestive heart failure require strict sodium restriction, few are able to diagnose sodium depletion in the very old. Diuretic-induced hyponatremia is usually insidious in its development and may be overlooked because the associated mental confusion is assumed to be caused by irreversible organic brain syndromes (Norregaard-Hansen *et al.*, 1986). Prolonged use of sodium-free tube feeding formulas (Isocal®) by elderly cardiacs on diuretics is most likely to cause severe sodium depletion (Stults, 1982).

Table IX. Drugs Causing Hyponatremia and Sodium Deficiency[a]

Hyponatremia	Hyponatremia and sodium deficiency
Chlorpropamide	Hydrochlorothiazide
Tolbutamide	Polythiazide
Vincristine	Spironolactone
Cyclophosphamide	Furosemide
Carbamazepine	Ethacrynic acid
Amitriptyline	
Thioridazine	
Clofibrate	
Captopril	

[a]Kimelman and Albert (1984) and Jamieson (1985).

Drugs having the potential to cause hyponatremia through changes in sodium distribution or hyperexcretion of sodium are shown in Table IX.

Potassium deficiency is recognized as likely to occur in frail elderly who are on diuretics and who concurrently consume low-potassium diets. Additional risk factors include intake of other drugs such as laxatives that cause potassium depletion. In cardiac patients on digitalis, potassium depletion provokes signs of digitalis toxicity with high risk of life-threatening cardiac arrhythmias. Digitalis toxicity is also associated with anorexia and nausea, which further increase the risk of inadequate potassium intake (Stults, 1982). Drugs that cause potassium depletion and therefore should be used cautiously or avoided in cardiac patients receiving digitalis are shown in Table X.

Magnesium deficiency, which can also cause cardiac arrhythmias in patients on digitalis, is frequently drug induced. Drugs frequently causing magnesium deficiency in the elderly are shown in Table XI.

In the subgroup of individuals on digitalis whose gut bacteria metabolize the drug, administration of antibiotics enhances the amount of unmetabolized drug that is ab-

Table X. Drugs That May Cause Potassium Depletion[a]

Furosemide
Ethacrynic acid
Bumetanide
Hydrochlorothiazide and other thiazides
Chlorthalidone
Albuterol
Corticosteroids
Phenolphthalein
Bisacodyl
Senna
Gentamicin

[a]Roe (1984c).

Table XI. Drugs That May Cause Magnesium Depletion[a]

Furosemide
Ethacrynic acid
Bumetanide
Hydrochlorothiazide and other thiazides
Neomycin
Gentamicin
Cephalothin
Cis-platinum

[a] Seelig (1981) and Roe (1981).

sorbed and hence increases the risk that digitalis toxicity may occur (Norregaard-Hansen *et al.*, 1986). Changes in the gut microflora because of diet may influence the ability for intestinal digitalis metabolism (Salyers, 1985).

3.1.2. Drug-Induced Cachexia

If unrecognized, anorexia, nausea, and vomiting, which are clinical signs of digitalis toxicity, lead to marked reductions in food intake with resultant development of protein–energy malnutrition (PEM) (digitalis cachexia). Clinical factors that increase the risk of digitalis toxicity and therefore the risk of these adverse nutritional outcomes include renal failure, chronic pulmonary disease, hypokalemia, hypomagnesemia, hypercalcemia, and quinidine administration (Smith, 1985).

In the elderly, digitalis cachexia may be thought to have other causation. Frequent therapeutic mismanagement of digitalis cachexia may then be by resorting to nasogastric tube feeding of these patients and not reducing their digitalis dosage. When elderly patients requiring digitalis do need to be formula fed via a tube, the drug should not be given via the tube with the formula running, since this practice can lead to blockage of the tube (Roe, 1985b). Instead, the infusion should be stopped before each digitalis dose, and then, before the drug is given, the tube should be flushed with water. This should be repeated after the drug is given, and then, after an hour, the formula infusion can be restarted.

3.1.3. Drug–Nutrient Interactions and Unwanted Metabolic Effects of Antihypertensive Drugs

These unwanted interactions and effects are commonly found in elderly patients. The unwanted outcomes of antihypertensive drugs can be subdivided into two categories: (1) drug–food interactions that result in loss of drug efficacy and (2) metabolic effects that lead to loss of disease control. In the former category, variations in the effectiveness of methyldopa provides an example. Reduction in the bioavailability of this drug may be explained by concurrent administration of high-protein liquid formula supplements, by administration of sulfates including sodium and magnesium sulfate, used as laxatives, or by ferrous sulfate (Roe, 1985b; Campbell *et al.*, 1985). The

Table XII. Drug–Nutrient Interactions and Their Effects on Elderly Patients on Antihypertensive Drugs[a]

Drug interaction		Metabolic and nutritional effects
Thiazides:	Potassium	Hypokalemia
	Sodium	Hyponatremia
	Magnesium	Hypomagnesemia
	Glucose	Hyperglycemia
	Uric acid	Hyperuricemia
	Calcium	Hypercalcemia
Triamterene:	Folic acid	Folate depletion
	Potassium	Hyperkalemia
Captopril:	Sodium	Hyponatremia
	Potassium	Hyperkalemia
Spironolactone:	Potassium	Hyperkalemia
Hydralazine:	Vitamin B_6	Vitamin B_6 deficiency

[a]Andersson (1984).

effects of high-protein feeding on methyldopa bioavailability are explained by the competitive absorption of methyldopa and diet-derived amino acids. The sulfate effect can be explained by intestinal sulfation of the drug, which affects drug disposition.

Unwanted metabolic effects of thiazides, which are commonly used as antihypertensive agents, include not only hypokalemia and hypomagnesemia but also hyperglycemia, hyperlipidemia, hypercalcemia, and hyperuricemia with precipitation of attacks of acute gout (Rapoport and Hurd, 1964; Ames and Peacock, 1984; Duarte *et al.*, 1971; Mudge, 1975). The seriousness of these events in the elderly is related to their underlying health problems such that, for example, thiazide-induced hyperglycemia in diabetics can cause significant hyperglycemia and thus loss of disease control.

Vitamin deficiencies can be associated with antihypertensive drugs. Hydralazine is a vitamin B_6 antagonist that can cause peripheral neuropathy (Kirkendall and Page, 1958). Triamterene, a mild diuretic often used as an adjuvant therapeutic agent in elderly hypertensives on thiazides, is a mild folate antagonist (Corcino *et al.*, 1970) that can produce chronic folate deficiency when given over extensive periods of time. Common drug–nutrient interactions occurring in patients on antihypertensive drugs are shown in Table XII.

3.2. *Drug–Nutrient Interactions in Elderly Patients with Chronic Respiratory Disease*

Chronic obstructive lung disease, including bronchitis, emphysema, and cor pulmonale, is more difficult to manage in the elderly than in younger people both because of the elderly's debility and because of their variable response to therapeutic measures. Management includes reduction of factors that exacerbate the condition including discouraging the patient from smoking, treatment of secondary infection, maintenance of an adequate airway, and nutritional support (Corcino *et al.*, 1970).

Treatment of secondary infection is either by using amoxicillin or ampicillin, by giving broad-spectrum antibiotics such as tetracycline, or by giving a trimethoprim–sulfa combination. When tetracycline is prescribed, it is essential to set times of drug administration so that these are at least 2 hr away from times when the patient consumes milk or other calcium-containing dairy foods or calcium, iron, or zinc supplements. When tetracycline is given with food or supplement sources of these divalent cations or with antacids containing aluminum hydroxide, it is inadequately absorbed (Bartelink, 1974). Trimethoprim is a mild folate antagonist and as such can reduce the efficiency of folate utilization and contribute to the development of folate deficiency (Kahn *et al.*, 1968).

Many elderly patients with chronic obstructive lung disease receive theophylline as a bronchodilator. Loss of the desired therapeutic effects of this drug may be explained by food effects on drug absorption or enhanced rates of drug metabolism brought about by high-protein feeding (Karim *et al.*, 1985; Hathcock, 1985). In frail elderly patients who are losing weight because their caloric intake is not commensurate with their high food-energy needs, it is difficult to maintain a safe and effective theophylline dosage level. Problems of theophylline dosing are related to the need to minimize the risk of toxicity, which is increased by lack of dose adjustment for those who are underweight and those whose protein intake is suddenly reduced (Krishnaswamy, 1985).

Corticosteroids may be prescribed for patients with obstructive lung disease of various etiologies. Although use of corticosteroids may be of short duration in patients with emphysema from smoking, prolonged corticosteroid treatment is used in systemic sclerosis. Prolonged therapy with corticosteroids in the elderly is associated with a high risk of acceleration of osteoporosis as well as risk of exacerbating the patient's catabolic state and producing hyperglycemia (Pohl, 1984).

Pulmonary tuberculosis is a significant cause of chronic obstructive lung disease in the elderly. Antituberculosis therapy commonly includes administration of isoniazid and rifampin with or without the use of ethambutol. Each of these drugs is likely to produce side effects that are linked to drug–nutrient interactions. Isoniazid is a vitamin B_6 antagonist that not only causes peripheral neuropathy but also can cause pellagra in patients whose niacin intake is low. This is explained by the fact that isoniazid, because of its anti-B_6 effects, blocks the conversion of tryptophan to niacin (Carlson *et al.*, 1956; DiLorenzo, 1967). Isoniazid also interferes with the utilization of vitamin D, which, in home- or hospital-bound elderly who are not exposed to sunlight, could contribute to the risk of osteomalacia (Brodie *et al.*, 1981).

Because of its effects on hepatic drug-metabolizing enzymes, rifampin can reduce blood and tissue concentrations of other drugs, including coumarin anticoagulants, which are vitamin K antagonists (Ramankiewicz and Ehrman, 1975).

Ethambutol is a zinc-chelating agent and it has been postulated that adverse ocular effects of the drug with diminution in visual acuity could result from zinc depletion (Roe, 1985c). Common drug–nutrient interactions occurring in patients with chronic respiratory disease are shown in Table XIII.

3.3. Drug–Nutrient Interactions in Elderly Neurological and Psychiatric Patients

Chronic diseases of the central nervous system are commonly treated by multiple-drug therapies. Therapeutic goals include seizure control, management of Parkinson's

Table XIII. Common Drug–Nutrient Interactions Occurring in Elderly Patients with Chronic Respiratory Disease[a]

Drug interaction		Effect on drug efficacy or nutritional status
Theophylline:	Protein	Loss of drug efficacy
Isoniazid:	Vitamin B_6	Vitamin B_6 deficiency
	Vitamin B_6, niacin	Pellagra
	Vitamin D	Osteomalacia

[a]Roe (1985c).

disease, and prevention of recurrence of cerebrovascular episodes. Other wanted effects of drug therapies include control of memory loss associated with organic brain syndromes including Alzheimer's disease.

Seizure control in the elderly is usually achieved with phenytoin, with or without phenobarbital. The bioavailability of phenytoin is affected by enteral formula and supplement composition. When phenytoin is given in a liquid formulation via nasogastric tubes, plasma levels of the drug are below the therapeutic range, and seizure control is not achieved. It has been variously suggested, based on *in vitro* experiments, that phenytoin absorption may be reduced by binding to protein in the formula or that magnesium salts in the formula reduce absorption or that the drug is bound to the plastic of the nasogastric tube, but there is no strong evidence to support any of these mechanisms (Bauer, 1982; Hooks *et al.*, 1986; Cacek *et al.*, 1986). However, it is generally agreed that when phenytoin is to be given via nasogastric tube, the formula flow should first be stopped and the drug given after adequate irrigation of the tube. Absorption of phenytoin is reduced when folic acid is given in doses greater than 5 mg (Lindenbaum, 1983).

Phenytoin and phenobarbital adversely affect folate, vitamin D, and vitamin K utilization (Reynolds *et al.*, 1966). When phenytoin or phenytoin plus phenobarbital is administered to elderly patients on a long-term basis, folate deficiency and osteomalacia may develop. Hemorrhage from vitamin K deficiency is unlikely to occur unless the patient additionally has cirrhosis or is taking anticoagulants (Solomon *et al.*, 1972).

Presently, treatment of Parkinson's disease is commonly with levodopa and carbidopa, which are given as one preparation. Levodopa is a vitamin B_6 antagonist. However, whereas formerly vitamin B_6 deficiency was seen in patients on levodopa, it is not seen as a clinical disorder in patients taking current doses of the levodopa–carbidopa preparation. Reduction in the risk of vitamin B_6 deficiency is explained by use of the carbidopa, a peripheral dopa decarboxylase inhibitor, which allows lower doses of levodopa to be used. Earlier guidelines for use of low-vitamin-B_6 diets in patients on levodopa are no longer recommended (Mars, 1974).

Elderly patients who have had transient ischemic attacks (minor strokes) are sometimes given coumarin anticoagulants. However, long-term anticoagulant drug therapy imposes a serious risk of cerebral hemorrhage, a risk that is increased by other factors contributing to the development of vitamin K deficiency (Millican, 1979).

The elderly with memory loss as a result of stroke or Alzheimer's disease may be

Table XIV. Tyramine Content of Foods and Beverages Contraindicated for Elderly Patients Taking MAOI Drugs[a]

Food or beverage	Tyramine content (μg/g or μg/ml)
Cheeses	
Cheddar	1416
Gruyere	516
Stilton	466
Camembert	86
Fish	
Pickled herring	3030
Beverages	
Chianti	25

[a]Modified from Overton and Lukert (1977).

prescribed so-called cerebral vasodilator drugs. One of these "drugs," niacin, is ineffective for treating memory loss but does cause marked flushing. Elderly patients with organic brain syndromes or with chronic psychoses receive psychotropic drugs that impose a major risk of drug–nutrient interactions. Phenothiazine tranquilizers and lithium salts are hyperphagic drugs that can lead to obesity in elderly patients on unrestricted food intake (Doss, 1979). Lithium blood levels are increased and the risk of lithium toxicity is increased by change to a sodium-restricted diet with or without concurrent use of diuretics (Platman and Fieve, 1969).

Antidepressant drugs include the monoamine oxidase inhibitors and tricyclic antidepressants. Monoamine oxidase inhibitors such as phenelzine can cause acute hypertensive crises when taken with or after foods or beverages high in tyramine. High-tyramine foods (listed in Table XIV) include cheese, particularly aged cheeses, as well as wines. When high-tyramine foods and beverages are ingested by people taking monoamine oxidase inhibitor drugs, tyramine (which is not oxidized) triggers the release of catecholamines, which cause the sudden rise in blood pressure. Because of the difficulty of assuring that the foods will not be consumed, and also because other drugs that are being taken interact with monoamine oxidase inhibitor drugs, it is rarely justifiable to prescribe these drugs in the elderly.

Common drug–nutrient interactions linked to the use of drugs affecting the central nervous system are listed in Table XV.

4. *Drug–Nutrient Interactions in Elderly Arthritic Patients*

Elderly arthritic patients include mainly those with osteoarthritis, gout, and rheumatoid arthritis. Important considerations in assessing the adverse nutritional effects of drugs in these arthritics are their drug-taking habits and the effects of their disease on their nutritional status. Most elderly with muscle and joint symptoms related to arthritis take analgesic drugs daily, some taking them at high dosages. The analgesics that are

Table XV. Drug–Nutrient Interactions Associated with Psychotropic and Other Central Nervous System Drugs[a]

Interaction		Adverse nutritional response or incompatibility reaction
Anticonvulsants		
Phenytoin:	Folic acid	Megaloblastic anemia or impaired drug absorption
	Vitamin D	Osteomalacia
	Warfarin	Vitamin K deficiency
Phenobarbital		As for phenytoin
Major tranquilizers		
Chlorpromazine and other phenothiazines		Hyperphagia and weight gain
Lithium carbonate		Hyperphagia and weight gain; toxicity with low-sodium diet
Antidepressants		
Phenelzine and other MAOI drugs		Tyramine reactions

[a]Roe (1984b).

favored by prescribing physicians and by patients are the nonsteroidal antiinflammatory agents (NSAIDs). The NSAIDs, including aspirin, indomethacin, naproxen, and other related drugs, can cause gastrointestinal bleeding, which, over time, leads to iron deficiency anemia (Hansten, 1985). These drugs can also produce other adverse effects including fluid retention leading to weight gain and hyperkalemia (USP, 1986). Risk of hyperkalemia in the elderly is greatest for those with impaired renal function and those concurrently taking potassium-sparing diuretics and/or potassium supplements (Favre *et al.*, 1982).

Elderly patients with recurrent attacks of gout are frequently prescribed colchicine, which may cause steatorrhea with malabsorption of nutrients that are absorbed in either the proximal or distal portions of the small intestine (Race *et al.*, 1970). However, since it is unusual to give colchicine over long periods of time, the risk of serious malnutrition caused by this drug is low.

Drugs given to elderly patients with rheumatoid arthritis carry the highest risk for causing adverse nutritional and metabolic effects. Penicillamine, which is a zinc chelator, can cause zinc deficiency, which is manifested by loss of appetite, resultant weight loss, dermatitis, and impaired wound healing. Because it also forms complexes with vitamin B_6 that are lost in the urine, penicillamine therapy can also lead to vitamin B_6 deficiency (Multicentre Trial Group, 1973). Corticosteroids, as previously mentioned, contribute to the risk of osteoporosis as well as preventing achievement of normoglycemia in elderly diabetics (Roe, 1985c; Hunder *et al.*, 1975).

Common drug–nutrient interactions in elderly arthritics are listed in Table XVI.

5. Drug–Nutrient Interactions in Elderly Diabetic Patients

5.1. Hyper- and Hypoglycemic Drugs

Elderly diabetics often take drugs for other health problems that may or may not be linked to their diabetes. Common reasons for their taking additional drugs include atherosclerotic heart disease, hypertension, cutaneous infections, arthritis, and colds

Table XVI. Drug–Nutrient Interactions in Elderly Arthritic Patients[a]

Interaction	Adverse nutritional response
Analgesics	
Indomethacin and other NSAIDs[b]	GI bleeding and iron deficiency anemia
	Hyperkalemia
	Fluid retention and weight gain
Antigout drugs	
Colchicine	Malabsorption syndrome
Antiarthritic drugs	
Penicillamine	Zinc deficiency
	Vitamin B_6 deficiency

[a]Roe (1985d).
[b]NSAIDs, nonsteroidal antiinflammatory drugs.

and coughs. Prescription and nonprescription drugs that they may take as well as alcohol in drug formulations and beverages can affect the metabolic control of their diabetes. These other drugs may cause hyper- or hypoglycemia. Hyperglycemic drugs include thiazide diuretics, corticosteroids, and ephedrine or ephedrinelike drugs in cold and cough medicines. Hypoglycemic drugs include alcohol, sulfa drugs, and aspirin. Other drugs that may have a hypoglycemic effect in some elderly diabetics include the hypocholesterolic agent gemfibrozil and β blockers such as propranolol (D'Arcy and Griffin, 1972). Whether or not these drugs actually cause loss of control of the patient's diabetes depends on the actual drug taken, the dose, the frequency, and on whether the patient is taking insulin or oral hypoglycemic agents. It is, however, important to consider that whether or not these drugs seriously affect diabetes control, they can interfere with the interpretation of blood sugar tests.

Alcohol has a hypoglycemic effect, particularly when drunk to excess by elderly who have not eaten. On the other hand, ingestion of alcoholic beverages can cause hyperglycemia both because the alcohol calories may contribute to food–energy overload and because alcohol shortens the period of action of oral antidiabetic agents such as tolbutamide (Arky *et al.*, 1968). Therapeutic doses of aspirin, as used in the treatment of arthritics, can cause hypoglycemia in diabetics on oral antidiabetic agents such as chlorpropamide. Sulfa drugs also enhance the hypoglycemic effects of tolbutamide and chlorpropamide (Larner and Haynes, 1975).

Drugs causing hyper- and hypoglycemia are summarized in Table XVII.

5.2. *Effects of Diabetic Diets on Drug Bioavailability*

The antifungal agent griseofulvin is better absorbed when taken after meals containing fat. In diabetics who are adhering to low-fat diets, failure to achieve drug control of common and widespread dermatophyte infection such as those induced by *Trichophyton rubrum* may be explained by inadequate absorption of the griseofulvin. Changes in the formulation of the drug, including reduction of particle size, have now improved the bioavailability of griseofulvin for those on low-fat diets, but the problem still exists when fat intake is minimal (Crounse, 1961).

Table XVII. Drugs Causing Hyperglycemia and Hypoglycemia in Diabetics[a]

Hyperglycemic drugs	Hypoglycemic drugs
Thiazides	Allopurinol[b]
Nifedipine	Salicylates
Corticosteroids	Sulfas
Epinephrine	Alcohol
Ephedrine	Anabolic steroids
Phenylephrine	
Phenylpropanolamine	
Pseudoephedrine	
Thyroid hormones	

[a]Dargaville (1985).
[b]Prolongs the duration of action of chlorpropamide.

5.3. Chlorpropamide–Alcohol Flush Reactions

Elderly diabetics receiving chlorpropamide as an oral antidiabetic agent should be warned that alcohol in beverages, foods, or other drugs may cause intense flushing. The chlorpropamide–alcohol flush reaction occurs in a subgroup of type II diabetics, who have been postulated to have a better prognosis relative to cardiovascular complications. Whether or not the chlorpropamide–alcohol flush reaction has any prognostic implications is presently unclear, but there is evidence that those diabetics displaying the flush can be identified genetically (Leslie *et al.*, 1979; Groop *et al.*, 1984).

6. Identifying the Risk and the Presence of Drug–Nutrient Reactions in the Elderly

The risk of drug–nutrient interactions may be identified by examination of patients' records and also by questioning patients about their use of nonprescription drugs and social drugs. Additional information that is required in assessing the risks of drug–food or drug–formula interactions includes knowledge of meal times and meal composition as well as of nutrient supplement use. In the elderly living at home, this information may be obtained from the patient or his/her relatives, friends, or caregivers. For elderly in acute care hospitals and nursing homes, it may be necessary to obtain the relevant information pertinent to drugs and diet not only from medical records but also from records kept in the dietary department.

Identifying the outcomes of drug–nutrient interactions requires information about symptoms, signs such as flush, and changes in the degree of disease control such as wheezing in patients whose chronic bronchitis was previously controlled by theophylline. Further, laboratory reports can provide evidence of change in nutritional or metabolic status that are attributable to drug therapies. However, it is essential to bear in mind that only the changes in the patient's condition that postdate the drug prescription or the dietary change leading to a drug–nutrient interaction can be responsible for the effect. It is also important to consider the Berkson bias when assessing the actual patient risk for and from drug–nutrient interactions. The Berkson bias is to the effect that hospital-based data cannot be extrapolated to nonhospital populations (Roberts *et al.*, 1978). In relation to the risk of drug–nutrient interactions, this should be interpreted to mean that the identification and the risk of drug–nutrient interactions is different for elderly with respect to their location.

Differences exist between elderly in the community and those in hospitals and nursing homes with respect to their drug usage patterns, dietary regimens, and disease states that explain differential risks of drug–nutrient interactions for those in older age groups.

7. Prevention and Treatment of Adverse Effects of Drug–Nutrient Interactions

7.1. Vitamin Supplements

Vitamin supplements are required by regular users of therapeutic drugs when a risk of progressive vitamin depletion exists as well as when a vitamin deficiency caused by the drug is present. Appropriate levels of the vitamins are listed in Table XVIII. In this table it is assumed that the drug user is already consuming the recommended dietary allowances (National Research Council, 1980) for these nutrients and that their needs for vitamins have not been altered by diseases that impair absorption or utilization of vitamins.

In the event that drug-related vitamin depletion (or risk of depletion) is complicated by dietary inadequacy or disease that induces vitamin depletion, the vitamin supplement should be moderately increased so that total vitamin intakes comprise basal requirements plus the increment required to overcome the nutrient depletion imposed by the drug. It is further recommended that the responses of drug users to vitamin supplements be monitored both by vitamin assays and by estimation of plasma levels of drugs. Failure to carry out such monitoring implies that the biochemical response of the

Table XVIII. Recommended Vitamin Intakes for Individuals Receiving Specific Drugs That Cause Malabsorption

Drug	Recommended total daily vitamin intake	
Phenytoin	Vitamin D	800–1200 IU
	Vitamin K	2–5 mg
	Folic acid	0.8–1.2 mg
	(not >2.0 mg/day)	
Sulfasalazine	Folic acid	0.8–1.2 mg
Cholestyramine	Vitamin A	5000–10,000 IU
Colestipol	Vitamin D	800–1200 IU
	Folic acid	0.8–1.2mg

elderly patient to vitamin supplements will be unknown, that early evidence of vitamin toxicity will be missed, and that reduction in plasma levels of drugs attributable to vitamin supplement administration will be overlooked (Roe, 1985c).

7.2. Mineral Supplements

Elderly patients who receive therapeutic drugs that can cause mineral depletion are not all in need of mineral supplements. Specific needs for mineral supplements exist when electrolyte imbalance is present as well as when there is a high risk that major mineral losses will occur as a consequence of drug usage. For example, calcium supplements are needed by patients requiring long-term corticosteroid therapy. The need for potassium supplements is present in elderly patients on loop diuretics who are hypokalemic as well as in those whose dietary intake of potassium is inadequate to meet their needs. It is important to monitor plasma levels of potassium in those receiving potassium supplements in order to reduce the risk of hyperkalemia (Roe, 1987).

8. References

Ames, R. P., and Peacock, P. B., 1984, Serum cholesterol during treatment of hypertension with diuretic drugs, *Arch. Intern. Med.* **144:**710–714.

Anderson, K. E., Conney, A. H., and Kappas, A., 1982, Nutritional influences on chemical biotransformations in humans, *Nutr. Report Internal.* **40:**161–172.

Andersson, O., 1984, The use of diuretics in modern antihypertensive therapy, *Acta Pharmacol. Toxicol.* **54**(Suppl. 1)**:**79–82.

Arky, R. A., Vevebrants, E. A., and Abramson, E. A., 1968, Irreversible hypoglycemia: A complication of alcohol and insulin, *J.A.M.A.* **206:**575–578.

Barr, R. S., Wilson, H. E., and Mazzaferri, E. L., 1975, Hypomagnesemic hypocalcemia secondary to renal magnesium wasting: A possible consequence of high-dose gentamicin therapy, *Ann. Intern. Med.* **82:**646–649.

Bartelink, A., 1974, Clinical drug interactions in the gastrointestinal tract in man, in: *Clinical Effects of Interaction Between Drugs* (L. E. Cluff and J. C. Petrie, eds.), Excerpta Medica, Amsterdam, p. 107.

Bauer, L. A., 1982, Interference of oral phenytoin absorption by continuous nasogastric feedings, *Neurology* **32:**570–572.

Becker, C. E., Roe, R. L., and Scott, R. A., 1974, *Alcohol as a Drug,* Williams & Wilkins, Baltimore, p. 23.

Benarde, M. A., 1971, *The Chemicals We Eat,* McGraw-Hill, New York, pp. 89–91.

Brodie, M. J., Boobis, A. R., Hillyard, C. J., Abeyasekara, G., Stevenson, J. C., MacIntyre, I., and Kevin Park, B., 1981, Effect of isoniazid on vitamin D metabolism and hepatic monooxygenase activity, *Clin. Pharmacol. Therp.* **30:**363–367.

Brown, W. J., and Brown, W. K., 1967, Thiazide induced alteration in carbohydrate tolerance in normal men, *Curr. Ther.* **9:**200–208.

Cacek, A. T., DeVito, J. M., and Koonce, J. R., 1986, *In vitro* evaluation of nasogastric administration methods for phenytoin, *Am. J. Hosp. Pharm.* **43:**689–692.

Campbell, N. R. C., Sundaram, R. S., Werness, P. G., Van Loon, R. M., and Weinshilboum, R. M., 1985, Sulfate and methyldopa metabolism: Metabolite patterns and platelet phenol sulfotransferase activity, *Clin. Pharmacol. Ther.* **37:**3088–3315.

Carlson, H. B., Anthony, E. M., Russell, W. F., Jr., and Middlebrook, G., 1956, Prophylaxis of isoniazid neuropathy with pyridoxine, *N. Engl. J. Med.* **255:**118–122.

Christopher, L. J., Ballinger, B. R., Shepherd, A. M. M., Ramsay, A., and Crooks, J., 1978, Drug prescribing patterns in the elderly: A cross-sectional study of inpatients, *Age Ageing* **7:**74–82.

Corcino, J., Waxman, S., and Herbert, V., 1970, Mechanism of triamterene-induced megaloblastosis, *Arch. Intern. Med.* **73:**419–424.

Crounse, R. G., 1961, Human pharmacology of griseofulvin: The effect of fat intake on gastrointestinal absorption, *J. Invest. Dermatol.* **37:**529–533.

Cusack, B., and Denham, M. J., 1984, Nutritional status and drug disposition in the elderly, in: *Drugs and Nutrition in the Geriatric Patient* (D. A. Roe, ed.), Churchill Livingstone, New York, pp. 71–91.

Cusack, B., Kelly, J. G., O'Malley, K., Noel, J., Lavan, J., and Horgan, J., 1979, Digoxin in the elderly: Pharmacokinetic consequences of old age, *Clin. Pharmacol. Ther.* **25:**772–776.

Cutie, A. J., Altman, E., and Lenkel, L., 1983, Compatibility of enteral products with commonly employed drug–drug additives, *J. Parent. Ent. Nutr.* **7:**186–191.

D'Arcy, P. F., and Griffin, J. P., 1972, *Iatrogenic Diseases*, Oxford University Press, London, pp. 95–100.

Dargaville, R., 1985, Drug interactions in treatment, in: *Diabetes Mellitus: A Guide to Treatment* (P. Taft, ed.), Adis Health Sciences Press, Boston, Sydney, pp. 7–83.

DiLorenzo, P. A., 1967, Pellagra-like syndrome associated with isoniazid therapy, *Acta Dermatol. Venereol.* **47:**318–322.

Doss, F. W., 1979, The effect of antipsychotic drugs on body weight; a retrospective review, *J. Clin. Psychiatry* **40:**528–530.

Duarte, G. C., Winnaker, J. L., Becker, K. L., and Pace, A., 1971, Thiazide-induced hypercalcemia, *N. Engl. J. Med.* **284:**828–830.

Eastwood, M. A., and Mitchell, W. D., 1976, Physical properties of fiber: A biological evaluation, in: *Fiber in Human Nutrition* (G. A. Spiller and R. J. Amen, eds.), Plenum Press, New York, pp. 109–129.

Favre, L., Glasson, P., and Vallotton, M. B., 1982, Reversible acute renal failure from combined triamterene and indomethacin: A study in healthy subjects, *Ann. Intern. Med.* **96:**317–320.

Feldman, C. H., Hutchinson, V. E., Pippenger, C. E., Blumenfeld, T. A., Feldman, B. R., and Davis, W. J., 1980, Effect of dietary protein and carbohydrate on theophylline metabolism in children, *Pediatrics* **66:**956–962.

Fichman, M. P., Vorherr, H., Kleeman, C. R., and Telfer, N., 1971, Diuretic-induced hyponatremia, *Ann. Intern. Med.* **75:**853–863.

Greenblatt, D. J., 1979, Reduced serum albumin level in the elderly: A report from the Boston Collaborative Drug Surveillance Program, *J. Am. Geriatr. Soc.* **27:**20–22.

Groop, L., Kosimies, S., and Tolpannen, E.-M., 1984, Characterization of patients with chlorpropamide–alcohol flush, *Acta Med. Scand.* **215:**141–149.

Hahn, T. J., and Halstead, L. R., 1979, Anticonvulsant drug-induced osteomalacia: Alterations in mineral metabolism and response to vitamin D_3 administration, *Calcif. Tissue Int.* **27:**13–18.

Hansten, P. D., 1985, *Drug Interactions,* 5th ed., Lea & Febiger, Philadelphia, pp. 336–337.

Hathcock, J. N., 1985, Nutrient and non-nutrient effects on drug metabolism, *Drug–Nutr. Interact.* **4:**217–234.

Hooks, M. A., Leon Longe, R., Taylor, T., and Francisco, G. E., 1986, Recovery of phenytoin from an enteral nutrient formula, *Am. J. Hosp. Pharm.* **43:**685–688.

Hunder, G. G., Sheps, S. G., Allen, G. L., and Joyce, J. W., 1975, Daily and alternate day corticosteroid regimens in treatment of giant cell arteritis. Comparison in a prospective study, *Ann. Intern. Med.* **82:**613–618.

Hyams, D. E., 1984a, Drug usage by the elderly, in: *Drugs and Nutrition in the Geriatric Patient* (D. A. Roe, ed.), Churchill Livingstone, New York, pp. 1–26.

Hyams, D. E., 1984b, Central nervous system antidepressants, in: *Geriatric Pharmacology and Therapeutics* (J. C. Blackwell, ed.), Science Publishers, Oxford, pp. 143–154.

Insogna, K. L., Bordley, D. R., Caro, J. F., and Lockwood, D. H., 1980, Osteomalacia and weakness from excessive antacid, *J.A.M.A.* **244:**2544–2546.

Jamieson, M. J., 1985, Hyponatraemia, *Br. Med. J.* **290:**1723–1728.

Kabasakalian, P., Katz, M., Rosenkrantz, B., and Townley, E., 1970, Parameters affecting absorption of griseofulvin using urinary metabolite excretion data, *J. Pharm. Sci.* **59:**595.

Kahn, S. B., Fein, S. A., and Brodsky, L., 1968, Effects of trimethoprim on folate metabolism in man, *Clin. Pharmacol. Ther.* **9:**550–560.

Kappas, A., Anderson, K. E., Conney, A. H., and Alvares, A. P., 1976, Influence of dietary protein and carbohydrate on antipyrine and theophylline metabolism in man, *Clin. Pharmacol. Ther.* **20:**643–653.

Karim, A., Burns, T., Janky, D., and Hurwitz, A., 1985, Food-induced changes in theophylline absorption from controlled-release formulations, Part II. Importance of meal composition and dosing time relative to meal intake in assessing changes in absorption, *Clin. Pharmacol. Ther.* **38**:642–647.

Kimelman, N., and Albert, S. G., 1984, Phenothiazine-induced hyponatremia in the elderly, *Gerontology* **30**:132–136.

Kirkendall, W. M., and Page, E. B., 1958, Polyneuritis occurring during hydralazine therapy: Report of two cases and discussion of adverse reactions to hydralazine, *J.A.M.A.* **167**:427–432.

Klotz, U., Avant, G. R., Hoyumpa, A., Schenker, S., and Wilkinson, G. R., 1975, The effects of age and liver disease on the disposition and elimination of diazepam in adult man, *J. Clin. Invest.* **55**:347–359.

Krishnaswamy, K., 1985, Nutrients/non-nutrients and drug metabolism, *Drug–Nutr. Meta.* **4**:235–247.

Lamy, P. P., 1986a, The elderly and drug interactions, *J. Am. Geriatr. Soc.* **34**:586–592.

Lamy, P. P., 1986b, Renal effects of non-steroidal antiinflammatory drugs. Heightened risk to the elderly? *J. Am. Geriatr. Soc.* **34**:361–367.

Larner, J., and Haynes, R. C., 1975, Insulin and oral hypoglycemic drugs: Glucagon, in: *The Pharmacological Basis of Therapeutics,* 5th ed. (L. S. Goodman and A. Gilman, eds.), Macmillan, New York, pp. 1521–1522.

Leikola, E., and Vartia, K. O., 1957, On penicillin levels in young and geriatric subjects, *J. Gerontol.* **12**:48–52.

Leslie, R. D. G., Barnett, A. H., and Pyke, D. A., 1979, Chlorpropamide alochol flushing and diabetic retinopathy, *Lancet* **1**:997–999.

Lindeman, R. D., 1986, Mineral metabolism, aging and the aged, in: *Nutrition, Aging and Health* (E. A. Young, ed.), Alan R. Liss, New York, pp. 187–210.

Lindenbaum, J., 1983, Drugs and vitamin B_{12} and folate metabolism, in: *Nutrition and Drugs* (M. Winick, ed.), John Wiley & Sons, New York, p. 79.

Lotz, M., Zisman, E., and Bartter, C., 1968, Evidence for a phosphorus depletion syndrome in man, *N. Engl. J. Med.* **278**:409–415.

MacLennan, W. J., Shepherd, A. N., and Stevenson, I. H., 1984, *The Elderly,* Springer-Verlag, New York, pp. 8–9, 149–150.

Mars, H., 1974, Levodopa, carbidopa and pyridoxine in Parkinson's disease. Metabolic interactions, *Arch. Neurol.* **30**:444–447.

Mattson, R. H., Gallagher, B. B., Reynolds, E. H., and Glass, D., 1973, Folate therapy in epilepsy. A controlled study, *Arch. Neurol.* **29**:78–81.

Mezey, E., 1978, Liver disease and nutrition, *Gastroenterology* **74**:770–783.

Millican, C. H., 1979, Anticoagulant therapy for prevention of stroke, *Med. Clin. North Am.* **63**:897–904.

Moser, M., 1984, Clinical trials, diuretics and the management of mild hypertension, *Arch. Intern. Med.* **144**:789–792.

Mudge, G. H., 1975, Diuretics and other agents employed in the mobilization of edema fluid, in: *The Pharmacological Basis of Therapeutics,* 5th ed. (L. S. Goodman and A. Gilman, eds.), Macmillan, New York, p. 832.

Multicentre Trial Group, 1973, Controlled trial of D(−)penicillamine in severe rheumatoid arthritis, *Lancet* **1**:275–280.

Murphy, M. B., Kohner, E., Lewis, P. J., Schumer, B., and Dollery, C. T., 1982, Glucose intolerance in hypertensive patients treated with diuretics; a 14-year follow-up, *Lancet* **2**:1293–1295.

National Research Council, 1988, *Recommended Dietary Allowances,* National Academy Press, Washington, D.C.

Neuvonen, P., Matilla, M., Gothini, R., and Hackman, R., 1971, Interference of iron and milk with absorption of tetracycline, *Scand. J. Clin. Lab. Invest.* **27**:76.

Norregaard-Hansen, K., Klitgaard, N. A., and Pedersen, K. E., 1986, The significance of the enterohepatic circulation on the metabolism of digoxin in patients with the ability of intestinal conversion of the drug, *Acta Med. Scand.* **220**:89–92.

Overton, M., and Lukert, B., 1977, *Clinical Nutrition: A Physiological Approach,* Yearbook Medical Publishers, Chicago, p. 161.

Petrick, R. J., and Kleinman, N. K., 1975, Meal interference with antibiotics administered orally in hospitals, *Am. J. Hosp. Pharm.* **32**:1008.

Platman, S. R., and Fieve, R. R., 1969, Lithium retention and excretion. The effect of sodium and fluid intake, *Arch. Gen. Psychiatry* **20**:285–289.

Pohl, J. E. F., 1984, Hormones, in: *Geriatric Pharmacology and Therapeutics* (J. C. Brocklehurst, ed.), Blackwell, Oxford, London, pp. 251–268.

Prescott, L. F., Steel, R. F., and Ferrier, W. R., 1970, The effects of particle size on the absorption of phenacetin in man: A correlation between plasma concentration and effects on the central nervous system, *Clin. Pharmacol. Ther.* **11**:496.

Race, T. F., Paes, I. C., and Faloon, W. W., 1970, Intestinal malabsorption induced by oral colchicine. Comparison with neomycin and cathartic agents, *Am. J. Med. Sci.* **259**:32–41.

Ramankiewicz, J. A., and Ehrman, M., 1975, Rifampin and warfarin: A drug interaction, *Ann. Intern. Med.* **82**:224–225.

Rapoport, M. I., and Hurd, H. F., 1964, Thiazide-induced glucose intolerance treated with potassium, *Arch. Intern. Med.* **113**:405–408.

Reynolds, E. H., Milner, G., Mathews, D. M., and Chanarin, I., 1966, Anticonvulsant therapy, megaloblastic haemopoiesis and folic acid metabolism, *Q. J. Med.* **35**:521–537.

Roberts, M. A., and Caird, F. I., 1976, Steady-state kinetics of digoxin in the elderly, *Age Ageing* **5**:214–223.

Roberts, R. S., Spitzer, W. O., Delmore, T., and Sackett, D. L., 1978, An empirical demonstration of Berkson's bias, *J. Chron. Dis.* **31**:119–128.

Robertson, D., 1984, Drug handling in old age, in: *Geriatric Pharmacology and Therapeutics* (J. C. Brocklehurst, ed.), Blackwell, Oxford, London, pp. 41–59.

Roe, D. A., 1981, Drug interference with the assessment of nutritional status, *Clin. Lab. Med.* **1**:647–664.

Roe, D. A., 1983, *Geriatric Nutrition,* Prentice-Hall, Englewood Cliffs, NJ, pp. 155–156.

Roe, D. A., 1984a, Food, formula and drug effects on the disposition of nutrients, *World Rev. Nutr. Diet.* **43**:80–94.

Roe, D. A., 1984b, Therapeutic significance of drug–nutrient interactions in the elderly, *Pharmacol. Rev.* **36**:109S–122S.

Roe, D. A., 1984c, Drug-induced mineral depletion in the elderly, in: *Drugs and Nutrition in the Geriatric Patient* (D. A. Roe, ed.), Churchill Livingstone, New York, pp. 105–119.

Roe, D. A., 1985a, Drug effects on nutrient absorption, transport, and metabolism, *Drug–Nutr. Interact.* **4**:117–135.

Roe, D. A., 1985b, Therapeutic effects of drug–nutrient interactions in the elderly, *J. Am. Diet. Assoc.* **85**:174–181.

Roe, D. A., 1985c, *Drug-Induced Nutritional Deficiencies,* 2nd ed., AVI, Westport, CT, pp. 288, 315.

Roe, D. A., 1985d, Pathologial changes associated with drug-induced malnutrition, in: *Nutritional Pathology: Pathobiochemistry of Dietary Imbalances* (H. Sidransky, ed.), Marcel Dekker, New York, pp. 357–379.

Roe, D. A., 1987, *Geriatric Nutrition,* 2nd ed., Prentice Hall, Englewood Cliffs, NJ, pp. 176–200.

Rowe, J. W., Andres, R., Tobin, J. D., Norris, A. H., and Shock, N. W., 1976, The effect of age on creatinine clearance in men: A cross-sectional and longitudinal study, *J. Gerontol.* **31**:155–163.

Salyers, A. A., 1985, Breakdown of polysaccharides by human intestinal bacteria, in: *Advances in Human Nutrition,* Volume 11 (E. J. Calabrese and G. H. Scherr, eds.), Chem-Orbital, Park Forest, IL, pp. 211–231.

Sattler, F. R., Weitekamp, M. R., and Ballard, J. O., 1986, Potential for bleeding with the new beta-lactam antibiotics, *Ann. Intern. Med.* **105**:924–931.

Seelig, M. S., 1981, Magnesium deficiency, in: *The Pathogenesis of Disease: Early Roots of Cardiovascular, Skeletal and Renal Abnormalities,* Plenum Medical, New York, p. 228.

Smith, T. W., 1985, New advances in the assessment and treatment of digitalis toxicity, *J. Clin. Pharmacol.* **25**:522–528.

Solomon, G. E., Hilgartner, M. W., and Kutt, H., 1972, Coagulation defects caused by diphenylhydantoin, *Neurology* **22**:1165–1171.

Stults, B. M., 1982, Digoxin use in the elderly, *J. Am. Geriatr. Soc.* **30**:158–164.

Thomas, T. P. L., 1984, The complications of systemic corticosteroid therapy in the elderly, *Gerontology* **30**:60–65.

Trier, J. S., 1962, Morphological alterations induced by methotrexate in the mucosa of human proximal intestine. 1. Serial observations by light microscopy, *Gastroenterology* **42**:295–305.
USP, 1986, *Drug Information for the Health Care Provider,* 6th ed., Volume 1, U.S. Pharmacopeial Convention, Rockville, MD, pp. 285–300, 869–876.
Viswanathan, C. T., and Welling, P. G., 1984, Food effects on drug absorption in the elderly, in: *Drugs and Nutrition in the Geriatric Patient* (D. A. Roe, ed.), Churchill Livingstone, New York, pp. 47–70.
World Health Organization, 1981, Health care in the elderly: Report of the technical group on the use of medicaments by the elderly, *Drugs* **22**:279–294.

Index

MIX
Papier aus verantwortungsvollen Quellen
Paper from responsible sources
FSC® C105338

If you have any concerns about our products,
you can contact us on
ProductSafety@springernature.com

In case Publisher is established outside the EU,
the EU authorized representative is:
Springer Nature Customer Service Center GmbH
Europaplatz 3, 69115 Heidelberg, Germany

Printed by Libri Plureos GmbH
in Hamburg, Germany